Pharmacognosy

Pharmacognosy

Eighth Edition

Varro E. Tyler, Ph.D.
Dean and Professor of Pharmacognosy,
Purdue University School of Pharmacy
and Pharmacal Sciences

Lynn R. Brady, Ph.D.
Professor of Pharmacognosy,
University of Washington School of
Pharmacy

James E. Robbers, Ph.D.
Professor of Pharmacognosy,
Purdue University School of Pharmacy
and Pharmacal Sciences

 LEA & FEBIGER • Philadelphia • 1981

Lea & Febiger
600 Washington Square
Philadelphia, PA   19106
U.S.A.

Library of Congress Cataloging in Publication Data

Tyler, Varro E.
   Pharmacognosy.

   Bibliography:
   Includes index.
   1. Pharmacognosy.   I. Brady, Lynn R., 1933–
II. Robbers, James E.   III. Title.   [DNLM:
1. Pharmacognosy.   QV 752 T984p]
RS160.T94   1981   615'.3   81-8162
ISBN 0-8121-0793-4   AACR2

First Edition, 1936

Second Edition, 1947
Reprinted, 1948, 1949

Third Edition, 1956
Reprinted, 1957, 1959

Fourth Edition, 1961
Reprinted, 1962

Fifth Edition, 1965
Reprinted, 1966, 1967, 1968

Sixth Edition, 1970
Reprinted, 1971, 1973, 1974

Seventh Edition, 1976
Reprinted, 1977

The use of portions of the text of USP XX and NF XV is by permission of the USP Convention. The convention is not responsible for any inaccuracy of quotation or for any false or misleading implication that may arise from separation of excerpts from the original context or by obsolescence resulting from publication of a supplement.

PRINTED IN THE UNITED STATES OF AMERICA

Print No.:   5   4   3   2   1

Preface

Changes in the practice of pharmacy and, concurrently, in the educational preparation for such practice have continued at an unprecedented rate since the appearance of the previous edition of this textbook. It is now universally recognized by physicians, patients, and pharmacy practitioners themselves that the transmittal of information concerning the appropriate use of drugs is the principal role of the pharmacist. Basic and applied science courses, which provide students with this knowledge, and clinical practice courses, which teach them how and when to communicate this knowledge, thus comprise the essentials of the pharmacy curriculum.

Pharmacognosy, "pharmacy's specific and peculiar contribution to the cause of science," has not only retained its position of importance in pharmaceutic studies, but, as a result of the increasing interest shown by consumers in such topics as herbal medicine and megadose vitamin therapy, has actually increased in significance. Pharmacists are the only members of the health-care team who are accessible to the general public on a daily basis. As such, they must be able to advise on a wide variety of drug-related matters ranging from the side effects of the newest antibiotic to the desirability or undesirability of consuming certain herbal teas.

This edition of *Pharmacognosy* has been revised to reflect these changes in the needs of pharmacists. The previously extensive "General Introduction" has been abridged to render it not only more concise, but also, it is hoped, more interesting. Obsolete drugs and references to them have been deleted, and new drugs have been added in most chapters. Some information of marginal interest, e.g., coverage of certain flavoring agents in the "Volatile Oils" chapter, has been reduced to tabular form. Tabular presentation of other, more significant drugs has also been introduced to facilitate comprehension and comparison of related groups, such as the penicillins. Because the study of biosynthetic details no longer forms a major part of most undergraduate courses in pharmacognosy, many of the diagrams depicting biosynthetic pathways and the accompanying explanations have been deleted. A number of the structures of chemical constituents have been redrawn to show the steric configuration of the molecules.

One entire chapter, "Pesticides," has

been eliminated. This does not reflect any reduction in the significance and utility of insecticides, herbicides, and related products. Instead, it recognizes the tremendous increase in their number and in the complexity of federal and state regulations governing their use. A single chapter can no longer provide adequate coverage. Rather than devote more space to a topic of marginal pharmaceutic interest, we decided to omit the topic entirely.

Popular demand for critical, scientific information on herbs and so-called "health foods" prompted inclusion in this edition of a new chapter devoted to this increasingly popular specialty. As many of the older, natural drugs were replaced by newer, more potent pharmaceuticals, authoritative information on them ceased to be available. Yet, the drugs themselves continued to be readily available, primarily in nondrug outlets, where they were accompanied by an enormous selection of advocacy literature presenting much misinformation on their safety and efficacy. Numerous requests for information led us to conclude that pharmacists today require an accurate, concise reference source that would enable them to provide counsel to patients desiring to self-medicate with herbs and related natural products. This source has been provided in the new chapter "Herbs and 'Health Foods'," which covers most of the better-known remedies.

These, then, are the principal changes incorporated in the text of the eighth edition of *Pharmacognosy*. We are hopeful that it, like its predecessors, will prove of interest and value to all those seeking information on the materials of plant, animal, and microbial origin used in the prevention and cure of illness.

West Lafayette, Indiana   Varro E. Tyler
and   Lynn R. Brady
Seattle, Washington   James E. Robbers

Contents

Chapter 1

General Introduction

WHAT IS PHARMACOGNOSY?

Pharmacognosy, which literally means a knowledge of drugs or pharmaceuticals, has been a part of the healing arts and sciences since mankind first began to treat illnesses. It has developed from ancient civilizations that used parts of plants and animals to concoct various potions to eliminate pain, control suffering, and counteract disease. Pharmacognosy has risen from the mysterious incantations of voodoo tribes and has survived the unwritten secret recipes of medicine men. It has progressed from an era of empiricism to the present age of specific therapeutic agents. Today, pharmacognosy is a highly specialized science that represents one of the major disciplines of pharmaceutic education. A number of the drugs used by the ancients are still employed in much the same manner by today's medical practitioners. Although it is true that extraction, separation, isolation, and identification of the component constituents of plant and animal drugs have occurred in relatively recent years, nevertheless the pur-

pose for which many of these medicinal substances are employed today parallels closely the use for which they were intended by our predecessors in the study of pharmacy and medicine.

Because of the interest it engenders in many of the scientists of today, pharmacognosy is a respected discipline which has no counterpart in the other professions. Perhaps because the lay public has heard little about the term "pharmacognosy," there is a lack of recognition and, further, a lack of association of the term with the specific subject matter it represents. However, an intuitive curiosity is inherent in the average person who reads or hears of opium, morphine, foxglove, insulin, reserpine, thyroid, penicillin, blood plasma, polio vaccine, and even the much maligned castor oil!

During the past few years, as a result of the intense concern with all aspects of ecology, there has been a renewed interest in so-called "natural" foods and drugs. The availability of an extremely wide variety of these products, ranging from foenugreek tea to ginseng chewing gum, has stimulated the public to learn more about them. Consequently, a vast literature on natural drugs written by laymen and intended to inform other laymen has come into existence. Much of this literature is relatively inaccurate, consisting of beliefs and opinions substituted for facts. The pharmacist must, of course, be aware of the existence of such pseudopharmacognostic writings, primarily to be able to caution his patients concerning them and to correct any factual misinformation gained from reading them. Chapter 16 in this text provides accurate, up-to-date information on these so-called "health foods" and herbs.

In order to gain proper perspective about a science that deals with plant and animal drugs and their constituents, it is exceedingly helpful to survey past records and to recognize those who have contributed to the subject matter that comprised the field of pharmacognosy in its beginning. By trial and error, primitive man must have acquired biologic knowledge that was useful in determining which plants and animals possessed food value and which were to be avoided because they were unpalatable, poisonous, or dangerous. His observations were handed down from one generation to another and were added to by his progeny. The healing powers of certain herbs, roots, and juices were undoubtedly discovered by accident; but once these attributes were learned, they were too important to be forgotten. The Babylonians made clay models of the human body, and early writings indicate that they were aware of the medicinal effects of a number of plants. It is a well-known fact that the ancient Egyptians were adept at embalming the dead and that they possessed an understanding of the human anatomy as well as a knowledge of the medicinal uses of many plants and animals, according to the *Papyrus Ebers*. This famous document, written in 1550 B.C., was found in the tomb of a mummy and is now preserved at the University of Leipzig.

Dioscorides, a Greek physician who lived in the first century A.D., wrote his "De Materia Medica" in 78 A.D. in which he described about 600 plants that were known to have medicinal properties. Of these, a surprisingly large number are still important in modern medicine. Aloe, belladonna, colchicum, ergot, hyoscyamus, and opium are a few that were used then in much the same manner as they are used today. Galen (131–200 A.D.) was a Greek pharmacist-physician who lived in Rome and who described the method of preparing formulas containing plant and animal drugs. He devoted considerable time to compiling this knowledge which was distributed throughout 20 books. As a tribute to his accuracy in recording his observations, the term "galenical" pharmacy was originated.

From this humble beginning, medicine and pharmacy gradually emerged along separate paths: the physician diagnosed the ailment and prescribed the remedy, and the apothecary or pharmacist specialized in the collection, preparation, and compounding of the substance. Thus, the term **materia medica,** meaning medicinal materials, was synonymous with the substances and products derived from natural sources and was employed by the physicians of that era.

The term **pharmacognosy** was introduced by C. A. Seydler, a medical student in Halle/Saale, Germany, in 1815. This name is formed from two Greek words, *pharmakon*, drug, and *gnosis*, knowledge. The most comprehensive idea of the scope of pharmacognosy was presented by Flückiger who stated that pharmacognosy "is the simultaneous application of various scientific disciplines with the object of acquiring knowledge of drugs from every point of view."

Pharmacognosy may be defined as "an applied science that deals with the biologic, biochemical, and economic features of natural drugs and their constituents." It is a study of drugs that originate in the plant and animal kingdoms. Modern aspects of the science include not only the crude drugs but also their natural derivatives. Digitalis leaf and its isolated glycoside, digitoxin; rauwolfia root and its purified alkaloid, reserpine; and thyroid gland with its extracted hormone, thyroxine, are all part of the subject matter of pharmacognosy.

In some instances drug constituents have been partially replaced in commerce by synthetic compounds of identical chemical structure and therapeutic properties; such **natural** and **synthetic substances** often can be distinguished by physical and chemical tests. For example, natural camphor is obtained from the camphor tree by steam distillation; it is dextrorotatory in its reaction to polarized light. In contrast, synthetic camphor may be manufactured by either of two methods: by *total synthesis* from vinyl chloride and cyclopentadiene (a completely synthetic process) or by *semisynthesis* from pinene derived from pine stumps (not entirely a synthetic process but a chemical modification of a natural product). Synthetic camphor is racemic and can be differentiated easily from the natural form.

Epinephrine, caffeine, codeine, ephedrine, menthol, penicillin, and other chemicals may also be obtained from either the natural source or by partial or total synthesis. They are considered a definite part of pharmacognosy.

In a broad sense, pharmacognosy embraces a knowledge of the history, distribution, cultivation, collection, selection, preparation, commerce, identification, evaluation, preservation, and use of drugs and economic substances that affect the health of man and other animals. Such economic substances extend beyond the category of crude drugs and their derivatives to include a variety of commercial and medicinal products often requiring complicated methods of preparation: al-

lergens, allergenic extracts, antibiotics, immunizing biologics, flavoring agents, and condiments. In a restricted sense, the definition of pharmacognosy implies a particular knowledge of methods of identification and evaluation of drugs.

As a part of the pharmaceutic curriculum, pharmacognosy forms an important link between **pharmacology** and **medicinal chemistry** on one hand and between **pharmacy** and **clinical pharmacy** on the other.

Pharmacology, like pharmacognosy, is an outgrowth of materia medica, the ancient science which dealt with all aspects of medicinal agents. Now, in this more specialized era, pharmacognosy deals primarily with information on the sources and constituents of natural drugs, and pharmacology is concerned with their actions and effects.

Methods of procurement and preparation affect the price of drugs; thus, insofar as economics are concerned, pharmacognosy is intimately associated with the phases of pharmacy administration that deal with prescription pricing. The relationship of pharmacognosy to dispensing pharmacy and clinical pharmacy is obvious when one considers the number of naturally derived drugs that are handled by the pharmacist in this age of drug specialties. Because of his knowledge of drug constituents, the pharmacist is able to predict not only the chemical and physical incompatibilities encountered in compounding, but also the therapeutic incompatibilities that the patient may encounter when utilizing a drug concomitantly with other prescribed or self-selected medications.

When supplying both prescription and over-the-counter (OTC) medication to patients, the pharmacist also provides information required for the safe and effective use of such drugs. The pharmacist further serves as an information source on all aspects of drugs to his colleagues in the medical, dental, and nursing professions. These advisory roles are made possible by the vast background of the pharmacist, the drug expert, in such fields as pharmacognosy, pharmacology, medicinal chemistry, and pharmaceutics.

Any treatise on plant and animal products encompasses a wide variety of uses inasmuch as natural substances are employed in almost every known industry. Although the pharmacist is mainly concerned with those substances having application to public health, he realizes that many of these therapeutic aids are also utilized as beverages, as spices and condiments, in confectioneries, and as technical products.

Coffee beans and tea leaves both yield caffeine, which has medicinal application, yet the original sources are mainstays in the diet of the American public. Wintergreen oil and ginger are used pharmaceutically, but a much greater quantity of each is utilized by the soft drink industry. Mustard seed and clove have definite therapeutic application, still they are in more demand in the spice and condiment trade. Cinnamon oil and peppermint oil are valuable carminatives; however, they enjoy an enviable reputation as popular flavoring agents in candies and chewing gums. Certain industries depend on large supplies of rosin, turpentine, linseed oil, acacia, pectin, and numerous other natural products that have a relatively limited application in the field of pharmacy.

CRUDE DRUGS

Crude drugs are vegetable or animal drugs that consist of natural substances that have undergone only the processes of collection and drying. The term, "**natural substances**," refers to those substances found in nature that comprise whole plants and herbs and anatomic parts thereof; vegetable saps, extracts, secretions, and other constituents thereof; whole animals and anatomic parts thereof; glands or other animal organs, extracts, secretions, and other constituents thereof; and that have not had changes made in their molecular structure as found in nature. The term, "**crude**," as used in relation to natural products, means any product that has not been advanced in value or improved in condition by shredding, grinding, chipping, crushing, distilling, evaporating, extracting, artificial mixing with other substances, or by any other process or treatment beyond that which is essential to its proper packing and to the prevention of decay or deterioration pending manufacture.

Crude drugs are used infrequently as therapeutic agents; more often, their chief principles are separated by various means and are employed in a more specific manner. These principles are known as **derivatives** or **extractives.** Regardless of whether the derivative or extractive is a single substance or a mixture of substances, it is considered as the **chief constituent** of the drug.

The process of drug extraction is a generally accepted method of obtaining these active principles. Extraction removes only those substances that can be dissolved in the liquid or liquid mixture referred to as the **solvent,** or, more specifically, as the **menstruum.** The undissolved portion of the drug that remains after the extraction process is completed is called the **marc.** The product of the extraction process is known as the **extractive** and is usually a mixture of substances. A large-scale drug extractor of the type currently used in the pharmaceutic industry is illustrated in Figure 1–1.

The **geographic source** and **habitat** are the region in which the plant or animal yielding the drug grows. Sometimes this term is applied erroneously to the drugs themselves. Drugs are collected in all parts of the world, though the tropics and sub-

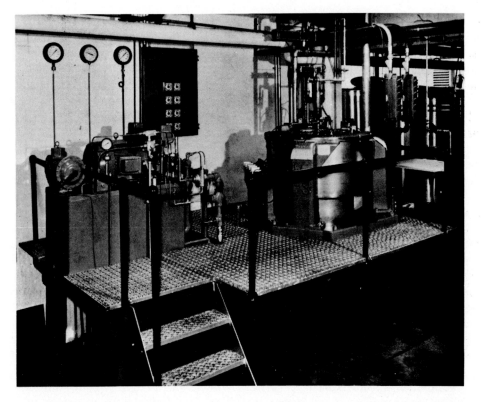

Fig. 1–1. A fully automatic industrial drug extractor. Its operating cycle, which involves pressures up to 2000 lbs per sq in and a centrifugal force of 1000 × g, can be programmed to meet process requirements. (Courtesy of Dr. Madis Laboratories, Inc.)

tropics, where plant species abound, yield more drugs than do the arctic and subarctic regions. The Mediterranean basin including Asia Minor yields more drugs than any other region of the world. However, India, the East Indies, central Europe, northern South America, Mexico, Central America, North America, and other regions yield numerous and valuable drugs.

Neither the **scientific name** of the plant nor the **commercial name** of the drug is necessarily an indication of the true habitat of drug plants. For example, the specific name of *Acacia senegal* seems to indicate that this plant, which yields gum arabic, is most abundant in Senegal. Actually, the bulk of the commercial gum now comes from trees cultivated in Sudan. In other cases, plants are common to a much larger territory than the specific name indicates, such as *Prunus virginiana.* Peru balsam, for example, does not come from Peru, but is produced in El Salvador, whereas most of the Spanish licorice now comes from Asia Minor.

Plants growing in their native countries are said to be **indigenous** to those regions, such as *Pinus palustris* in the southern United States, *Aconitum napellus* in the mountainous regions of Europe, and others. Plants are said to be **naturalized** when they grow in a foreign land or in a locality other than their native homes, such as *Datura stramonium,* which was introduced into the United States from Europe. Some of these plants may have

been introduced with the seeds of cultivated plants, some by birds or ocean currents, others by ballast of ships, and so on.

Drugs can be collected from wild plants,
or plants can be cultivated for the production of drugs.

Cultivated medicinal plants have been
propagated for centuries in China, India,
Europe, and many other lands. Plant cultivation was known to the people of ancient
civilizations inasmuch as sculptures and
drawings depict hand pollination of the
date palm by the Assyrians in 9000 B.C. and
cultivation of rice and barley by the
Chinese and Egyptians in 5000 B.C.

In Europe, medicinal plant gardens of
the monasteries date back to the early
Christian era. Since shortly after the discovery of America and continuing to the
present, many countries have made definite attempts to cultivate drug and economic plants. Thus, vanilla, which is native to Mexico and Central America, is now
produced at such distances from its original habitat as the islands of Réunion,
Tahiti, and Mauritius. Cocoa, another native of Mexico, is now produced in large
quantities in Nigeria and Ghana, in Sri
Lanka, and in Indonesia.

Cinchona, native to the South American
Andes, was developed as a crop in Indonesia. By 1900, the South American
production was practically nil, owing to
the wanton destruction of wild trees; thus,
the Dutch in the Netherlands East Indies
held a world monopoly on cinchona. A
similar situation existed with coca,
another South American plant transported
to that area.

In many instances plants have been cultivated in their native habitats, either because of dwindling natural supply or to
improve the quality of the drug. Before
World War II, the Japanese had established
large plantations of camphor trees in For-
mosa and held a virtual monopoly in natural camphor. Other drugs, such as Ceylon

cinnamon and opium, are produced entirely from cultivated plants.

Extensive cultivation of certain drug
plants is conducted in specific geographic
areas of the United States. Louisiana produces castor oil from cultivated plants.
Occasionally, however, some circumstances will completely eliminate a certain
section as a drug-producing region. Formerly, mints were extensively cultivated
in southwestern Michigan and northern
Indiana. Peppermint, spearmint, and other
mints were grown in mile-long rows, particularly near Mentha, Michigan. In the
early 1950s, a fungus blight invaded the
fields of that area and within a few years it
was considered uneconomical to attempt
further cultivation. At present, Washington and Oregon have assumed leadership
in the production of mints and mint oils
although both Michigan and Indiana have
relocated their areas of cultivation. In recent years the state of California has spon-
sored drug and oil plant cultivation among
the farms in the southern part of the state,
and this section now produces several million dollars' worth of drugs and economic
products annually, all from cultivated
plants.

It is important to ascertain that plants
cultivated in a certain geographic area will
develop the desired type and amount of
constituents. The differences in the relative amounts of volatile constituents often
determine the character of the oil and, consequently, the demand for that particular
oil. California orange oil is marketed at
more than twice the price of Florida oils.
The preference for Michigan peppermint
oils over Washington and Oregon oils is
owing to the types of constituents
developed—the Michigan oils taste better.

COMMERCE IN DRUGS

The **commercial origin** of a drug refers
to its production and its channels of trade.

Drugs frequently bear a geographic name indicating the country or region in which they are collected, the country or city from which they are shipped, or their variety. These names do not necessarily reflect the area where the plant grows. English hyoscyamus leaves are gathered from plants growing in England and are principally consumed in that country; Indian rhubarb is the product of plants growing in various parts of India; Spanish licorice is a botanic variety of *Glycyrrhiza glabra*, originally produced in Spain but now produced elsewhere; and Oregon grape root is a species of *Mahonia* and may or may not come from Oregon. The commercial origin may change in the course of time as with cinchona, vanilla, and coca previously mentioned.

Since World War II, most of the drug items have been shipped directly from the producing areas to New York City. Although many drug collectors and dealers conducted their business through a governmental agency in the past, little drug commerce now passes through such an agency. The exceptions are the communist countries and their European satellites where governmental agencies control all commerce.

PREPARATION OF DRUGS FOR THE COMMERCIAL MARKET

COLLECTION

Collection of drugs from cultivated plants always insures a true natural source and a reliable product. This may, or may not, be the case when drugs are collected from wild plants. Carelessness or ignorance on the part of the collector can result in complete or partial substitution. This is especially true when drugs are difficult to collect or the natural source is scarce. Many drugs are collected from wild plants, sometimes on a fairly extensive scale

(tragacanth, senna) when collection is the vocation of the gatherer, and sometimes on a limited scale when collection is an avocation (podophyllum, hydrastis). Because drugs come from all over the world, collection areas are almost universal, and collectors may vary from uneducated natives to highly skilled botanists.

Certain areas of the United States are particularly noteworthy as collection areas. White pine, podophyllum, ginseng, and many other native American drugs are collected in the Blue Ridge Mountain region, of which Asheville, North Carolina, is one of the important collection areas. Native American drugs are usually collected by individuals, such as farm children and part-time agricultural laborers.

The proper time of harvesting or collecting is particularly important because the nature and quantity of constituents vary greatly in some species according to the season. The most advantageous collection time is when the part of the plant that constitutes the drug is highest in its content of active principles and when the material will dry to give the maximum quality and appearance.

HARVESTING

The mode of harvesting varies with each drug produced and with the pharmaceutic requirements of each drug. Some drugs may be collected by hand labor; however, when the cost of labor is an important factor, the use of mechanical devices is often more successful in economic production of the drug. With some drugs, where the skillful selection of plant parts is an important factor (digitalis), mechanical means cannot replace hand labor.

DRYING

By drying the plant material, one removes sufficient moisture to insure good keeping qualities and to prevent molding, the action of enzymes, the action of bacteria, and chemical or other possible changes. Drying fixes the constituents, facilitates grinding and milling, and converts the drug into a more convenient form for commercial handling. Proper and successful drying involves two main principles: control of temperature and regulation of air flow. Control of the drying operation is determined by the nature of the material to be dried and by the desired appearance of the finished product. The plant material can be dried either by the sun or by the use of artificial heat.

With some natural products, such as vanilla, processes of fermentation or sweating are necessary to bring about changes in the constituents. Such drugs require special drying processes, usually called "curing."

GARBLING

Garbling is the final step in the preparation of a crude drug. Garbling consists of the removal of extraneous matter, such as other parts of the plant, dirt, and added adulterants. This step is done to some extent during collection, but should be carried out after the drug is dried and before the drug is baled or packaged. Although garbling may be done by mechanical means in some cases, it is usually a semiskilled operation.

PACKAGING, STORAGE, AND PRESERVATION

The packaging of drugs depends on their final disposition. In commerce, if transportation, storage, and ultimate use for manufacturing purposes are involved, it is customary to choose the type of packaging that provides ample protection to the drug and gives economy of space. Leaf and herb material is usually baled with power balers

into a solid compact mass that is then sewn into a burlap cover. Bales that are shipped overseas weigh from 100 to 250 pounds. Senna leaves from India come in bales of 400 pounds; stramonium from Argentina in bales of 700 pounds. Drugs that are likely to deteriorate from absorbed moisture (digitalis, ergot) are packed in moisture-proof cans. Gums, resins, and extracts are shipped in barrels, boxes, or casks.

Packaging is often characteristic for certain drugs. The standard package for all grades of aloe is a 55-gallon steel drum, and this type of container is also employed for balsam of Peru. Matting-covered packages of cinnamon from the Far East, seroons (bales covered with cowhide) containing sarsaparilla from South America, lead flasks with oil of rose from Bulgaria, and many other odd forms of packaging are noted in the drug trade.

Proper storage and preservation are important factors in maintaining a high degree of quality of the drug. Hard-packed bales, barks, and resinous drugs usually reabsorb little moisture. But leaf, herb, and root drugs that are not well packed tend to absorb amounts of moisture that reach 10, 15, or even 30% of the weight of the drug. Excessive moisture not only increases the weight of the drug, thus reducing the percentage of active constituents, but also favors enzymatic activity and facilitates fungal growth.

Light adversely affects drugs that are highly colored, rendering them unattractive and possibly causing undesirable changes in constituents. The oxygen of the air increases oxidation of the constituents of drugs, especially when oxidases are present. Therefore, the warehouse should be cool, dark, and well ventilated with dry air.

The protection of drugs against **attacks by insects** must not be overlooked. The insects that infest vegetable drugs belong

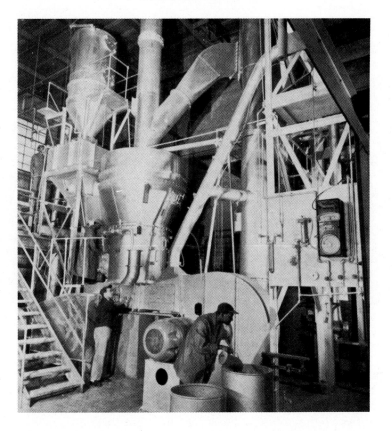

Fig. 1–2. A grinding mill used in large-scale commercial production of crude drugs. (Courtesy of S. B. Penick and Company.)

chiefly to the orders *Lepidoptera, Coleoptera,* and *Diptera.*

For destruction of insects and prevention of their attacks, a number of methods have been employed. The simplest method is to expose the drug to a temperature of 65°C. This method is probably the most efficient not only in preventing insect attacks, but in preventing many other forms of deterioration. For the fumigation of large lots of crude drugs, such as those stored in warehouses and manufacturing plants, the use of methyl bromide has met with considerable success.

Small lots of drugs may readily be stored in tight, light-resistant containers. Tin cans, covered metal bins, or amber glass containers are the most satisfactory. Drugs should not be stored in wooden boxes or in drawers and never in paper bags. Not only is deterioration hastened, but odors are communicated from one drug to another, attacks by insects are facilitated, and destruction by mice and rats may occur. If drugs in small quantities are stored in tight containers, insect attack can be controlled by adding to the container a few drops of chloroform or carbon tetrachloride from time to time. In the case of digitalis and ergot, whose low moisture content must be maintained at all times, the insertion of a suitable cartridge or device containing a nonliquefying, inert, dehydrating substance may be introduced into the tight container.

Because high temperatures accelerate all

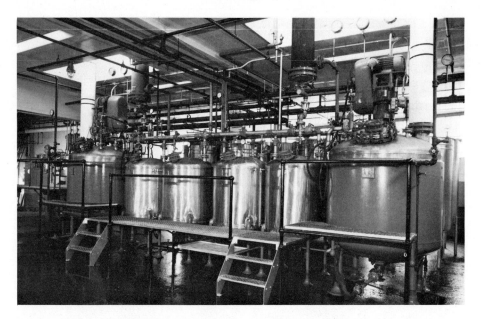

Fig. 1–3. Semiautomatic vacuum and atmospheric reflux reactors used to produce various kinds of resins, enzymes, and extracts. (Courtesy of Dr. Madis Laboratories, Inc.)

chemical reactions, including those involved in deterioration, drugs must always be stored at as low a temperature as possible. The ideal temperature is just above freezing, but since this is impractical in most cases, the warehouse or other storage place should be as cool as possible. Certain drugs, such as the biologics, must be stored at a temperature between 2° and 8°C.

ANIMAL DRUGS

Animal drugs are produced from wild or domesticated animals. Wild animals must be hunted (whale, musk deer) or fished for (cod and halibut), and thus, in a sense, their collection parallels the collection of vegetable drugs. Many animal drugs, however, are produced from domesticated animals and, therefore, correspond to the cultivated vegetable drugs. When drugs consist of insects, the drugs are either collected from wild insects (cantharides) or definite attempts are made to cultivate

them, i.e., to furnish the insects with food and shelter and to maintain optimum conditions for their propagation (honeybee).

Drugs such as lanolin and milk products, as well as hormones, endocrine products, and some enzymes, are obtained from domesticated hogs, sheep, or cattle. The slaughterhouse is the usual source of glandular products and enzymes, and the larger packing establishments have departments for the recovery and refinement of these therapeutic agents and pharmaceuticals. Processing and purification of the animal drugs vary with the individual drug.

EVALUATION OF DRUGS

To evaluate a drug means to identify it and to determine its quality and purity.

The identity of a drug can be established by actual collection of the drug from a plant or animal that has been positively identified. Research investigators must be absolutely certain of the origin of their samples; hence, "drug gardens" are frequently established by institutions engaged in pharmacognostic research. Another method of identification is the comparison of a representative unknown sample to a published description of the drug and to authentic drug samples.

Quality refers to the intrinsic value of the drug, i.e., the amount of medicinal principles or active constituents present. These constituents are classified into groups of nonprotoplasmic cell contents and can be found in the section of this chapter on "Classification of Drugs." These groups include: carbohydrates, glycosides, tannins, lipids, volatile oils, resins and resin-combinations, steroids, alkaloids, peptide hormones, enzymes and other proteins, vitamins, antibiotics, biologics, allergens, and others.

A high grade of quality in a drug is of primary importance, and effort should be made to obtain and maintain this high quality. The evaluation of a drug involves a number of methods that may be classified as follows: (1) organoleptic, (2) microscopic, (3) biologic, (4) chemical, (5) physical (Fig. 1–4).

Organoleptic (lit. "impression on the organs") refers to evaluation by means of the organs of sense and includes the macroscopic appearance of the drug, its odor and taste, occasionally the sound or "snap" of its fracture, and the "feel" of the drug to the touch.

The microscope is not only essential to the study of adulterants in powdered plant and animal drugs, but is indispensable in the identification of the pure powdered drug. Powdered drugs possess few macroscopic features of identification other than color, odor, and taste; hence, the microscopic characteristics are important.

The pharmacologic activity of certain drugs has been applied to their evaluation and standardization. Assays on living animals as well as on intact or excised organs often indicate the strength of the drug or its preparations. Because living organ-

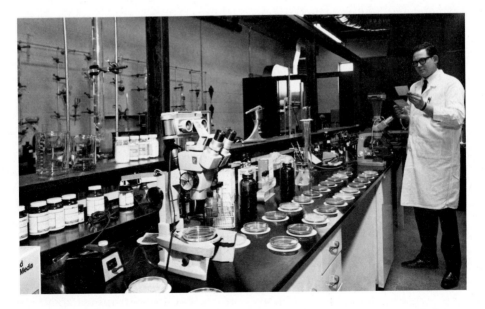

Fig. 1–4. A drug quality-control laboratory where chemical, physical, microbiologic, and pharmacognostic tests are carried out on natural drug products. (Courtesy of Dr. Madis Laboratories, Inc.)

isms are used, the assays are called biologic assays or bioassays.

Because the active constituents of many natural drugs have been determined, chemical methods of evaluating crude drugs and their products are useful and, consequently, are widely employed. For many drugs, the chemical assay represents the best method of determining the official potency.

The application of typical physical constants to crude drugs is rare. However, physical constants are extensively applied to the active principles of drugs, such as alkaloids, volatile oils, fixed oils, and others.

CLASSIFICATION OF DRUGS

In pharmacognosy, drugs may be classified according to (1) their morphology, (2) the taxonomy of the plants and animals from which they are obtained, (3) their therapeutic applications, and (4) their chemical constituents. Each of these methods of classification has advantages and disadvantages, and the emphasis depends on the ultimate goal of the individual. If a person is expected to identify specific drugs and to ascertain their adulterants, a **morphologic** classification is applicable. In this system, the drugs are grouped according to the part of the plant or animal represented, such as roots, leaves, organs, or glands. However, the form of the commercial article is not always distinguishable and cannot be readily placed in its proper category.

Consideration of the natural relationship or phylogeny among plants and among animals gives rise to a **taxonomic** classification. With the present-day knowledge of the evolutionary development of living organisms, this arrangement has served adequately for many years. A large number of plant families have certain distinguishing characteristics

that permit drugs from these families to be studied at one time; thus, drugs consisting of cremocarp fruits (anise, fennel, caraway) are considered with other members of the Umbelliferae, drugs obtained from plants having alternate leaves, cymose flowers, and fruits that are capsules or berries (belladonna, hyoscyamus, stramonium) are considered with the Solanaceae, and drugs possessing square stems, opposite leaves, and bilabiate flowers (peppermint, spearmint, thyme) are considered with the Labiatae. This type of arrangement is sometimes called the botanic arrangement for plant drugs or the zoologic arrangement for animal drugs. In the latter case, all arthropods are grouped, as are all mammals, fish, and other natural phylogenetic types.

Inasmuch as drugs are employed medicinally because of their therapeutic effects, a third method of study is the **pharmacologic** or **therapeutic** classification. All of the cathartic drugs are associated with this classification regardless of morphology, taxonomy, or chemical relation. Thus, cascara sagrada, senna, podophyllum, and castor oil are considered at one time because of their action on the intestinal tract. Similarly, digitalis, strophanthus, and squill are grouped together because they affect cardiac muscle. This type of consideration forms the basis for the science of pharmacology.

Because the activity and therapeutic use of drugs are based on chemical constituents, it would appear that a **chemical** classification is the preferred method of study. Most drugs contain a variety of constituents, some therapeutically active, others only chemically active, and still others antagonistic to each other. Certain plant families exhibit definite types of chemical principles; for example, mydriatic alkaloids (atropine, scopolamine) characterize the Solanaceae, volatile oils represent the Umbelliferae, and oleoresins abound in the Pinaceae. By studying at one time all drugs containing alkaloids, it is possible to establish relationships between them. In a like manner, drugs containing volatile oils, or resins, or tannins, or glycosides can be classified in their respective phytochemical groups.

The pharmacist no longer gathers his own plant and animal drugs, he rarely finds it necessary to identify and determine the purity of crude drugs, and he is never called on to examine powdered drugs microscopically. However, he is expected to know the chemical nature of his drugs, regardless of their natural or synthetic origin, so that he might predict incompatibilities, solubility, palatability, and therapeutic and toxic effects. The modern pharmacist is a "drug specialist," and in that capacity he is consulted by other members of the health professions.

Modern pharmacognosy is built on the significant aspects of cell physiology and biochemistry as they affect the biosynthetic development of the constituents of plants and animals. Our expanding knowledge of the chemical constituents of plants has revealed the existence of a close relationship between these chemicals and the taxonomic position of the plants themselves. In other words, certain chemical compounds have been found to characterize certain botanic groupings (taxa).

Depending on its relative biosynthetic complexity, the compound may be characteristic of a limited number of species, an entire family, or even a whole class or order of plants. The biosynthetically complex alkaloid, morphine, occurs only in 2 species of the genus *Papaver* (*P. somniferum* and *P. setigerum*), but the somewhat simpler protopine is found in all plants of the poppy family. Compounds that are biosynthetically simple are so widely distributed that they lack systematic significance. Nicotine, for example, with its close relationship to the ubiquitous nicotinic acid, has been found in many remotely related plants, such as the club mosses and the composites.

Nearly 3 centuries ago, the London apothecary James Petiver published the results of his experiments that demonstrated that closely related plants frequently possess similar physiologic activities, or, as he put it, "herbs of the same make . . . have like virtue." Today his findings are not surprising, for it is recognized that plants containing similar or identical chemical constituents also have similar medicinal properties. Thus, because all species of *Cinchona* contain quinine, all are useful in the treatment of malaria. Similarly, in lists of plants used by native people, the same genera and families occur repeatedly. This is true for botanics used for everything from contraception to arrow poisons, indeed, for any purpose that is an expression of the plants' physiologic activity.

Understanding of these facts has led to the development of a relatively new branch of science known as chemotaxonomy or biochemical systematics. Comprised of nearly equal parts of chemistry and biology, this discipline attempts to utilize chemical facts to obtain a more exact understanding of biologic evolution and natural relationships. Its principles and findings are of particular interest to the student of pharmacognosy who may apply them to determine potential sources of known drugs or to explore those areas of the biologic kingdom in which new ones are most likely to be discovered. Tyler's compilations of chemical characteristics of plant families of medicinal importance provide a useful starting point.

CHEMISTRY OF DRUGS

The living organism may be considered a biosynthetic laboratory not only for chemical compounds (carbohydrates, proteins, fats) that are utilized as food by man and animals, but also for a multitude of compounds (glycosides, alkaloids, volatile oils) that exert a physiologic effect. These chemical compounds give plant and animal drugs their therapeutic properties. Drugs are used as such in their crude form or they may be extracted, the resulting principles being employed as medicinal agents. It is obvious, therefore, that any study of pharmacognosy must embrace a thorough consideration of these chemical entities. The usual term for these entities is **constituents;** but because the plant or animal is composed of many chemical compounds, it is common practice to single out those compounds that are responsible for the therapeutic effect and to call them **active constituents.**

These active constituents are differentiated from **inert constituents,** which also occur in plant and animal drugs. Cellulose, lignin, suberin, and cutin are usually regarded as inert matter in plant drugs; in addition, starch, albumin, coloring matters, and other substances may have no definite pharmacologic activity and also are considered inert constituents. In animal drugs, keratin, chitin, muscle fiber, and connective tissue are regarded as inert. Often the presence of inert substances may modify or prevent the absorbability or potency of the active constituents. To eliminate the undesirable effects of inert matter in the crude drug or its preparations, active principles are extracted, crystallized, and purified for therapeutic use. These constituents have been referred to as "secondary" plant substances. No completely satisfactory explanation has been advanced for their presence in a great number of plant families; nevertheless, their occurrence in related genera and their chemical relationships indicate that they may play roles of some significance in plant metabolism.

Active constituents may be divided into two classes: **pharmaceutically active** and **pharmacologically active.** Pharmaceutically active constituents may cause precipitation or other chemical changes in a medicinal preparation. For instance, neither cinchona bark nor its extracts could be used in formulating preparations containing iron salts because the cinchotannic acid would combine with these salts and cause precipitation. Cinchotannic acid, then, is a pharmaceutically active constituent. The use of quinine hydrochloride obviates this incompatibility because it is a purified crystalline compound that does not contain the slightest trace of cinchotannic acid. In contrast, the rheotannic acid present in rhubarb serves as an astringent to prevent the griping action usually associated with anthraquinone drugs of that type. In this case, rheotannic acid is one of the pharmacologically active constituents. Depending on the particular activity of the constituent and on the other constituents or ingredients with which it is associated, certain principles may be placed in one or the other category.

Pharmacologically active constituents are responsible for the therapeutic activity of the drug. They may be either single chemical substances or mixtures of principles, the separation of which is neither practical nor advantageous. The single chemicals are exemplified by sugars, starches, plant acids, enzymes, glycosides, steroids, alkaloids, proteins, hormones, and vitamins. The mixtures include fixed oils, fats, waxes, volatile oils, resins, oleoresins, oleo-gum-resins, and balsams.

The secondary constituents of drug plants are influenced by 3 principal factors: heredity (genetic composition), ontogeny (stage of development), and environment. Genetic effects induce both quantitative and qualitative changes, but those caused by environmental influences are primarily quantitative. Plants of the same species that resemble one another closely in form and structure (phenotypically) may, nevertheless, be quite different in genetic composition (genotypically). This often results in distinct differences in chemical composition, particularly with reference to secondary constituents. Such plants are said to belong to different chemical races.

Perhaps the best-known pharmacognostic examples of chemical races are found in the ergot fungus, *Claviceps purpurea*. Individual strains have been isolated representing chemical races that produce superior yields of single desired alkaloids, e.g., ergotamine, instead of the usual small concentrations of complex mixtures of alkaloids. Other examples include chemical races of certain species of *Eucalyptus* that exhibit large variations in the content of cineole and related constituents in their volatile oils. Chemical races of *Strophanthus sarmentosus* differing markedly in their content of glycosides and sapogenins have also been reported.

Ontogeny also plays a significant role in the nature of the active constituents found in medicinal plants. Although it might be expected that the concentration of secondary metabolites would increase with the age of the plant, it is not generally appreciated that the identity of these constituents may also vary according to the stage of development. The cannabidiol content of *Cannabis sativa* reaches a peak early in the growing season and then begins to decline. When this decline occurs, the concentration of tetrahydrocannabinol begins to increase reciprocally and continues until the plant approaches maturity. Old plants, as well as stored plant material, are characterized by high concentrations of cannabinol. In the opium poppy, *Papaver somniferum*, the morphine content of the capsules is highest 2 to 3 weeks after flowering. If the latex is harvested earlier, related alkaloids such as thebaine and codeine predominate. On the other hand, if harvesting is delayed too long, the morphine decomposes.

Environmental factors that can produce variations in secondary plant constituents include soil, climate, associated flora, and methods of cultivation. Because all these factors are more or less related, they are difficult to evaluate individually. For example, many alkaloid-containing plants accumulate higher concentrations of such constituents in moist regions than in arid lands. However, this may actually be related to the soil, which is usually poor in nitrogen in arid regions, and rich nitrogen sources are usually required for good yields of alkaloids. This is not necessarily the case with volatile-oil-bearing plants because excess nitrogen does not necessarily cause an increase in their yields. Indeed, such plants abound in dry areas as opposed to moister habitats.

One phase of pharmacognosy that has assumed a role of importance in recent years is the study of the biochemical pathways leading to the formation of secondary constituents used as drugs. This study is commonly referred to as **drug biosynthesis** or **biogenesis.** Just as an understanding of the chemical synthesis of phenobarbital or other synthetic drugs is of fundamental importance to the student of medicinal chemistry, a knowledge of the biochemical synthesis of drugs of natural origin is of equal importance to the student of pharmacognosy (Fig. 1–5).

Any discussion of crude drugs and their derivatives must necessarily begin with the plant or animal that formed them by an inherent **biosynthetic process.** The biosynthesis of many plant constituents is often complex and sometimes still not completely known. More information about this interesting phase of plant physiology will be presented in subsequent chapters as the individual types of constituents are discussed. The biosynthetic processes whereby animal cells form hormones, pro-

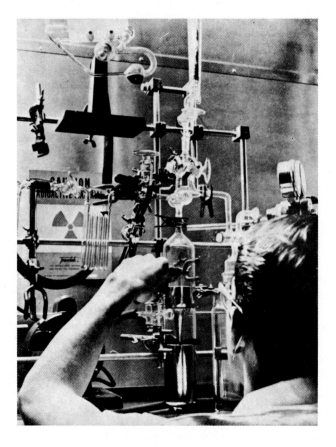

Fig. 1–5. Radioactive carbon used in drug metabolism study at the radiochemistry laboratory, Pfizer Medical Research Laboratories, Groton, Connecticut. Drugs labeled with radioactive materials reveal information concerning biosynthesis, molecular structure, and other phases of plant and animal metabolism. (Courtesy of Charles Pfizer and Company, Inc.)

teins, and enzymes are also under investigation by research workers.

Early experiments devoted to the elucidation of such chemical pathways were fraught with difficulty and often yielded equivocal results. Because suitable experimental methods were unavailable, researchers turned to speculation and the formulation of hypothetic reaction sequences. Some of these "paper chemistry" hypotheses have proved to be remarkably accurate predictions of actual metabolic pathways in the living organism. For example, as early as 1912, the Swiss chemist, G. Trier, proposed that amino acids and their simple derivatives, which were widely distributed in nature, served as precursors of structurally complex alkaloids. Nearly 40 years passed before this brilliant insight could be verified experimentally.

Within the last 4 decades, isotopically labeled organic compounds have become generally available. These so-called "tracer" substances can be administered to a plant or animal and their subsequent metabolism can be followed to determine whether the compound functions as a precursor or moiety of the metabolite in question. The classic example of such experimentation is the use of $^{14}CO_2$ by Melvin Calvin and his associates at the University of California to determine the path of carbon during photosynthesis. In recent years numerous studies of the biosynthetic pathways of medicinally important plant and animal constituents have been carried out, and scientific papers devoted to this topic are appearing at such a rapid rate that any detailed review of the subject would be outdated before it could be published. Fortunately, the basic steps in the pathways leading to most types of primary and secondary biologic constituents have been elucidated.

Some of these fundamental reaction sequences leading to the different types of secondary constituents used as drugs will be presented in the chapters dealing with the individual drugs and their constituents, but to facilitate a general understanding of the pathways involved and their interrelationships, they are summarized in Fig. 1—6. Emphasis is placed on the pharmaceutically important secondary constituents because the student has already acquired a knowledge of the biosynthesis of most primary constituents (sugars, fats, amino acids, etc.) in prerequisite courses in biochemistry. However,

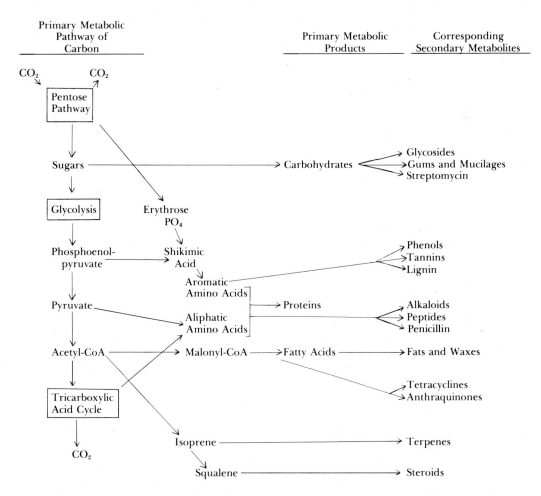

Fig. 1—6. Interrelationships of biosynthetic pathways leading to secondary constituents in plants.

basic pathways of primary metabolism are reviewed briefly in the appropriate sections to give some indication of the relationships of the secondary pathways to the more fundamental biochemical processes.

In Chapters 2 through 14, drugs and drug constituents are discussed individually. Drugs that are official now, were official in the past, or have been used medicinally without official recognition are listed in each chapter. The nomenclature, history, preparation for the commercial market, descriptions, constituents, standards, uses, dose preparations, prescription specialties (if any), and other pertinent information for each are featured. Because pharmacognosy is a subject concerned with natural products, emphasis remains on the biologic aspects of these drugs. Although the chemical classification is employed, the drugs must still be considered the results of plant and animal metabolism.

The chapters devoted to these active constituents and the drugs containing them are:

2. **CARBOHYDRATES AND RELATED COMPOUNDS.** Compounds composed of carbon, hydrogen, and oxygen as polyhydroxy aldehyde or ketone alcohols: sucrose, lactose, starch, acacia, tragacanth, agar, pectin.

3. **GLYCOSIDES.** Substances that on hydrolysis yield one or more sugars among the products of the reaction: barbaloin, glycyrrhizin, vanillin, salicin, amygdalin.

Also included are **TANNINS,** a group of complex phenolic compounds capable of combining with proteins: hamamelitannin, gallotannic acid.

4. **LIPIDS.** Compounds comprising fixed oils, fats, and waxes.

FIXED OILS AND FATS. Glyceryl esters of fatty acids that are saponified by alkalies: olive oil, peanut oil, sesame oil, castor oil.

WAXES. Esters of fatty acids with high-molecular-weight monohydric alcohols: beeswax, spermaceti, carnauba wax.

5. **VOLATILE OILS.** Essential oils that represent the odoriferous principles of plants: peppermint oil, clove oil, cinnamon oil, anise oil, rose oil.

6. **RESINS AND RESIN COMBINATIONS.** Compounds comprising resins, oleoresins, oleo-gum-resins, and balsams.

RESINS. Solid or semisolid amorphous products of complex chemical nature: rosin, podophyllum resin, jalap resin.

OLEORESINS. Resins and volatile oils in homogeneous mixtures: turpentine, copaiba.

OLEO-GUM-RESINS. Oleoresins and gums in homogeneous mixtures: asafetida, myrrh.

BALSAMS. Resins with mixtures of aromatic substances such as benzoic acid, cinnamic acid, or both: benzoin, tolu balsam, Peru balsam, styrax.

7. **STEROIDS.** Derivatives of cyclopentenophenanthrene: estrogens, androgens, adrenal cortex hormones, cardioactive aglycones, bile acids, cholesterol, ergosterol.

8. **ALKALOIDS.** Nitrogenous crystalline or oily compounds, usually basic in character: atropine, morphine, quinine, cocaine, reserpine.

9. **PEPTIDE HORMONES.** Active principles secreted by certain endocrine glands: glucagon, insulin, oxytocin, vasopressin, ACTH.

10. **ENZYMES AND OTHER PROTEINS.** Organic catalysts produced by living organisms: pepsin, pancreatin, rennin, papain, trypsin.

Nitrogenous organic substances composed of amino acid units: gelatin, heparin, protamine.

11. **VITAMINS.** Chemical compounds necessary for normal growth and function of animals: thiamine, riboflavin, cyanocobalamin, ascorbic acid, tocopherol.

12. **ANTIBIOTICS.** Chemical entities produced biosynthetically that are destructive or inhibitory to microorganisms: penicillin, streptomycin, erythromycin, bacitracin, tyrothricin, polymyxin, tetracycline,

oleandomycin, kanamycin, griseofulvin, gentamicin.

13. **BIOLOGICS.** Products composed of antigenic matter or antibody preparations capable of developing a state of immunity in the patient: adsorbed diphtheria toxoid, smallpox vaccine, poliomyelitis vaccines, immune globulins, diphtheria antitoxin; also biologics related to human blood: albumin human, antihemophilic factor.

14. **ALLERGENS.** Substances, usually protoplasmic in origin, that cause unusual responses in hypersensitive individuals: pollen grains, mold spores, feathers, animal dander, poison ivy.

Two additional chapters are included in this text. They are devoted to drug-related topics of considerable significance to many practicing pharmacists.

15. **POISONOUS PLANTS.** Higher plants and fungi that produce toxic effects when introduced into the human body: jimson weed, nightshade, water hemlock, amanita, inocybe.

16. **HERBS AND "HEALTH FOODS."** Products of natural origin used by the laity in the self-treatment of disease states or less-than-optimal health conditions. Many are without therapeutic effect, and some are toxic.

READING REFERENCES

Bennett, H.: *Industrial Waxes*, Vols. I–II, New York, Chemical Publishing Co., Inc., 1963.

Bernfeld, P., ed.: *Biogenesis of Natural Compounds*, 2nd ed., New York, Pergamon Press, Inc., 1967.

Boyer, P. D., ed.: *The Enzymes*, 3rd ed., Vols. I–XIII, New York, Academic Press, Inc., 1970–1976.

Briggs, M. H., and Brotherton, J.: *Steroid Biochemistry and Pharmacology*, New York, Academic Press, Inc., 1970.

Camp, J.: *Magic, Myth and Medicine*, New York, Taplinger Publishing Co., 1974.

Chemical Technology, Vol. V, *Natural Organic Materials and Related Synthetic Products*, New York, Barnes & Noble Books, 1972.

Davis, P. H., and Heywood, V. H.: *Principles of Angiosperm Taxonomy*, Princeton, N.J., D. Van Nostrand Co., Inc., 1965.

Farnsworth, N. R.: Drugs from Higher Plants, Tile and Till, *55*(2):32, 1969.

Farnsworth, N. R.: Immunizing Biologicals, Tile and Till, *56*(1):3; (2):20; (3):52; (4):62, 1970.

Gibbs, R. D.: *Chemotaxonomy of Flowering Plants*, Vols. I–IV, Montreal, McGill-Queen's University Press, 1974.

Gibson, M. R.: Botanicals: A Factor in 50% of Drug Products! Am. Prof. Pharm., *35*(2):44, 1969.

Goodwin, T. W., and Mercer, E. T.: *Introduction to Plant Biochemistry*, Oxford, Pergamon Press Ltd., 1972.

Guenther, E.: *The Essential Oils*, Vols. I–VI, New York, D. Van Nostrand Co., Inc., 1949–1952.

Guthrie, R. D.: *Introduction to Carbohydrate Chemistry*, 4th ed., Oxford, Clarendon Press, 1974.

Harris, K. L., ed.: *Microscopic-Analytical Methods in Food and Drug Control*, Food and Drug Technical Bulletin No. 1, Washington, D.C., U.S. Department of Health, Education, and Welfare, Food and Drug Administration, 1960.

Harrison, R. H.: *Healing Herbs of the Bible*, Leiden, E. J. Brill, 1966.

Heftmann, E.: *Steroid Biochemistry*, New York, Academic Press, Inc., 1970.

Hegnauer, R.: *Chemotaxonomie der Pflanzen*, Vols. I–VI, Basel and Stuttgart, Birkhäuser Verlag, 1962–1973.

Heywood, V. H., ed.: *Modern Methods in Plant Taxonomy*, New York, Academic Press, Inc., 1968.

Hilditch, T. P., and Williams, P. N.: *The Chemical Constitution of Natural Fats*, 4th ed., New York, Barnes & Noble, Inc., 1964.

Howes, F. N.: *Vegetable Tanning Materials*, London, Butterworth Scientific Publications, 1953.

Jackson, B. P., and Snowdon, D. W.: *Powdered Vegetable Drugs*, New York, American Elsevier Publishing Co., Inc., 1968.

Joklik, W. K., and Willett, H. P., eds.: *Zinsser Microbiology*, 16th ed., New York, Appleton-Century-Crofts, 1976.

Karrer, W.: *Konstitution und Vorkommen der organischen Pflanzenstoffe (exclusive Alkaloide)*, Basel and Stuttgart, Birkhäuser Verlag, 1958.

Karrer, W., Cherbuliez, E., and Eugster, C. H.: *Konstitution und Vorkommen der organischen Planzenstoffe (exclusive Alkaloide)*, Ergänzungsband 1, Basel and Stuttgart, Birkhäuser Verlag, 1977.

Kreig, M. B.: *Green Medicine*, Chicago, Rand McNally & Co., 1964.

Manske, R. H. F., ed.: The Alkaloids, Vols. I–XVII, New York, Academic Press, Inc., 1950–1979.

Meister, A.: *Biochemistry of the Amino Acids*, 2nd ed., Vols I–II, New York, Academic Press, Inc., 1965.

Miller, L. P., ed., *Phytochemistry,* Vols. I–III, New York, Van Nostrand Reinhold Co., 1973.

Newman, A. A., ed.: *Chemistry of Terpenes and Terpenoids,* London, Academic Press, Inc. (London) Ltd., 1972.

Patterson, R.: *Allergic Diseases,* Philadelphia, J. B. Lippincott Co., 1972.

Pigman, W. W., and Horton, D. eds.: *The Carbohydrates,* 2nd ed., Vols. I–II, New York, Academic Press, Inc., 1970–1972.

Quimby, E. H., Feitelberg, S., and Gross, W.: *Radioactive Nuclides in Medicine and Biology,* 3rd ed., Philadelphia, Lea & Febiger, 1970.

Rainbow, C., and Rose, A. H.: *Biochemistry of Industrial Micro-organisms,* New York, Academic Press, Inc., 1963.

Schery, R. W.: *Plants for Man,* 2nd ed., Englewood Cliffs, N.J., Prentice-Hall, Inc., 1972.

Smith, P. M.: *The Chemotaxonomy of Plants,* London, Edward Arnold (Publishers) Limited, 1976.

Sonnedecker, G., ed.: *Kremers and Urdang's History of Pharmacy,* 3rd ed., Philadelphia, J. B. Lippincott Co., 1963.

Stahl, E.: *Drug Analysis by Chromatography and Microscopy,* Ann Arbor, Mich., Ann Arbor Science Publishers, 1973.

Steinegger, E., and Hänsel, R.: *Lehrbuch der Pharmacognosie,* 3rd ed., Berlin, Springer-Verlag, 1972.

Taylor, N.: *Plant Drugs That Changed the World,* New York, Mead & Co., 1965.

Templeton, W.: *An Introduction to the Chemistry of the Terpenoids and Steroids,* London, Butterworth & Co. (Publishers) Ltd., 1969.

Tétényi, P.: *Infraspecific Chemical Taxa of Medicinal Plants,* New York, Chemical Publishing Co., Inc., 1970.

Tooley, P.: *Fats, Oils, and Waxes,* London, John Murray, 1971.

Trease, G. E., and Evans, W. C.: *Pharmacognosy,* 11th ed., London, Baillière Tindall, 1978.

Tyler, V. E., Jr., and Abou-Chaar, C. I.: Chemical Characteristics of Plant Families of Medicinal Importance. I. Dicotyledons, Pharmazie, *15*(11):628, 1960.

Tyler, V. E., Jr.: Chemical Characteristics of Plant Families of Medicinal Importance, II. Pteridophytes, Gymnosperms and Monocotyledons, Lloydia, *24*(2):57, 1961.

Tyler, V. E., and Schwarting, A. E.: *Experimental Pharmacognosy,* 3rd ed., Minneapolis, Burgess Publishing Co., 1962.

Wallis, T. E.: *Textbook of Pharmacognosy,* 5th ed., London, J. & A. Churchill Ltd., 1967.

Whistler, R. L., and BeMiller, J. N.: *Industrial Gums,* 2nd ed., New York, Academic Press, Inc., 1973.

Chapter 2

Carbohydrates and Related Compounds

Carbohydrates are aldehyde or ketone alcohols containing carbon, hydrogen, and oxygen in which the hydrogen and oxygen are in generally the same ratio as in water. Because carbohydrates are the first products formed in photosynthesis, they are a convenient starting point for any discussion of constituents of vegetable drugs. Moreover, carbohydrates are the products from which, by subsequent organic reactions, the plant synthesizes a great number of other constituents.

Carbohydrates may be classified into 2 broad groups: sugars and polysaccharides. Sugars are monosaccharides, i.e., compounds that cannot be hydrolyzed to simpler sugars; disaccharides, which yield 2 monosaccharide molecules on hydrolysis; trisaccharides, which yield 3; tetrasaccharides, which yield 4; and so forth. Monosaccharides are classified by the number of carbon atoms in the molecule. Those with 3 carbon atoms are trioses; 4 carbon atoms, tetroses; 5 carbon atoms, pentoses; 6 carbon atoms, hexoses; and others. Sugars are crystalline, soluble in water, and sweet tasting.

The more complex, high-molecular-weight polysaccharides are represented by starch (page 35), inulin (page 39), and the celluloses (page 40). These polysaccharides can usually be hydrolyzed to a component hexose and are therefore called hexosans; starch, which yields glucose, is known as a glucosan; and inulin, which yields fructose, is known as a fructosan. Sugars and starch are important products in the economy of mankind. They are extensively used as foods and pharmaceuticals.

The plant also builds its structural skeleton from carbohydrate material. Cellulose, a polysaccharide composed of glucose units joined by β-1,4 linkages, forms the primary cell walls in plants. Other substances also occur with cellulose, for example, the hemicelluloses. These are also high-molecular-weight polysaccharides but are considerably more soluble and more easily hydrolyzed than cel-

lulose. Closely related to the hemicelluloses are the gums and mucilages (page 43), which constitute an important group of drugs both from the pharmaceutic and the therapeutic viewpoint. Also associated with cellulose are the pectins (page 53), which have some pharmaceutic application.

No summary of the carbohydrates is complete without mentioning the pentoses and pentosans. The name pentose is applied to a group of sugars that has the general formula $C_5H_{10}O_5$ (arabinose, xylose, ribose). The pentoses are products resulting from the hydrolysis of the pentosans. Xylan, which occurs in the wood of deciduous trees, is an example of a pentosan. Pentoses also result from the hydrolysis of gums and mucilages.

MONOSACCHARIDES. A simple sugar is chemically defined as a substance belonging to the carbohydrate group that is a ketonic or aldehydic substitution product of a polyhydroxy alcohol. The simplest of these is a diose $HO-CH_2-CHO$ (hydroxyacetaldehyde), which does not occur free in nature. An aldehydic and a ketonic triose do exist (glyceraldehyde and dihydroxyacetone), usually in the form of phosphate esters. Moreover, certain organisms can oxidize glycerin to dihydroxyacetone. The tetroses also are not found in the free state. Pentoses, however, occur commonly in nature, usually as products of hydrolysis of hemicelluloses, gums, and mucilages.

Hexoses are by far the most important monosaccharides found in plants. They are the first detectable sugars synthesized by plants and form the units from which most of the polysaccharides are constructed. There are 16 possible aldohexoses and 8 ketohexoses which, if we consider both the *alpha* and *beta* forms, permit 48 isomers. Of these, only 2 occur in the free state in plants: they are D-fructose (levulose) and D-glucose (dex-

trose). Both are found in sweet fruits, honey, and invert sugar. When starch is hydrolyzed it yields glucose, whereas inulin yields fructose.

Glucose is an aldohexose, that is, a polyhydroxy alcohol having an aldehyde group whereas fructose, which has a ketone group, is a ketohexose. These groups explain the reducing properties of the monosaccharides and account for the commonly applied term "reducing sugars." The hexoses may be considered as 6-membered, open-chain compounds. Five of the carbon atoms have alcohol substituents, and the sixth carbon is part of an aldehyde or ketone group. Such an aliphatic formula readily illustrates and explains stereoisomerism, but many of the other properties of the hexoses can only be explained on the basis of a ring structure.

Evidence indicates that glucose and other hexoses often exist in cyclic forms as well as in straight chain structures. Glucose generally forms a 6-membered pyranose ring that may be written in either of 2 ways. (See diagram that follows.)

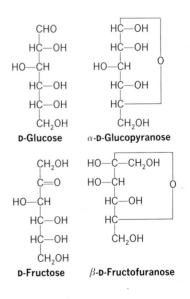

D-Glucose α-D-Glucopyranose

D-Fructose β-D-Fructofuranose

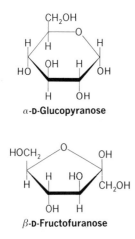

α-**D-Glucopyranose**

β-**D-Fructofuranose**

Fructose is more complex because it can exist in 2 cyclic forms. Fructopyranose is the structure of the crystalline sugar, and the furanose structure (5-membered ring) seems to occur when fructose is present in oligosaccharides and polysaccharides.

Phosphate esters of certain heptoses (7-carbon sugars) are of vital importance in the glucose metabolism of animals and in the photosynthetic process of plants. A few years ago, an 8-carbon sugar was isolated from crushed avocado pulp. This unusual sugar was named D-glycero-D-manno-octulose; it has also been isolated from species of the rock-garden plant, *Sedum*.

DISACCHARIDES. Sucrose (α-D-glucopyranosyl-β-D-fructofuranoside) is the only disaccharide that occurs abundantly in the free state in plants, although maltose has been reported as occasionally present in the cell sap. Sucrose occurs in fruit juices, sugar cane, sugar beet, the sap of certain maples and in many other plants. Upon hydrolysis sucrose yields *invert sugar*, which consists of equimolecular quantities of glucose and fructose. Sucrose is a nonreducing sugar.

Maltose (4-0-α-D-glucopyranosyl-D-glucopyranose), although seldomly occurring in the free state in nature, is pro-

duced in large quantities by the hydrolysis of starch during the germination of barley and other grains (diastatic fermentation). It is a reducing sugar and, upon hydrolysis, yields 2 molecules of glucose.

Glucose, fructose, sucrose, and maltose are the sugars most commonly occurring in vegetable drugs. Certain other sugars, however, occur to a limited extent in nature, either in the free state or in glycosidal combination. Among these are the monosaccharides: mannose (occurring in mannosans) and galactose (a constituent of lactose and raffinose); and the disaccharides: trehalose (widely distributed in the fungi) and lactose (milk sugar). Lactose possesses a functional aldehyde group and is a reducing sugar. Trehalose is a nonreducing sugar.

BIOSYNTHESIS OF CARBOHYDRATES

PRODUCTION OF MONOSACCHARIDES BY PHOTOSYNTHESIS. Carbohydrates are products of photosynthesis, a biologic process that converts electromagnetic energy into chemical energy. In the green plant, photosynthesis consists of 2 classes of reactions. One class comprises the so-called light reactions that actually convert electromagnetic energy into chemical potential. The other class consists of the enzymatic reactions that utilize the energy from the light reactions to fix carbon dioxide into sugar. These are referred to as the dark reactions. The results of both of these types of reactions are most simply summarized in the following equation:

$$2H_2O + CO_2 + light \xrightarrow{\text{chlorophyll}} (CH_2O) + H_2O + O_2$$

Although this equation summarizes the overall relationships of the reactants and products, it gives no clue as to the nature of the chemical intermediates involved in the process. The elucidation of the reactions by which carbon dioxide is accepted

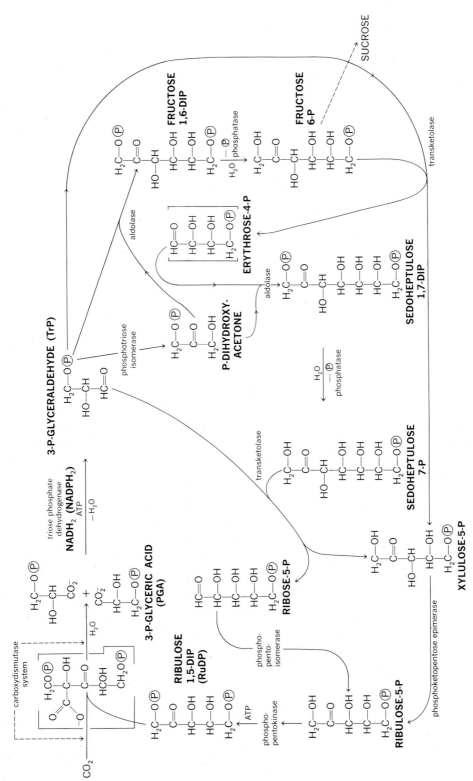

Fig. 2–1.   The path of carbon dioxide fixation in photosynthesis.

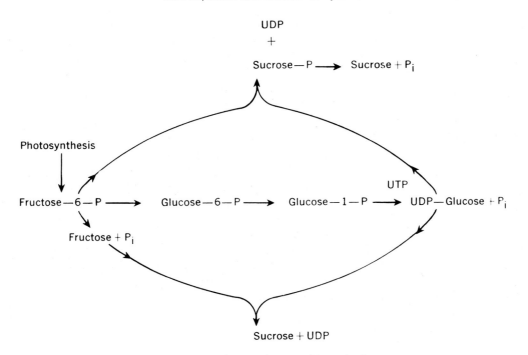

Fig. 2–2. Pathways of sucrose biosynthesis.

into an organic compound and ultimately into sugars with regeneration of the carbon dioxide acceptor was a major achievement in biosynthetic research. The pathway of carbon in photosynthesis, as worked out primarily by Calvin and co-workers, is presented in Figure 2–1.

PRODUCTION OF SUCROSE. Sucrose is of considerable metabolic importance in higher plants. Studies have shown that sucrose is not only the first sugar formed in photosynthesis but also the main transport material. Newly formed sucrose is, therefore, probably the usual precursor for polysaccharide synthesis. Although an alternative pathway consisting of a reaction between glucose 1-phosphate and fructose is responsible for sucrose production in certain microorganisms, the biosynthesis of this important metabolite in higher plants apparently occurs as shown in Figure 2–2.

Fructose 6-phosphate, derived from the photosynthetic cycle, is converted to glu-cose 1-phosphate which, in turn, reacts with UTP to form UDP-glucose. UDP-glucose either reacts with fructose 6-phosphate to form first sucrose phosphate and ultimately sucrose, or with fructose to form sucrose directly. Once formed, the free sucrose may either remain in situ or may be translocated via the sieve tubes to various parts of the plants. A number of reactions, e.g., hydrolysis by invertase or reversal of the synthetic sequence, convert sucrose to monosaccharides from which other oligosaccharides or polysaccharides may be derived.

SUGARS AND SUGAR-CONTAINING DRUGS

SUCROSE

Sucrose is a sugar obtained from *Saccharum officinarum* Linné (Fam. Gramineae), *Beta vulgaris* Linné (Fam.

Chenopodiaceae), and other sources. It contains no added substances.

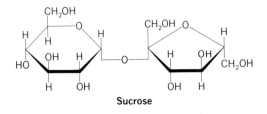

Sucrose

Sucrose is also known as **saccharum** or **sugar** and is widely distributed in plants. It is obtained commercially from sugar cane and sugar beets, but it can be obtained from the sugar maple (*Acer saccharum*, Fam. Aceraceae), from various palms, and other sources. Cane sugar is produced in Cuba, Puerto Rico, Louisiana, the Philippines, Hawaii, Indonesia, and India, while beet sugar is largely produced in Germany, Austria, Russia, France, and the United States. The enormous total world production is about equally divided between cane sugar and beet sugar.

Sugar cane is native to India and was introduced into Europe by the Venetians during the Crusades. In the fifteenth and sixteenth centuries, sugar cane found its way into most European colonies in the tropics.

Sugar beets are grown in places other than tropical and semitropical countries. In Michigan, California, and other states, the cultivation and harvesting of sugar beets represent an important industry (Fig. 2–3).

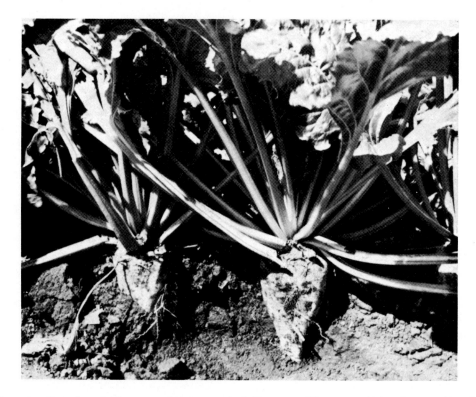

Fig. 2–3.   Sugar beets with stems and leaves attached. (Courtesy of Farmers and Manufacturers Beet Sugar Association, Saginaw, Michigan.)

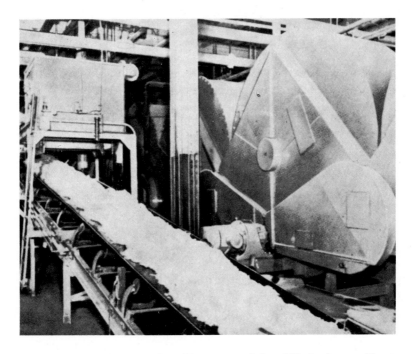

Fig. 2–4. Sugar beet cossettes being conducted by conveyor belt to diffusion battery. (Courtesy of Farmers and Manufacturers Beet Sugar Association, Saginaw, Michigan.)

PRODUCTION. The juice is obtained from sugar cane by crushing the stems between a series of heavy iron rollers. It is boiled with lime to neutralize the plant acids, which would otherwise change the sucrose to invert sugar, and to coagulate albumins. The latter rise to the top as a scum and are removed. The juice is filtered, sometimes decolorized with sulfur dioxide, concentrated, and crystallized. When crystals of sugar are no longer obtainable, the residual, dark-colored syrup is **molasses,** which is extensively used in foods, prepared animal foods, and in the manufacture of ethyl alcohol.

Sucrose is obtained from sugar beets in a somewhat different manner. The beets are dug, washed, and sliced into small, limp slivers known as "cossettes" (Fig. 2–4). Sucrose and other soluble constituents are extracted from the plant material with hot water. The crude sugar-containing solution is then subjected to the purification process.

USES. Sugar is a pharmaceutic necessity for syrups; it is also a demulcent and a nutrient. In sufficient concentration in aqueous solution, sugar is bacteriostatic and preservative. Sugar masks disagreeable tastes in troches and tablets and retards oxidation in certain preparations.

DEXTROSE

Dextrose, α-D(+)-glucopyranose or D-glucose is a sugar usually obtained by the hydrolysis of starch. Dextrose occurs naturally in grapes and other fruits and may be obtained either from these sources or by the hydrolysis of certain natural glucosides. It is also referred to as D-glucose and is usually prepared in a manner similar to that of liquid glucose. The conversion takes place after heating at 45 pounds pressure for about 35 minutes. The sugar is crystallized, washed, and dried to yield a dextrose of 99.5 to 100% purity.

Dextrose is the usual pharmaceutic title of this compound and is widely used in commerce and industry. However, the accepted scientific name, glucose, is employed in the chemical and biochemical literature.

Uses. Dextrose is a nutrient and may be given by mouth, by enema, by subcutaneous injection, or by intravenous injection, as required. It is an ingredient in dextrose injection and in dextrose and sodium chloride injection. It also is present in anticoagulant citrate dextrose solution and in anticoagulant citrate phosphate dextrose solution, each of which is an anticoagulant for the storage of whole blood. Dextrose, frequently in the form of liquid glucose, is used commercially in the manufacture of candy, carbonated beverages, ice cream, bakery products, and in the canning industry.

LIQUID GLUCOSE

Liquid glucose is a product obtained by the incomplete hydrolysis of starch. It consists chiefly of dextrose, but also contains dextrins, maltose, and water.

In the United States, liquid glucose is usually made from cornstarch (see page 38). The washed starch is mixed with diluted hydrochloric acid and heated for 22 minutes at about 30 pounds pressure, the acid is neutralized, and the neutral liquid is centrifuged and filtered until clear. This clear liquid is then evaporated to the syrupy condition.

Unfortunately, the name glucose applies to this product and to dextrose.

Description and Properties. Liquid glucose is a colorless or yellowish, thick, syrupy liquid that is nearly odorless and tastes sweet.

Uses. Liquid glucose is a pharmaceutic necessity. It is employed as a sweetening agent, as a substitute for sucrose in syrups, and as a tablet binder and coating agent.

Calcium gluconate is the calcium salt of gluconic acid. Gluconic acid is obtained by the oxidation of dextrose, either with chlorine or electrolytically in the presence of a bromide. It can also be obtained by fermentation. Calcium gluconate is soluble in cold water and less irritating for parenteral use than is calcium chloride. An electrolyte replenisher, calcium gluconate is used to obtain the therapeutic effects of calcium. The usual dose is 1 g orally 3 or more times a day or by intravenous infusion at intervals of 1 to 3 days.

Calcium gluceptate and calcium levulinate are calcium salts of 7- and 5-carbon acids that are prepared semisynthetically from readily available carbohydrates. Glucoheptonic acid is prepared from glucose via a cyanohydrin intermediate, and levulinic acid can be prepared from starch or cane sugar by boiling with hydrochloric acid. The salts are calcemic and are used parenterally to obtain the therapeutic effects of calcium.

Ferrous gluconate is the ferrous salt of gluconic acid. It is classed as a hematinic and is employed in iron deficiency anemia. The usual dose is 300 mg 3 times a day. It causes less gastric distress than do inorganic ferrous salts.

Proprietary Products. Entron®, Fergon®, and Ferralet®.

FRUCTOSE

Fructose, D-fructose, levulose, β-D (−)-fructopyranose, β-D (−)-fructofuranose, or fruit sugar is a sugar usually obtained by the inversion of aqueous solutions of sucrose and the subsequent separation of fructose from glucose. When sucrose is hydrolyzed, fructose and dextrose are formed in equal quantities. Fructose is a ketone sugar that occurs naturally in most sweet fruits (hence, the name fruit sugar) and in honey. It may be obtained also by the hydrolysis of inulin.

DESCRIPTION AND PHYSICAL PROPERTIES. Fructose occurs as colorless crystals or as a white, crystalline or granular, odorless powder that has a sweet taste. It is freely soluble in water.

USES. Fructose is used as a food for diabetic people and may be of particular benefit in diabetic acidosis. Infant feeding formulas often contain fructose. When given parenterally, it produces less urinary secretion than glucose.

Fructose is an ingredient in fructose injection and fructose and sodium chloride injection. These preparations are fluid, nutrient, and electrolyte replenishers and are administered either intravenously or subcutaneously, as required.

COMMERCIAL PRODUCT. Frutabs®.

LACTOSE

Cow's milk is the fresh, unpasteurized or pasteurized milk of *Bos taurus* Linné (Fam. Bovidae), without modification. It complies with the legal standards of the state or community in which it is sold.

Cow's milk is a white, opaque liquid that is an emulsion of minute fat globules suspended in a solution of casein, albumin, lactose, and inorganic salts. It has a slight but pleasant odor and an agreeable sweet taste. Cow's milk has a specific gravity between 1.029 and 1.034 and contains from 80 to 90% of water in which are dissolved about 3% of casein, about 5% of lactose, and from 0.1 to 1% of mineral salts. Milk contains from 2.5 to 5% of fat (butter) and is rich in vitamins. When milk is allowed to stand a few hours, the fat globules (cream) rise to the top. Each is surrounded by an albuminous layer.

When churned, the fat globules unite to form **butter,** leaving a liquid known as **buttermilk.** The milk left after separation of the cream is known as **skimmed milk** which, if treated with rennin, forms a coagulum. Upon proper treatment, this coagulum is made into **cheese.** The liquid separated from the coagulum is known as **whey** and contains lactose and inorganic salts. **Condensed milk** is prepared by partial evaporation of milk in a vacuum and consequent sterilization in hermetically sealed containers by autoclaving. **Malted milk** is prepared by evaporating milk with an extract of malt. Low heat and vacuum are used to prevent the destruction of enzymes.

Milk is a nutrient. It is the source of lactose, yogurt, and kumyss (fermented milk). Casein and sodium caseinate are employed in culture media.

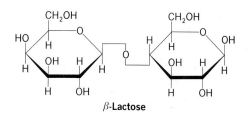

β-Lactose

Lactose or milk sugar is a sugar obtained from milk. The sugar is crystallized from the whey obtained in the manufacture of cheese. These impure crystals are redissolved in water, decolorized with charcoal, and recrystallized.

DESCRIPTION. Lactose is a nutrient and a pharmaceutic necessity. It is odorless and has a faintly sweet taste. Lactose is stable in air, but readily absorbs odors. Upon hydrolysis, lactose yields D-glucose and D-galactose. It reduces Fehling's solution, undergoes mutarotation, and forms an osazone. Lactose is hydrolyzed by the specific enzyme, lactase. It is not hydrolyzed by maltase, sucrase, or diastase and differs markedly from the other sugars because it easily undergoes lactic and butyric acid fermentations.

Uses. Lactose is a tablet diluent. It is less sweet than sucrose and is more easily hydrolyzed. It is used, therefore, as a nutrient in infant's food; it also has a minor role in establishing the intestinal microflora because it provides the preferred substrate for lactobacilli. Its principal pharmaceutic use is as an inert diluent for other drugs.

Lactulose is a semisynthetic sugar prepared by alkaline epimerization of lactose. It yields fructose and galactose upon hydrolysis. Lactulose is poorly absorbed, and most orally ingested lactulose reaches the colon unchanged. Bacteria in the colon metabolize the disaccharide to acetic and lactic acids, and sufficient accumulation of these irritating acids causes a laxative effect.

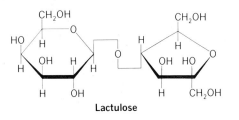

Lactulose

Although a daily dosage of 10 to 20 g of lactulose is effective in chronic constipation, the most significant therapeutic use of this sugar is to decrease the blood ammonia concentration in portal-systemic encephalopathy. The acidified stools trap ammonia as the ammonium ion; reabsorption is thus prevented, and blood ammonia levels may be decreased by 25 to 50%. The usual dosage regimen is 20 to 30 g of lactulose as a syrup 3 or 4 times a day.

PRESCRIPTION PRODUCTS. Cephulac® and Duphalac®.

XYLOSE

Xylose, D-xylose, or wood sugar is a pentose obtained by boiling corn cobs, straw, or similar materials with dilute acid to hydrolyze the xylan polymer. Xylose has a sweet taste and is normally absorbed from the small intestine, but it is not metabolized to a significant extent by mammalian enzymes. The latter properties have led to its approval by FDA for use as a diagnostic agent to evaluate intestinal absorption. The relative excretion of xylose in the urine is indicative of intestinal malabsorption states that may accompany such conditions as celiac disease, sprue, Crohn's diease (regional ileitis), pellagra, radiation enteritis, and surgical resection.

PRESCRIPTION PRODUCT. Xylo-Pfan®.

CARAMEL

Caramel or burnt sugar coloring is a concentrated solution of the product obtained by heating sugar or glucose until the sweet taste is destroyed and a uniform dark brown mass results; a small amount of alkali, alkaline carbonate, or a trace of mineral acid is added while heating.

DESCRIPTION. Caramel is a thick, dark brown liquid having the characteristic odor of burnt sugar and a pleasant, bitter taste. The specific gravity is not less than 1.30 at 25°C. Caramel mixes with water in all proportions and is soluble in dilute alcohol up to 55% by volume. One part in 1000 of distilled water yields a clear, yellowish orange solution.

USE. Caramel is used in coloring certain pharmaceutic preparations.

DRUGS CONTAINING COMPOUNDS METABOLICALLY RELATED TO SUGARS

PRODUCTS OF GLYCOLYTIC AND OXIDATIVE METABOLISM

Because the catabolism of carbohydrates provides the basic metabolic framework upon which all of the cell's activities depend, these reactions are usually examined in great detail in textbooks of biochemistry. For this reason, only a brief summary is presented here.

Certain important pharmaceutic products, such as ethanol and citric acid, are produced by the cellular respiration of carbohydrates, especially glucose. Ordinarily the reactions involved are considered to comprise several consecutive systems. The first reactions involve the anaerobic conversion of glucose to pyruvic acid by glycolysis (Embden-Meyerhof pathway, Fig. 2–5). Subsequently, in the absence of air, the pyruvic acid may be converted to lactic acid or to ethanol, depending on the identity of the biologic sys-

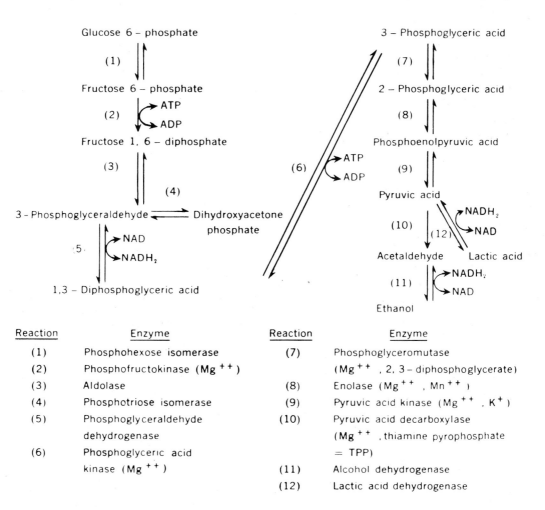

Reaction	Enzyme	Reaction	Enzyme
(1)	Phosphohexose isomerase	(7)	Phosphoglyceromutase
(2)	Phosphofructokinase (Mg^{++})		(Mg^{++}, 2, 3 – diphosphoglycerate)
(3)	Aldolase	(8)	Enolase (Mg^{++}, Mn^{++})
(4)	Phosphotriose isomerase	(9)	Pyruvic acid kinase (Mg^{++}, K^+)
(5)	Phosphoglyceraldehyde dehydrogenase	(10)	Pyruvic acid decarboxylase (Mg^{++}, thiamine pyrophosphate = TPP)
(6)	Phosphoglyceric acid kinase (Mg^{++})	(11)	Alcohol dehydrogenase
		(12)	Lactic acid dehydrogenase

Fig. 2–5. Reactions of glycolysis.

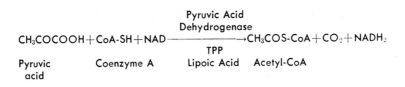

$$CH_3COCOOH + CoA\text{-}SH + NAD \xrightarrow[\text{TPP}]{\text{Pyruvic Acid Dehydrogenase}} CH_3COS\text{-}CoA + CO_2 + NADH_2$$

Pyruvic   Coenzyme A   Lipoic Acid   Acetyl-CoA
acid

Fig. 2–6.   Oxidative decarboxylation of pyruvic acid.

tem involved. In the second series of reactions, pyruvic acid undergoes oxidative decarboxylation to yield acetyl coenzyme A (acetyl-CoA or "active acetate," Fig. 2–6), which can be utilized in a variety of reactions including the acetylation of aromatic amines and alkaloids or the biosynthesis of fatty acids or steroids. However, most of the acetyl-CoA undergoes condensation with oxaloacetate to form citrate, thereby entering the tricarboxylic acid cycle where it is ultimately oxidized to carbon dioxide and water with the liberation of energy (Fig. 2–7).

Although some alternative mechanisms for glucose dissimilation are known, e.g.,

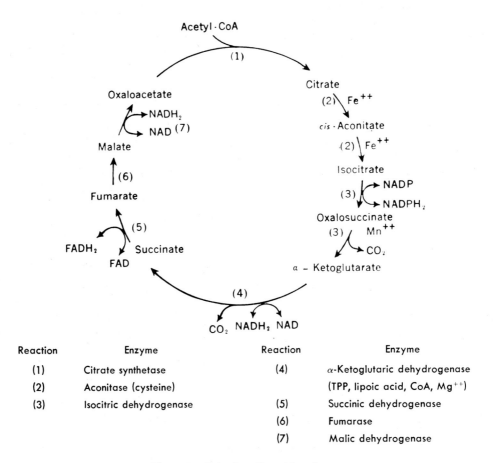

Reaction	Enzyme	Reaction	Enzyme
(1)	Citrate synthetase	(4)	α-Ketoglutaric dehydrogenase
(2)	Aconitase (cysteine)		(TPP, lipoic acid, CoA, Mg^{++})
(3)	Isocitric dehydrogenase	(5)	Succinic dehydrogenase
		(6)	Fumarase
		(7)	Malic dehydrogenase

Fig. 2–7.   Tricarboxylic acid cycle.

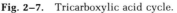

hexose monophosphate shunt, the aforementioned are the principal reaction sequences. They are summarized in Figures 2–5, 2–6, and 2–7, starting with glucose 6-phosphate, which may derive directly from the photosynthetic cycle or from the phosphorolysis of polysaccharide.

CHERRY JUICE

Cherry juice or succus cerasi is the liquid expressed from the fresh, ripe fruit of *Prunus cerasus* Linné (Fam. Rosaceae).

The cherries are washed, stemmed but not pitted, and coarsely ground to break the pits without mashing the kernels. The mixture is preserved with 0.1% benzoic acid and allowed to stand at room temperature (possibly for several days) until the addition of one-half its volume of alcohol to a small portion of the juice produces a clear solution that does not become cloudy within 30 minutes. This test indicates that the pectin in the juice has been destroyed by enzymatic action and that the juice or the syrup made from the juice can be used in medicinal preparations without causing cloudiness owing to the presence of alcohol. The pectin-free juice is pressed from the mixture and filtered to a clear liquid.

Cherry juice contains not less than 1% of malic acid.

Cherry juice is used in the preparation of **cherry syrup,** a flavored vehicle that serves as a pleasant disguising agent in pharmaceutic mixtures, especially those of an acidulous nature.

ACIDS

Plant acids, such as citric, lactic, and tartaric acids, find wide application in the formulation of foods and medicines. These acids function as acidulants or components of buffer systems to control acidity. They are nearly ideal substances for such purposes. The organic acids cause less irritation than do comparable quantities of inorganic acids. They are also nontoxic, a property that would be anticipated for a primary biologic metabolite such as citric acid.

Citric acid was first isolated in crystal form from lemon juice by Scheele in 1784. It is present in many fruits and plants and is obtained commercially from lemons, limes, or pineapples, but mostly by fermentation of sucrose. Citric acid appears as colorless, odorless, translucent crystals and is readily soluble in water and alcohol.

This tricarboxylic acid is particularly useful in buffering systems. Citric acid is used as an acidulant in effervescent formulations and in a variety of other products. It is an ingredient in sodium citrate and citric acid solution, a systemic alkalizer, and in anticoagulant citrate dextrose solution and anticoagulant citrate phosphate dextrose solution.

Lactic acid is available as a colorless or yellowish, nearly odorless, syrupy liquid. It is miscible with water, alcohol, and ether and consists of a mixture of lactic acid and lactic acid lactate equivalent to a total of not less than 85% and not more than 90% by weight of lactic acid. It is obtained by the lactic fermentation of sugars or is prepared synthetically.

Lactic acid is used as an acidulant, especially in infant feeding formulas. Sodium lactate injection is a fluid and electrolyte replenisher. Calcium lactate is a calcium replenisher; the usual oral dose is 1 to 5 g 3 times a day.

Tartaric acid is a dicarboxylic acid obtained as a by-product of the wine industry. It is soluble in water and freely soluble in alcohol. Tartaric acid is used as a substitute for citric acid in buffer systems and in effervescent formulations.

Ferrous fumarate is a hematinic agent that is comparable to ferrous gluconate. The usual therapeutic dose is 200 mg 3 or 4 times a day.

Eldofe®, Feostat®, Ferranol®, Fumasorb®, Fumerin®, Ircon®, Laud-Iron®, Palmiron®, and Toleron®.

ALCOHOL

Alcohol or ethanol is a liquid containing not less than 92.3% by weight, corresponding to 94.9% by volume, of ethanol at 15.56° C. As a 70% w/v solution, alcohol is used as a local anti-infective.

Diluted alcohol is a mixture of alcohol and water in which the percentage of ethanol, by volume at 15.56° C, is 48.4 to 49.5. Diluted alcohol is employed as a solvent.

The natural processes of fermentation have been utilized since earliest historic times to make alcoholic beverages. Beer made from fermented grain is mentioned in the *Papyrus Ebers* (about 1500 B.C.), and fermented grape juice or wine was probably known earlier. Natural fermentation produces a concentration of alcohol in the fermenting liquid that rarely exceeds 14% by volume because the fermentative organisms are usually inhibited at such a concentration.

The process of distillation, by which the alcohol in the fermented liquid can be concentrated in the distillate, was not known until the eighth century A.D. Only in modern times has the process been so perfected that pure alcohol results. By distillation, brandy (from wine), whiskey (from fermented malted grain), and rum (from fermented molasses) are produced on a commercial basis. Each usually contains from 40 to 55% of alcohol. Wine is sometimes used medicinally as a mild stimulant and tonic, and brandy and whiskey are properly classed as central depressants.

PRODUCTS OF REDUCTIVE METABOLISM

Dulcitol, mannitol, sorbitol, and other sugar alcohols are widely distributed in plants, but enzymes or enzyme systems capable of reducing a sugar to a sugar alcohol have never been isolated from a higher plant source.

However, evidence gained from studies conducted with microbial enzymes indicates that sugar alcohol (glycitol) phosphates may be formed by reduction of ketose phosphates in reactions utilizing NAD or NADP as the hydrogen carrier. The free glycitols are subsequently produced by the action of specific phosphatases. Examples of reactions catalyzed by enzymes, (1) mannitol phosphate dehydrogenase and (2) mannitol 1-phosphatase, follow:

$$\text{(1)}$$
$$\text{Fructose-6-P} + \text{NADH}_2 \rightleftharpoons \text{Mannitol-1-P} + \text{NAD}$$

$$\text{(2)}$$
$$\text{Mannitol-1-P} \rightleftharpoons \text{Mannitol} + \text{Pi}$$

In certain fungi, mannitol is formed directly from D-fructose by the action of mannitol dehydrogenase:

$$\text{Fructose} + \text{NADPH}_2 \rightleftharpoons \text{Mannitol} + \text{NADP}$$

MANNITOL

Mannitol or D-mannitol is a hexahydric alcohol obtained by reduction of mannose or by isolation from manna. Manna is the dried saccharine exudate of *Fraxinus ornus* Linné (Fam. Oleaceae) and contains 50 to 60% of mannitol; manna has also been used for its laxative properties.

Mannitol is a white, crystalline powder that is odorless and sweet tasting. It crystallizes in orthorhombic prisms or in aggregates of fine needles and is freely soluble in water and boiling alcohol, but almost insoluble in cold alcohol.

Mannitol is not absorbed from the gastrointestinal tract. When it is administered parenterally, it is not metabolized and is eliminated readily by glomerular filtration (approximately 80% of a 100 g dose appears in the urine in 3 hours). The latter properties have led to the use of mannitol as a diagnostic aid and as an osmotic diuretic. Some tubular reabsorption of mannitol (less than 10%) introduces an uncontrolled variable when this substance is used for diagnostic purposes.

The usual diagnostic dose of mannitol injection is 200 mg per kg of body weight in a 15 to 25% solution administered intravenously in 3 to 5 minutes. The usual diuretic dose is 50 to 100 g daily in a 5 to 20% solution by intravenous infusion at a rate adjusted to maintain a urine flow of at least 30 to 50 ml per hour; either mannitol injection or mannitol and sodium chloride injection is used for diuretic purposes.

PRESCRIPTION PRODUCT. Osmitrol®.

SORBITOL

Sorbitol or D-glucitol is a hexitol that was originally obtained from the ripe berries of the mountain ash, *Sorbus aucuparia* Linné (Fam. Rosaceae). It also occurs in many fruits but is generally prepared from glucose by hydrogenation or by electrolytic reduction. It is also known as **D-sorbitol.**

Sorbitol is a well-known hexahydric sugar alcohol that has received wide acceptance in pharmaceutic and commercial fields. This compound was developed during World War I when mannitol hexanitrate was introduced as a substitute for mercury fulminate, which was in short supply. Mannitol was obtained from glucose, and substantial quantities of sorbitol remained as a by-product. At that time there were few known markets for sorbitol. At present, sorbitol is widely used in both crystalline and soluble forms. Sorbitol is readily soluble and compatible with syrup, alcohol, and other polyols.

Sorbitol tastes approximately half as sweet as sucrose, has humectant properties, is not absorbed on oral ingestion, and is not metabolized readily. These properties make sorbitol a particularly useful ingredient in toothpastes, chewing gums, and various dietetic products. Sorbitol must be used in conjunction with saccharin or some other noncaloric sweetener in dietetic beverages because it acts as an osmotic laxative when taken in large amounts. Solutions of this hexitol are also used for urologic irrigation.

PROPRIETARY PRODUCT. Sorbo®.

RELATED PRODUCT. Sorbitol is an ingredient in Probilagol®.

Iron sorbitex injection is a solution consisting of a complex of iron, sorbitol, and citric acid. It is used intramuscularly as a hematinic in patients with iron deficiency anemia that is not amenable to oral iron therapy.

PRESCRIPTION PRODUCT. Jectofer®.

POLYSACCHARIDES AND POLYSACCHARIDE-CONTAINING DRUGS

STARCH

Probably no other single organic compound is as widely distributed in plants as is starch. It is produced in large quantities in green leaves as the temporary storage form of photosynthetic products. As a permanent reserve food material for the plant, starch occurs in seeds and in the pith, medullary rays, and cortex of the stems and roots of perennials and other plants. It constitutes from 50 to 65% of the dry weight of cereal seeds and as much as 80% of the dry matter of potato tubers.

In the United States alone, more than 3 billion pounds of pure starch are marketed annually; of this amount, more than 95% is made from corn. Although starch is widely distributed in the plant kingdom, relatively few plants provide starch on a large scale. Corn and other cereals, such as rice and wheat, contribute to the world's supply. Commercial starch is also obtained from potato tubers, maranta rhizomes, and cassava roots. Starch occurs in granules (or grains) that have characteristic striations. These striations and the size and shape of the granules are more or less characteristic in many species of plants and may be used as a microscopic means of identifying the botanic origin of the starch. In this manner, the identity of many food and drug products of vegetable origin may be established.

CHEMISTRY AND PROPERTIES OF STARCH. Starch is generally a mixture of two structurally different polysaccharides. One component, termed **amylose,** is a linear molecule composed of 250 to 300 D-glucopyranose units uniformly linked by α-1,4 glucosidic bonds, which tend to cause the molecule to assume a helixlike shape. The second component, **amylopectin,** consists of 1000 or more glucose units that are also connected with α-1,4 linkages. However, a number of α-1,6 links also occur at branch points. These links amount to about 4% of the total linkages, or 1 for approximately every 25 glucose units.

Because of these structural differences, amylose is more soluble in water than is amylopectin, and this characteristic may be used to separate the two components. More efficient separations are effected by complexing and precipitating the amylose with suitable agents, including various alcohols or nitroparaffins. Amylose reacts with iodine to form a deep blue complex; amylopectin gives a blue-violet or purple color.

Most starches have a similar ratio of amylose to amylopectin, averaging about 25% of the former to 75% of the latter. Certain waxy or glutinous starches contain either no amylose or small amounts (less than 6%).

α-**amylase** (α-1,4-glucan 4-glucanohydrolase), an enzyme present in pancreatic juice and saliva, hydrolyzes starch by a random splitting of α-1,4-glucosidic linkages. Amylose thus gives rise to a mixture of glucose, maltose, and amylopectin, a mixture of branched and unbranched oligosaccharides containing α-1,6 bonds.

β-**amylase** (α-1,4-glucan maltohydrolase) produces its effect by removing maltose units from the nonreducing ends of polysaccharide molecules. The endproduct in the case of amylose is nearly pure maltose. The hydrolytic action of β-amylase on the α-1,4 linkages of amylopectin continues until a branch point is approached. Because the enzyme lacks the capacity to hydrolyze α-1,6 bonds, the reaction stops, leaving polysaccharide fragments known as dextrins as the product of incomplete hydrolysis.

Hydrolysis of starch by mineral acids ultimately produces glucose in nearly quantitative yields. The course of hydrolysis may be conveniently followed by the iodine reaction, which changes successively from blue-black to purple to red to no reaction.

Starches generally form colloidal sols rather than true solutions. If a suspension of starch in cold water is added to boiling water while stirring, the opaque granules swell and finally rupture to give a translucent sol. If this sol is somewhat concentrated, it sets to a firm jelly when cooled. Cold, concentrated aqueous solution of the caustic alkalies, of chloral hydrate, of ammonium thiocyanate, or of hydrochloric acid also cause the swelling and ultimate rupture of the starch granules to form pastes.

BIOSYNTHESIS OF STARCH. Synthesis of the amylose fraction of starch is effected by enzymes known as transglycosylases. The reaction involves the lengthening of priming chains of identical composition by the addition of single glucose residues. In certain microorganisms, glucose 1-phosphate is the glucose donor, and the enzyme that catalyzes the transfer is phosphorylase.

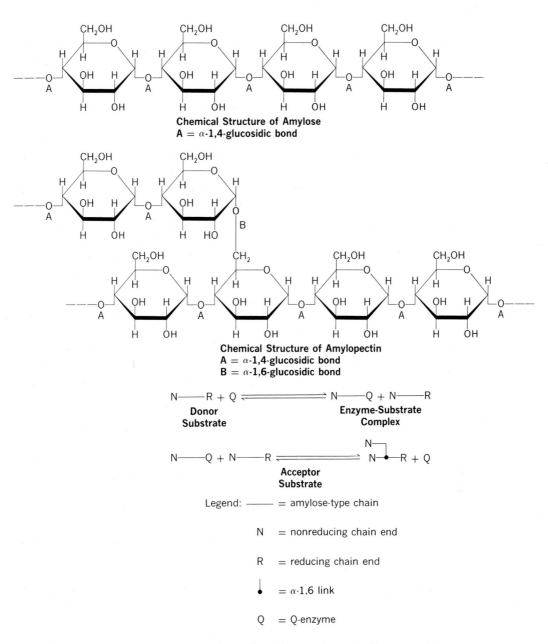

Chemical Structure of Amylose
A = α-1,4-glucosidic bond

Chemical Structure of Amylopectin
A = α-1,4-glucosidic bond
B = α-1,6-glucosidic bond

N———R + Q ⇌ N———Q + N———R
Donor   Enzyme-Substrate
Substrate   Complex

N———Q + N———R ⇌ N—N—•—R + Q
Acceptor
Substrate

Legend: ——— = amylose-type chain

N   = nonreducing chain end

R   = reducing chain end

↓•   = α-1,6 link

Q   = Q-enzyme

Fig. 2–8.   Formation of α-1,6 branch in amylopectin (diagrammatic).

Various sugar nucleotides, such as UDP-glucose and ADP-glucose, function as glycosyl donors in higher plants. Primer is essential to the reaction and must be a chain of at least 3 α-1,4-linked glucose units. The following equations illustrating this reaction show UDP-glucose as the source of the glucose residues:

$$(\text{Glucose})_n + \text{UDP-glucose} \rightarrow (\text{Glucose})_{n+1} + \text{UDP}$$

$$(\text{Glucose})_{n+1} + \text{UDP-glucose} \rightarrow (\text{Glucose})_{n+2} + \text{UDP, etc.}$$

Amylopectin, the branched component of starch, is formed from amylose by the action of a transglycosylase designated Q-enzyme. This enzyme effects the splitting of a monosaccharide chain containing at least 40 glucose units into 2 fragments. The fragment that carries the newly exposed reducing end first forms an enzyme-substrate complex and, in this form, is transferred to an appropriate acceptor chain, establishing an α-1,6 branch. This is illustrated diagrammatically in Figure 2–8.

CORN, WHEAT, AND POTATO STARCHES

Starch, as the term is used in pharmaceutic circles, consists of granules separated from the mature grain of corn, *Zea mays* Linné (Fam. Gramineae), the mature grain of wheat, *Triticum aestivum* Linné (Fam. Gramineae), or from tubers of the potato, *Solanum tuberosum* Linné (Fam. Solanaceae). Granules of cornstarch are polygonal, rounded, or spheroidal and are about 35 μm in diameter. Wheat and potato starches are less uniform in composition, each containing 2 distinct types of granules. Wheat starch contains large lenticular granules 20 to 50 μm in diameter and small spheric granules 5 to 10 μm in diameter; potato starch consists of irregularly ovoid or spheric granules 30 to 100 μm in diameter and subspheric granules

10 to 35 μm in diameter. Starches obtained from different botanic sources may not exhibit identical properties for specific pharmaceutic purposes, such as tablet disintegration, and they should not be interchanged unless performance equivalency has been ascertained.

Preparation of starch involves disruption of the plant cells to release the starch granules, and appropriate manipulations are necessary in the case of corn and wheat to eliminate tacky proteins (glutens), which impede free flow of the starch and lipids from the embryo (germ), causing the embryo to become rancid. The separated embryos contain vitamin E (see page 320) and can be processed to yield useful oils. Figure 2–9 illustrates the products that can be obtained from corn and the procedures that are involved.

Starch is used as an ingredient in dusting powders and as a pharmaceutic aid. The latter applications include use as a tablet filler, binder, and disintegrant. Purified **starch amylose** is also particularly useful for such purposes. A starch suspension may be swallowed as an antidote for iodine poisoning, and starch glycerite is used as an emollient and as a base for suppositories. Starch has many commercial uses, such as paper sizing, cloth sizing, and laundry starching. It is the starting material from which liquid glucose (corn syrup), dextrose, and dextrins are made.

Pregelatinized starch is starch that has been chemically or mechanically processed to rupture all or part of the granules in the presence of water. It is subsequently dried. The material may be modified further to enhance compressibility and flow characteristics. Pregelatinized starch is slightly soluble to soluble in cold water and is used as a tablet excipient.

Hetastarch is a semisynthetic material that is prepared in such a manner that the material is approximately 90% amylopec-

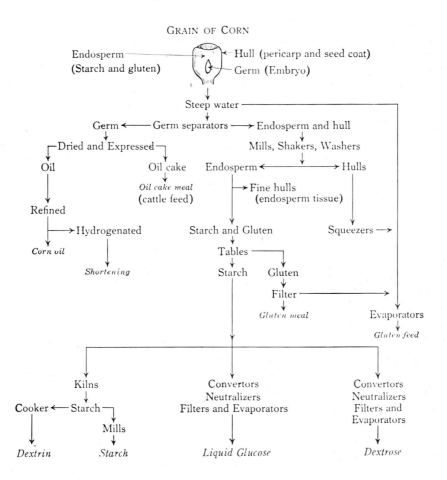

Fig. 2–9. Products obtained from *Zea mays*.

tin and 7 or 8 hydroxyethyl substituents are present for each 10 glucose units. A 6% solution of hetastarch is used as a plasma expander.

It is adjunct therapy in treatment of shock caused by hemorrhage, burns, surgery, sepsis, or other trauma. The duration of the improved hemodynamic status is 24 to 36 hours. The polymer is degraded, and molecules with molecular weights of less than 50,000 are eliminated rapidly by renal excretion.

PRESCRIPTION PRODUCT. Volex®.

INULIN

Inulin or hydrous inulin is a D-fructo-furanose polymer whose residues are linked in linear fashion by β-2,1 bonds. It is obtained from the subterranean organs of members of the family Compositae. It is particularly abundant in taraxacum, inula (elecampane), lappa (burdock root), echinacea (cone flower), triticum (couch grass or dog grass), and chicory (succory or blue dandelion root). Inulin occurs in the cell sap and, by immersing the fresh rhizome or root in alcohol for some time, the inulin usually crystallizes in sphaerite aggregates. Inulin is used in culture media as a fermentative identifying agent for certain bacteria and in special laboratory methods for the evaluation of renal function. It is filtered only by the glomeruli and is neither excreted nor reabsorbed by the tubules. The usual dose is 10 g dissolved in 100 ml of sodium chloride injection by intravenous infusion.

DEXTRAN

Dextran is an α-1,6-linked polyglucan that is formed from sucrose by the action of a transglucosylase enzyme system (dextran sucrase) present in *Leuconostoc mesenteroides*. This reaction can be summarized in the following equation:

$$n\,\text{Sucrose} + (\text{Glucose})_x \rightarrow (\text{Glucose})_{x+n} + n\,\text{Fructose}$$
$$\text{Primer} \qquad\qquad \text{Dextran}$$

Dextrans of the desired size are prepared by controlled depolymerization (acid hydrolysis, fungal dextranase, or ultrasonic vibration) of native dextrans or by controlled fermentation, including use of a cell-free enzyme system. At present, dextrans with clinical utility have molecular weights of 40,000, 70,000, and 75,000. The two large dextrans are used in 6% solutions as plasma expanders in cases of shock or pending shock caused by hemorrhage, trauma, or severe burns; dextran is not a substitute for whole blood when the latter is indicated. These dextran preparations are well suited for their intended uses because their osmolarity and viscosity resemble those of plasma, they are serologically indifferent and relatively nontoxic, and their effectiveness is prolonged by the slow metabolic cleavage of the 1,6-glucosidic linkage.

The low-molecular-weight dextran crosses extravascular space and is excreted

readily, but a 10% solution can be used as an adjunct in the treatment of shock. It is also employed to reduce blood viscosity and to improve microcirculation at low flow states. Dextrans interfere with some laboratory tests and may significantly increase clotting time.

PRESCRIPTION SPECIALTIES. Gentran®, LMD®, Macrodex®, and Rheomacrodex®.

Iron dextran injection is a sterile, colloidal solution of ferric hydroxide in complex with partially hydrolyzed dextran of low molecular weight in water for injection. It is a hematinic preparation that is administered by intramuscular or intravenous injection. Iron dextran injection is particularly useful when oral iron preparations are not well tolerated.

PRESCRIPTION PRODUCTS. Feostat®, Ferrodex®, Hematran®, Hydextran®, Imferon®, K-FeRON®, and Norferan®.

CELLULOSE

PURIFIED COTTON

Purified cotton is the hair of the seed of cultivated varieties of *Gossypium hirsutum* Linné, or of other species of *Gossypium* (Fam. Malvaceae), that is freed from adhering impurities, deprived of fatty matter, bleached and sterilized in its final container. Purified cotton is also referred to as **absorbent cotton.** *Gossypium*, the ancient name for the cotton plant, is from the Arabic *gos* meaning a soft silky substance; *hirsutum* is from the Latin meaning rough or hairy.

G. hirsutum, as cultivated in the southern United States, is an annual herb that attains a maximum height of about 4 feet and yields most of the commercial cotton known as American Upland Cotton; *G. barbadense*, a somewhat larger plant, is cultivated in South Carolina and Georgia along the sea coast and yields Sea Island Cotton.

The plants produce capsules (bolls) (Fig. 2–10) that open along longitudinal sutures when ripe and reveal a mass of white hairs attached to the brownish seeds. The mass of hairs (cotton fibers) and seeds are collected and "ginned," a machine process for removing the seeds. To render cotton absorbent and suitable for surgical use, it is first carded (combed) to remove gross impurities and short hairs (linters). The cotton is then washed with weak alkali solution to remove fatty materials, bleached with chlorinated soda, washed with weak acid, washed with water, and finally dried and recarded into flat sheets. After the absorbent cotton is packaged, it is usually sterilized.

Cotton for textiles is spun into thread and then woven; or, it may be treated with various chemicals, thereby yielding such fabrics as mercerized cotton, rayons, and others. The United States produces about half the world's supply of cotton. Cotton is also produced in Egypt and other tropical parts of Africa, India, the West and East Indies, and South America.

Cotton has been known since remotest antiquity. It has been cultivated in India for more than 3000 years. Egypt had a well-developed cotton industry 4000 years ago. It has been found in the mounds of the Aztecs in Mexico.

DESCRIPTION. Purified cotton occurs as white, soft, fine filamentlike hairs that appear under the microscope as hollow, flattened, and twisted bands that are striate and slightly thickened at the edges. The hairs are unicellular and nonglandular, ranging from 2.5 to 4.5 cm in length and from 25 to 35 μ in diameter. Cotton is nearly odorless and practically tasteless.

Purified cotton should be free from alkali, acid, fatty matter, dyes, and water-soluble substances. Such cotton consists almost exclusively of cellulose, a β-linked linear glucopyranosyl polymer. The β-linkage is not hydrolyzed by mammalian enzyme systems, an important considera-

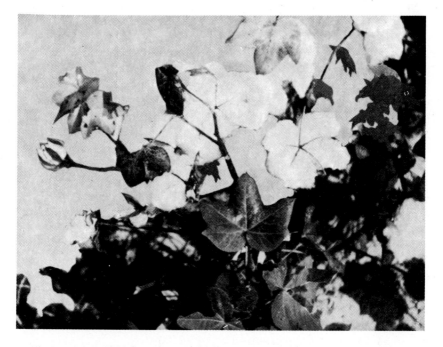

Fig. 2–10. Cotton plant showing both mature and immature capsules (bolls).

tion in the application of many cellulose derivatives, but is hydrolyzed by cellulase, which is produced by many microorganisms including the rumen microflora of herbivorous animals.

USES. Purified cotton is employed as a surgical dressing; it serves as a mechanical protection to absorb blood, mucus, or pus, and to keep bacteria from infecting wounds. Commercially, cotton is employed for textiles and is a source of pure cellulose in the manufacture of explosives, cellulose acetate, and other materials. Absorbent gauze, microcrystalline cellulose, purified rayon, and such cellulose derivatives as carboxymethylcellulose, cellulose acetate phthalate, ethylcellulose, hydroxypropyl methylcellulose, methylcellulose, oxidized cellulose, and pyroxylin find special applications in pharmacy and medicine.

Powdered cellulose is purified, mechanically disintegrated cellulose prepared by processing α-cellulose obtained as a pulp from fibrous plant materials. It exists in various grades and exhibits degrees of fineness ranging from a free-flowing dense powder to a coarse, fluffy, nonflowing material. It is used as a self-binding tablet diluent and disintegrating agent.

Microcrystalline cellulose is a purified, partially depolymerized cellulose prepared by treating α-cellulose, obtained as a pulp from fibrous plant material, with mineral acids. It is used as a diluent in the production of tablets.

Purified rayon is a fibrous form of bleached, regenerated cellulose. It is used as a surgical aid and may not contain more than 1.25% of titanium dioxide.

CELLULOSE DERIVATIVES

Methylcellulose is a methyl ether of cellulose containing not less than 27.5% and not more than 31.5% of methoxy groups. It is obtained by the reaction of cellulose with caustic soda and methyl chloride and consists of a white, fibrous powder or granules. In water methylcellulose swells to produce a clear to opalescent, viscous, colloidal suspension. Methylcellulose is a bulk laxative and a suspending agent. The usual cathartic dose is 1 to 1.5 g with water 2 to 4 times a day. Ophthalmic solutions (0.5 and 1.0%; Visculose®) of methylcellulose are used as topical protectants; these products are marketed as "artificial tears" or contact lens solutions.

PROPRIETARY PRODUCTS. Hydrolose®, Odrinex®, and Melozets®. (NOTE: Melozets® and Odrinex® are used to control excessive appetite in obesity.)

Ethylcellulose is an ethyl ether of cellulose containing not less than 44% and not more than 51% of ethoxy groups. It is a free-flowing white powder. Ethylcellulose is a tablet binder.

Hydroxypropyl methylcellulose is the propylene glycol ether of methylcellulose in which both hydroxypropyl and methyl groups are attached to the anhydroglucose rings of cellulose by ether linkages. It contains not less than 19% and not more than 30% of methoxy groups and not less than 3% and not more than 12% of hydroxypropyl functions. It occurs as a white, fibrous or granular powder. Hydroxypropyl methylcellulose is used as a suspending agent, a thickening agent, and a tablet excipient. Ophthalmic solutions (0.2 to 2.5%; aqua-FLOW®, Bro-lac®, Goniosol®, Isopto®, Lacril®, Lyteers®, Tearisol®, and Ultra Tears®) of this hydrophilic polymer are used as topical protectants or artificial tears for contact lenses.

Pyroxylin or soluble guncotton is a product obtained by the action of a mixture of nitric and sulfuric acids on cotton. It is a mixture of cellulose nitrates. Pyroxylin is a pharmaceutic aid used in the preparation of collodion and flexible collodion, topical protectants.

Oxidized cellulose contains not less

than 16% and not more than 24% of carboxyl groups. It is usually available in the form of sterile pads, pledgets, and strips and is used as a local hemostatic.

SPECIALTY PRODUCTS. Oxycel®, Surgicel®.

Cellulose acetate phthalate is a reaction product of phthalic anhydride and a partial acetate ester of cellulose. It contains not less than 19% and not more than 23.5% of acetyl groups and not less than 30% and not more than 36% of phthalyl groups. It is a free-flowing, white powder and is used as a tablet-coating agent.

Sodium carboxymethylcellulose is the sodium salt of a polycarboxymethyl ether of cellulose. It is a hygroscopic powder that is used as a suspending agent, a thickening agent, a tablet excipient, and a bulk laxative. It is also used in varying proportions with microcrystalline cellulose to give suspending agents with different viscosities. The usual cathartic dose of sodium carboxymethylcellulose is 1.5 g with water 3 times a day.

PROPRIETARY PRODUCTS. Dialose® and Disoplex®.

Carboxymethylcellulose and its sodium salt are used as bulking agents, usually combined with other drug substances, in products intended for appetite suppression. Representative products include Anorexin®, Appedrine®, Diet-Trim®, Spantrol®, and Diet-Aid®.

GUMS AND MUCILAGES

Gums are natural plant hydrocolloids that may be classified as anionic or nonionic polysaccharides or salts of polysaccharides. They are translucent, amorphous substances that are frequently produced in higher plants as a protective after injury. Useful hydrocolloids are also contained in some seed embryos or other plant parts (in the case of pectins), are extracted from various marine algae, and are produced by selected microorganisms.

A number of semisynthetic cellulose derivatives (see page 42) are used for their hydrophilic properties, and they can be considered as specialized hydrocolloid gums.

Gums are typically heterogenous in composition. Upon hydrolysis, arabinose, galactose, glucose, mannose, xylose, and various uronic acids are the most frequently observed components. The uronic acids may form salts with calcium, magnesium, and other cations; methyl ether and sulfate ester substituents further modify the hydrophilic properties of some natural polysaccharides.

Gums find diverse applications in pharmacy. They are ingredients in dental and other adhesives and in bulk laxatives. But, their most frequent contribution is as agents of pharmaceutic necessity. These hydrophilic polymers are useful as tablet binders, emulsifiers, gelating agents, suspending agents, stabilizers, and thickeners. When problems are encountered in the utilization of hydrocolloids, some alteration in the hydration of the polymer is usually involved; for example, gums are precipitated from solution by alcohol and by lead subacetate solution.

An effort has been made to distinguish between mucilages and gums on the basis that gums readily dissolve in water whereas mucilages form slimy masses. Other investigators have tried to distinguish between them on the basis that mucilages are physiologic products and gums are pathologic products. However, these classifications have not been successful. Knowledge of the nature of the polysaccharide polymers is increasing, and it now seems advantageous to abandon extensive use of such designations and to focus on those features that are associated with useful physical properties. The hydrocolloids may be linear or branched, and they may have acidic, basic, or neutral characteristics. Basic polymers have limited commercial importance; acidic and neutral hydrocolloids are widely used, and some generalizations can be made about their properties.

Gums consisting of linear polymers are less soluble than those with branched constituents, and linear hydrocolloids yield solutions with greater viscosity. These features are related to the increased possibility for good alignment and considerable intermolecular hydrogen bonding among linear molecules. This tendency for intermolecular associations also explains why solutions of linear polysaccharides are less stable (tend to precipitate), especially with reductions in temperature, than solutions of branched molecules. This observation could significantly influence the shelf life of product formulations. When linear polymers contain uronic acid residues, coulombic repulsion reduces intermolecular associations and gives more stability to solutions. However, hydrocolloids with acid groups also have the potential for anionic-cationic interaction to give precipitation or to alter the hydrophilic properties in another manner.

Branched hydrocolloids form gels rather than viscous solutions at higher concentrations. They tend to be tacky when moist, a feature that is advantageous for adhesive purposes, and to rehydrate more readily than linear hydrocolloids, a property of importance in drug formulations that must be reconstituted immediately before use.

The sources of commercially useful gums or hydrocolloids can be summarized as follows:

1. Shrub or tree exudates—acacia, karaya, tragacanth
2. Marine gums—agar, algin, carrageenan
3. Seed gums—guar, locust bean, psyllium
4. Plant extracts—pectins
5. Starch and cellulose derivatives—hetastarch (see page 38), car-boxymethylcellulose, ethylcellulose, hydroxypropyl methylcellulose, methylcellulose, oxidized cellulose (page 42)
6. Microbial gums—dextrans (page 40), xanthan

Plant exudates have been the traditional gums for pharmaceutic purposes, and they still find significant application; however, these gums are labor intensive and carry a premium price, and their use will probably continue to decline. Marine gums are widely used as utility gums at the present time, and their competitive position appears stable. Guar gum is obtained from an annual legume that is adaptable to modern agricultural practices and will likely join various cellulose derivatives and the microbial gums as those hydrocolloids whose applications are expanding.

TRAGACANTH

Tragacanth is the dried, gummy exudate from *Astragalus gummifer* Labillardière, or other Asiatic species of *Astragalus* (Fam. Leguminosae). It is commonly known as **gum tragacanth.** The name tragacanth is from the Greek *tragos* (goat) and *akantha* (horn) and probably refers to the curved shape of the drug; *astragalus* means milkbone and refers to the exuding and subsequent hardening of the drug; *gummifer* is from the Latin and means gum-bearing. The plants are thorny branching shrubs about 1 meter in height and are abundant in the highlands of Asia Minor, Iran, Syria, the Soviet Union, and Greece. When the plant is injured, the cell walls of the pith and then of the medullary rays are gradually transformed into gum. The gum absorbs water and creates internal pressure within the stem, thus forcing the gum to the surface through the incision that caused the injury. When the gum strikes the air, it gradually hardens owing to the evaporation of the water. The nature of the incision governs the shape of the final product. The gum exuding from natural injuries is more or less wormlike and is twisted into coils (formerly known as **vermiform tragacanth**) or is shaped like irregular tears (formerly known as **tragacanth sorts**) of a yellowish or brownish color. The better grade comes from transverse incisions made with a knife in the main stem and older branches. The gum from such incisions is known as **ribbon gum** and **flake gum** depending on the shape of the solidified exudate. The gum usually shows longitudinal striations caused by small irregularities in the incision. The metamorphosis occurs only at night, and the tragacanth ribbons exhibit transverse striations that show the amount that exudes each night. The shorter the drying time, the whiter and more translucent the ribbons. This form of tragacanth is graded commercially by numbers: No. 1 is almost colorless (white) and nearly translucent, No. 2 and No. 3 have more color and opacity. Tragacanth was known to Theophrastus (300 B.C.) and Dioscorides and seems to have been used during the Middle Ages. It was not until recent times, however, that the natives learned to clean the bases of the bushes and incise the bark with a knife, thus producing the clean, white, semitransparent product of present-day commerce.

Tragacanth contains 60 to 70% of bassorin, a complex of polymethoxylated acids, that swells in water but does not dissolve. Bassorin has an elongated molecular shape and forms a viscous solution. Tragacanthin, which is probably demethoxylated bassorin, comprises about 30% of the gum and is the more water-soluble component.

Tragacanth is employed pharmaceutically as a suspending agent for insoluble powders in mixtures, as an emulsifying agent for oils and resins, and as an adhesive. Tragacanth is the most resistant of the hydrocolloids to acid hydrolysis and thus is preferred for use in highly acidic conditions. It is employed in cosmetics (hand lotions) as a demulcent and an emollient and in cloth printing, confectionery, and other processes.

ACACIA

Acacia is the dried, gummy exudate from the stems and branches of *Acacia senegal* (Linné) Willdenow or of other related African species of *Acacia* (Fam. Leguminosae). It is commonly known as **gum arabic.** *Acacia* is from the Greek *akakia*, coming from *ake*, meaning pointed and referring to the thorny nature of the plant; *senegal* refers to its habitat. The name "gum arabic" seems to be a misnomer because little acacia is produced on the Arabian peninsula and none is exported. The name may reflect the drug's extensive use by the early Arabian physicians.

Acacia plants are thorny trees about 6 meters in height that grow in the Sudan and in Senegal. Most of the official drug comes from cultivated trees in Kordofan. The trees are tapped by making a transverse incision in the bark and peeling the bark both above and below the cut (Fig. 2–11), thus exposing an area of cambium 2 to 3 feet in length and 2 to 3 inches in breadth. In 2 or 3 weeks, the tears of gum formed on this exposed surface are collected; the average annual yield of gum per tree is 900 to 2000 g. The formation of the gum may be caused by bacterial action or by the action of a ferment. No trace of metamorphosed cell walls is found in the gum; therefore, the gum must be formed from cell contents. The gum is occasionally exposed to and bleached by the sun. Numerous minute cracks often form in the outer portion of the tears during the bleaching process, thus giving them a semiopaque appearance. The tears are gar-

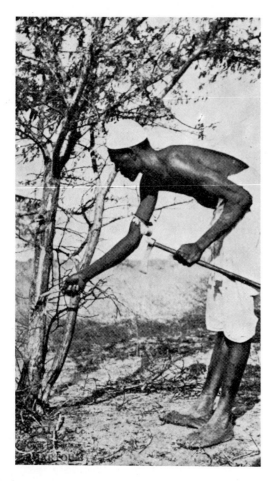

Fig. 2–11.   Bark is peeled from the stems of *Acacia senegal* growing in the Sudan. (Photo, courtesy of Boxall and Company, Ltd., Khartoum and P. S. Busschaert Company, Inc., New York.)

key. The West African gum (Senegal) was imported by the Portuguese during the fifteenth century.

Acacia consists principally of arabin, which is a complex mixture of calcium, magnesium, and potassium salts of arabic acid. Arabic acid is a branched polysaccharide that yields L-arabinose, D-galactose, D-glucuronic acid, and L-rhamnose on hydrolysis. 1,3-Linked D-galactopyranose units form the backbone chain of the molecule, and the terminal residues of the 1,6-linked side chains are primarily uronic acids. Acacia contains 12 to 15% of water and several occluded enzymes (oxidases, peroxidases, and pectinases) that can cause problems in some formulations.

Acacia is unusually soluble for a hydrocolloid and can form solutions over a wide range of concentrations. It remains in solution at alcohol concentrations below 60%, a property that is useful in some drug formulations. Solutions of acacia have low viscosity and good stability over the pH range of 2 to 10; these properties contribute to the gum's use as an excellent emulsifying agent.

Acacia is also used as a suspending agent. It possesses useful demulcent and emollient properties and finds application as an adhesive and binder in tablet granulations.

Ghatti gum or Indian gum is a product that is sometimes used as a substitute for acacia. It is an exudate from *Anogeissus latifolia* (Fam. Combretaceae), a tree indigenous to India and Sri Lanka. It is a branched hydrocolloid and readily forms dispersions with cold water; the dispersions are more viscous than those of acacia.

KARAYA GUM

Karaya gum or sterculia gum is the dried, gummy exudate from *Sterculia urens* Roxburgh, *S. villosa* Roxburgh, *S.*

bled and graded by hand, then packed and shipped via Port Sudan.

Acacia has been an article of commerce since remote times. The tree and heaps of gum are pictured during the reign of Ramses III and in later inscriptions. It was exported from the Gulf of Aden 1700 years before Christ. Theophrastus mentioned it in the third century B.C. under the name of "Egyptian gum." During the Middle Ages, acacia was obtained from Egypt and Tur-

tragacantha Lindley, or other species of *Sterculia* Linné (Fam. Sterculiaceae), or from *Cochlospermum gossypium* DeCandolle or other species of *Cochlospermum* Kunth (Fam. Bixaceae). These trees are native to India and are widely scattered in the Indian forests. They may attain a height of 10 meters, but the trunks are large, soft, and corky. Sterculia is from the Latin *Sterculius*, the deity that presided over manuring, and refers to the fetid odor of the trees.

The gum exudes naturally or from incisions made to the heartwood and is collected throughout the year, mostly from March to June. The incisions produce knoblike masses of gum that are collected frequently for 9 months. The tree should then be allowed to rest for 2 to 3 years. Three commercial grades are collected in the central provinces of India and exported from Bombay; the various meshes of granular and powdered karaya are produced in the United States.

Karaya gum consists of an acetylated, branched heteropolysaccharide with a high component of D-galacturonic acid and D-glucuronic acid residues. Varying amounts of pigmented impurities are also present in commercial grades of this gum; its color ranges from pale yellowish to pinkish brown. Karaya gum is one of the least soluble of the exuded plant gums. It absorbs water, swells to several times its original bulk, and forms a discontinuous type of mucilage.

Karaya gum is used as a bulk laxative, as an agent for forming emulsions and suspensions, and as a dental adhesive. It is used extensively in wave set solutions and in skin lotions, in the textile and printing industries, in the preparation of food products, and in the preparation of composite building materials.

Specialty Products. Karaya gum is an ingredient in Hydrocil®, Imbicoll®, and Saraka®.

SODIUM ALGINATE

Sodium alginate or algin is the purified carbohydrate product extracted from brown seaweeds by the use of dilute alkali. It is chiefly obtained from *Macrocystis pyrifera* (Turn.) Ag. (Fam. Lessoniaceae). Algin is found in all species of brown seaweeds (Class Phaeophyceae), and some commercial algin has been obtained from, among other sources, species of *Ascophyllum*, *Ecklonia*, *Laminaria*, and *Nereocystis*. *Macrocystis pyrifera* is harvested from several temperate zones of the Pacific Ocean; the area off Southern California is a major producing site.

Algin consists chiefly of the sodium salt of alginic acid, a linear polymer of L-guluronic acid and D-mannuronic acid. Mannuronic acid is the major component, but there is some variation with the algal source. The alginic acid molecule appears to be a copolymer of 1,4-linked mannopyranosyluronic acid units, of 1,4-linked gulopyranosyluronic acid units, and of segments where these uronic acids alternate with 1,4-linkages.

Sodium alginate occurs as a nearly odorless and tasteless, coarse or fine powder and is yellowish white in color. It is readily soluble in water forming a viscous, colloidal solution. It is insoluble in alcohol, ether, chloroform, and strong acid.

Sodium alginate (Kelgin®) is a suspending agent. It is also used in the food industry (ice cream, chocolate milk, salad dressings, icings, confectionery), for suspending cosmetic preparations, as a sizing, and for other industrial purposes. Algin is metabolized by the body and has a caloric value of approximately 1.4 calories per g. The caloric value of the small amount used in most manufactured products is insignificant.

Alginic acid is relatively insoluble in water, but it is used as a tablet binder and thickening agent. Useful gel-forming properties are associated with salts of various polyvalent cations and alginic acid. Calcium alginate has found application for a number of gelation purposes, including the formation of a firm gel for preparing dental impressions. The propylene glycol ester of algin has been prepared and is especially useful in formulations that require greater acid stability than that possessed by the parent hydrocolloid.

AGAR

Agar is the dried, hydrophilic, colloidal substance extracted from *Gelidium cartilagineum* (Linné) Gaillon (Fam. Gelidiaceae), *Gracilaria confervoides* (Linné) Greville (Fam. Sphaerococcaceae), and related red algae (Class Rhodophyceae). Agar is sometimes referred to as **Japanese isinglas.**

These algae grow along the eastern coast of Asia and the coasts of North America and Europe. Most of the commercial supply comes from Japan, Spain, Portugal, and Morocco. Mexico, New Zealand, South Africa, and the United States are also significant producers.

Agar is prepared in California as follows: the fresh seaweed is washed for 24 hours in running water, extracted in steam-heated digesters with dilute acid solution and then with water for a total period of about 30 hours. The hot aqueous extract is cooled and then congealed in ice machines. The water from the agar almost completely separates as ice. The 300-pound agar ice block (containing about 5 pounds of dry agar) is crushed, melted, and filtered through a rotary vacuum filter. The moist agar flakes are dried by currents of dry air in tall cylinders. The fully dried product can be reduced to a fine powder.

Agar usually occurs as bundles consisting of thin, membranous, agglutinated strips or in cut, flaked, or granulated forms.

It may be weak yellowish orange, yellowish gray to pale yellow, or colorless. It is tough when damp, brittle when dry, odorless or slightly odorous, and has a mucilaginous taste. Agar is insoluble in cold water, but if one part of agar is boiled for 10 minutes with 65 times its weight of water, it yields a firm gel when cooled.

Agar is predominantly the calcium salt of strongly ionized, acidic polysaccharides. It can be resolved into 2 major fractions, agarose and agaropectin. The structures of these constituents have not been fully established, and they are probably variable. The primary carbohydrate component appears to consist of alternating, 1,3-linked D-galactopyranosyl and 3,6-anhydro-L-galactopyranosyl units. Most of the anhydrogalactose residues in agaropectin have a sulfate ester substituent, but agarose is characterized by a low sulfate content.

Agar hydrates to form a smooth, nonirritating bulk that favors normal peristalsis and is used as a laxative. Agar is also used as a suspending agent, an emulsifier, a gelating agent for suppositories and surgical lubricants, and a tablet excipient and disintegrant. It is extensively used as a gel in bacteriologic culture media and as an aid in food processing and other industrial processes.

PROPRIETARY PRODUCTS. Agoral® and Petrogalar®.

Agarose also finds special application in clinical diagnostics. It is used as a matrix for immunodiffusion, for electrophoretic separation of globulin and other proteins, and for techniques involving gel filtration and gel chromatography.

CARRAGEENAN

Carrageenan is a term referring to closely related hydrocolloids that are obtained from various red algae or seaweeds. *Chondrus crispus* (Linné) Stackhouse and

Gigartina mamillosa (Goodenough et Woodward) J. Agardh (Fam. Gigartinaceae) are major sources of carrageenan; these algae are commonly known as chondrus or Irish moss.

These plants are common along the northwestern coast of France, the British Isles, and the coast of Nova Scotia (Fig. 2–12). The plants are collected chiefly during June and July, spread out on the beach and bleached by the action of the sun and dew, then treated with salt water, and finally dried and stored. The chief points of collection in the United States are located 15 to 25 miles south of Boston where *Chondrus crispus* is gathered and used in the manufacture of carrageenan. *Gigartina mamillosa* is most abundant north of the *Chondrus crispus* region; thus, it rarely occurs in the drug collected in the United States, though it is not unusual in the imported chondrus.

Chrondrus is an allusion to the cartilagelike character of the dry thallus; *Gigartina* is an allusion to the fruit bodies that appear as elevated tubercles on the thallus. The specific name, *crispus*, pertains to the curled fronds; *mamillosa* to the small breastlike, stalked fruit bodies or cystocarps.

The carrageenan hydrocolloids are galactans with sulfate esters and physically resemble agar. The carrageenans differ chemically from agar because they have a higher sulfate ester content. Carrageenans can be separated into several

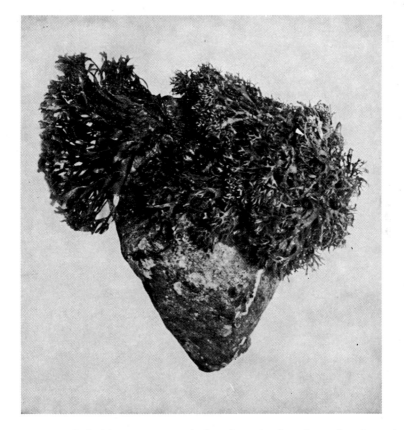

Fig. 2–12. Specimen of *Chondrus crispus* attached to the rock where it was found growing along the Massachusetts coast.

components, including k-carrageenan, i-carrageenan, and λ-carrageenan.

There are some differences in the specific properties and applications of the individual carrageenans. For example, k- and i-carrageenans tend to orient in stable helices when in solution, but λ-carrageenan does not. Consistent with these properties, k- and i-carrageenans are good gelating agents, and the nongelling λ-carrageenan is a more useful thickener.

Carrageenans are widely used to form gels and to give stability to emulsions and suspensions. The firm texture and good rinsability of these hydrocolloids are particularly desirable in toothpaste formulations. They are also used as a demulcent, a bulk laxative, and an ingredient in many food preparations.

PROPRIETARY PRODUCT. Chondrus is an ingredient in the laxative preparation, Kondremul®.

Furcellaria fastigiata (Huds.) Lamour., a red alga, yields an extract called furcellaran or Danish agar. This hydrocolloid is similar to k-carrageenan, and it finds some use, expecially in Europe, as a gelating and suspending agent.

PLANTAGO SEED

Plantago seed, psyllium seed, or plantain seed is the cleaned, dried, ripe seed of *Plantago psyllium* Linné or of *P. indica* Linné (*P. arenaria* Waldstein et Kitaibel), known in commerce as Spanish or French psyllium seed; or of *P. ovata* Forskal, known in commerce as blonde psyllium or Indian plantago seed (Fam. Plantaginaceae) (Fig. 2–13). *Plantago* is from the Latin and means sole of the foot, referring to the shape of the leaf; *psyllium* is from the Greek and means flea, referring to the color, size, and shape of the seed (fleaseed); *arenaria* is from the Latin *arena* and means sand, referring to the sandy habitat of the plant. *Ovata* refers to the ovate shape of the leaf.

P. psyllium is an annual, caulescent, glandular, pubescent herb native to the Mediterranean countries and extensively

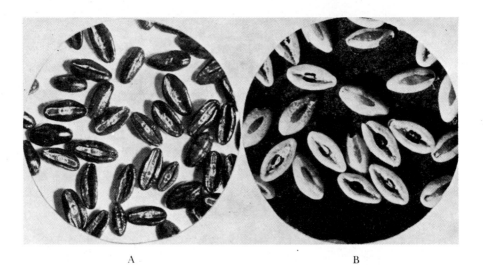

A   B

Fig. 2–13.   Psyllium seed: *A*, French psyllium seed *(Plantago psyllium)*. *B*, Indian plantago seed *(Plantago ovata)*.

cultivated in France, which yields the bulk of the American imported psyllium seed.

P. ovata is an annual, acaulescent herb native to Asia and the Mediterranean countries. The plant is cultivated extensively in Pakistan.

In France, the seeds are planted in March and harvested in August when they are about three-quarters mature. The fields are mowed about dawn, when the dew is heaviest, to prevent scattering of the seed. The plants, partially dried in the sun, are threshed, and the seeds are cleaned and bagged and allowed to dry fully. In Europe, the seeds have been a domestic remedy since the sixteenth century, but only since 1930 have they been extensively used in America as a popular remedy for constipation.

Commercially, the most important plantago product is the husk of the seed of *P. ovata*. It is produced in Pakistan and further purified and processed in the United States.

Plantago seeds contain 10 to 30% of hydrocolloid, which is localized in the outer seed coat. The hydrocolloid material can be separated into acidic and neutral polysaccharide fractions, and, upon hydrolysis, L-arabinose, D-galactose, D-galacturonic acid, L-rhamnose, and D-xylose are obtained. The exact compositions of the polymers have not been determined. Solutions of the purified gum are thixotropic; the viscosity decreases as shear rate increases, a property that is of potential value.

STANDARDS AND TESTS. When psyllium seed is placed in water, the radial and outer walls of the epidermal cells swell to form layers of mucilage about the seed (Fig. 2–14). The following test for quality has been devised:

Place 1 g of plantago seed in a 25-ml graduated cylinder, add water to the 20-ml mark, and shake the cylinder at intervals during 24 hours; allow the seeds to settle

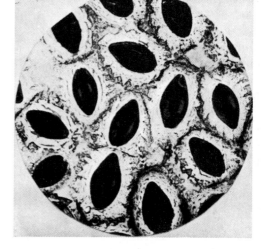

Fig. 2–14. Seeds of *Plantago psyllium* placed in water show the swelling of the mucilage.

for 12 hours and note the total volume occupied by the swollen seeds: the seeds of *P. psyllium* occupy a volume of not less than 14 ml, those of *P. ovata* not less than 10 ml, and those of *P. indica* not less than 8 ml.

USE AND DOSE. Plantago seed is a cathartic. Its action is caused by the swelling of the mucilaginous seed coat, thus giving bulk and lubrication. The seeds should be taken with a considerable amount of water. Usual dose is 7.5 g.

The mucilaginous layer of the seed coat is separated by a physicochemical process and is known in commerce as "psyllium seed husks." Combined with various chemicals such as powdered anhydrous dextrose, sodium bicarbonate, monobasic potassium phosphate, citric acid, and others, the husks are used as an adjunct in the treatment of constipation.

PROPRIETARY PRODUCTS. Psyllium seed or husks are an ingredient in a number of laxative preparations including: Casyllium®, Effersyllium®, Hydrocil®, Metamucil®, Mucilose®, Plova®, Serutan®, Siblin®, Syllact®, and Syllamalt®.

Cydonium or quince seed is the ripe seed of *Cydonia vulgaris* Persoon (Fam. Rosaceae). These seeds possess a mucilaginous epithelium equivalent to approximately 20% of their weight. This mucilage is composed of cellulose suspended in a more soluble polysaccharide that yields L-arabinose and a mixture of aldobiouronic acids. The hydrocolloid forms viscous solutions with thixotropic properties, and it is used as an ingredient in some wave setting lotions. Economic considerations preclude many other potential uses of this hydrocolloid.

GUAR GUM

Guar gum or guaran is the powdered endosperm of the seed of *Cyamopsis tetragonolobus* (Linné) Taubert (Fam. Leguminosae), an annual plant that is readily cultivated in dry climates. Texas is a major producing area. Use of this gum is expanding rapidly, and there is no practical limit on the amount of gum that can be produced by modern agricultural practices to meet the demand.

The hydrocolloid is a galactomannan. 1,4-Linked D-mannopyranosyl units form a linear chain; single 1,6-linked D-galactopyranosyl residues are attached to alternate mannose moieties. This molecular structure gives properties that are intermediate between those typically associated with branched and linear hydrocolloids. The gum hydrates in cold water and is stable in acidic formulations.

Guar gum is used as a bulk-forming laxative and as a thickening agent, a tablet binder, and a disintegrator in pharmaceuticals. However, the food processing and paper industries are the largest users of this gum.

PROPRIETARY PRODUCT. Gentlax®.

LOCUST BEAN GUM

Locust bean gum is the hydrocolloid-containing powdered endosperm of the seed of *Ceratonia siliqua* Linné (Fam.

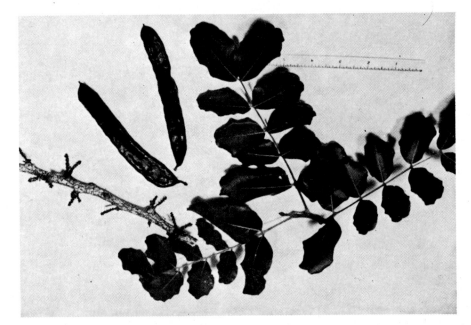

Fig. 2–15. Carob *(Ceratonia siliqua)* showing the compound leaves, also the pods containing seeds from which locust bean gum is obtained. (Photo, courtesy of Dr. Julia F. Morton, Director, Morton Collectanea, University of Miami.)

Chapter 3

Glycosides and Tannins

Glycosides are compounds that yield one or more sugars among the products of hydrolysis. The most frequently occurring sugar is β-D-glucose although rhamnose, digitoxose, cymarose, and other sugars are components of glycosides. When the sugar formed is glucose, the substance may be called a glucoside; however, because other sugars may be developed during the hydrolysis, the term glycoside is applied.

Chemically, the glycosides are acetals in which the hydroxyl of the sugar is condensed with a hydroxyl group of the nonsugar component, and the secondary hydroxyl is condensed within the sugar molecule itself to form an oxide ring. More simply, glycosides may be considered as sugar ethers. The nonsugar component is known as the **aglycone;** the sugar component is called the **glycone.** Both *alpha* and *beta* glycosides are possible, depending on the stereoconfiguration of the glycosidic linkage. However, one should note that only *beta* forms occur in plants. It should be noted also that emulsin and most other natural enzymes hydrolyze only the *beta* varieties.

From the biologic viewpoint, glycosides play an important role in the life of the plant and are involved in its regulatory, protective, and sanitary functions. Among such a wide variety of compounds one finds many therapeutically active agents. In fact, the group contributes to almost every therapeutic class. Some of our most valuable cardiac specifics are glycosides from digitalis, strophanthus, squill, convallaria, apocynum, and others (see page 170). Laxative drugs, such as senna, aloe, rhubarb, cascara sagrada, and frangula contain emodin and other anthraquinone glycosides; sinigrin, a glycoside from black mustard, yields allyl isothiocyanate, a powerful local irritant; and gaultherin from wintergreen yields methyl salicylate, an analgesic.

The classification of glycosides is a difficult matter. If the classification is based on the sugar group, a number of rare sugars are involved, the structures of which are not too well known; if the aglycone group is used as a basis of classification, one encounters groups from probably all classes of plant constituents: tannins, sterols, carotenoids, anthocyanins, and many others, including several whose structures are as yet unknown. A therapeutic classification, although excellent from a pharmaceutic viewpoint, omits many glycosides of pharmacognostic interest.

Some glycosides contain more than one saccharide group, possibly as di- or trisaccharides. Upon proper conditions of hydrolysis, one or more of the saccharide groups can be removed from such compounds, resulting in glycosides of simpler structure (see amygdalin, page 70). The most common sugar present is D-glucose, although the presence of other sugars, such as rhamnose, is quite possible. Occasionally, rare sugars are found as components of glycosides, such as digitoxose, digitalose, and cymarose.

All natural glycosides are hydrolyzed into a sugar and another organic compound by boiling with mineral acids; however, they vary widely in the ease with which this hydrolysis is performed. In most cases, the glycoside is easily hydrolyzed by an enzyme that occurs in the same plant tissue, but in different cells from those that contain the glycoside. Injury to the tissues, the germination process, and perhaps other physiologic activities of the cells bring the enzyme in contact with the glycoside, and the hydrolysis of the latter takes place. A large number of enzymes have been found in plants. Many of these enzymes hydrolyze only a single glycoside; however, 2 enzymes, namely **emulsin** of almond kernels and **myrosin** of black mustard seeds, each hydrolyze a considerable number of glycosides. Glycosides that are derivatives of rhamnose require a special enzyme known as rhamnase for their hydrolysis.

BIOSYNTHESIS OF GLYCOSIDES

Consideration of glycoside (heteroside) biosynthesis necessarily consists of 2 parts. The general reactions couple a sugar residue to an aglycone. Presumably this transfer reaction is similar in all biologic systems. This contrasts with the pathways for biosynthesis of the various types of aglycones, which tend to be diverse and must be considered individually.

Available evidence indicates that the principal pathway of glycoside formation involves the transfer of a uridylyl group from uridine triphosphate to a sugar 1-phosphate. Enzymes catalyzing this reaction are referred to as uridylyl transferases (1) and have been isolated from animal, plant, and microbial sources. Phosphates of pentoses, hexoses, or various sugar derivatives may participate. The subsequent reaction, mediated by glycosyl transferases (2), involves the transfer of the sugar from uridine diphosphate to a suitable acceptor (aglycone), thus forming the glycoside.

$$\text{(1)}$$
$$\text{UTP + Sugar-1-P} \rightleftharpoons \text{UDP-Sugar + PPi}$$

$$\text{(2)}$$
$$\text{UDP-Sugar + Acceptor} \rightleftharpoons \text{Acceptor-Sugar + UDP}$$
$$\text{(Glycoside)}$$

Once such a glycoside is formed, other enzymes may transfer another sugar unit to the monosaccharide moiety, converting it to a disaccharide. Enzymes occur in various glycoside-containing plants that are capable of producing tri- and tetrasaccharide moieties of the glycosides by analogous reactions.

To illustrate the biosynthesis of an aglycone moiety and the stereospecificity that can be involved in the glycosyl transferase reaction, the formation of cyanogenic glycosides is an interesting case to note. The process of glycoside formation is shown in Figure 3–1 for prunasin, a cyanogenic glucoside. The amino acid

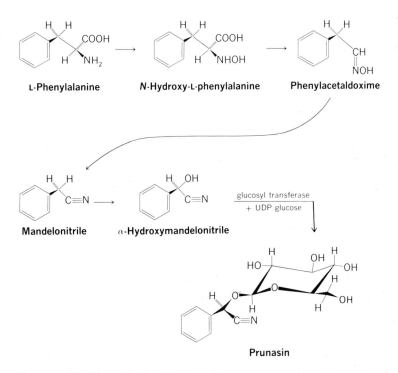

Fig. 3–1. The biosynthetic pathway for the cyanogenic glycoside, prunasin.

phenylalanine, which arises from the shikimate pathway (see page 112), is the starting precursor. An aldoxime, a nitrile, and a cyanohydrin are involved as intermediates in the pathway. The presence of a chiral center in mandelonitrile provides the opportunity for 2 β-glucosides to occur. In wild cherry, *Prunus serotina*, prunasin (D-mandelonitrile glucoside) is formed. The isomeric sambunigrin (L-mandelonitrile glucoside) is formed in *Sambucus nigra*. Apparently, these compounds do not occur in the same species, further confirming the stereospecificity of the glycosyl transferases that catalyze their formation.

When the chemical nature of the aglycone group is used as a basis of systematization, the classification of the glycoside-containing drugs follows this scheme: (1) cardioactive group (see page 170); (2) anthraquinone group; (3) saponin group; (4) cyanophore group; (5) isothiocyanate group; (6) flavonol group; (7) alcohol group; (8) aldehyde group; (9) lactone group; (10) phenol group; and (11) tannins.

ANTHRAQUINONE GLYCOSIDES

A number of glycosides with aglycones related to anthracene are present in such drugs as cascara sagrada, frangula, aloe, rhubarb, senna, and chrysarobin. With the exception of chrysarobin (which is too irritating), these drugs are employed as cathartics. The glycosides, upon hydrolysis, yield aglycones that are di-, tri-, or tetrahydroxyanthraquinones or modifications of these compounds. A typical example is frangulin, which hydrolyzes to form emodin (1,6,8-trihydroxy-3-methylanthraquinone) and rhamnose. The structural formula of a glycoside yielding emodin and those yielding chrysophanic acid (1,8-dihydroxy-3-methylanthraquinone), aloe-emodin (1,8-dihydroxy-3-hydroxymethylanthraquinone), and rhein (1,8-dihydroxyanthraquinone-3-carboxylic acid) are shown in Figure 3–2. Glycosides of anthranols and anthrones, reduced derivatives of anthraquinones, also occur in the plant materials, and they make significant contributions to the therapeutic action of these natural products.

The free anthraquinone aglycones exhibit little therapeutic activity. The sugar residue facilitates absorption and translocation of the aglycone to the site of action. The anthraquinone and related glycosides are stimulant cathartics and exert their action by increasing the tone of the smooth muscle in the wall of the large intestine. Glycosides of anthranols and anthrones elicit a more drastic action than do the corresponding anthraquinone glycosides, and a preponderance of the former constituents in the glycosidic mixture can cause discomforting griping action.

Biosynthesis of Anthraquinone Glycosides. Much of our knowledge of the biosynthesis of anthraquinones has been obtained from studies of microorganisms. Feedings of labeled acetate to *Penicillium islandicum*, a species that produces several anthraquinone derivatives, have revealed that the distribution of radioactivity in these compounds is consistent with formation via a head-to-tail condensation of acetate units. A poly-β-ketomethylene acid intermediate is probably first produced and then gives rise to the various oxygenated aromatic compounds following intramolecular condensations. Anthranols and anthrones are likely intermediates in the formation of anthraquinones. Presumably, the emodin-like anthraquinones are formed in higher plants by a similar pathway. The transglycosylation reaction, which creates a glycoside, probably occurs at a late stage in the pathway after the anthraquinone nucleus has been formed.

CASCARA SAGRADA

Cascara sagrada or rhamnus purshiana is the dried bark of *Rhamnus purshianus* DeCandolle (Fam. Rhamnaceae). The species epithet was formerly spelled *purshiana*, and that form is retained in one of the titles applied to the drug. It

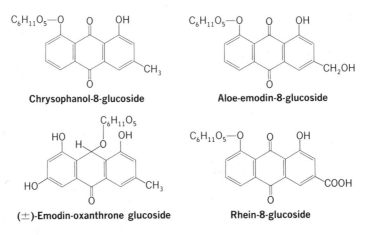

Chrysophanol-8-glucoside

Aloe-emodin-8-glucoside

(±)-Emodin-oxanthrone glucoside

Rhein-8-glucoside

Fig. 3–2.   Representative structures of anthraquinone glycosides.

should be aged for at least 1 year prior to use in medicinal preparations. Reduced forms of the emodin-type glycosides are present in the fresh bark; during the minimum 1-year storage period, these glycosides are converted to monomeric oxidized glycosides, which exhibit a milder cathartic activity.

The name cascara sagrada is Spanish for sacred bark; *Rhamnus* is the ancient classic name for buckthorn; *purshianus* was given in honor of the German botanist, Friedrich Pursh. The plant is a tree that attains a height of 10 meters and is indigenous to the Pacific Coast of North America. Most of the present-day market supply comes from Oregon, Washington, and southern British Columbia. Collections are made during the summer, beginning at the end of May and continuing until the rainy season starts. The wild trees are scattered in the native forests on the mountains. The bark is stripped from the tree by making longitudinal incisions (see Fig. 3–3) and peeling off sections that tend to roll into large quills. The trees are often felled and the bark is removed from the larger branches. The bark is sacked and conveyed to suitable places, often sawmill platforms, for sun drying. The inner surface is not exposed to the sun, however, in order to retain the yellow

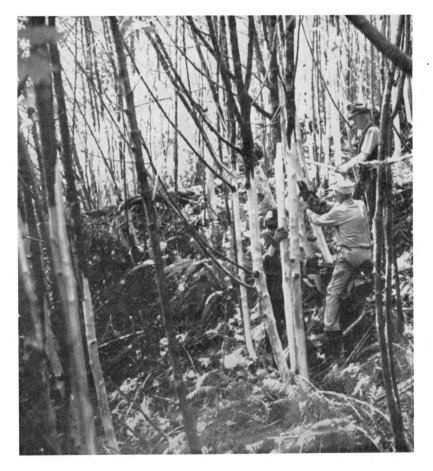

Fig. 3–3. Collecting cascara bark in Oregon forest. (Courtesy of S. B. Penick and Company.)

color. After the large quills are dried, they are run through a "breaker" and broken into small transversely curved pieces.

Two types of anthracene compounds have been reported: normal O-glycosides (based on emodin), about 10 to 20%, and aloinlike C-glycosides, representing about 80 to 90% of the total. About a dozen such compounds have been identified. Two of the C-glycosides are barbaloin and deoxybarbaloin (chrysaloin). Four additional compounds of this type are designated as cascarosides A, B, C, and D. Cascarosides A and B are based on optical isomers of barbaloin and cascarosides C and D on optical isomers of chrysaloin. All 4 of the cascarosides, being primary glycosides of barbaloin and chrysaloin, are actually both O- and C-glycosides. The remaining 4 to 6 anthracene derivatives identified in the drug are normal O-glycosides, based mostly on emodin. Hydrolysis of the total glycosides yields rhamnose and glucose in an approximate ratio of 1:1.

USE AND DOSE. Cascara sagrada is a cathartic. Its principal use is in the correction of habitual constipation where it not only acts as a laxative but restores natural tone to the colon. The bitter taste and the activity is considerably reduced by treating cascara sagrada extracts with alkaline earths or magnesium oxide. The usual dose of cascara sagrada fluidextract (bitter cascara) is 1 ml; of aromatic cascara sagrada fluidextract (sweet cascara), 5 ml; of cascara sagrada extract, 300 mg.

SPECIALTY PRODUCTS. Cascara sagrada is the active ingredient in Cas-Evac® and a number of generic products.

Many preparations containing cascara sagrada have appeared on the market. The extract has been combined with such laxative ingredients as (1) phenolphthalein—Oxothalein®, (2) phenolphthalein and bile salts—Caroid® and Bile Salts with Phenol-phthalein, (3) phenolphthalein, bile salts, and aloin—Amlax®, (4) aloe—Nature's Remedy®, (5) psyllium husks and prune powder—Casyllium®, (6) karaya gum—Imbicoll® with Cascara Sagrada, (7) agar, sodium alginate, and mineral oil—Petrogalar® with Cascara Sagrada, and (8) dioctyl sodium sulfosuccinate—Stimulax®.

Casanthranol is a purified mixture of the anthranol glycosides extracted from cascara sagrada. It is marketed as Peristim Forte®, which has a usual dose of 90 mg. Casanthranol is also combined with surfactant drugs and/or hydrocolloids; such formulations include Afko-Lube Lax®, Casa-Laud®, Comfolax Plus®, Constiban®, Dialose Plus®, Diothron®, Disanthrol®, Disolan®, Hydrocil Fortified®, and Peri-Colace®.

Frangula or buckthorn bark is the dried bark of *Rhamnus frangula* Linné. This plant is a shrub that grows in Europe and western Asia. The composition and activity of frangula bark correspond to those of cascara sagrada, and it finds a comparable use in Europe and the Near East. Products from the dried, ripe fruits of *R. catharticus* Linné are also used in these areas for their cathartic action. Other *Rhamnus* species contain anthraquinone glycosides, but are not employed in medicine.

Saraka® contains frangula and karaya gum.

ALOE

Aloe or aloes is the dried latex of the leaves of *Aloe barbadensis* Miller (*A. vera* Linné), known in commerce as Curaçao aloe (Fig. 3–4), or of *A. ferox* Miller and hybrids of this species with *A. africana* Miller and *A. spicata* Baker, known in commerce as Cape aloe (Fam. Liliaceae).

Aloe yields not less than 50% of water-soluble extractive.

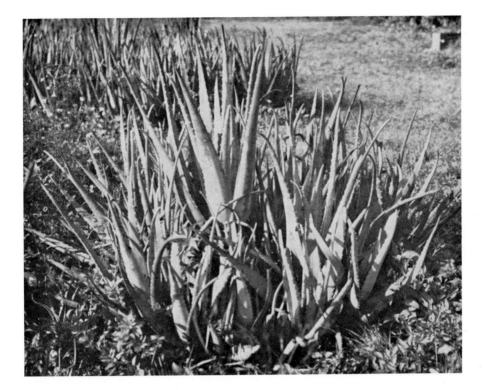

Fig. 3—4. Typical cluster of *Aloe barbadensis (Aloe vera)*, the plant yielding Curaçao aloe. (Photo, courtesy of Dr. Julia F. Morton, Director, Morton Collectanea, University of Miami.)

Aloe is from the Arabic *alloeh* or the Hebrew *halal*, meaning a shining, bitter substance; *vera* is from the Latin *verus*, meaning true. *Barbadensis* refers to the Barbados Islands; *ferox* is from the Latin meaning wild or ferocious; *africana* refers to the habitat of the plant, southern Africa; and *spicata* refers to the flowers in spikes.

About 300 species of *Aloe* are known, most of which are indigenous to Africa. Many have been introduced into the West Indies and Europe. The aloes are typical xerophytic plants that have fleshy leaves, usually have spines at the margins, and resemble to some extent the agave or century plant (*Agave americana* Linné, Fam. Amaryllidaceae).

Aloe barbadensis is a native of northern Africa, but was introduced into the Barbados Islands in the seventeenth century. *A. chinensis*, a variety of *A. barbadensis* (*A. vera*), was introduced into Curaçao from China in 1817. The drug was cultivated to a considerable extent in Barbados until the middle of the nineteenth century, but since that time the industry apparently has died out. Curaçao aloe, which is often called Barbados aloe, comes from the Dutch islands of Aruba and Bonaire. The leaves are cut in March and April and placed cut-end downward on a V-shaped trough, the latter being inclined so that the latex can be led into a vessel (Fig. 3—5). The latex is evaporated in a copper kettle and, when of the proper consistency, is poured into metal containers and allowed to har-

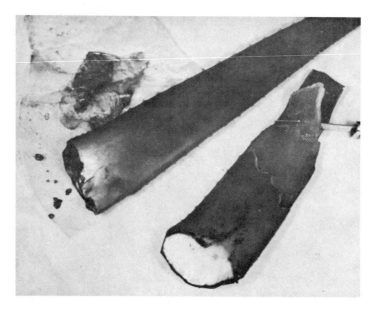

Fig. 3–5. Cut, fleshy, white-based leaves of *Aloe barbadensis* showing: *left*, darkened juice and *right*, mucilaginous interior. (Photo, courtesy of Dr. Julia F. Morton, Director, Morton Collectanea, University of Miami.)

den. At the present time, the principal areas of production are Aruba, Bonaire, Haiti, Venezuela, and South Africa. Curaçao aloe is the most important form occurring in the United States.

Aloe occurs on the market as opaque masses that range from reddish black to brownish black to dark brown in color. The taste of each variety of aloe is nauseating and bitter. The odor is characteristic and disagreeable.

Aloe contains a number of anthraquinone glycosides, the principal one of which is barbaloin (aloe-emodin anthrone C-10 glucoside).

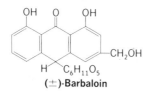

(±)-**Barbaloin**

O-glycosides of barbaloin with an additional sugar have also been isolated from certain samples of Cape aloe. These compounds have been designated aloinosides. Free (nonglycosidal) aloe-emodin and a free and combined anthranol are also present. Chrysophanic acid has been detected in certain types of the drug.

The active constituents of aloe vary qualitatively and quantitatively according to the species from which the drug is obtained. Analyses have revealed that Curaçao aloe is superior to Cape aloe because it contains two-and-one-half times as much aloe-emodin. Curaçao aloe also contains an appreciable amount of free and combined chrysophanic acid not present in the other types.

In addition to these physiologically active compounds (10 to 30%), aloe contains inactive ingredients including large amounts (16 to 63%) of a resinous material plus a volatile oil.

USES AND DOSE. Aloe is a pharmaceutic aid for compound benzoin tincture and a cathartic. When used as a cathartic, it acts chiefly on the large intestine, but it has been largely replaced for this purpose by aloin. Aloe glycosides elicit a relatively drastic cathartic action, and some authorities advocate a preferential use of other cathartic substances. Aloe is available with cascara sagrada in Nature's Remedy® and with podophyllum in Carter's Little Pills®.

The fresh mucilaginous juice of the leaves of *Aloe barbadensis (A. vera)* has been used for centuries in the treatment of burns, abrasions, and other skin irritations by the natives of the countries in which this plant grows. The Seminole Indians split aloe leaves and apply them directly to injuries and wounds to promote healing. In 1935, the juice was recommended in treating third-degree X-ray burns and, more recently, has been advocated in treating atomic radiation burns.

The variable nature of this mucilaginous juice made it extremely difficult to incorporate into a stabilized type of preparation. At present, the application of the fresh gel has been supplanted by the use of ointments in which the components of the juice are the principal ingredients. The cellular composition of the leaf necessitates the puncture of each cell that contains the mucilage. The gel must be forcefully removed from the leaf tissue and, to remove cellular impurities, must be passed through stainless steel strainers because of the acid pH of the juice.

This extracted gel is then blended with a special lanolin base. The ointment is recommended for the treatment of sunburns, deep thermal burns, and radiation burns. It affords relief from pain and itching and tends to minimize keratosis and ulceration.

PROPRIETARY PRODUCT. Alo®-Ointment.

Aloin is a mixture of active principles obtained from aloe. It varies in chemical composition and in physical and chemical properties according to the variety of aloe from which it is derived. Essentially, it represents the active water-soluble glycosides and related constituents of aloe that are separated from the inert, water-insoluble resinous matter.

The usual cathartic dose of aloin is 15 mg. Aloin is combined with other cathartics such as cascara sagrada and phenolphthalein.

SPECIALTY PRODUCTS. Alophen®, Amlax®.

RHUBARB

Rhubarb, rheum, or Chinese rhubarb consists of the dried rhizome and root that are deprived of periderm tissues of *Rheum officinale* Baillon (Fig. 3–6), of *R. palmatum* Linné, of other species (except *R. rhaponticum* Linné, the common garden rhubarb plant), or of hybrids of *Rheum* Linné (Fam. Polygonaceae) and are grown in China.

Indian rhubarb or Himalayan rhubarb consists of the dried rhizome and root of *R. emodi* Wallich, of *R. webbianum* Royle, or of some related *Rheum* species that are native to India, Pakistan, or Nepal.

Rheum is from the Latin *Rha*, the name of the Volga River near which species of *Rheum* grow. *Palmatum* refers to the large spreading leaves, *emodi* refers to the emodin content, and *webbianum* refers to an Indian taxonomist.

The principal constituents of medicinal rhubarbs are rhein anthrones. Rhubarb has been used in cathartic preparations; the cathartic action is relatively drastic, and the use of other cathartic substances has been largely adopted.

PROPRIETARY PRODUCT. Rhubetts®.

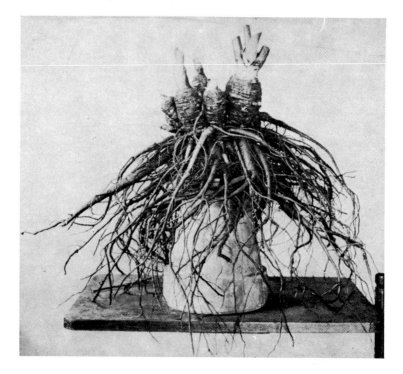

Fig. 3–6. *Rheum officinale* root system, showing large distinctive rhizomes and relatively small roots.

SENNA

Senna or senna leaves consists of the dried leaflet of *Cassia acutifolia* Delile, known in commerce as Alexandria senna, or of *C. angustifolia* Vahl, known in commerce as Tinnevelly senna (Fam. Leguminosae). The name *Senna* is from the Arabic *sena*, the native name of the drug; *Cassia* is from the Hebrew *qetsiah*, meaning to cut off, and refers to the fact that the bark of some of the species was once peeled off and used (the application of the name *cassia* to cinnamon barks should be noted); *acutifolia* is Latin and refers to the sharply pointed leaflets; and *angustifolia* means narrow leaved (Fig. 3–7). The plants are low-branching shrubs; *C. acutifolia* grows wild near the Nile River from Aswan to Kordofan and *C.*

angustifolia grows wild in Somalia, the Arabian peninsula, and India. Most of the commercial supply of the drug is collected from plants cultivated in southern India (Tinnevelly); some material is also produced in the Jammu district of India and in Northwest Pakistan.

Alexandria senna is harvested in April and in September by cutting off the tops of the plants about 15 cm above the ground and drying them in the sun. Afterward, the stems and pods are separated from the leaflets by using sieves. The portion that passes through the sieves is then "tossed." The leaves work to the surface and the heavier stalk fragments sink to the bottom. The leaves are then graded and baled or packed in bags. This process of collection and separation accounts for the large number of broken leaves in

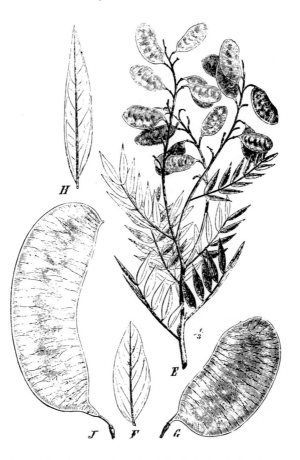

Fig. 3–7. *Cassia acutifolia: E,* fruiting branch; *F,* single leaflet; *G,* pod. *Cassia angustifolia: H,* single leaf; *J,* pod.

Alexandria senna. This drug was formerly shipped via Alexandria but is now distributed through Port Sudan on the Red Sea.

Tinnevelly senna is gathered by hand and dried in the sun, then carefully baled and shipped primarily from the port of Tuticorin. It is cultivated in nearby areas to which the term "Tinnevelly" is applied. Senna is cultivated on wet lands resembling rice paddies; in fact, rice is often one crop of the season, and senna is a later crop of the same season. The poorer grades of senna are grown on dry land without irrigation. Senna is graded according to the size of the leaf and the color of the leaflets: blue-green leaves are best, yellowish leaves are poorest.

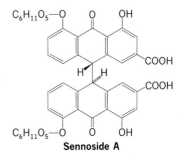

Sennoside A

Senna was introduced into European medicine in the ninth or tenth century by the Arabians. Its native use seems to ante-date historic record. According to Isaac Judaeus, a native of Egypt who lived about 850 to 900 A.D., senna was brought to Egypt from Mecca.

The principal active constituents of senna are dimeric glycosides whose agly-cones are comprised of aloe-emodin and/or rhein. Those present in greatest concentration are sennosides A and B, a pair of optical isomers whose aglycones are rhein dianthrone (sennidin A and B). Sennosides C and D are minor con-stituents having dimeric aglycones com-prised of 1 molecule of rhein and 1 molecule of aloe-emodin. Small quantities of monomeric glycosides and free an-thraquinones are also present. Senna pods also contain useful, active glycosides; some of the primary glycosides in the pods have as many as 10 sugar molecules attached to a rhein dianthrone nucleus.

USE AND DOSE. Senna is a cathartic. Usual dose is 2 g.

PROPRIETARY PRODUCTS. Black Draught®, Dr. Caldwell's Senna Laxative®, Fletcher's Castoria®, Swiss Kriss®, X-Prep®.

A concentrate of the active constituents and an isolated mixture of sennosides, which may be prepared from either the leaves or the pods, are used in various products, some of which contain a senna component combined with a hydrocolloid or a surfactant. Such products include Gentlax®, Glysennid®, Senokap®, and Senokot®.

CHRYSAROBIN

Chrysarobin is a mixture of neutral principles obtained from Goa powder, a substance deposited in the wood of *Andira araroba* Aguiar (Fam. Leguminosae). *Andira* is of Portuguese origin; *araroba* is the Latinized East Indian name of the bark, *aroba*; *Chrysarobin* is from the Greek *Khrysos*, meaning gold, and from *aroba*.

Goa is the former Portuguese colony on the Malabar Coast to which the plant was imported in 1852. This is a large tree found in the provinces of Bahia and Ser-gipe in Brazil.

Goa powder arises in the living cells of the wood of the stems. The cell walls metamorphose and finally disintegrate, forming large lacunae in which the al-tered products are deposited in the form of a yellowish brown powder. This pow-der is more or less admixed with the tissues of the bark and wood. The trees are hewn and cut into convenient pieces and the Goa powder is scraped out. The crude article is purified by sifting it free from fragments of wood, drying, and powder-ing. At present, Goa powder is a scarce item in drug markets.

Goa powder is light yellow when fresh, but, on exposure to air, becomes dark brown or brownish purple. It contains from 50 to 75% of a neutral principle, chrysarobin; about 2% of resin; 7% of bitter extractive; and a small amount of chrysophanic acid.

Chrysarobin is prepared by extracting Goa powder with hot benzene, evaporat-ing the solution to dryness, and powder-ing. It is a brown to orange-yellow mi-crocrystalline powder that is odorless and tasteless, but irritating to the mucous membranes.

A representative sample of chrysarobin contains approximately 30 to 40% of chryso-phanolanthrone or chrysophanolanthranol, 20% of emodinanthrone-monomethyl ether, and 30% of dehydro-emodinanthrone-monomethyl ether. These compounds are related to the anthraquinones; thus, chrysarobin has a laxative action although it is not suitable for internal use.

USES. Chrysarobin is a keratolytic agent employed in the treatment of psoriasis, trichophytosis, and chronic eczema. It is used topically in the form of an ointment or a solution (0.1 to 0.2%), but because of its irritating properties it should not be used on the face or scalp. Variable composition of chrysarobin and lack of adequate standardization procedures have created problems in insuring reproducible therapeutic effects. Anthralin, a synthetic anthracenetriol, has largely replaced the use of chrysarobin; prescription products of anthralin include Anthra-Derm®, Anthera®, and Lasan® Unguent.

DANTHRON

Danthron or chrysazin is 1,8-dihydroxyanthraquinone. It occurs as an orange-colored crystalline powder that is practically insoluble in water, but soluble in alcohol, ether, benzene, and other solvents.

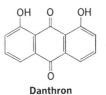

Danthron

Although 1,8-dihydroxyanthraquinone is a natural constituent in certain drugs, it is difficult to isolate in a pure state; thus, danthron is prepared synthetically from 1,8-anthraquinone potassium disulfonate.

Uses and Dose. Danthron is a cathartic drug and is an important intermediate in the manufacture of anthralin and of alizarin and indanthrene dyestuffs. Usual dose is 75 to 150 mg.

Proprietary Products. Dorbane®, Modane®, Tonelax®. Danthron is also combined with a surfactant in a number of products, including Doctate-P®, Dorbantyl®, Doxan®, Doxidan®, and Magcyl®.

SAPONIN GLYCOSIDES

This group of glycosides is widely distributed in the higher plants. Saponins form colloidal solutions in water that foam upon shaking; they have a bitter, acrid taste, and drugs containing them are usually sternutatory and otherwise irritating to the mucous membrane. They destroy red blood corpuscles by hemolysis and are toxic, especially to cold-blooded animals. Many saponins are used as fish poisons. Upon hydrolysis they yield an aglycone known as a "sapogenin." The sapogenins form readily crystallizable compounds upon acetylization. This process can be used to purify sapogenins. The more poisonous saponins are often called "sapotoxins." Glycyrrhiza and sarsaparilla (see page 68) are among the drugs containing saponins. Plants such as the California soap plant, *Chlorogalum pomeridianum* (DC.) Kunth. (Fam. Liliaceae), which yields amolonin, are sources of saponins that are used extensively for industrial purposes.

Much of the research conducted on the saponin-containing plants was motivated by the attempt to discover precursors for cortisone (see page 183). This substance was originally isolated from the adrenal cortex and later synthesized from certain bile acids of cattle. Because these sources limit the supply of cortisone, academic, industrial, and governmental research agencies have examined many species of plants, particularly those containing steroidal sapogenins.

The determination of the initial desirability of any given steroid compound as a cortisone precursor is based on whether it has hydroxyl groups in the 3- and 11-positions on the molecule or has the ability to be converted readily to this structure. It would appear that the most outstanding plant steroids for cortisone production are:

diosgenin and botogenin from the genus *Dioscorea*

hecogenin, manogenin, and gitogenin from species of *Agave*

sarsasapogenin and smilagenin from the genus *Smilax*

sarmentogenin from the genus *Strophanthus*

sitosterol from crude vegetable oils.

Members of the Liliaceae, Amaryllidaceae, and Dioscoreaceae show the presence of sapogenins among the monocotyledons; however, the genus *Strophanthus* in the Apocynaceae was formerly thought to be the most promising of the dicotyledons. Most of the investigative work for the development of cortisone from plant precursors has centered about the sapogenins in the 3 monocotyledonous families named previously.

Biosynthesis of Saponin Glycosides. Saponin glycosides are divided into 2 types based on the chemical structure of their aglycones (sapogenins). The so-called neutral saponins are derivatives of steroids with spirochetal side chains; the acid saponins possess triterpenoid structures. Biogenesis of the steroid nucleus will be discussed in the chapter on steroids. Less is known about triterpenoid biosynthesis than is known about the steroids, but labeled acetate and mevalonate have been incorporated into such compounds. Therefore, the main pathway leading to both types of sapogenins is similar and involves the head-to-tail coupling of acetate units. However, a branch occurs, probably after the formation of the triterpenoid hydrocarbon, squalene, that leads to steroids in one direction and to cyclic triterpenoids in the other (Fig. 3–8).

GLYCYRRHIZA

Glycyrrhiza is the dried rhizome and roots of *Glycyrrhiza glabra* Linné, known in commerce as Spanish licorice, or of *G. glabra* Linné var. *glandulifera* Waldstein et Kitaibel, known in commerce as Russian licorice, or of other varieties of *G. glabra* Linné that yield a yellow and sweet wood (Fam. Leguminosae). *Glycyrrhiza* is of Greek origin and means sweet root; *glabra* means smooth and refers to the

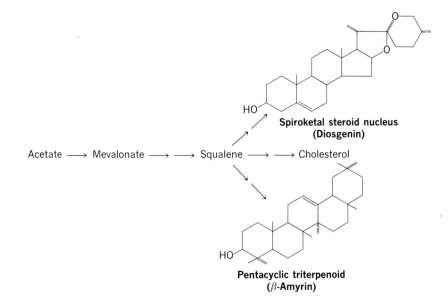

Fig. 3–8.   Biosynthesis of sapogenins.

smooth, podlike fruit of this species. The fruit in the variety *glandulifera* has glandlike swellings. Glycyrrhiza is also called **licorice root.**

Propagation of the variety *typica* is generally done by rhizome cuttings that are planted in rows about 1.3 meters apart. At the end of the third or fourth year, the rhizome and roots are dug, preferably in the autumn and from plants that have not borne fruit, thereby insuring maximum sweetness of the sap. The washed material is air dried (4 to 6 months) and packed into bales or cut and tied into short cylindric bundles (see Fig. 3–9). The large thick roots of Russian licorice are peeled before drying. In Turkey, Spain, and Israel, a considerable amount of the crop is extracted with water, the liquid is clarified and evaporated, and the resulting extract is molded into sticks or other forms.

Glycyrrhiza contains a saponinlike glycoside, glycyrrhizin (glycyrrhizic acid), which is 50 times as sweet as sugar. Upon hydrolysis, the glycoside loses its sweet taste and is converted to the aglycone glycyrrhetic acid plus 2 molecules of glucuronic acid. Glycyrrhetic acid is a pentacyclic triterpene derivative of the β-amyrin type. Other constituents include flavonoid glycosides (liquiritin, isoliquiritin, liquiritoside, isoliquiritoside, rhamnoliquiritin, and rhamnoisoliquiritin), coumarin derivatives (herniarin and umbelliferone), asparagine, 22,23-dihydrostigmasterol, glucose, mannitol, and about 20% of starch. Reports of estrogens in the plant appear to be based on low-level estrogenlike activity of other constituents.

Glycyrrhiza is considered to possess demulcent and expectorant properties. It is used considerably as a flavoring agent and is frequently employed to mask the taste of such bitter drugs as aloe, ammonium chloride, quinine, and others; the surfactant property of the saponins may also facilitate absorption of poorly absorbed drugs, such as the anthraquinone glycosides. Commercially, licorice is added to chewing gums, chocolate candy, cigarettes, smoking mixtures, chewing tobacco, and snuff; when it is added to beer, it increases the foaminess; when it is added to root beer, stout, and porter, it imparts a bitter taste.

Pharmacologic studies of licorice have been extensive in recent years, particularly in Europe. As a result, glycyrrhetic acid is utilized there in dermatologic practice for its anti-inflammatory properties, and licorice root extract is employed in the treatment of peptic ulcer and of Addison's disease (chronic adrenocortical insufficiency).

Glycyrrhizin increases fluid and sodium retention and promotes potassium depletion. Persons with cardiac problems and hypertension should avoid consumption of significant quantities of licorice.

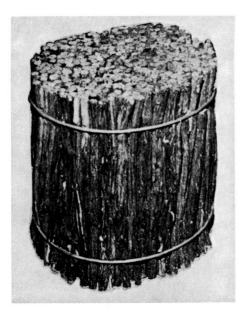

Fig. 3–9. A bundle of Spanish licorice root.

Pure glycyrrhiza extract or pure licorice root extract is prepared from glycyrrhiza and is a black pilular mass having a characteristic sweet taste. It is an ingredient in aromatic cascara sagrada fluidextract.

Glycyrrhiza fluidextract is prepared by extracting coarsely ground licorice root with warm water, rendering the extractive alkaline with ammonium hydroxide, concentrating, and bringing it to final volume with alcohol and water. It is a pharmaceutic aid.

DIOSCOREA

Yam is a popular name for several of the edible species of *Dioscorea* and is sometimes incorrectly applied to certain varieties of the sweet potato. Various species of *Dioscorea* known as Mexican yams represent rich sources of the principles used as cortisone precursors. Botogenin and diosgenin are obtained from the root of *Dioscorea spiculiflora*, a cultivated species. The steroid nucleus of botogenin was altered by transferring an oxygen atom from the 12- to the 11-position of the polycyclic molecule before it could be utilized as an intermediate in the production of cortisone. Diosgenin, obtained upon hydrolysis of dioscin, is now the major precursor of glucocorticosteroids, which are prepared by processes that involve microbial transformation (see page 184).

A Mexican yam derived from *D. floribunda* is considered by the U.S. Department of Agriculture as the best source of steroids.

CYANOPHORE GLYCOSIDES

Several glycosides yielding hydrocyanic acid as one of the products of hydrolysis are commonly found in rosaceous plants. They are sometimes designated as cyanogenic glycosides. Perhaps the most widely distributed of these is amygdalin. (Note that another of the hydrolytic products is benzaldehyde; thus, amygdalin-containing drugs may also be classified in the aldehyde glycoside group.)

The common cyanophore glycosides are derivatives of mandelonitrile (benzaldehyde-cyanohydrin). The group is represented by amygdalin, which is found in large quantities in bitter almonds, in kernels of apricots, cherries, peaches, plums, and in many other seeds of the Rosaceae, and also by prunasin, which occurs in *Prunus serotina*. Both amygdalin and prunasin yield D-mandelonitrile as the aglycone. Sambunigrin from *Sambucus nigra* liberates L-mandelonitrile as its aglycone.

When amygdalin is hydrolyzed, it forms 2 molecules of glucose (Fig. 3–10). Although these are usually written as linked in apparent disaccharide form, one should note that a disaccharide sugar has never been broken off from the molecule by any known means of hydrolysis. Amygdalin is therefore a true glucoside rather than a maltoside. The hydrolysis of amygdalin takes place in 3 steps, which are briefly as follows:

1. Most hydrolyzing agents break the molecule first to liberate 1 molecule of glucose and 1 molecule of mandelonitrile glucoside.

2. The second molecule of glucose is liberated with the formation of mandelonitrile.

3. The mandelonitrile then breaks down with the formation of benzaldehyde and hydrocyanic acid.

The enzyme emulsin, as obtained from almond kernels, consists of a mixture of 2 enzymes: amygdalase, which causes the first step in the hydrolysis, and prunase, which causes the second step. (It is said

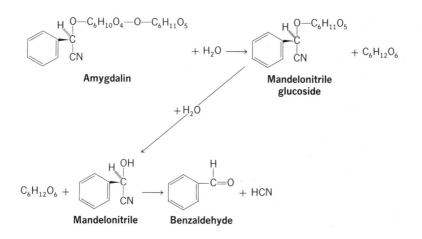

Fig. 3–10. Hydrolysis of amygdalin.

that emulsin consists of at least 4 enzymes.)

Preparations from plant materials containing cyanogenic glycosides are widely employed as flavoring agents. Anticancer claims have also been made for an amygdalin-containing preparation known as laetrile or vitamin B_{17}, and the possibility for control of sickle cell anemia with cyanogenic glycosides has been noted. The FDA has not recognized the efficacy of laetrile for treatment of cancer although some states have legalized its sale (see page 472).

WILD CHERRY

Wild cherry is the carefully dried stem bark of *Prunus serotina* Ehrhart (Fam. Rosaceae). *Prunus* is the classic name of the plum tree; *serotina* means late or backward, referring to the time of flowering and fruiting of the species. Wild cherry is known as **prunus virginiana** and as **wild black cherry tree.**

The plant is a tree that grows to a height of 30 meters or more in the eastern United States and Canada. The commercial supplies of the drug come chiefly from Tennessee, Mississippi, Virginia, and North Carolina (Fig. 3–11).

Wild cherry bark was used by the Indians, and no doubt the early settlers learned its use from them. It has long enjoyed popular usage in domestic medicine.

Wild cherry bark contains a cyanogenic glycoside, prunasin (D-mandelonitrile glucoside), a compound formed by the partial hydrolysis of amygdalin (see Fig. 3–10). Other constituents include the hydrolytic enzyme, prunase, p-coumaric acid, trimethyl gallic acid, starch, and traces of a volatile oil. A resin that yields scopoletin on hydrolysis is also present. The yield of hydrocyanic acid varies from 0.23 to 0.32% in inner bark, 0.03% in trunk bark, and varies even in bark of the same thickness from the same tree. When the exposure is such that the chloroplastids are abundant in the cells of the bark, the percentage of the D-mandelonitrile glucoside is higher. When the exposure is such that the cells do not take an active part in photosynthesis, the percentage of the glucoside is lower. In the latter case the bark is yellowish brown.

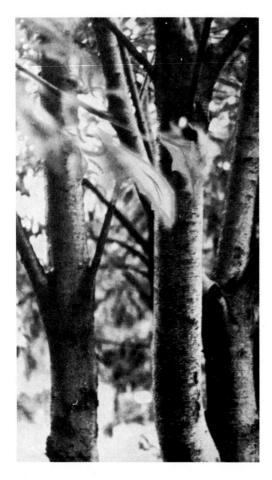

Fig. 3–11. Photograph of the trunks of wild cherry trees showing the characteristic transverse lenticels of the bark. (Courtesy of S. B. Penick and Company.)

Wild cherry, in the syrup form, is employed as a flavored vehicle, especially in cough remedies. It has been considered a sedative expectorant.

ISOTHIOCYANATE GLYCOSIDES

The seeds of several cruciferous plants contain glycosides, the aglycones of which are isothiocyanates. These aglycones may be either aliphatic or aromatic derivatives. Principal among these glycosides are sinigrin from black mustard, sinalbin from white mustard, and gluconapin from rape seed. When hydrolyzed by the enzyme myrosin, they yield the mustard oils. Although the fixed oil content of these seeds exceeds the amount of the volatile oil developed on hydrolysis, the activity is caused by the latter.

MUSTARD

Black mustard, sinapis nigra, or brown mustard is the dried ripe seed of varieties of *Brassica nigra* (Linné) Koch or of *B. juncea* (Linné) Czerniaew or of varieties of these species (Fam. Cruciferae). The term, Cruciferae, is from the Latin, meaning cross bearing, and refers to the shape of the flowers whose petals are arranged in the form of a Maltese cross; *sinapis* is from the Celtic *nap*, meaning turnip; *Brassica* is from the Celtic *bresic*, meaning cabbage; *juncea* is from the Latin, meaning rush or reed; and *nigra* is from the Latin, meaning black. The term *mustard* is believed to be derived from the use of the seeds as a condiment. The sweet *must* of old wine was mixed with crushed seeds to form a paste called "mustum ardens" (hot must), hence the name "mustard."

The plants are annual herbs that have slender erect stems, yellow flowers, pinnatifid leaves, and somewhat four-sided siliques with short stalks. They are native to Europe and southwestern Asia, but are naturalized and cultivated in temperate climates in many countries and show considerable variations in form. *B. nigra* is cultivated in England and on the continent, and *B. juncea* is cultivated in India. Black mustard is mentioned in an edict of Diocletian (301 A.D.) as a condiment, and both Theophrastus and Pliny mention its use in medicine. During the Middle Ages it was an accompaniment to salted meats. The popularity of mustard as a condiment has by no means diminished.

Although black mustard contains fixed oil (30 to 35%), its principal constituent is the glycoside, sinigrin (potassium myronate), which is accompanied (probably in adjacent cells) by the enzyme, myrosin. Upon the addition of water to the crushed or powdered seeds, the myrosin effects the hydrolysis of the sinigrin as shown below.

The allyl isothiocyanate produced is volatile; it is commonly called volatile mustard oil.

Black mustard is a local irritant and an emetic. Externally, the drug is a rubefacient and vesicant. Commercially, it is used as a condiment.

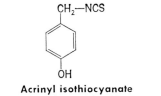

Acrinyl isothiocyanate
(Parahydroxybenzyl isothiocyanate)

than allyl isothiocyanate. It also contains 20 to 25% of fixed oil.

FLAVONOL GLYCOSIDES

The flavonol glycosides and their aglycones are generally termed flavonoids. A large number of different flavonoids occur in nature, and these yellow pigments are widely distributed throughout the higher plants. Rutin, quercitrin, and the citrus bioflavonoids (including hesperidin, hesperetin, diosmin, and naringen) are among the best known flavonoid constituents.

Rutin and hesperidin have been called vitamin P or permeability factors. They have been used in the treatment of various conditions characterized by capillary bleeding and increased capillary fragility. Claims have also been advanced for the value of citrus bioflavonoids in treating symptoms of the common cold. Evidence for the therapeutic efficacy of rutin, citrus

$$C_3H_5-\underset{\underset{N-O-SO_3K}{\|}}{C}-S-C_6H_{11}O_5 + H_2O \longrightarrow S=C=N-CH_2-CH=CH_2 + KHSO_4 + C_6H_{12}O_6$$

Sinigrin + (Myrosin) $\longrightarrow$ Allyl isothiocyanate + Pot. acid + Glucose
(Mustard oil)   sulfate

White mustard or sinapis alba consists of the dried, ripe seeds of *Brassica alba* (Linné) Hooker filius (Fam. Cruciferae). White mustard is as commercially important as black mustard. The plant resembles that of *B. nigra* but is usually considerably shorter and its siliques are more rounded and tapered. Like black mustard, it is cultivated in temperate climates all over the world.

White mustard contains the enzyme, myrosin, and a glucoside, sinalbin, which, upon hydrolysis, yield acrinyl isothiocyanate, a pungent-tasting but almost odorless oil that is much less volatile

bioflavonoids, and related compounds is not conclusive, and products containing them are no longer marketed for medicinal purposes in the United States. They are included in some preparations as dietary supplements.

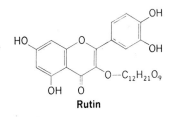

Rutin

ALCOHOL GLYCOSIDES

SALICIN

Salicin is a glycoside obtained from several species of *Salix* and *Populus*. Most willow and poplar barks yield salicin, but the principal sources are *Salix purpurea* and *S. fragilis*. The glycoside, populin (benzoylsalicin), is also associated with salicin in the barks of the Salicaceae.

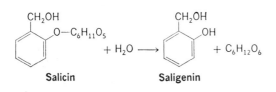

Salicin   Saligenin

Salicin is hydrolyzed into D-glucose and saligenin (salicyl alcohol) by emulsin. Salicin has antirheumatic properties (1-g dose). Its action closely resembles that of salicylic acid and is probably oxidized to salicylic acid in the human system. Recognition of the properties of salicin clarifies many folkloric uses of poplar and willow barks.

ALDEHYDE GLYCOSIDES

Vanilla is a drug that has an aldehydic aglycone as its chief constituent. **Vanillin** is the aglycone developed during the curing of vanilla beans. Vanillin is methyl-protocatechuic aldehyde.

VANILLA

Vanilla or vanilla bean is the cured, full-grown, unripe fruit of *Vanilla planifolia* Andrews, often known in commerce as Mexican or Bourbon vanilla, or of *V. tahitensis* J. W. Moore, known in commerce as Tahiti vanilla (Fam. Orchidaceae). *Vanilla* is from the Spanish *vania*, a sheathlike pod, and *illa*, meaning small; *planifolia* is from the Latin *planus*, meaning flat, and *folium*, meaning leaf; *tahitensis* refers to Tahiti, its adopted home.

The plants are perennial, climbing, dioecious epiphytes attached to the trunks of trees by means of aerial rootlets. The plant is native to the woods of eastern Mexico but is cultivated in tropical countries where the temperature does not fall below 18°C and where the humidity is high.

The plant is usually propagated by means of cuttings and, after 2 or 3 years, reaches the flowering stage. The plant continues to bear fruit for 30 or 40 years. The flowers, approximately 30 on each plant, are hand pollinated, thus producing larger and better fruits. The fruits are collected as they ripen to a yellow color, 6 to 10 months after pollination, and are cured by dipping in warm water and repeated sweating between woolen blankets in the sun during the day and packing in wool-covered boxes at night. This requires about 2 months, during which the pods lose from 70 to 80% of their original weight and take on the characteristic color and odor of the commercial drug. The pods are then graded, tied into bundles of about 50 to 75, and sealed in tin containers for shipment.

The Spaniards found that the Aztecs of Mexico used vanilla as a flavor for cocoa and consequently introduced its use into Europe. Cultivation began in Réunion and Madagascar (now the Malagasy Republic) in 1839, and shortly after, other countries adopted this practice.

Green vanilla contains two glycosides, glucovanillin (avenein) and glucovanillic alcohol. Glucovanillin is hydrolyzed by an enzyme during the curing process into glucose and vanillin, and glucovanillic alcohol is similarly hydrolyzed into glucose and vanillic alcohol, which is, in turn, oxidized to vanillic aldehyde (vanillin).

Vanillin is the principal flavoring constituent. Vanilla also contains about 10% of sugar, 10% of fixed oil, and calcium oxalate.

Uses. Vanilla, in the form of vanilla tincture, is used as a flavoring agent and as a pharmaceutic aid. It is a source of vanillin.

COMMERCIAL VARIETIES:

Mexican or Vera Cruz vanilla is the best grade on the market; the pods frequently attain a length of 30 to 35 cm. The supply is largely consumed in Mexico and the United States.

Bourbon vanilla is produced on the island of Réunion and shipped from the Malagasy Republic. It resembles the Mexican variety but is about two-thirds as long, blacker in color, usually covered with a sublimate of needle-shaped vanillin crystals, and possesses a coumarinlike odor.

Tahiti vanilla, grown in Tahiti and Hawaii, is reddish brown in color, about as long as the Mexican variety, but sharply attenuated and twisted in the lower portion. The odor is somewhat unpleasant, and the variety is less suitable for flavoring.

Vanilla splits and cuts represent the more mature fruits in which dehiscence has taken place. They are cut into short lengths.

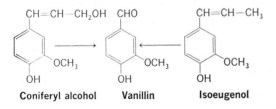

Coniferyl alcohol   Vanillin   Isoeugenol

Vanillin is 4-hydroxy-3-methoxybenzaldehyde or methylprotocatechuic aldehyde. It may be obtained from vanilla or prepared synthetically from other sources:

(1) coniferin, a glycoside present in the cambium sap of pine trees; (2) eugenol, a phenol present in clove oil; and (3) lignin, a by-product of the pulp industry. Most of the vanillin in commerce is made from lignin.

Vanillin consists of fine, white to slightly yellow, needlelike crystals that have an odor and a taste resembling vanilla. It is slightly soluble in water and glycerin and is freely soluble in alcohol, chloroform, and ether. Vanillin is employed as a flavoring agent.

LACTONE GLYCOSIDES

Although **coumarin** is widely distributed in plants, glycosides containing coumarin as such are rare. Several glycosides of hydroxylated coumarin derivatives, however, occur in plant materials; these glycosides include skimmin in Japanese star anise, aesculin in various parts of the horse chestnut tree, daphnin in mezereum, fraxin in ash bark, scopolin in belladonna, and limettin in citrus trees. None of the hydroxycoumarin glycosides is of particular medicinal importance.

Some use has been made of natural, nonglycosidic coumarin and other lactone substances. Coumarin and **tonka beans,** coumarin-containing seeds of *Dipteryx odorata* (Aublet) Willdenow and *D. oppositifolia* (Aublet) Willdenow (Fam. Leguminosae), were formerly used pharmaceutically as flavoring agents. Some coumarin derivatives still find application for their anticoagulant properties. The antispasmodic activity of the barks of *Viburnum prunifolium* Linné (blackhaw) and *V. opulus* Linné (true cramp bark) (Fam. Caprifoliaceae) has been attributed to scopoletin (6-methoxy-7-hydroxycoumarin) and other coumarins. Preparations of these plant drugs were used at one time as uterine sedatives. Other lactone-containing natural products include **cantharidin,** which is used for dermatologic purposes, and **santonin,** which is obtained from the unexpanded flowerheads of *Artemisia cina* Berg, *A. maritima* Linné, and several other *Artemisia* species (Fam. Compositae). Santonin was formerly used as an anthelmintic, but its use has been discontinued in the United States owing to its potential toxicity.

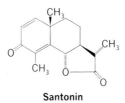

Santonin

COUMARIN

Coumarin is the lactone of *o*-hydroxycinnamic acid. It occurs as colorless, prismatic crystals and has a characteristic fragrant odor and a bitter, aromatic, burning taste. It is soluble in alcohol. Coumarin can be synthesized readily.

Coumarin is rather widely distributed in nature. In addition to its occurrence in tonka beans (1 to 3%), it has been isolated from sweet vernal grass (*Anthoxanthum odoratum* Linné, Fam. Gramineae), sweet clover [*Melilotus albus* Medicus and *M. officinalis* (Linné) Lamarck, Fam. Leguminosae], sweet-scented bedstraw (*Galium triflorum* Michaux, Fam. Rubiaceae), and red clover (*Trifolium pratense* Linné, Fam. Leguminosae).

Coumarin and extracts of tonka beans were formerly used as flavoring agents. However, coumarin-drug interactions occur with a number of therapeutic substances, and the FDA has banned the use of coumarin and coumarin-containing materials for flavoring purposes.

Bishydroxycoumarin or dicumarol is a drug related to coumarin. It was obtained originally from improperly cured leaves and flowering tops of *Melilotus officinalis*

(Linné) Lamarck (Fam. Leguminosae), but is now prepared synthetically.

Dicumarol is an anticoagulant. The usual dose is 200 to 300 mg initially, then 25 to 200 mg once a day, as indicated by prothrombin-time determinations. A number of synthetic analogs of bishydroxycoumarin also are used in anticoagulant therapy; these include warfarin salts (Athrombin-K®, Coumadin®, Panwarfin®) and phenprocoumon (Liquamar®).

CANTHARIDES

Cantharides, Spanish flies, Russian flies, or blistering flies consists of the dried insect, *Cantharis vesicatoria* (Linné) De Geer (Fam. Meloidae). *Cantharis* is Greek and means beetle, *vesicatoria* is from the Latin *vesica*, meaning a bladder and refers to the blistering qualities. This insect is found on certain shrubs of the Caprifoliaceae and Oleaceae that grow in southern and central Europe. The mature insects, which are brilliant green with a metallic luster, usually appear in June or July. In the early morning, when the insects are still sluggish from the cold night air, the shrubs are shaken or beaten with poles, and the insects are collected on cloths spread on the ground. The insects are killed by plunging into dilute vinegar, by exposure to the fumes of hot vinegar, ammonia, or sulfur dioxide, or by means of chloroform, ether, or similar drugs. After the insects are killed, they are carefully dried at a temperature not higher than 40°C. The drug should be stored in tight containers, and a few drops of chloroform or carbon tetrachloride should be added

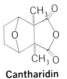

Cantharidin

occasionally to preserve the drug from attack by other insects.

Cantharides contains as its chief constituent the vesicating principle, cantharidin (0.6 to 1.0%), which is the lactone or anhydride of cantharidic acid. In addition, about 12% of a fat is associated with the cantharidin in the soft body tissues of the insect.

Uses. Cantharides is an irritant, a vesicant, and rubefacient. If taken internally, it is excreted by the kidney, irritates the urinary tract, and can result in priapism. This accounts for the drug's popular reputation as an aphrodisiac. Internal administration of cantharides is potentially dangerous, however, and deaths have been reported. Topical application of a solution of cantharidin is effective in the removal of certain types of warts; a preparation containing 0.7% cantharidin in collodion (Cantharone®) is available for this purpose.

PHENOL GLYCOSIDES

The aglycone groups of many of the naturally occurring glycosides are phenolic in character. Thus, arbutin, found in uva ursi, chimaphila, and other ericaceous drugs, yields hydroquinone and glucose upon hydrolysis. Hesperidin, which occurs in various citrus fruits (page 73) and is included with the flavonol group, may be classified as a phenol glycoside. Phloridzin, found in the root bark of rosaceous plants, baptisin from baptisia, and iridin from *Iris* species are additional examples of phenol glycosides.

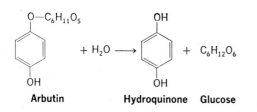

| Arbutin | Hydroquinone | Glucose |

UVA URSI

Uva ursi or bearberry is the dried leaf of *Arctostaphylos uva-ursi* (Linné) Sprengel or its varieties *coactylis* or *adenotricha* Fernald and MacBride (Fam. Ericaceae). The plant is a procumbent evergreen shrub indigenous to Europe, Asia, and the northern United States and Canada.

In addition to the glycoside, arbutin, the leaves contain corilagin, pyroside, several esters of arbutin, quercitin, gallic acid, elagic acid, and ursolic acid.

Uva ursi has a long history of use for its diuretic and astringent properties. Extract of uva ursi was formerly an ingredient in some proprietary formulations, but its use in prescription medications has been replaced by more effective diuretic agents. The inclusion of uva ursi and other diuretic materials in various products intended for weight reduction is without recognized merit.

TANNINS

Tannins comprise a large group of complex substances that are widely distributed in the plant kingdom; almost every plant family embodies species that contain tannins. When tannins occur in appreciable quantities, they are usually localized in specific plant parts, such as leaves, fruits, barks, or stems.

Chemically, tannins are complex substances; they usually occur as mixtures of polyphenols that are difficult to separate because they do not crystallize. Some authors prefer to use the term "tannin extracts" rather than "tannins." Recently, the use of chromatographic methods has enabled research workers not only to confirm the complicated nature of tannin extracts but also to identify the simple polyphenols present in small amounts in such mixtures. Determination of the latter is important because complex tannins are generally considered to have arisen from simple polyphenols by polymerization. Many condensed tannins have never been isolated or characterized; thus, their biogenetic development is not positively known.

Tannins are customarily divided into 2 chemical classes based on the identity of the phenolic nuclei involved and on the way they are joined. Members of the first class consist of gallic acid or related polyhydric compounds esterified with glucose. Because such esters are readily hydrolyzed to yield the phenolic acids and the sugar, they are referred to as **hydrolyzable tannins.**

Nonhydrolyzable or condensed tannins comprise the second class. Basically, these tannins contain only phenolic nuclei, but frequently are linked to carbohydrates or proteins. Most such tannins result from the condensation of 2 or more flavan-3-ols, such as catechin, or of flavan-3,4-diols, such as leucocyanidin. When treated with hydrolytic agents, these tannins tend to polymerize, yielding insoluble, usually red-colored products known as phlobaphenes.

Both classes of tannin are widely distributed in nature. It must be emphasized that, in many species, both types are present, although one type generally tends to predominate in any particular plant part.

Tannins are noncrystallizable compounds that, with water, form colloidal solutions possessing an acid reaction and a sharp "puckering" taste. They cause precipitation of solutions of gelatin as well as of alkaloids, they form dark blue or greenish black soluble compounds with ferric salts, they produce a deep red color with potassium ferricyanide and ammonia, and they are precipitated by salts of copper, lead, and tin and by strong aqueous potassium dichromate (or 1% chromic acid) solutions. In alkaline solutions, many of their derivatives readily absorb oxygen.

Tannins precipitate proteins from solution and can combine with proteins, rendering them resistant to proteolytic enzymes. When applied to living tissues, this action is known as an "astringent" action and forms the basis for therapeutic application of tannins. Tannin-bearing drugs, such as hamamelis and nutgall, as well as partially purified tannins (tannic acid) and their derivatives (acetyltannic acid), are employed in medicine as astringents in the gastrointestinal tract and on skin abrasions. In the treatment of burns, the proteins of the exposed tissues are precipitated and form a mildly antiseptic, protective coat under which the regeneration of new tissues may take place.

Considerable epidemiologic and experimental evidence suggests that prolonged utilization of certain tannin-rich plant materials may be hazardous owing to their carcinogenetic potential. The habitual chewing of betel nut (*Areca catechu*), an alkaloid-containing drug that is also rich in condensed catechin tannin, has been linked to high rates of oral and esophageal cancer in India and South Africa. Even the drinking of ordinary tea (leaves of *Camellia sinensis*) has been implicated. Apparently, the British, who add milk to their tea, thereby binding the tannin, have a much lower incidence of esophageal "obstruction" than do the Dutch, who formerly drank large quantities of tea without milk. Experimentally, the subcutaneous injection into rats of aqueous extracts of tannin-rich *Areca catechu* and *Rhus copallina* produced a significant number of malignant mesenchymal tumors.

The ability of tannins to precipitate proteins is also utilized in the process of vegetable tanning, which converts animal hides to leather. The tannin not only affects the pliancy and toughness of the leather, but also acts as a preservative because of its antiseptic qualities. Various types of tannins produce a variety of leathers; thus, certain hydrolyzable types form a "bloom" whereas the nonhydrolyzable types produce the "tanner's red." The deeply colored compounds obtained with iron salts have been used on a commercial scale in the manufacture of inks. Because of their precipitating qualities, solutions of tannins are utilized in the laboratory as reagents for the detection of gelatin, proteins, and alkaloids. In the antidotal treatment of alkaloidal poisoning, tannin solutions are extremely valu-

able for inactivating the alkaloid by the formation of insoluble tannate.

TANNIN-CONTAINING PLANT MATERIALS

HAMAMELIS LEAF

Hamamelis leaf or witch hazel leaves is the dried leaf of *Hamamelis virginiana* Linné (Fam. Hamamelidaceae).

Hamamelis is from the Greek *hama*, meaning at the same time and *melis* meaning a fruit; *virginiana* indicates that the plant is found in Virginia, although the actual habitat ranges from New

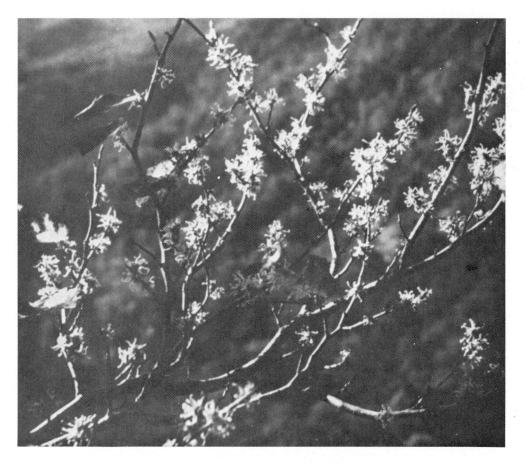

Fig. 3–12. Autumn flowers of the witch hazel tree.

Brunswick to Minnesota and extends southward to Florida and Texas. The plant is a shrub or small tree that attains a height of 8 meters and is found particularly in low, damp woods. The flowers (Fig. 3–12) appear in the fall as the fruits of the previous year ripen. The leaves are collected throughout the summer and are dried in the open air, preferably under shade to preserve the green color. The commercial supply comes from the Blue Ridge Mountain region, chiefly from Virginia, North Carolina, and Tennessee. The decoction or infusion of witch hazel leaves has been commonly used since the days of the early colonists who learned of the drug from the American Indians.

CONSTITUENTS. Hamamelis leaf contains hamamelitannin and a second tannin that appears to be derived from gallic acid; a hexose sugar, a volatile oil, a bitter principle, gallic acid, and calcium oxalate. Hamamelis leaf possesses astringent and hemostatic properties.

PRODUCT. Hamamelis leaf fluidextract is commercially available.

NUTGALL

Nutgall is the excrescence obtained from the young twigs of *Quercus infectoria* Olivier and allied species of *Quercus* (Fam. Fagaceae). The galls are obtained principally from Aleppo in Asiatic Turkey.

The excrescence (gall) is caused by the puncture of a hymenopterous insect, *Cynips tinctoria*, and the presence of the deposited ovum. Several stages in the development of the gall correspond to the development of the insect:

1. When the larva begins to develop and the gall begins to enlarge, the cells of the outer and central zones contain numerous small starch grains.

2. When the chrysalis stage is reached, the starch near the middle of the gall is replaced in part by gallic acid, but the peripheral and central cells contain masses of tannic acid.

3. As the winged insect develops, nearly all of the cells contain masses of tannic acid with a slight amount of adhering gallic acid.

4. When the insect emerges from the gall, a hole to the central cavity is formed. Thus, the tannic acid, owing to the presence of moisture and air, may be oxidized in part into an insoluble product, and the gall becomes more porous, thereby constituting the so-called **white gall** of commerce.

The technical and medicinal use of galls was known to the ancient Greeks (450 B.C.). Since the Crusades, great quantities of galls have been exported from Asia Minor.

CONSTITUENTS. The principal constituent is tannic acid, which is found to the extent of 50 to 70%; the drug also contains gallic acid, 2 to 4%; ellagic acid; starch; and resin.

Nutgall, the chief source of tannic acid, is used in the tanning and dyeing industry and, formerly, in the manufacture of ink. Medicinally, it has astringent properties.

ALLIED PRODUCTS. **Japanese and Chinese galls** are formed on *Rhus chinensis* Mill. (Fam. Anacardiaceae) owing to the stings of certain plant lice *(Aphis)*. These galls are rich in tannin and, as they contain less coloring matter than the oak galls, are used in the manufacture of gallic acid.

TANNIC ACID

Tannic acid, gallotannic acid, or tannin is a tannin usually obtained from nutgall. The powdered galls are extracted with a mixture of ether, alcohol, and water and the liquid separates into 2 layers. The aqueous layer contains gallotannin and the ethereal layer contains the free gallic acid present in the gall. After separation, the solution of gallotannin is evaporated and the tannin is purified in various ways.

COMPOSITION. Tannic acid is not a single homogeneous compound, but is a mixture of esters of gallic acid with glucose whose exact composition varies according to its source. The tannin from Chinese galls analyzes entirely as octa- or nonagalloylglucose and yields, on hydrolysis, methyl gallate and 1,2,3,4,6-pentagalloylglucose. Turkish tannin, which is a mixture of hexa- or heptagalloylglucoses, hydrolyzes to form methyl gallate and a mixture of 1,2,3,6- and 1,3,4,6-tetragalloylglucose. Both types of tannic acid yield, on milder treatment, methyl m-digallate, indicating the presence of an m-trigalloyl group in each.

DESCRIPTION. Tannic acid occurs as an amorphous powder, glistening scales, or spongy masses that are light brown to yellowish white. The odor is faint and the taste is strongly astringent. Tannic acid is soluble in water, alcohol, and acetone and insoluble in ether, chloroform, and benzin.

USES AND DOSES. Tannic acid is an astringent. It was formerly used in the treatment of burns, but this application has been discontinued. Its topical use is now restricted to the treatment of bed sores, minor ulcerations, and the like. As an alkaloidal precipitant, it has been employed in cases of alkaloidal poisoning.

PROPRIETARY PRODUCTS. Topical preparations that incorporate tannic acid as an astringent include Amertan®, Tanac®, Tanicaine®, and Tanurol®.

Gallic acid is 3,4,5-trihydroxybenzoic acid that crystallizes with 1 molecule of water. It occurs in nutgall and can be prepared from tannic acid by hydrolysis with dilute acids. Bismuth subgallate is used by ostomates to help to control odors.

READING REFERENCES

Coursey, D. G.: *Yams: An Account of the Nature, Origins, Cultivation, and Utilization of the Useful Members of the Dioscoreaceae*, New York, Humanities Press, 1968.

Endres, H., Howes, F. N., and Von Regel, C.: *Gerbstoffe Tanning Materials*, Lfg. 1, *Die Rohstoffe des Pflanzenreichs*, 5th ed., Weinheim, Germany, J. Cramer, 1962.

Fairbairn, J. W.: *Anthraquinone Laxatives*, New York, John Wiley & Sons, Inc., 1977.

Harborne, J. B., Mabry, T. J., and Mabry, H., eds.: *The Flavonoids*, London, Chapman and Hall Ltd., 1975.

Haslam, E.: *Chemistry of Vegetable Tannins*, New York, Academic Press, Inc., 1966.

Haworth, R. D.: The Chemistry of Tannins, Adv. Sci., 19 (81):396, 1963.

Kefford, J. F., and Chandler, B. V.: *The Chemical Constituents of Citrus Fruits*, New York, Academic Press, Inc., 1970.

Lorenzetti, L. J., Salisbury, R., Beal, J. L., and Baldwin, J. N.: Bacteriostatic Property of *Aloe vera*, J. Pharm. Sci., 53 (10):1287, 1964.

Mabry, T. J., Markham, K. R., and Thomas, M. B.: *The Systematic Identification of Flavonoids*, New York, Springer-Verlag New York, Inc., 1970.

Miller, L. P., ed.: *Phytochemistry*, Vols. I–III, New York, Van Nostrand Reinhold Co., 1973.

Morton, J. F.: Folk Uses and Commercial Exploitation of Aloe Leaf Pulp, Econ. Botany, 15 (4):311, 1961.

Patai, S., ed.: *The Chemistry of the Quinonoid Compounds*, New York, Interscience Publishers, 1974.

Piras, R., and Pontis, H. G., eds.: *Biochemistry of the Glycosidic Linkage*, New York, Academic Press, Inc., 1972.

Schofield, M.: The Genus Vanilla versus Synthetic Vanillin, Perfumery Essent. Oil Record, 59 (8):582, 1968.

Sim, S. K.: *Medicinal Plant Glycosides*, Toronto, University of Toronto Press, 1967.

Takeda, K.: The Steroidal Sapogenins of the Dioscoreaceae, Prog. Phytochem., 3:287, 1972.

Thompson, R. H.: *Naturally Occurring Quinones*, 2nd ed., New York, Academic Press, Inc., 1971.

Chapter 4

Lipids

Lipids (fixed oils, fats, and waxes) are esters of long-chain fatty acids and alcohols, or of closely related derivatives. The chief difference between these substances is the type of alcohol; in fixed oils and fats, glycerol combines with the fatty acids; in waxes, the alcohol has a higher molecular weight, e.g., cetyl alcohol.

Fats and fixed oils are obtained from either plants (olive oil, peanut oil) or animals (lard). Their primary function is food (energy) storage. The fixed oils and fats are important products used pharmaceutically, industrially, and nutritionally. Waxes may also be of plant or animal origin. Many drugs contain fixed oils and fats as their principal constituents; the fixed oils and fats are often separated from the crude vegetable drugs (by expression) or the crude animal drugs (by rendering or extraction) and are employed as drugs in the refined state.

Fixed oils and fats differ only as to melting point; those that are liquid at normal temperatures are known as fatty or fixed oils whereas those that are semisolid or solid at ordinary temperatures are known as fats. Although most vegetable oils are liquid at ordinary temperatures and most animal fats are solid, there are notable exceptions such as cocoa butter, which is a solid vegetable oil, and cod liver oil, which is a liquid animal fat (see page 301).

The United States Pharmacopeia includes several tests that determine the identity, quality, and purity of fixed oils. These tests are based on the chemical constitution of the fatty acids. The **acid value** or **acid number** (the number of milligrams of potassium hydroxide required to neutralize the free fatty acids in 1 g of the substance) indicates the amount of free fatty acids present in the oil; the **saponification value** indicates the number of milligrams of potassium hydroxide required to neutralize the free acids and saponify the esters contained in 1 g of the substance; the **Reichert-Meissl number** is the number of milliliters of 0.1N potassium hydroxide solution required to neutralize the volatile water-soluble acids obtained by the hydrolysis of 5 g of the fat; and the **iodine number** (the number of grams of iodine absorbed, under prescribed conditions, by 100 g of the substance) indicates the degree of unsaturation. Other physical constants, such as melting point, specific gravity, and refractive index, also serve as identity, purity, and quality tests.

Fixed oils and fats of vegetable origin are obtained by expression in hydraulic presses. If the expression is carried out in the cold, the oil is known as a "virgin oil" or a "cold-pressed oil." In contrast, if the expression is carried out in heat, the oil is known as a "hot-pressed oil." Sometimes organic solvents are used for the extraction of oils. Animal fats are separated from other tissues by rendering with steam, with or without pressure. The heat melts the fat, which rises to the top and may be separated by decantation. Oils may be further clarified by filtration and bleached with ozone. Stearins are often removed by chilling and filtration.

Vegetable oils and fats may occur in various parts of the plant but, as a general rule, seeds contain larger quantities of fats and oils than do other plant parts. Seeds are the usual source of fixed oils and, as a few

glycerides of fatty acids that have the general formula:

$$
\begin{array}{l}
CH_2-O-CO-R \\
| \\
CH-O-CO-R' \\
| \\
CH_2-O-CO-R''
\end{array}
$$

If R, R', and R'' are the same fatty acid radical, the compound is called triolein, tripalmitin, tristearin, and so forth. If R, R', and R'' are different fatty acids, a mixed glyceride results. The composition of the glycerides in any fixed oil or fat is influenced by the amounts of various fatty acids that are present during formation. Thus, the composition of fixed oils and fats from any source can vary within certain limits.

Usually, the glycerides of unsaturated fatty acids are liquid whereas the glycerides of saturated fatty acids of sufficient chain length are solid. The predominance of either type in an oil determines whether the mixture is liquid or solid. Some of the more common fatty acids are:

Caproic	$CH_3(CH_2)_4COOH$
Caprylic	$CH_3(CH_2)_6COOH$
Capric	$CH_3(CH_2)_8COOH$
Lauric	$CH_3(CH_2)_{10}COOH$
Myristic	$CH_3(CH_2)_{12}COOH$
Palmitic	$CH_3(CH_2)_{14}COOH$
Stearic	$CH_3(CH_2)_{16}COOH$
Arachidic	$CH_3(CH_2)_{18}COOH$
Oleic	$CH_3(CH_2)_7CH:CH(CH_2)_7COOH$
Linoleic	$CH_3(CH_2)_4CH:CHCH_2CH:CH(CH_2)_7COOH$
Linolenic	$CH_3CH_2CH:CHCH_2CH:CHCH_2CH:CH(CH_2)_7COOH$
Ricinoleic	$CH_3(CH_2)_5CHOHCH_2CH:CH(CH_2)_7COOH$

examples, the following might be mentioned: cottonseed, linseed, sesame seed, hemp seed, coconut, castor beans, almond, and others. In a few instances, other plant parts yield considerable quantities of fixed oil (pericarp of the olive). In certain fungi (e.g., ergot), fat is the characteristic reserve food material.

Chemically, the fixed oils and fats are

BIOSYNTHESIS OF LIPIDS

For many years, the synthesis of fats and fixed oils by living organisms was believed to be effected simply by a reversal of the reactions responsible for their degradation. Specifically, these include the hydrolysis of the glycerol-fatty acid esters by the enzyme lipase and the subsequent removal of 2-carbon units as acetyl-CoA from the fatty acid chain by β-oxidation. Biosynthetic studies indicate that the formation of these lipids utilizes different chemical pathways.

The biosynthesis of the fatty acid moieties is carried out by a series of reactions involving 2 enzyme complexes plus ATP, $NADPH_2$, Mn^{++}, and carbon dioxide.

Acetate first reacts with CoA, and the acetyl-CoA thus formed is converted by reaction with carbon dioxide to malonyl-CoA. This, in turn, reacts with an additional molecule of acetyl-CoA to form a

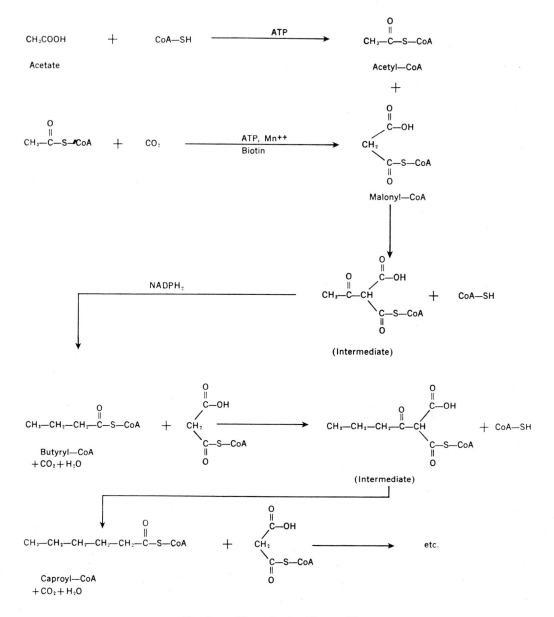

Fig. 4–1. Biosynthesis of fatty acids.

5-carbon intermediate, which undergoes reduction and elimination of carbon dioxide to produce butyryl-CoA. Malonyl-CoA again reacts with this compound to form a 7-carbon intermediate, which is reduced to caproyl-CoA. Repetition of the reaction results in a fatty acid containing an even number of carbon atoms in its chain (Fig. 4–1). Thus, the malonyl portion of malonyl-CoA, a 3-carbon compound, is actually the source of the 2-carbon biosynthetic units of the fatty acids.

Pathways of biosynthesis of unsaturated, branched-chain, odd-numbered, and otherwise modified fatty acids have not been established in detail. There is evidence that the first step in the production of a mono-unsaturated acid is the formation of the acyl-CoA derivative of its saturated analog. This is followed by enzymatic desaturation. Hydroxylation appears to be independent or to follow desaturation. Apparently, hydroxylation is not involved as an intermediate step in the desaturation process. Evidence suggests that the saturated acyl group of the acyl-CoA derivative is transferred to the 2-position of phosphatidyl glycerol before the desaturation and additional reactions.

Enzymes present in certain fractions of unripe castor seeds (*Ricinus communis*, Fam. Euphorbiaceae) can hydroxylate oleic acid to produce ricinoleic acid. The probable sequence for the formation of the latter compound is summarized by the reaction sequence in the opposite column.

The glycerol moiety utilized in lipid biosynthesis derives mainly from the L-isomer of α-glycerophosphate (L-α-GP). Reactions involved in the formation of a typical triglyceride are summarized in Figure 4–2.

L-α-GP, which may derive either from free glycerol or from the glycolysis intermediate, dihydroxyacetone phosphate, reacts successively with 2 molecules of fatty

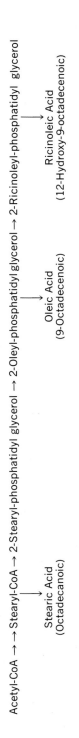

Acetyl-CoA → → Stearyl-CoA → 2-Stearyl-phosphatidyl glycerol → 2-Oleyl-phosphatidyl glycerol → 2-Ricinoleyl-phosphatidyl glycerol

Stearic Acid
(Octadecanoic)

Oleic Acid
(9-Octadecenoic)

Ricinoleic Acid
(12-Hydroxy-9-octadecenoic)

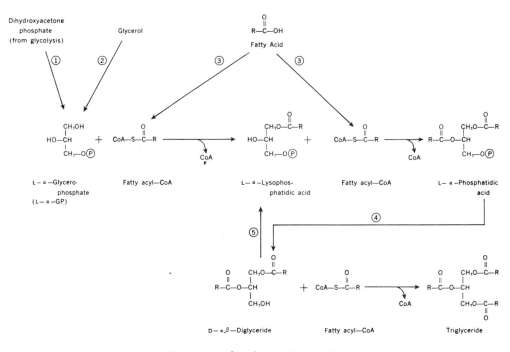

Enzymes and Cofactors Required

1. L-α-GP dehydrogenase + NADH₂
2. Glycerokinase + ATP
3. Acetyl-CoA + ATP
4. Phosphatidic acid phosphatase
5. Diglyceride kinase + ATP

Fig. 4–2. Biosynthesis of a triglyceride.

acyl-CoA to form first L-α-lysophosphatidic acid and then L-α-phosphatidic acid. The latter compound is converted to an α, β-diglyceride, which can either cycle back to the phosphatidic acids or react with another fatty acyl-CoA to form a triglyceride.

Relatively little is known about the biosynthetic pathways leading to other pharmaceutically important lipids. The higher alcohol esters of waxes are probably formed from smaller fatty acid units in a manner analogous to fatty acid biosynthesis. Hydrocarbon components of lipids may arise by reduction of squalene or a metabolic equivalent.

Fixed oils are sometimes classified into **drying oils, semidrying oils,** and **nondry-** ing oils. This classification is based on their ability to absorb oxygen from the air. Oxygen saturates the double bonds to form oxides that may polymerize to form hard films. This property of drying oils is of great importance in the paint industry. The double bonds in the unsaturated fatty acids also take up hydrogen under the proper conditions. **Hydrogenation** of the liquid oils produces semisolid fats that are extensively used as cooking fats and shortenings.

Fixed oils may be **hydrogenated** by passing hydrogen, in the presence of nickel or palladium, through the oil heated to 160 to 200°C. The unsaturated glycerides are more or less converted to saturated glycerides, which are solid at room temperature and stable. Many such oils are used for culinary purposes.

Sulfated or sulfonated oils are obtained by reacting sulfuric acid with the oil, keeping the temperature down by chilling. The oil is then washed and neutralized. If the oil contains an olefinic linkage, the acid molecule adds onto the double bond. The compound formed is a sulfate of the fat. These materials have surfactant properties that find industrial application.

Fixed oils and fats are employed in pharmaceuticals for their emollient properties. They may also serve, either in their natural form or in emulsions, as vehicles for other medicaments. A few, such as castor oil, have special therapeutic properties; the prostaglandins are other lipid metabolites that have recently attracted considerable attention for their physiologic properties and therapeutic potential. In the arts and in industry, fats and oils are used in the manufacture of soaps (sodium and potassium salts of the fatty acids), as drying oils in the manufacture of paints and varnishes, and as lubricants. Lipids also form an important class of foods; their high caloric value and low osmotic pressure have prompted interest in some plant oils as parenteral nutrients in hyperalimentation regimens (Intralipid®).

Sodium morrhuate, the sodium salts of fatty acids obtained from cod liver oil, is used as a sclerosing agent to obliterate varicose veins. Other fatty acids are used as topical antifungal agents, dietary supplements, and agents of pharmaceutic necessity.

The oil-soluble vitamins are lipids by nature and could be included in this chapter according to a strictly chemical classification. However, to achieve uniformity of types of subject matter, they are considered with the water-soluble vitamins in Chapter 11.

Numerous studies are being conducted to screen the fixed oils obtained from the seeds of many plants. Physical properties, pharmacologic activity, and chemical components are being determined in the search for new therapeutic agents and commercially important lipids. In addition, investigations are being undertaken to ascertain the most advantageous types of antioxidants to prevent or to retard rancidity of fixed oils and fats.

FIXED OILS

CASTOR OIL

Castor bean or castor oil seed is the ripe seed of *Ricinus communis* Linné (Fam. Euphorbiaceae). *Ricinus* is Latin and means a tick or a bug, referring to the seed's resemblance to some bugs in shape and markings.

The plant is an annual in temperate climates, or a tree, attaining the height of 15 meters, in the tropics. There are many forms of the plant with variations in the shape of the leaves and the color, size, and markings of the seeds. The fruit is a 3-celled spiny capsule (Fig. 4–3), each cell containing an ovoid albuminous seed. The plant is indigenous to India. It is extensively cultivated in India, Brazil, other South and Central American countries, the Soviet Union, various parts of Africa, southern Europe, and southern United States. The seeds have been found in Egyptian tombs. The oil apparently had only technical use until the eighteenth century when its medicinal use began.

The seed is anatropous, elliptical-ovoid, somewhat compressed, from 8 to 18 mm in length, and from 4 to 7.5 mm in thickness. Externally, the seed is mottled grayish and brown, but varies considerably in color. It is smooth, with a prominent whitish caruncle at the somewhat pointed end from which the raphe extends, on the flat or ventral side, to the chalazal end. Its seed coat is thin and brittle and the endosperm

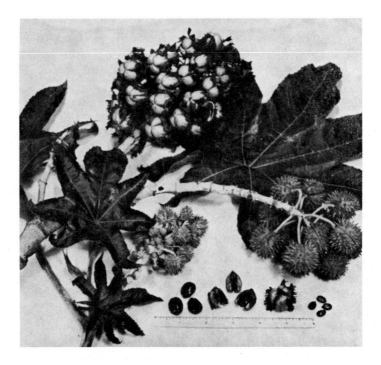

Fig. 4–3. Castor bean *(Ricinus communis)* showing large palmate leaves, immature and mature fruits, and (lower center) large black seeds contrasted with (lower right) smaller seeds of brown-speckled variety. (Photo, courtesy of Dr. Julia F. Morton, Director, Morton Collectanea, University of Miami.)

is large, white, oily, and bears 2 thin foliaceous cotyledons, one on either side of a central, lenticular cavity, and connected with the short caulicle and radicle, the latter directed toward the micropyle (Fig. 4–4).

Castor seeds contain from 45 to 55% of fixed oil; about 20% of protein substances consisting of globulin, albumin, nucleoalbumin, glycoprotein, and **ricin** (a toxalbumin); an alkaloid, ricinine; and several enzymes. The seed coat yields 10% of ash; the kernel yields about 3.5%. The toxalbumin, ricin, is not removed in the extraction of the castor oil, but remains in the **oil cake.** Ricin is poisonous to cattle, but does not affect poultry.

Castor bean pomace contains an allergen that causes allergic reactions in hypersensitive individuals. This powerful allergen is in the nontoxic protein polysaccharide fraction (see page 431).

Deactivation of toxic substances and removal of the allergenic fraction are problems that must be solved in the future.

Castor oil is the fixed oil obtained from the seed of *Ricinus communis*. It is prepared by passing the seeds through a decorticator, which has rollers with sharp cutting edges that break the testae but do not injure the kernel. The testae are then separated by sieves and compressed air, and the kernels are subjected to pressure. The oil is steamed to destroy albumins, is filtered, and is bleached.

The yield of the "cold-pressed" oil separated by hydraulic pressure is 60% and represents a light-colored, good grade. The

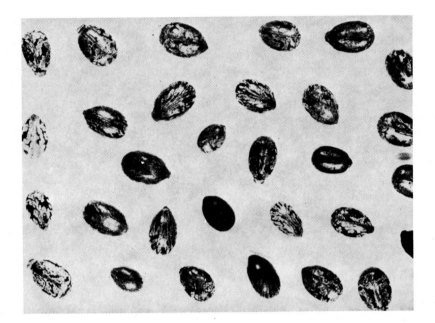

Fig. 4—4. Castor beans.

remainder of the oil from the seeds is solvent extracted, yielding a darker, lower-grade oil.

Castor oil is a pale yellowish or almost colorless, transparent, viscid liquid. It has a faint, mild odor and a bland, characteristic taste.

Castor oil is composed of a mixture of triglycerides, about 75% of which is triricinolein. The remainder consists of diricinoleoglycerides with the third acyl group, representing either oleic, linoleic, dihydroxystearic, or a saturated (palmitic or stearic) acid. Triricinolein is hydrolyzed by lipases in the duodenum to release ricinoleic (12-hydroxy-octadec-9-enoic) acid, which exerts a cathartic effect.

USES AND DOSE. Castor oil is a stimulant cathartic with a usual dose of 15 to 60 ml. The oil is also used as a plasticizer in flexible collodion. Ricinoleic acid is an ingredient (0.5 to 0.7%) in vaginal jellies (Aci-Jel®, Lanteen®) for restoration and maintenance of vaginal acidity. Commer-

cially, castor oil is employed in the manufacture of soaps and as a lubricant for internal combustion engines.

OLIVE OIL

Olive oil is the fixed oil obtained from the ripe fruit of *Olea europaea* Linné (Fam. Oleaceae). Olive oil is sometimes called **sweet oil.** The generic name *Olea* is from the Latin *oliva*, meaning olive or from the Greek *elaion*, meaning oil.

The olive tree is a small evergreen tree that attains a great age, but seldom exceeds 10 meters in height. It was apparently a native of Palestine and has been widely cultivated in the Mediterranean countries from remote antiquity. It is now also cultivated in the southwestern United States and many other subtropical localities. There are a large number of cultivated varieties of the olive, the fruits of which vary widely in size, color, and yield of oil.

The fruit is a drupe, usually purple when ripe. The full-grown but green fruit, as well as the ripe fruit, when pickled in brine, are widely used as a condiment. The olive "stone" or endocarp enclosing the seed has been finely comminuted and used as an adulterant of spices and certain powdered drugs.

Olive oil is offered on the market in several grades of purity. **Virgin oil** is obtained by gently pressing the peeled pulp free from the endocarp. First and second grades of edible oil are pressed from crushed pulp, the first grade with less pressure, the second grade from the same pulp with more pressure. Hand-picked olives are used, and the oil is obtained promptly before decomposition produces fatty acids. Finally, the pulp, mixed with hot water, is pressed again for technical oil; or, the pulp is extracted with carbon disulfide to obtain "sulfur" olive oil of inferior quality. The fallen, decomposed, or refuse olives that are allowed to ferment furnish a low grade "tournant oil," which contains large amounts of free fatty acids.

Olive oil is a pale yellow or light greenish yellow, oily liquid whose odor is slight but characteristic and whose taste is bland to faintly acrid. Olive oil is miscible with ether, carbon disulfide, and chloroform and slightly soluble in alcohol. Its specific gravity is 0.910 to 0.915 at 25° C. Upon chilling, olive oil tends to become cloudy, and at 0° C, it usually forms a whitish granular mass.

Although the composition of olive oil seems to vary rather widely, 2 major types are recognized based on the relative concentrations of the component acids of the glycerides. The Turkish variety contains about 75% of oleic acid, 10% of palmitic acid, and 9% of linoleic acid, with lesser amounts of stearic, myristic, hexadecenoic, and arachidic acids. The Italian variety contains only about 65% of oleic

acid, 15% each of palmitic and linoleic acids, and other minor component acids.

Uses. Olive oil is classed as a pharmaceutic aid. It is used as a setting retardant for dental cements and in the preparation of soaps, plasters, and liniments. It is also a demulcent, an emollient, and a laxative. Olive oil is a nutrient and is widely used as a salad oil.

PEANUT OIL

Peanut is the ripe fruit or seed of *Arachis hypogaea* Linné (Fam. Leguminosae). The plant is a low annual herb with imparipinnate leaves and yellow papilionaceous flowers. It is native to Brazil, but is extensively cultivated in the southern United States, Gambia, Nigeria, and other localities with similar climates. The fruit is not a true nut because the immature pod penetrates into the soil and ripens underground. It contains from 1 to 6 reddish brown seeds. When ripe, the plants with the fruits are raked from the soil into windrows. When dry, the pods are machine separated and sacked for shipment, or the dried plants are threshed to separate and clean the seeds. For human consumption, the fruits are roasted, passed between rollers, and the seeds are separated. The kernels contain about 45% of fixed oil, 20% of protein, and a high content of thiamine; hence, they are highly nutritious and are extensively used as food, both whole and when ground to a paste **(peanut butter).**

Peanut oil is the refined fixed oil obtained from the seed kernels of one or more of the cultivated varieties of *A. hypogaea*. Peanut oil is sometimes referred to as **arachis oil.**

It is a colorless or a yellowish liquid with a slightly nutlike odor and a bland taste.

Peanut oil consists of a mixture of glycerides with component acids of the following approximate composition: oleic

(50 to 65%); linoleic (18 to 30%); palmitic (8 to 10%); stearic, arachidic, behenic, and lignoceric acids (together, 10 to 12%). It closely resembles olive oil and is used as a pharmaceutic aid. Its principal use is as a food oil. It is nondrying and therefore has no value in paints but does have value as a lubricant. The oil saponifies slowly but yields an excellent, firm, white soap.

Use. Peanut oil is a solvent for intramuscular injections.

Peanut oil cake, the residue following expression of the fixed oil, is a valuable livestock food.

SOYBEAN OIL

Soybean is the ripe seed of *Glycine soja* Siebold et Zuccarini (Fam. Leguminosae), an important food and forage crop. The plant is an annual with trifoliate, hairy leaves, rather inconspicuous, pale blue to violet flowers, and broad pods containing 2 to 5 seeds. The seeds are more or less compressed, spheroidal or ellipsoidal, and vary in color from nearly white to yellowgreen or brownish black. The seeds contain about 35% of carbohydrates, up to 50% of protein substances, up to 20% of fixed oil, and the enzyme, urease.

Soybeans are used medicinally as a food in diabetes and as a general food for humans and livestock.

Soybean oil is the refined, fixed oil obtained from the seeds of the soya plant. The oil is obtained by pressure, and the yield seldom exceeds 10%. It consists of a mixture of glycerides with the following component acids: linoleic (50%); oleic (30%); linolenic (7%); saturated, chiefly palmitic and stearic (14%). It is a drying oil with an iodine value between 120 and 141 and is not useful as a cooking oil.

Soybean oil is an ingredient in a parenteral nutrient (Intralipid®) and is a source of lecithin. Lecithin is an ingredient in a number of proprietary products that are useful in controlling deranged lipid and cholesterol metabolisms. Stigmasterol, obtained from the lipid fraction of soybeans, can be used as a precursor for steroidal hormones (see page 185). The oil is used extensively in the manufacture of varnishes, insulators, and other products.

Soybean cake, the residue after pressing out the oil, has a high value as a livestock food. It not only contains a large amount of protein and some oil, but the 5% of ash consists largely of potassium and phosphorus.

Soybean meal is the flour sifted from the decorticated, ground seed of *Glycine soja* deprived of fat. It can be used for the detection of urea nitrogen in blood serum by the enzymatic action of the urease in the soybean meal.

COTTONSEED OIL

Cottonseed oil is the refined, fixed oil obtained from the seed of cultivated plants of various varieties of *Gossypium hirsutum* Linné or of other species of *Gossypium* (Fam. Malvaceae). The cottonseed, after ginning off the fibers, is decorticated and cleaned of hulls. The kernels are steamed and pressed at about 1500 pounds pressure to yield about 30% of oil. The oil, thus obtained, is turbid and reddish in color. It is refined by filtering, decolorizing, and "winter chilling," which removes the stearin.

Cottonseed oil is a pale yellow, oily liquid. It is odorless and has a bland taste.

The oil consists of a mixture of glycerides with the following component acids: linoleic (45%), oleic (30%), palmitic (20%), myristic (3%), stearic and arachidic (1% of each).

Uses. Cottonseed oil is employed pharmaceutically as a solvent for a number of injections. A considerable quantity is hydrogenated and used to make substitutes for lard. A large amount is also used in the manufacture of soap.

Cottonseed cake contains about 0.6% of a toxic principle, gossypol, which occurs in secretory cavities in all parts of the plant. It is present in cold-pressed oil and can be removed by treatment with alkalies.

SESAME OIL

Sesamum seed or sesame seed is the seed of one or more cultivated varieties of *Sesamum indicum* Linné (Fam. Pedaliaceae).

Sesamum is from the Greek *sesamon*, the original name of the plant; *indicum* refers to its habitat, India. The plant is an annual herb attaining the height of about 1 meter. It is native to southern Asia but is cultivated from Africa to the East Indies, in the West Indies, and in the southern United States.

The seeds are small, flattened, oval or ovate, smooth and shiny, and whitish, yellow, or reddish brown. Their taste is sweet and oily. They contain 45 to 55% of fixed oil, 22% of proteins (aleurone), and 4% of mucilage. These seeds are nutritious and form an important food in India. In Europe and America they are used like poppy seeds on bread and rolls. The fixed oil is obtained by expression.

Sesame oil is the refined, fixed oil obtained from the seed of one or more cultivated varieties of S. *indicum*. It is also referred to as **teel oil or benne oil.** The oil is a pale yellow, oily liquid, almost odorless and bland tasting.

Sesame oil consists of a mixture of glycerides with the following component acids: approximately equal parts of oleic and linoleic (about 43% of each), palmitic (9%), stearic (4%). The excellent stability of the oil is owing to the phenolic con-

stituent, sesamol, which is produced by hydrolysis of sesamolin, a lignan present in the unsaponifiable fraction of the oil.

Uses. Sesame oil is classed as a pharmaceutic aid and is used as a solvent for intramuscular injections. It has nutritive, laxative, demulcent, and emollient properties. Sesamolin, contained in the unsaponifiable fraction of the oil, is an effective synergist for pyrethrum insecticides.

ALMOND OIL

Sweet almond and bitter almond consist of the ripe seeds of different varieties of *Prunus amygdalus* Batsch (Fam. Rosaceae).

Prunus is the classic name of the plum tree; *amygdalus* is from the Greek *amygdolos,* meaning almond tree; *amara* and *dulcis*, the variety designations, are Latin and mean bitter and sweet, respectively.

The tree is native to Asia Minor, Iran, and Syria and is cultivated and naturalized in all tropical and warm-temperate regions. The presence of amygdalin in the bitter almond and its bitter taste distinguish it from sweet almond. Commercial products are obtained mostly from Sicily, southern Italy, southern France, northern Africa, and California. In commerce, the yellowish, more or less porous, fibrous, and brittle endocarp may be present (Fig. 4–5).

Both bitter and sweet almonds are expressed for their fixed oil (45 to 50%). Practical economic considerations favor the use of bitter almonds or sweet almonds of inferior quality. Bitter almonds, after maceration to permit hydrolysis of amygdalin, also yield a volatile oil that is used as a flavoring agent. Sweet almonds are extensively used as a food, but bitter almonds are not suitable for this purpose. The seeds of the bitter almond were known to be

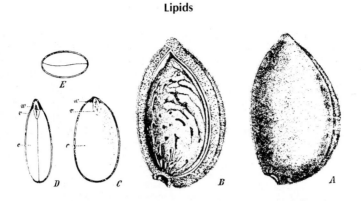

Fig. 4–5. Drupelike fruit of almond *(Prunus amygdalus)*; *A*, whole fruit with distinct suture; *B*, longitudinal section showing fibrous sarcocarp and thin-shelled endocarp; *C, D, E*, sections of the seed; *c*, cotyledons; *w*, hypocotyl; *v*, epicotyl or plumule.

poisonous in the days of antiquity. The sweet almond is mentioned early in the Old Testament (Genesis 43:11) as one of the fruits Israel commanded his sons to carry from Palestine as a gift to Egypt. Theophrastus makes several references to the almond. Charlemagne (812 A.D.) introduced the tree on the imperial farms, and, in the fourteenth century, the almond was an important item of Venetian trade.

Almond oil, expressed almond oil, or sweet almond oil is the fixed oil obtained by expression from the kernels of varieties of *P. amygdalus*.

Almond oil consists of a mixture of glycerides with component acids of the following approximate composition: oleic (77%), linoleic (17%), palmitic (5%), myristic (1%).

Uses. Expressed almond oil is an emollient and an ingredient in cosmetics.

PERSIC OIL

Persic oil, apricot kernel oil, or peach kernel oil is the oil expressed from the kernels of varieties of *P. armeniaca* Linné (apricot kernel oil) or from the kernels of varieties of *P. persica* Siebold et Zuccarini (peach kernel oil) (Fam. Rosaceae).

Persic oil is prepared in the same manner as is expressed almond oil. Its characteristics closely resemble those of expressed almond oil, and it is used as a vehicle and pharmaceutic necessity.

COCONUT OIL

Coconut oil is the fixed oil obtained by expression or extraction from the seed kernels of the coconut palm, *Cocos nucifera* Linné (Fam. Palmae). This tall, stately tree rises to a height of 30 meters, has a tuft of leaves at the top, and bears 100 or more fruits (coconuts) each year (Fig. 4–6). The oil consists of a mixture of glycerides in which 80 to 85% of the acids are saturated; it is a semisolid at 20° C. Lauric (50%) and myristic (20%) are the major fatty acids. These low-molecular-weight acids give the oil a high saponification value, and coconut oil yields quality soaps and shampoos.

Coconut oil also contains glycerides of caprylic and capric acids (C_8 and C_{10} saturated fatty acids). A lipid fraction contain-

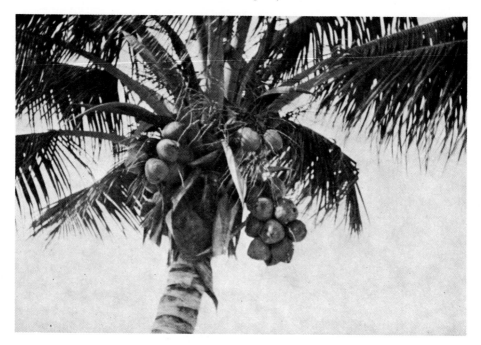

Fig. 4–6. Habit of growth of the fruits of *Cocos nucifera*.

ing these medium chain triglycerides (MCT®) is used when conventional food fats are not well digested or absorbed.

CORN OIL

Corn oil is the refined oil obtained from the embryo of *Zea mays* Linné (Fam. Gramineae).

After the cracked corn leaves the attrition mills (see preparation of starch, page 38), the germs (embryos) are separated by floating out in deep, rectangular tanks. After washing free from starch and gluten, the germs are subjected to pressure and heat, which expresses the oil. The **germ oil cake** that remains is ground and sold as cattle feed **(oil cake meal)**. The crude oil is clarified by filtering and settling and refined by removing the fatty acids, refrigerating, filtering, and sterilizing. Corn oil is a clear, light yellow, oily liquid that has a faint characteristic odor and taste.

The oil consists of a mixture of glycerides with component acids of the following approximate composition: linoleic (50%), oleic (37%), palmitic (10%), stearic (3%).

Corn oil is used as a solvent for injections; it is also a solvent for irradiated ergosterol. It is an edible oil and, as such, is used in salads and in the preparation of food. An emulsion containing 67% of corn oil is used as a high-calorie dietary supplement (Lipomul Oral®). When hydrogenated, the oil becomes semisolid and is used as a shortening for baking.

SAFFLOWER OIL

Safflower seed oil is the fixed oil obtained from the seeds of *Carthamus tinctorius* Linné (Fam. Compositae).

The oil consists of a mixture of glycerides whose component acids are largely unsaturated. A typical sample contains linoleic acid (75%), oleic acid (18%), and a mixture of saturated acids totaling about 6%. The claims that ingestion of quantities of polyunsaturated fatty acids in various forms, e.g., margarines, oil-filled capsules, and others, results in a decreased blood cholesterol level are based on insubstantial evidence. Further, there is no indication that a combination of choline, pyridoxine, or other lipotropic substances with unsaturated fatty acids possesses any therapeutic advantage over the substances themselves. Although a number of safflower oil preparations, especially capsules of various sizes, are presently marketed, their use as antilipemics without adequate dietary adjustments is not rational therapy.

IODIZED OIL INJECTION

Iodized oil is an iodine addition product of vegetable oil or oils. Poppy seed oil is frequently used. Iodized oil contains not less than 38% and not more than 42% of organically combined iodine. It is a thick, viscous, oily liquid with an alliaceous odor. It decomposes when exposed to air and sunlight, becoming dark brown in color. Iodized oil is packaged in a sterile form for parenteral use.

Iodized oil is radiopaque and is used as a diagnostic aid in such procedures as hysterosalpingography, sialography, and bronchography. The usual dose is 1 to 30 ml by special injection, depending on the procedure.

SPECIALTY PRODUCT. Lipiodol®.

FATS AND RELATED COMPOUNDS

THEOBROMA OIL

Cacao seeds or cacao beans are the roasted seeds of Theobroma cacao Linné (Fam. Sterculiaceae). Theobroma is Greek and means "food of the gods"; cacao is from the Aztec name of the tree; "chocolate" is from the Nahuatl. It has long been highly esteemed by the Aztecs, the Mexicans, and later by the Europeans, who explored the Americas.

The plant is a tree attaining the height of about 12 meters and is indigenous to Mexico, but widely cultivated in tropical countries. The flowers arise from the older branches or trunk and develop into large, ovoid, fleshy fruits that are 10-furrowed longitudinally, are yellow or reddish, and contain 5 rows of seeds, 10 or 12 in each row (Fig. 4–7). Cacao was known to Columbus and Cortez. Most of the cacao seed on the market is obtained from Ecuador (the Guayaquil variety is especially valuable), Curaçao, Mexico, Trinidad, Central America, Brazil, West Africa (Nigeria and Ghana), Sri Lanka, and the Philippine Islands.

The seeds are separated from the pod and allowed to ferment. During the process, they change from white to dark reddish brown. They are then roasted (not above 140° C) to lose water and develop their characteristic odor and taste. The roasted seeds are passed through a "nibbling" machine to crack the seed coats **(cacao shells),** which are separated from the kernels by winnowing. The broken kernels are called "nibs," and, when ground between hot rollers, they yield a paste containing up to 50% of fat, **cacao butter.** The paste congeals at room temperature to form **bitter chocolate. Sweet chocolate** is bitter chocolate to which sugar and vanilla or other flavoring substances have been added. After expressing cacao butter, the marc, which retains some oil, is powdered and is known as **prepared cacao** or **breakfast cocoa.** Some brands of cocoa contain alkali to render it "soluble"; it is, of course, not soluble, but the alkali partially saponifies the fat at the surface of each minute particle, resulting in a

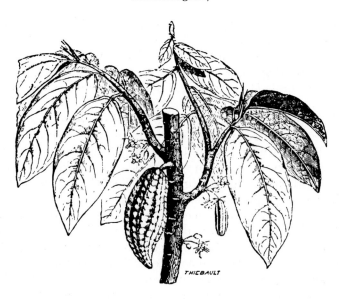

Fig. 4–7.   Cacao tree (*Theobroma cacao*) showing the peculiar habit of the fruits in developing on the main axis as well as on the branches.

smoother and more complete suspension of the cocoa in water or milk.

Cacao seeds or cacao beans are often found on the market as such. The seed is irregularly ellipsoidal or ovoid, somewhat flattened, and 15 to 30 mm in length. Externally, it is reddish brown to dark brown and the seed coat is thin and shell-like, readily separable from the cotyledons. The latter are fleshy, much folded, and connected with a stout radicle that is situated at the hilum portion of the seed. Their odor is chocolatelike, and taste is slightly bitter.

The seeds contain 35 to 50% of a fixed oil, about 15% of starch, 15% of proteins, 1 to 4% of theobromine, 0.07 to 0.36% of caffeine. The red color of the seed is owing to a principle known as cacao-red, which is formed by the action of a ferment on a glycoside. When the seeds are roasted, the theobromine in the kernel passes into the shell. The shell is the commercial source of this xanthine derivative.

Cocoa is a powder prepared from the roasted, cured kernels of the ripe seed of *Theobroma cacao*. It occurs as a weak red-dish to purplish brown to moderate brown powder that has a chocolatelike odor and a taste that is not sweet.

Uses. Cocoa is employed in making **cocoa syrup,** which is a flavored vehicle. Cocoa, also known as "breakfast cocoa," is a popular beverage and usually contains more than 22% of "fat" (nonvolatile ether-soluble extractive). NOTE: Cocoa containing not more than 12% of nonvolatile ether-soluble extractive is preferred for cocoa syrup; it yields a syrup that has a minimum tendency to separate.

Theobroma oil or cocoa butter is the fat obtained from the roasted seed of *T. cacao*. It is a yellowish white solid that has a faint, agreeable odor and a bland, chocolatelike taste. It melts between 30 and 35° C.

Theobroma oil consists of a mixture of glycerides with component acids of the following approximate composition: oleic (37%), stearic (34%), palmitic (26%), linoleic (2%). The relatively sharp melting point of the fat and its comparative brittleness and nongreasiness are owing to its peculiar glyceride structure. Mono-oleodisaturated glycerides, chiefly oleo-palmitostearin, are its major constituents.

Cocoa butter is used pharmaceutically as a suppository base.

HYDROGENATED VEGETABLE OIL

Hydrogenated vegetable oil is refined, bleached, hydrogenated, and deodorized vegetable oil stearins and consists mainly of the triglycerides of stearic and palmitic acids. It is a fine, white powder at room temperature and melts between 61 and 66° C to give a pale yellow, oily liquid. It is used as a tablet lubricant.

LANOLIN

Lanolin is the purified, fatlike substance from the wool of the sheep, *Ovis aries* Linné (Fam. Bovidae). It contains between 25 and 30% of water and therefore is commonly called **hydrous wool fat.**

Lanolin is a yellowish white, ointment-like mass that has a slight, characteristic odor. When heated on a steam bath, it separates at first into 2 layers. Continued heating with frequent stirring drives off the water that makes up the lower layer.

The chief constituents are cholesterol and isocholesterol. Lanolin also contains the esters of lanopalmitic, lanoceric, carnaubic, oleic, myristic, and other fatty acids.

Uses. Lanolin is used as a water-absorbable ointment base. It is employed for the external administration of remedies locally or by inunction. Lanolin is an ingredient in many skin creams and cosmetics. As such, however, it may act as an allergenic contactant in hypersensitive persons (see page 433).

ANHYDROUS LANOLIN

Anhydrous lanolin is lanolin that contains not more than 0.25% of water. After lanolin has been purified and bleached, it is dehydrated. Anhydrous lanolin is usually referred to as **wool fat.**

Uses. Anhydrous lanolin is a water-absorbable ointment base. It is more readily absorbed through the skin than any other known fat and is therefore valuable as a base for therapeutic agents that are administered by inunction. In addition, it possesses emollient properties.

FATTY ACIDS

A number of fatty acids and their salts and derivatives are employed as agents of pharmaceutic necessity. These acids are usually obtained by hydrolysis of fats or oils. The materials are usually mixtures, and the composition can vary with the source. Some acids are used in topical antifungal preparations; sodium morrhuate is a sclerosing agent, and linoleic and linolenic acids are used as a dietary supplement.

STEARIC ACID

Stearic acid of pharmaceutic quality contains not less than 40% of stearic acid and not less than 40% of palmitic acid; the sum of these 2 acids is not less than 90%. **Purified stearic acid** contains not less than 90% stearic acid, and the total content of stearic and palmitic acids is not less than 96%. These materials are hard, white or faintly yellow solids or powders and are practically insoluble in water. Stearic acid is used as an emulsion adjunct and a tablet lubricant.

Calcium stearate and magnesium stearate are used as tablet lubricants, zinc stearate is used in dusting powders, sodium stearate is used as an emulsifying and stiffening agent, and aluminum monostearate is used as a suspending agent. Glyceryl monostearate and propylene glycol monostearate are employed as emulsifying agents.

OLEIC ACID

Oleic acid is obtained from edible fats and fixed oils. It is often obtained as a by-product in the production of stearic acid. Oleic acid consists chiefly of cis-9-octadecenoic acid and is a colorless to pale yellow, oily liquid. It is practically insoluble in water, but is miscible with alcohol. It gradually absorbs oxygen and darkens when exposed to air.

Oleic acid is used as an emulsion adjunct. Ethyl oleate is used as a pharmaceutic vehicle, and oleyl alcohol is employed as an emollient and emulsifying agent.

LINOLEIC AND LINOLENIC ACIDS

Linoleic and linolenic acids are polyunsaturated octadecenoic acids. These fatty acids are essential for human nutrition and have been called vitamin F. A mixture of essential unsaturated fatty acids that contains primarily linoleic and linolenic acids can be obtained from soybean oil and other suitable vegetable oils. This mixture of acids is used as a dietary supplement.

UNDECYLENIC ACID

Undecylenic acid is 10-undecenoic acid. It is prepared by pyrolysis of ricinoleic acid, which is obtained from castor oil. Undecylenic acid has antifungal properties and is an ingredient, often combined with zinc undecylenate or other agents, in ointments and powders for topical application to treat athlete's foot (Desenex®). Calcium undecylenate is used in powders for diaper rash and similar skin irritations.

Caprylate and propionate salts are also used in topical formulations (e.g., Sop-ronol®) for control of fungal infections. The antifungal activity of glyceryl triacetate (Enzactin®), another dermatologic agent, is related to the gradual release of acetic acid; the acid is released in a concentration that is nonirritating.

SODIUM MORRHUATE

Sodium morrhuate is the sodium salts of the fatty acids of cod liver oil. It is available as a sterile solution and is used as a sclerosing agent to obliterate varicose veins. The usual dose, administered intravenously by special injection, is 1 ml of a 5% solution to a localized area. Sodium morrhuate injection may show a separation of solid material on standing; it should not be used if any such material does not dissolve completely when warmed.

WAXES

Waxes are usually defined as esters resulting from the condensation of high-molecular-weight, straight-chain acids and high-molecular-weight, primary, straight-chain alcohols. Such esters, of course, exist in waxes, but, in reality, waxes are better defined as mixtures of different molecular weight acids and alcohols. In addition, waxes may also contain paraffins.

In plants, waxes are found in connection with the outer cell walls of epidermal tissue, particularly in fruits and leaves. The function of wax appears to be protection against the penetration or loss of water. Insects also secrete waxes for various purposes. Carnauba wax and bayberry wax are examples of vegetable waxes, and lac wax and beeswax are examples of insect waxes.

Waxes are employed in pharmaceuticals to ''harden'' ointments and cosmetic creams. They are also used in the preparation of cerates. In industry and the arts, waxes are used for protective coatings.

SYNTHETIC SPERMACETI

Spermaceti, a waxy substance obtained from the head of the sperm whale [*Physeter macrocephalus* Linné (Fam. Physeteridae)], was formerly recognized as a quality emollient and a desirable ingredient in cold creams and other cosmetics. However, the sperm whale is an endangered species, and spermaceti is no longer available. Efforts to find a substitute for spermaceti have led to the use of a synthetic spermaceti or of jojoba oil.

Spermaceti consisted of a mixture of hexadecyl esters of fatty acids. Hexadecyl dodecanoate (cetyl laurate), hexadecyl tetradecanoate (cetyl myristate), hexadecyl hexadecanoate (cetyl palmitate), and hexadecyl octadecanoate (cetyl stearate) comprised at least 85% of the total esters.

Synthetic spermaceti or cetyl esters wax is a mixture consisting primarily of esters of saturated fatty alcohols (C_{14} to C_{18}) and saturated fatty acids (C_{14} to C_{18}).

Cetyl alcohol is a mixture of solid alcohols consisting chiefly of cetyl alcohol or 1-hexadecanol. It is used as an emulsifying aid and as a stiffening agent in pharmaceutic preparations.

JOJOBA OIL

Jojoba oil is a liquid wax expressed from seeds of *Simmondsia chinensis* (Link) Scheider (Fam. Buxaceae). The plant is a bushy shrub native to the arid regions of northern Mexico and to the southwestern United States.

Jojoba seeds contain 45 to 55% of an ester mixture (not triglycerides) that is a liquid at ambient temperatures. The major components identified upon hydrolysis of the mixture are 35% of eicosenoic acid (a C_{20} unsaturated acid), 22% of eicosenol (a C_{20} unsaturated alcohol), and 21% of docosenol (a C_{22} unsaturated alcohol). Hydrogenation of the oil yields a crystalline wax that has the appearance and properties of spermaceti.

Jojoba oil and its hydrogenated derivatives are useful emollients and agents of pharmaceutic necessity.

BEESWAX

Yellow wax or beeswax is the purified wax from the honeycomb of the bee, *Apis mellifera* Linné (Fam. Apidae). Wax is secreted in cells on the ventral surface of the last 4 segments of the abdomen of the worker bees. The wax excretes through pores in the chitinous plates and is employed by the young worker bees in the construction of the comb.

The honeycomb, after separation from the honey, is melted in water, then cooled and remelted, and finally strained and allowed to harden in molds.

Beeswax is a solid varying in color from yellow to grayish brown. It has an agreeable honeylike odor and a faint, characteristic taste. When cold, beeswax is somewhat brittle and exhibits a dull, granular, noncrystalline fracture.

The wax consists principally of alkyl esters of fatty and wax acids (about 72%), chiefly myricyl palmitate; free wax acids (about 14%), especially cerotic acid and its homologs; hydrocarbons (12%); and other minor constituents including moisture, pollen, and propolis (bee glue). The latter 2 materials are responsible for most of the color of the wax.

Uses. Yellow wax is a stiffening agent and is an ingredient in yellow ointment. It is also used as a base for cerates and plasters. Commercially, it is contained in a number of polishes.

White wax is bleached, purified wax from the honeycomb of the bee, *A. mellifera* Linné (Fam. Apidae). The bleaching process is accomplished by allowing the melted wax to flow slowly over revolving wetted cylinders upon which it hardens in thin ribbonlike layers. These layers are removed and exposed to sunlight and air until they are bleached. (The process usually is repeated.) The bleached wax is finally melted and cast into cakes of various shapes. White wax is sometimes referred to as bleached beeswax. A rapid, reliable, and inexpensive method of detecting the presence of certain adulterants of natural beeswax is known as the saponification cloud test.

USES. White wax is employed pharmaceutically in ointments and in cold creams.

CARNAUBA WAX

Carnauba wax is obtained from the leaves of *Copernicia prunifera* (Mueller) H. E. Moore [*C. cerifera* (Arruda da Camara) Martius] (Fam. Palmae), a palm growing from northern Brazil to Argentina. The wax consists of alkyl esters of wax acids (80%), chiefly myricyl cerotate; free monohydric alcohols (10%); a lactone; resin; and other minor constituents. It is used in the manufacture of candles, wax varnishes, leather and furniture polishes, and in place of beeswax.

PROSTAGLANDINS

Prostaglandins are C_{20} lipid metabolites formed in the body from essential, unsaturated fatty acids of the diet. Prostaglandins apparently occur in nearly all mammalian tissues, but they are present in low concentrations. The major prostaglandins have been grouped into 4 main classes designated as prostaglandins A, B, E, and F. All prostaglandins (PG) have a cyclopentane ring with 2 aliphatic side chains. Subscripts indicate the number of double bonds in the side chains and the stereochemistry of members of each group.

Details of the physiologic roles of prostaglandins remain to be clarified. Attention was initially attracted to these substances in 1930 when it was observed that constituents in human semen could produce contraction and relaxation of the human uterus. A large body of biologic knowledge, especially regarding members of the PGE and PGF series, has been accumulated. Mammalian cells and tissues may respond differently (stimulation or inhibition of a biologic process) to individual prostaglandins; in some instances, this response may be a concentration factor. Prostaglandins appear to act at the level of the cell membrane, and they may modulate the transmission of hormonal or other extracellular stimuli into cyclic AMP for the internal regulation of cellular functions. Actions of this type seem consistent with the pharmacologic effects that have been noted with the prostaglandins. Pharmacologic effects of these compounds involve contraction or, in some cases, relaxation of smooth muscles of the female reproductive system, of the cardiovascular system, of the intestinal tract, and of the bronchi. They also influence gastric secretion and renal function.

Securing a feasible source of the various prostaglandins was a major deterrent to the early exploration of their biologic properties and therapeutic potential. Much of the explosion of knowledge about these compounds during the past decade is a result of several achievements that have resolved the supply problem. Key accomplishments include the development of an enzymatic synthesis that uses prostaglandin synthetase from sheep seminal vesicles, the discovery of prostaglandin materials in *Plexaura homomalla* (sea fan or sea whip), which is a coral found in reefs off the Florida coast, and the development of several procedures for total chemical synthesis.

The prostaglandins have diverse pharmacologic effects, and some enthusiasts believe that their therapeutic potential transcends that of the steroids. The use of PGE$_2$ or PGF$_{2\alpha}$ for termination of second trimester pregnancy is the only application that has received FDA approval at this time. However, experimental studies have revealed potential for therapeutic use of various prostaglandins, including use to induce labor at term (PGE$_2$ and PGF$_{2\alpha}$), to prevent premature labor (PGE), to induce menstruation (PGE), to increase fertility in certain conditions (PGE), to manage some types of hypertension (PGA$_1$ and PGE$_2$), to control certain cardiac arrhythmias (PGF$_{2\alpha}$), to correct some defects in red blood cells (PGE), to exert antithrombogenic and thrombolytic activity (PGE$_1$), to control asthmatic seizures (PGE$_1$), to inhibit gastric secretions in the treatment of peptic ulcers (PGE), and to treat several other conditions. The multiple effects of the prostaglandins and the diverse response to individual prostaglandins by various body tissues are factors that give above-average chances for undesirable side effects in any therapeutic use of these compounds; this appears to be a problem, but its full significance remains to be evaluated in most situations. Because prostaglandins are formed in situ in most body tissues, the potential for use of prostaglandin synthetase inhibitors is also receiving investigational attention.

PROSTAGLANDIN F$_{2\alpha}$

Prostaglandin F$_{2\alpha}$, PGF$_{2\alpha}$, or dinoprost is available as the tromethamine salt for use in terminating second trimester pregnancy. It stimulates contractions of the gravid uterus that are similar to the contractions of the term uterus at labor. Side effects are usually related to the contractile effect of PGF$_{2\alpha}$; the action may extend to smooth muscle of the gastrointestinal tract, producing vomiting and/or diarrhea, and to smooth muscle of the vascular system, causing elevation in blood pressure.

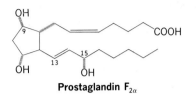

Prostaglandin F$_{2\alpha}$

PGF$_{2\alpha}$ is rapidly inactivated (serum half-life of 10 minutes or less) in the lungs and other body tissues. Two metabolic processes have been identified as participating in the inactivation of this prostaglandin: reduction of the unsaturated bond at position 13 and oxidation of the 15-hydroxyl group to a keto function. A short duration of action is usually considered desirable for oxytocic agents, but it could present a problem in other potential therapeutic applications. In the latter situations, the 15-methyl analog of PGF$_{2\alpha}$ may be indicative of future developments. This analog has been prepared synthetically and exhibits approximately 400 times the activity and 4 times the biologic half-life of the parent compound.

The usual dose of PGF$_{2\alpha}$ is 40 mg by slow injection into the amniotic sac. If the abortion process has not been established or completed within 24 hours, an additional dose of the drug may be administered.

PRESCRIPTION PRODUCT. Prostin F2 Alpha®.

PROSTAGLANDIN E$_2$

Prostaglandin E$_2$, PGE$_2$, or dinoprostone is another uterine stimulant that has been approved for termination of second trimester pregnancy. PGE$_2$ differs from PGF$_{2\alpha}$ only in that the 9-oxygen substituent is a keto group. PGE$_2$ is available as a vaginal suppository that should be stored at a temperature below $-20°$ C.

A 20-mg suppository is inserted intravaginally every 3 to 5 hours until abortion occurs, but the maximum dose should not exceed 240 mg. The pharmacologic effects of PGE_2 are similar to those of $PGF_{2\alpha}$. Frequently encountered adverse reactions include vomiting, pyrexia, diarrhea, nausea, headache, and chills.

PRESCRIPTION PRODUCT. Prostin E2®.

READING REFERENCES

Bennett, H.: *Industrial Waxes*, 2nd ed., Vols. I–II, New York, Chemical Publishing Co., Inc., 1975.

Brown, J. H.: Jojoba Liquid Wax—Substitute for Spermaceti, Manuf. Chem. Aerosol News, 50(6):47, 1979.

Cook, L. R.: *Chocolate Production and Use*, New York, Books for Industry, Inc., 1972.

Curtis-Prior, P. B.: *Prostaglandins: An Introduction to Their Biochemistry, Physiology, and Pharmacology*, New York, North-Holland Publishing Co., 1976.

Goodwin, T. W., ed.: *Biochemistry of Lipids*, Baltimore, University Park Press, 1974.

Goodwin, T. W., ed.: *Biochemistry of Lipids II*, Baltimore, University Park Press, 1977.

Hitchcock, C., and Nichols, B. W.: *Plant Lipid Biochemistry*, New York, Academic Press, Inc., 1971.

Kahn, R. H., and Lands, W. E. M., eds.: *Prostaglandins and Cyclic AMP: Biological Actions and Clinical Applications*, New York, Academic Press, Inc., 1973.

Karim, S. M. M., ed.: *Prostaglandins and Reproduction*, Baltimore, University Park Press, 1975.

Karim, S. M. M., ed.: *Prostaglandins: Chemical and Biochemical Aspects*, Baltimore, University Park Press, 1976.

Karim, S. M. M., ed.: *Prostaglandins: Physiological, Pharmacological and Pathological Aspects*, Baltimore, University Park Press, 1976.

Kolattukudy, P. E., ed.: *Chemistry and Biochemistry of Natural Waxes*, New York, Elsevier Scientific Publishing Co., 1976.

Mead, J. F., and Fulco, A. J.: *The Unsaturated and Polyunsaturated Fatty Acids in Health and Disease*, Springfield, Illinois, Charles C Thomas, Publishers, 1976.

Meng, H. C., and Wilmore, D. W.: *Symposium on Fat Emulsions in Parenteral Nutrition*, Chicago, American Medical Association, 1976.

Paoletti, R., Jacini, G., and Porcellati, G., eds.: *Lipids*, Vols. I–II, New York, Raven Press, 1975.

Robinson, H. J., and Vane, J. R., eds.: *Prostaglandin Synthetase Inhibitors*, New York, Raven Press, 1974.

Samuelsson, B., and Paoletti, R., eds.: *Advances in Prostaglandin and Thromboxane Research*, Vols. I–V, New York, Raven Press, 1976–1978.

Synder, F., ed.: *Lipid Metabolism in Mammals*, New York, Plenum Press, 1977.

Swern, D., ed.: *Bailey's Industrial Oil and Fat Products*, 4th ed., Vol. I, New York, Wiley-Interscience, 1979.

Thompson, S. W.: *The Pathology of Parenteral Nutrition with Lipids*, Springfield, Illinois, Charles C Thomas, Publishers, 1974.

Chapter 5

Volatile Oils

Volatile oils are the odorous principles found in various plant parts. Because they evaporate when exposed to the air at ordinary temperatures, they are called **volatile oils, ethereal oils,** or **essential oils.** The last term is applied because volatile oils represent the "essences" or odoriferous constituents of the plants. Volatile oils are colorless as a rule, particularly when they are fresh, but on long standing they may oxidize and resinify, thus darkening in color. To prevent this darkening, they should be stored in a cool, dry place in tightly stoppered, preferably full (not half-emptied), amber glass containers.

Depending on the plant family, volatile oils may occur in specialized secretory structures such as glandular hairs (Labiatae), modified parenchyma cells (Piperaceae), oil-tubes called vittae (Umbelliferae), or in lysigenous or schizogenous passages (Pinaceae, Rutaceae). They may be formed directly by the protoplasm, by decomposition of the resinogenous layer of the cell wall, or by the hydrolysis of certain glycosides. In the conifers, volatile oils may occur in all tissues; in the rose, they appear in appreciable quantities only in the petals; in cinnamon, only in the bark and the leaves; in the umbelliferous fruits, only in the pericarp; in the mints, only in the glandular hairs of the stems and leaves; and in the orange, one kind of oil occurs only in the flower petals and another kind only in the rind. Volatile oils may act as repellents to insects, thus preventing the destruction of the flowers and leaves; or they may serve as insect attractants, thus aiding in cross-fertilization of the flowers.

Chemical constituents of volatile oils may be divided into 2 broad classes, based on their biosynthetic origin: (1) terpene derivatives formed via the acetate-mevalonic acid pathway, and (2) aromatic compounds formed via the shikimic acid-phenylpropanoid route. The biosynthesis of relatively few of these compounds has been investigated in any detail. Most experimental studies have merely demonstrated that a particular precursor, e.g., acetate, is incorporated into a terpene molecule in a particular pattern, and little attention has been devoted to the interconversion of the numerous terpene derivatives themselves. Selected examples of biosyntheses that have been demonstrated experimentally with labeled precursors follow in the appropriate sections.

Although volatile oils differ greatly in their chemical constitution, they have a number of physical properties in common. They possess characteristic odors, they are characterized by high refractive indices, most of them are optically active, and their specific rotation is often a valuable diagnostic property. As a rule, volatile oils are immiscible with water, but they are sufficiently soluble to impart their odor to water. The aromatic waters are dependent on this slight solubility. Volatile oils, however, are soluble in ether, alcohol, and most organic solvents.

Several points of differentiation exist between volatile oils and fixed oils. Volatile oils can be distilled from their natural sources; they do not consist of glyceryl esters of fatty acids; hence, they do not leave a permanent grease spot on paper and cannot be saponified with alkalies. Volatile oils do not become rancid as do the fixed oils, but instead, on exposure to light and air, they oxidize and resinify.

Practically all volatile oils consist of chemical mixtures that are often quite complex; they vary widely in chemical composition. Almost any type of organic compound may be found in volatile oils (hydrocarbons, alcohols, ketones, aldehydes, ethers, oxides, esters, and others), and only a few possess a single component in a high percentage (volatile mustard oil yields not less than 93% of allylisothiocyanate; clove oil contains not less than 85% of phenolic substances, chiefly eugenol).

METHODS OF OBTAINING VOLATILE OILS

Volatile oils are usually obtained by distillation of the plant parts containing the oil. The method of distillation depends on the condition of the plant material. Three

types of distillation are used by industrial firms: (1) water, (2) water and steam, and (3) direct steam.

Water distillation is applied to plant material that is dried and not subject to injury by boiling. Turpentine oil is obtained in this manner. The crude turpentine oleoresin, comprised of plant exudate, rainwater, wood chips, pine needles, and other components (see page 153), is introduced into the distilling chamber and subjected to heat until all volatile matter, both oil and water, is condensed in the condensing chamber. Turpentine oil, consisting almost entirely of terpenes, is not affected by this amount of heat.

Water and steam distillation is employed for either dried or fresh substances that may be injured by boiling. In the case of dried material (cinnamon, clove), the drug is ground and then covered with a layer of water. Steam is passed through the macerated mixture. Because the oil could be impaired by direct boiling, the steam is generated elsewhere and is piped into the container holding the drug. The oily layer of the condensed distillate is separated from the aqueous layer, and the oil may be marketed with or without further processing.

In the method of **direct steam distillation,** applicable to fresh plant drugs (peppermint, spearmint), the crop is cut and placed directly into a metal distilling tank on a truck bed. The truck is driven to a distilling shed where steam lines are attached to the bottom of the distilling tank. The plant material is still green and contains considerable natural moisture, therefore maceration is unnecessary. Steam is forced through the fresh herb and carries the oil droplets through a vapor pipe attached at the top of the tank to the condensing chamber.

During steam distillation (Fig. 5–1) certain components of a volatile oil tend to hydrolyze whereas other constituents are

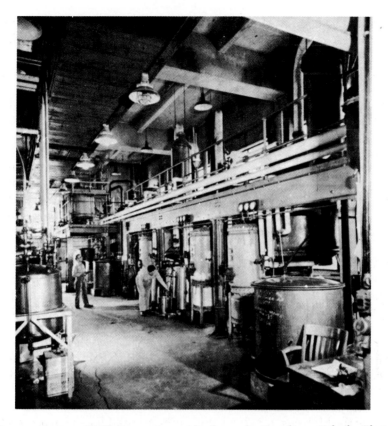

Fig. 5–1. Large-scale steam distillation equipment for the production of essential oils. (Photo, courtesy of Fritzsche Brothers, Inc., New York.)

decomposed by the high temperatures. Ideal distillation methods utilizing steam should provide for the highest possible diffusion rate of steam and water through plant membranes and should thus keep the hydrolysis and decomposition at a minimum.

Glycosidic volatile oils (mustard oil) are obtained by enzymatic hydrolysis of the glycosides. In black mustard seeds, the glycoside, sinigrin, is hydrolyzed by myrosin with the production of volatile mustard oil (see page 73).

Some volatile oils cannot be distilled without decomposition and are usually obtained by **expression** (lemon oil, orange oil) or possibly by other mechanical means. In the United States, the general method for obtaining citrus oils involves puncturing the oil glands by rolling the fruit over a trough lined with sharp projections that are long enough to penetrate the epidermis and pierce the oil glands located in the outer portion of the peel (**ecuelle** method). A pressing action on the fruit removes the oil from the glands, and a fine spray of water washes the oil from the mashed peel while the juice is extracted through a center tube that cores the fruit. The resulting oil-water emulsion is separated by centrifugation. A variation in this process is to remove the peel from the fruit before the oil is extracted.

Often the volatile oil content of fresh plant parts (flower petals) is so small that oil removal is not commercially feasible by the aforementioned methods. In such instances, an odorless, bland fixed oil or fat is spread in a thin layer on glass plates. The flower petals are placed on the fat for a few hours; then a new layer of petals is introduced. After the fat has absorbed as much fragrance as possible, the oil may be removed by extraction with alcohol. This process is known as **enfleurage** and was formerly used extensively in the production of perfumes and pomades.

In the perfume industry, most of the modern essential oil production is accomplished by **extraction,** using solvent systems based on such volatile solvents as petroleum ether or benzene. The chief advantage of extraction over distillation is that uniform temperatures (usually 50° C) can be maintained during most of the process. As a result, extracted oils have a more natural odor that is unmatched by distilled oils, which may have undergone altered chemical constitution by the high temperatures. This feature is of considerable importance to the perfume industry; however, because of the high cost involved, the extraction process probably will not be adopted by firms producing volatile oils. The established distillation method is a low-cost operation compared to the cost of the extraction process.

Destructive distillation is a means of obtaining **empyreumatic** oils. When the wood or resin of members of the Pinaceae or Cupressaceae is heated without access of air, a decomposition takes place, and a number of volatile compounds are driven off. The resultant mass is charcoal. The condensed volatile matter usually separates into 2 layers: an aqueous layer containing wood naphtha (methyl alcohol) and pyroligneous (crude acetic) acid, and a tarry liquid in the form of pine tar, juniper tar, or other tars depending on the wood introduced. This dry distillation is usually conducted in retorts, and if the wood is chipped or coarsely ground and the heat applied rapidly, the yield of tar represents about 10% of the wood used.

MEDICINAL AND COMMERCIAL USES

Many crude drugs are used medicinally because of their volatile oil content; however, in numerous cases, the volatile oils separated from the drugs are used as drugs themselves. Similarly, various crude drugs are powdered and are employed as spices and condiments (anise, clove, nutmeg). The volatile oil drugs and the separated oils are most commonly used for flavoring purposes. They possess a carminative action, but a few (eucalyptus oil, wintergreen oil) possess additional therapeutic properties. In addition to their pharmaceutic uses, the volatile oils are employed widely as flavors for foods and confections and in the spice, perfume, and cosmetic trades.

The fabrication of **perfumes** is a multimillion dollar industry. Perfumery materials such as volatile oils are not only used directly for perfumes and cosmetics, but are essential for the manufacture of soaps, toiletries, and deodorizers and for masking or providing odor to household cleaners, polishes, and insecticides.

Fine perfumes are considered as works of art. They have been defined as judicious blends of odorants, each having its own particular odor, but whose combined odor is itself characteristically unique. The formulas for these perfumes are generally well-guarded secrets, and the perfumer must have an intimate knowledge of perhaps 1000 aromatic substances when formulating a perfume. Perfume formulation has been compared to the creation of a musical composition; the various odorants can be classified like musical notes into top, medium, and base notes. Most perfumes contain elements of all 3 categories, which are blended to provide a unique, harmonious odor. The top notes are the most volatile products. They leave the skin rapidly and include lemon, lavender, and anise oils. Odorants with intermediate volatility and tenacity are classified as middle notes and include thyme, neroli, and rose oils. Base notes are products with low volatility and high tenacity and are also described as fixatives because they provide staying power for the perfume. Common examples are vanillin (see page 75); musk, the dried secretion from the preputial follicles of the male musk deer of Asia; civet, a glandular secretion appearing in an outwardly discharging pocket underneath the posterior appendage of both the male and female civet cats; and ambergris, one of the most valuable materials used by the perfumer and a pathologic product formed in the stomach of the sperm whale when it is feeding on squid or cuttlefish. It is thought that the indigestible beaks of these animals irritate the whale's stomach, which in turn stimulates the formation of the ambergris.

Because volatile oils are mixtures of a number of constituents, one may assume that more than one constituent possesses physiologic activity. Volatile oils generally consist of an **eleoptene,** the hydrocarbon portion of the oil, which is liquid, and one or more **stearoptenes,** the oxidized hydrocarbon portions of the oil, which are usually solid (although exceptions to this are not rare). Thus, peppermint herb owes its activity to the volatile oil; the oil in turn owes its properties to the stearoptene, menthol. Menthol is not the only constituent present; menthyl acetate, limonene, menthone, cineol, and several others have been isolated and identified. Nevertheless, peppermint oil is used for different purposes than is menthol. Stearoptenes are generally obtained by freezing the oil or by other methods. Menthol, thymol, and anethole are solid stearoptenes; eucalyptol, eugenol, and methyl salicylate are liquid oxygenated hydrocarbons.

Many volatile oils possess antiseptic properties; the antibacterial, antimicrobial, and antifungal activities of essential oils and perfume oils have been the subject of a series of investigations. This bacteriostatic effect may have been responsible for the high value placed on certain spices of the Babylonian period and is probably why they were "worth their weight in gold." Thus, because of their preservative qualities, as well as their fragrance, spices were mixed with foodstuffs in early historic times. Undoubtedly, the presence of the antiseptic oils in the spices prevents excessive growth of bacteria, resulting in less food spoilage.

CHEMISTRY OF VOLATILE OILS

In only a few cases, as previously noted, do volatile oils consist of a single chemical compound in a state of comparative purity. In most cases, they are mixtures containing compounds of diverse types. These compounds may be separated in various ways: (1) low temperatures, which crystallize out the stearoptenes, (2) fractional distillation, (3) fractional crystallization from poor solvents, (4) gas chromatography, and (5) removal by chemical action. In the last group, compounds with free acidic groups may be removed from the oil with sodium carbonate, basic compounds may be removed with hydrochloric acid, phenols with sodium hydroxide, aldehydes with sodium bisulfite, and so forth.

In recent years, advances in analytic instrumentation, particularly in the area of chemical separation techniques based on gas-liquid and high-pressure liquid chromatography, coupled with spectroscopy, such as infrared, nuclear magnetic resonance, and mass spectrometry, have led to the precise identification of the components of volatile oils, including trace constituents.

Many volatile oils consist largely of **ter-**

penes. Terpenes are defined as natural products whose structure may be divided into isoprene units. These units arise from acetate via mevalonic acid and are branched-chain, 5-carbon units containing 2 unsaturated bonds.

$$CH_2=\overset{\overset{\displaystyle CH_3}{|}}{C}-CH=CH_2$$

Isoprene
C_5H_8

During the formation of terpenes, the isoprene units are linked in a head-to-tail fashion, and the number of units incorporated into a particular terpene serves as a basis for the classification of these compounds (Fig. 5–2). Monoterpenes are composed of 2 isoprene units and have the molecular formula, $C_{10}H_{16}$. Sesquiterpenes, $C_{15}H_{24}$, contain 3 isoprene units. Diterpenes, $C_{20}H_{32}$, have 4 isoprene units, and triterpenes, $C_{30}H_{48}$, are composed of 6 isoprene units. The terpenes found most often in volatile oils are monoterpenes. They can occur in acyclic, monocyclic, and bicyclic forms as hydrocarbons and as oxygenated derivatives, such as alcohols, aldehydes, ketones, phenols, oxides, and esters.

Another major group of volatile-oil constituents are the **phenylpropanoids.** These compounds contain the C_6 phenyl ring with an attached C_3 propane side chain. Figure 5–3 illustrates examples of these natural products. Many of the phenylpropanoids found in volatile oils are phenols or phenol ethers. In some cases, the propane side chain has been abridged to give a C_6–C_1 structure, such as in methyl salicylate and vanillin, or a C_6–C_2 structure, as in phenylethyl alcohol.

Because the various constituents of vol-

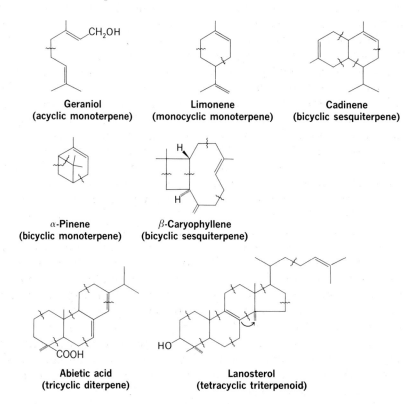

Geraniol
(acyclic monoterpene)

Limonene
(monocyclic monoterpene)

Cadinene
(bicyclic sesquiterpene)

α-Pinene
(bicyclic monoterpene)

β-Caryophyllene
(bicyclic sesquiterpene)

Abietic acid
(tricyclic diterpene)

Lanosterol
(tetracyclic triterpenoid)

Fig. 5–2. Representative terpenes showing the isoprene units in each molecule.

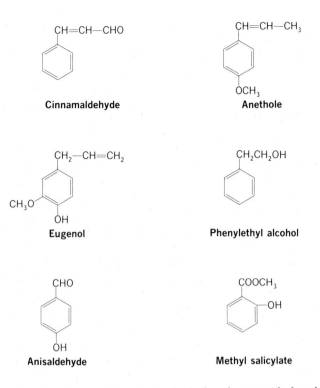

Cinnamaldehyde

Anethole

Eugenol

Phenylethyl alcohol

Anisaldehyde

Methyl salicylate

Fig. 5–3. Representative phenylpropanoids and abridged phenylpropanoids found as constituents of volatile oils.

atile oils are responsible for the characteristic odors, flavors, and therapeutic properties of the oils, a chemical classification of the oils should be based on their principal chemical constituents. However, because the types of constituents are so diverse and so numerous, the assignment of the oil or the oil-bearing drug to a definite place in such a classification is often difficult. For example, unoxygenated terpenes sometimes account for a large percentage of the oil. The stearoptene, which is present in smaller quantity, represents the constituent that is chiefly responsible for imparting the characteristic odor or flavor. The following are the divisions in which volatile oils and volatile-oil-containing drugs are placed: (1) hydrocarbons, (2) alcohols, (3) aldehydes, (4) ketones, (5) phenols, (6) phenolic ethers, (7) oxides, and (8) esters.

In addition to the molecular structure, the **stereochemistry** of the constituents of volatile oils markedly determines the type of olfactory response evoked by the compounds. Geometric isomers, whether *ortho/meta/para* or *cis/trans*, are in most cases readily distinguished both as to quality and strength of odor. An interesting stereochemical feature of many terpenes is the fact that both **enantiomers** (optically active isomers) exist in nature. In some cases, a plant species produces only one of the enantiomers whereas a different species may produce both. Among the monoterpenes that occur as the (+) form in certain species and as the (−) enantiomeric form in others are limonene, α-terpineol, α-fenchol, borneol, menthone, carvone, and linalool. Limonene, α-terpinol, α-fenchol, carvone, and camphor, as well as many others, can be found in plants as the racemic mixture.

As with many other natural product compounds that exist in enantiomeric forms, such as alkaloids and amino acids, the physiologic responses elicited by each isomer can differ. For example, (+)-carvone has an odor of caraway, whereas (−)-carvone produces a spearmint odor. These observations lend support to the stereochemical theory of olfaction which proposes that different kinds of olfactory receptor sites are in the nose. Odorant molecules could lodge on these sites and would have shapes and sizes that were complementary to the shape and size of the particular receptor. A proper fit at the receptor would be required to initiate a nerve impulse that would register in the brain the perception of the odor.

BIOSYNTHESIS OF VOLATILE OIL CONSTITUENTS

The biosynthetic building blocks for **terpenes** are isoprene units. The so-called biosynthetically active isoprene units are isopentenyl pyrophosphate and dimethylallyl pyrophosphate, compounds that arise from acetate via mevalonic acid (see page 166). Geranyl pyrophosphate is the C-10 precursor of the terpenes and is believed to play a key role in the formation of monoterpenes. It is formed by the condensation of one unit each of isopentenyl pyrophosphate and dimethylallyl pyrophosphate. As seen from Figure 5–4, geranyl pyrophosphate is believed to be the direct precursor to acyclic monoterpenes. However, it must be isomerized to neryl pyrophosphate before the cyclic monoterpenes can be formed because the trans isomer does not have the correct stereochemistry for cyclization. Another possibility is the formation of neryl pyrophosphate from isopentenyl pyrophosphate and dimethylallyl pyrophosphate independent of a geranyl pyrophosphate step. The intermediates in the formation of the cyclic terpenes are shown as carbonium ions; however, the true species are probably pyrophosphate esters or enzyme-bound intermediates.

The principal precursors for **phenylpropanoid** compounds, which are found in volatile oils, are cinnamic acid and p-hydroxycinnamic acid, also known as p-coumaric acid. In plants, these compounds arise from the aromatic amino acids phenylalanine and tyrosine, respectively, which in turn are synthesized via the shikimic acid pathway (Fig. 5–5). This biosynthetic pathway has been elucidated in microorganisms by using auxotrophic mutants of Escherichia coli and Enterobacter aerogenes that required the aromatic amino acids for growth. In the biosynthesis, 2 glucose metabolites, erythrose 4-phosphate and phosphoenolpyruvate, react to yield a phosphorylated 7-carbon keto sugar, DAHP. This compound cyclizes to 5-dehydroquinic acid which is then converted to shikimic acid. Shikimic acid, through a series of phosphorylated intermediates, yields chorismic acid, which is an important branch-point intermediate. One branch leads to anthranilic acid and then to tryptophan. The other leads to prephenic acid, the last nonaromatic compound in the sequence. Prephenic acid can be aromatized in 2 ways. The first proceeds by dehydration and simultaneous decarboxylation to yield phenylpyruvic acid, the direct precursor of phenylalanine. The second occurs by dehydrogenation and decarboxylation to yield p-hydroxyphenylpyruvic acid, the precursor of tyrosine.

The phenylpropanoid precursor, cinnamic acid, is formed by the direct enzymatic deamination of phenylalanine,

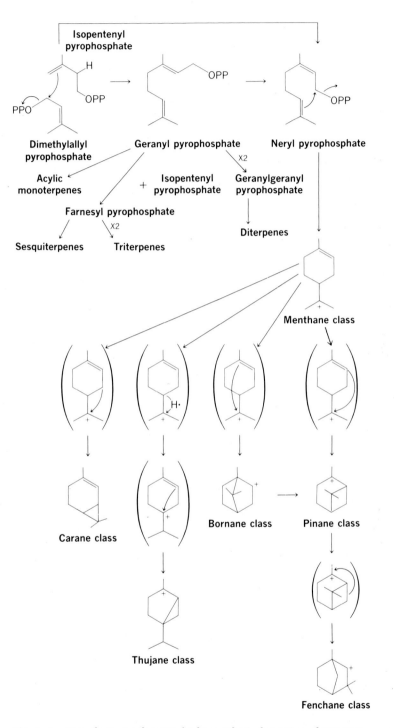

Fig. 5–4. Hypothetic mechanism for biosynthetic formation of terpenes.

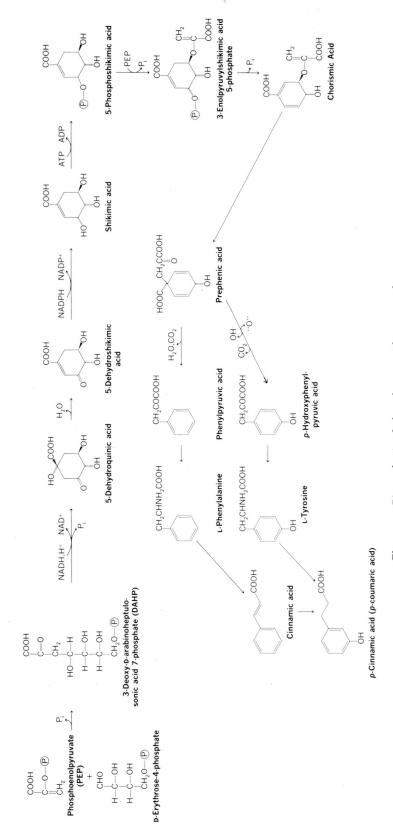

Fig. 5–5. Biosynthesis of phenylpropanoid compounds.

and p-coumaric acid can originate in an analogous way from tyrosine or by hydroxylation of cinnamic acid at the *para* position.

HYDROCARBON VOLATILE OILS

Hydrocarbons occur in practically all volatile oils. Limonene is probably the most widely distributed of the monocyclic terpenes (see Fig. 5–2). It occurs in citrus, mint, myristica, caraway, myrcia, pine needle, cardamom, coriander, juniper, and many other oils. Another important monocyclic hydrocarbon monoterpene is p-cymene, which is found in coriander, thyme, cinnamon, and myristica oils. Pinene (see Fig. 5–2), a dicyclic monoterpene, is also widely distributed. It is found in many conifer oils, as well as in lemon, anise, eucalyptus, thyme, fennel, coriander, orange flower, and myristica oils. Sabinene, a dicyclic monoterpene of the thujane class, is distributed in cubeb, cardamom, and lemon oils. Acyclic monoterpene hydrocarbons are rather rare, but myrcene from myricia, juniper, thyme, lemon, and myristica oils may be cited as an example. Cadinene (see Fig. 5–2), occurring in cubeb and juniper tar, is a typical sesquiterpene hydrocarbon. β-Caryophyllene (see Fig. 5–2), which is found in wormwood, peppermint, cinnamon, and clove oils, is an example of a sesquiterpene with a more unusual chemical structure.

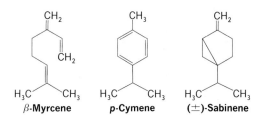

β-Myrcene   p-Cymene   (±)-Sabinene

Volatile oil drugs that are composed chiefly of hydrocarbons are cubeb and turpentine oil (Table 5–1).

Rectified turpentine oil is turpentine oil rectified by distillation from an aqueous solution of sodium hydroxide. It is dispensed when turpentine oil is required for internal use. It is a local irritant and is used as an expectorant, diuretic, urinary antiseptic, and anthelmintic. Usual dose is 0.3 ml.

Terpin hydrate or terpinol is formed by the action of nitric acid on rectified turpentine oil in the presence of alcohol. It is cis-p-menthane-1,8-diol hydrate ($C_{10}H_{18}(OH)_2 \cdot H_2O$).

Terpin hydrate is a stimulant to the mucous membrane; therefore, it is used as an expectorant in the form of terpin hydrate elixir. The usual dose of terpin hydrate is 85 mg.

ALCOHOL VOLATILE OILS

Alcohols found in volatile oils may be classified into (1) acyclic alcohols, (2) monocyclic alcohols, and (3) dicyclic alcohols. Methyl, ethyl, isobutyl, isoamyl, hexyl, and the higher aliphatic alcohols occur in volatile oils but, because they are soluble in water, they are washed away in the process of steam distillation. Many natural oils, however, contain acyclic alcohols that are terpene derivatives. Among

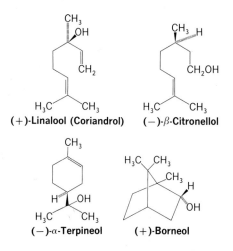

(+)-Linalool (Coriandrol)   (−)-β-Citronellol

(−)-α-Terpineol   (+)-Borneol

Table 5–1. Hydrocarbon Volatile Oil Drugs

Name	Part Used	Botanical Origin	Geographic Origin	Important Constituents	Use
Cubeb	nearly full-grown unripe fruit	a woody climber, *Piper cubeba* (Piperaceae)	Indonesia	(+)-sabinene, 1,4-cineole, (−)-cadinene, terpineol	antiseptic and stimulating expectorant in the OTC drug, Medicated Throat Discs®
Turpentine oil (spirits of turpentine)	volatile oil distilled from the oleoresin	the tree, *Pinus palustris* and other species of *Pinus* (Pinaceae)	Southeastern United States	64% α-pinene, 33% β-pinene	Counterirritant in the OTC drugs, Vicks Vaporub®, Mentholatum Deep Heating®, and Sloan's Liniment®

Table 5–2. Alcohol Volatile Oil Drugs

Name	Part Used	Botanical Origin	Geographic Origin	Important Constituents	Use
Cardamom oil (Fig. 5–6)	volatile oil distilled from the dried, ripe seed	a perennial herb, *Elettaria cardamomum* (Zingiberaceae)	Malabar Coast of India, Sri Lanka, Laos, Guatemala, El Salvador	26–40% cineole, 28–34% α-terpinyl acetate, 2–14% limonene, 3–5% sabinene, 2–8% linalyl acetate	flavor, carminative
Coriander oil (Fig. 5–7)	volatile oil distilled with steam from the dried, ripe fruit	an annual herb, *Coriandrum sativum* (Umbelliferae)	Soviet Union, India, Morocco, Poland, Rumania, Yugoslavia, Argentina	60–70% (+)-linalool, limonene, α-pinene, γ-terpinene, *p*-cymene	flavor, carminative
Rose oil (otto of rose)	volatile oil distilled with steam from the fresh flowers	perennial herbs or shrubs, *Rosa gallica, R. damascena, R. alba, R. centifolia* and varieties of these species (Rosaceae)	Bulgaria, southern France, Turkey, Morocco, Italy	geraniol, (−)-citronellol, phenylethyl alcohol, nerol	perfume
Orange flower oil (neroli oil)	volatile oil distilled from the fresh flowers	a tree, *Citrus aurantium* (Rutaceae)	southern France, Algeria, Sicily, Spain, Tunisia, Morocco	30% (−)-linalool, (+)-α-terpineol, geraniol, geranyl acetate, pinene, 7% linalyl acetate, limonene	perfume, flavor
Juniper oil	volatile oil distilled with steam from the dried, ripe fruit	small evergreens, *Juniperus communis* and its variety *depressa* (Cupressaceae)	Italy, Yugoslavia	α-pinene, β-pinene, myrcene, limonene, α-terpineol	flavor, diuretic in the OTC drug, Odrinil®
Pine oil	volatile oil obtained by extraction and fractionation or by steam distillation of the wood	the tree, *Pinus palustris* and other species of *Pinus* (Pinaceae)	southeastern United States, China	65% α-terpineol, 10% methyl chavicol and related phenol ethers, 9% borneol, 8% fenchol, 4% menthols	disinfectant, deodorant

the more important of these are geraniol (see Fig. 5–2), linalool, and citronellol. Among the more important monocyclic alcohols are menthol (from peppermint) and α-terpineol; borneol is a dicyclic terpene alcohol from Borneo camphor. Sesquiterpene alcohols include zingiberol (see page 156).

Among the important alcohol volatile oil drugs are peppermint, cardamom oil, coriander oil, rose oil, orange flower oil, juniper oil, and pine oil (Table 5–2).

PEPPERMINT

Peppermint consists of the dried leaf and flowering top of *Mentha piperita* Linné (Fam. Labiatae). *Mentha* is from the Greek *Mintha,* the name of a mythical nymph metamorphosed into this plant; *piperita* is from the Latin *piper,* meaning pepper, and alludes to the aromatic and pungent taste of peppermint.

The plant is a perennial herb indigenous to Europe and naturalized in the northern

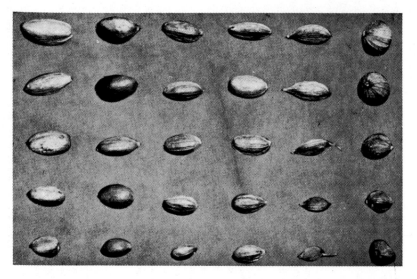

Fig. 5–6. Commercial cardamoms: from top to bottom, "longs," "short-longs," "mediums," "shorts," "tiny."

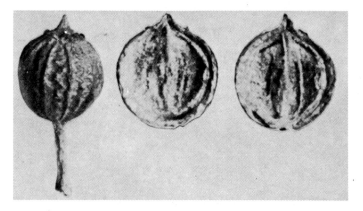

Fig. 5–7. Coriander fruit, magnified 6 times.

United States and Canada. It is extensively cultivated in areas where the fertile soil has high water-holding capacity. If rainfall is not sufficient, an irrigation system is essential. Peppermint requires a daytime length of 15 to 16 hours and as much sunlight as possible. To obtain good field crops, clean planting stock must be used because disease control measures have not yet been fully developed. The plants are propagated by rhizome cuttings. When in flower, they are cut with a mowing machine, raked into windrows, dried for a few hours in the sun, and hauled to the still house. If the plant is to be used as a drug, it is carefully dried and preserved. Several varieties of peppermint are cultivated in the United States; but, whereas the American peppermint oil is all derived from M. piperita, the Japanese peppermint oil is obtained from M. arvensis Linné var. piperascens. Peppermint was described by John Ray in his Historia Plantarum (1704). It was extensively cultivated in England as early as 1750.

Peppermint contains volatile oil (about 1%), resin, and tannin.

Commercial dried peppermint usually consists of the dried herb though it should contain not more than 2% of stems over 3 mm in diameter. It loses some volatile oil during drying and more during storage; the usual commercial sample has suffered 95% deterioration and yields no volatile oil upon steam distillation. However, the distillate water may be aromatic.

Uses. Peppermint is a carminative and a flavor. As a medicine, it has been largely replaced by peppermint oil.

Peppermint oil is the volatile oil distilled with steam from the fresh overground parts of the flowering plant of Mentha piperita Linné (Fam. Labiatae) (Fig. 5–8), rectified by distillation and neither partially nor wholly dementholized. It yields not less than 5% of esters, calculated as menthyl acetate ($C_{12}H_{22}O_2$),

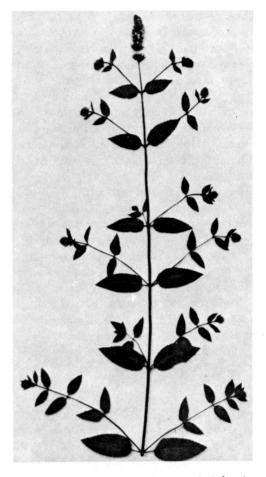

Fig. 5–8. Mentha piperita (peppermint) showing opposite, petiolate leaves and dense, terminal inflorescences. (Photo, courtesy of A. M. Todd Company, Kalamazoo, Michigan.)

and not less than 50% of total menthol ($C_{10}H_{20}O$), free and as esters.

The American production of peppermint oil has increased tremendously in the past century; in 1844, 88,000 pounds were produced, in 1944, 867,000 pounds were produced, and, in 1976, 3,700,000 pounds were produced and valued at $55 million; $31 million of this total represented the value of exported oil. About 90% of the oil is obtained from Washington, Oregon, and Idaho, principally from the Willamette river valley and Madras areas of Oregon, the Columbia river basin of Washington, and portions of the Snake river valley in Idaho. The remainder of the oil is produced in Wisconsin and Indiana. A few years ago, southern Michigan was the major area of mint cultivation in the United States, but a fungus blight (*Verticillium* wilt) infected crops and caused abandonment of thousands of acres of formerly productive land. In recent years, wilt-resistant strains of peppermint have been developed by using the technique of irradiation-induced mutations, thereby eliminating the threat to the industry of fungal blight. In 1978, approximately 17,000 acres were under cultivation in Washington and yielded an average of 70 pounds of oil to the acre.

DESCRIPTION. Peppermint oil is a colorless or pale yellow liquid that has a strong, penetrating odor of peppermint and a pungent taste that is followed by a sensation of cold when air is drawn into the mouth.

American peppermint oil contains from 50 to 78% of free (−)-menthol and from 5 to 20% combined in various esters such as the acetate. It also contains (+)-menthone, (−)-menthone, cineole, (−)-limonene, (+)-isomenthone, (+)-neomenthone, and (−)-β-caryophyllene.

Because of the commercial importance of the mint oils, the interconversions of the various terpene constituents of the oils have been studied more extensively than those of other volatile oil plants. Incorporation of $^{14}CO_2$ into the various menthane derivatives that characterize different *Mentha* species has allowed precursor relationships to be deduced (Fig. 5–9). Several of the proposed steps were directly demonstrated by isolating radioactively labeled monoterpenes and feeding them back to leaf slices or foliage. Cell-free extracts from *Mentha* leaves with pulegone-^{14}C have confirmed the pule-gone→menthone→menthol portion of the pathway and have established that $NADPH_2$ is an essential cofactor in these reduction reactions. An enzyme preparation from *Mentha* leaves has also been shown to reduce the isopropylidene double bond of piperitenone to yield piperitone. Small amounts of menthone and menthol were also formed with piperitenone as the substrate, indicating that the cyclohexene double bond of the precursor was reduced.

A key step in the biosynthesis of the p-menthane monoterpenes appears to be the dehydration of α-terpineol to terpinolene and limonene (see Fig. 5–9). The steps leading to the formation of α-terpineol from mevalonic acid are common to several different species of mints. The pathways then diverge where α-terpineol is dehydrated to limonene in spearmint and to terpinolene in peppermint. The next step in the sequence is hydroxylation and subsequent dehydrogenation to produce either the carvone series of monoterpenes found in spearmint or the piperitenone series of monoterpenes found in peppermint. Breeding experiments with the mints indicate that a single dominant gene produces the carvone series whereas the homozygous recessive genotype produces the piperitenone series. Apparently, the gene that differentiates between these series may be the gene that governs the enzyme that dehydrates α-terpineol to either limonene or terpinolene.

The influence of environmental factors on essential oil composition has been apparent to commercial producers for many years. Plants of the same species and genotype may produce oils of different quality when grown in different areas. The long days of northern latitudes favor the production of a peppermint oil that contains relatively small amounts of menthone and menthofuran and large amounts of

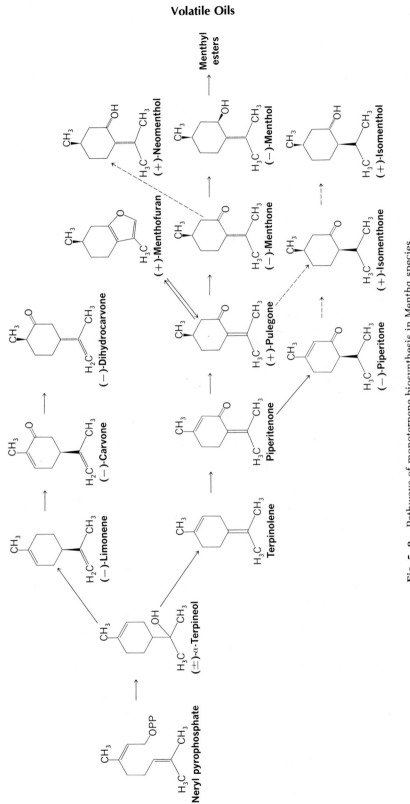

Fig. 5–9. Pathways of monoterpene biosynthesis in *Mentha* species.

menthol, whereas plants subjected to short day illumination produce an oil that contains small amounts of menthol and relatively large amounts of menthofuran.

Sequential studies with $^{14}CO_2$ have suggested that pulegone is the predominant terpene in young tissues of peppermint, where it is accompanied by menthofuran. Menthone, which is found in older tissues, also gradually disappears while menthol accumulates and is replaced, in turn, by menthyl acetate.

This sequence of biogenetic events helps to explain why peppermint oils obtained from plants containing relatively large amounts of young tissue are inferior. High concentrations (up to 30% in some cases) of menthofuran in such oils impart a disagreeable cloying odor to products in which they may be incorporated. The reaction pulegone → menthofuran is apparently reversible, and the concentration of both of these compounds decreases in favor of menthone, menthol, and menthyl acetate as the plant ages. Consequently, oils of good quality can be obtained only from plants containing a high percentage of mature tissues.

The problem of obtaining mature tissues is particularly acute in the Yakima valley of central Washington where environmental conditions favor early and luxuriant flowering of mint plants with concomitant production of a large proportion of relatively young tissues. Careful control of the time of harvest enables growers in that area to produce oils of satisfactory quality.

Uses. Peppermint oil is a pharmaceutic aid (flavor). It has been used as a carminative, a stimulant, and a counterirritant. Its chief commercial importance is as a flavor for confections, especially for chewing gum.

It was estimated in 1972 that the domestic use of peppermint oil was as follows: chewing gum, 55%; toothpaste, mouthwash, and pharmaceuticals, 34%; confec-tionary products, 10%; and other products, 1%. In recent years, about one third of our national production has found its way into export trade, which has increased more than 400% since the 1940s.

NONPRESCRIPTION PRODUCTS. Peppermint oil is used as a flavoring agent in Medicated Throat Discs® and Listerine Mouthwash® and as a carminative and flavoring agent in the antacid products BiSoDol®, Gelusil®, Phillips' Milk of Magnesia®, and Tums®.

Japanese peppermint oil or mentha arvensis oil is obtained by steam distillation from *Mentha arvensis* Linné var. *piperascens*. This oil is considerably higher in menthol content, but is inferior in flavor to peppermint oil. It is, therefore, solely employed as a source of menthol. The plant is indigenous to Japan and is the source of Japanese menthol. Some years ago the plant was introduced into southern California and Brazil; both areas now produce considerable amounts of menthol.

Menthol or menthan-3-ol is an alcohol obtained from diverse mint oils or prepared synthetically. Menthol may be levorotatory [(−)-menthol], from natural or synthetic sources, or racemic [(±)-menthol], produced synthetically.

Menthol is usually prepared from Japanese peppermint oil by refrigeration (−22° C) during which the menthol crystallizes. The liquid portion is poured off, and the crystallized menthol is pressed between filter papers and subsequently purified by recrystallization. Synthetic racemic menthol is produced by hydrogenation of thymol. Menthol may also be prepared from pinene.

Menthol occurs as colorless, hexagonal crystals that are usually needlelike, as fused masses, or as a crystalline powder. It has a pleasant, peppermintlike odor.

Uses. Menthol is a topical antipruritic. It has been used on the skin or mucous membranes as a counterirritant, an antiseptic, and a stimulant; internally, menthol has a depressant effect on the heart. Menthol is topically applied as 0.1 to 2% preparations for use on the skin.

NONPRESCRIPTION PRODUCTS. Menthol is used as an antipruritic in such burn and sunburn preparations as Noxzema Medicated Cream®, Solarcaine®, and Unguentine®; in preparations to treat poison ivy rash, Ivy Dry Cream® and Rhulicream®; in douche powders, Stomaseptine® and Zonite®; in diaper rash preparations, Johnson and Johnson Medicated Powder®; and in preparations to treat athlete's foot, NP27 Powder®. It is used as a counterirritant in external analgesic preparations that include Absorbine Jr.®, Analgesic Balm®, Ben-Gay®, Mentholatum®, Minit-Rub®, and Vicks Vaporub®.

ALDEHYDE VOLATILE OILS

Aldehydes occurring in volatile oils may be divided into acyclic and cyclic. Included among the former are citral, which is a 3:1 mixture of geranial to neral, and citronellal, the aldehyde corresponding to citronellol. The aromatic aldehydes include cinnamaldehyde (see Fig. 5–3), vanillin (vanilla, benzoin, tolu and Peru balsams), and anisaldehyde (see Fig. 5–3).

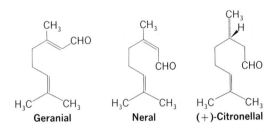

| Geranial | Neral | (+)-Citronellal |

Biosynthesis of such aromatic aldehydes as benzaldehyde and vanillin takes place from phenylpropanoid precursors. Because these compounds comprise the aglycones of certain glycosides, their formation was discussed under that heading.

The terpene aldehydes derive from acetate metabolism, as illustrated in Figure 5–4.

Among the important drugs in this class are cinnamon, cinnamon oil, orange oil, lemon peel, lemon oil, hamamelis water, and citronella oil (Table 5–3).

CINNAMON

Cinnamon or Saigon cinnamon is the dried bark of *Cinnamomum loureirii* Nees (Fam. Lauraceae).

An important cinnamon in U.S. commerce is **Ceylon cinnamon,** the dried inner bark of shoots of coppiced trees of C. *zeylanicum* Nees (Fam. Lauraceae) (Fig. 5–10).

Cassia cinnamon is the dried bark of C. *cassia* (Nees) Nees ex Blume.

Cinnamon may be from the Arabic, *kinnamon;* the Malay, *kayu manis,* sweet wood; or the Hebrew, *ginnamon. Loureirii* is in honor of the French botanist *Loureiro; zeylanicum* signifies Ceylon; *Cassia* is from the Greek *kassia,* meaning to strip off the bark.

Cinnamon is named as a spice in the books of Moses, by the ancient Greek and Latin historians, and in Chinese herbals as early as 2700 B.C. Its cultivation in Ceylon probably dates from 1200 A.D.

The wild cinnamon trees seldom exceed 9 meters in height. The leaves are coriaceous, green, and glossy; the flowers are in terminal panicles; and the fruit is fleshy and ovoid.

Practically all commercial cinnamon is now obtained from cultivated trees in Sri Lanka (Ceylon), southeastern China, Vietnam, Laos, Indonesia, the West Indies and many other localities. However, cinnamon from southeastern Asia and adjacent islands is superior in quality.

The bark is gathered from young trees usually less than 6 years old and, in Sri Lanka, mostly from coppice shoots 18 to 36

Table 5–3.   Aldehyde Volatile Oil Drugs

Name	Part	Botanical Origin	Geographic Origin	Important Constituents	Use
Orange oil	volatile oil obtained by expression from the fresh peel of the ripe fruit	a tree, *Citrus sinensis* (Rutaceae)	California, Florida, Algeria, Tunisia, Morocco, Spain, Israel	1–2% decanal, more than 90% limonene	flavor
Citronella oil	volatile oil distilled with steam from freshly cut or partially dried leaves	the grass, *Cymbopogon winterianus* and *C. nardus* (Gramineae)	Sri Lanka, Indonesia, China, Taiwan, Central America	32–45% (+)-citronellal 12–18% geranial 11–15% (+)-citronellol	perfume insect repellant
Hamamelis water (distilled witch hazel extract)	hydroalcoholic solution of the volatile oil prepared by steam distillation of the recently cut and partially dried dormant twigs	the tree, *Hamamelis virginiana* (Hamamelidaceae)	eastern United States and Canada	9.7% 2-hexen-1-al, 3.2% acetaldehyde, 3.5% α-ionone, 1.0% β-ionone, 0.2% safrole	astringent in the OTC drugs, Dr. Hands Teething Lotion and Gel®, and the hemorrhoid preparations, Tucks®, Rantex®, Mediconet®, Hazel-Balm® and Gentz-Wipes®

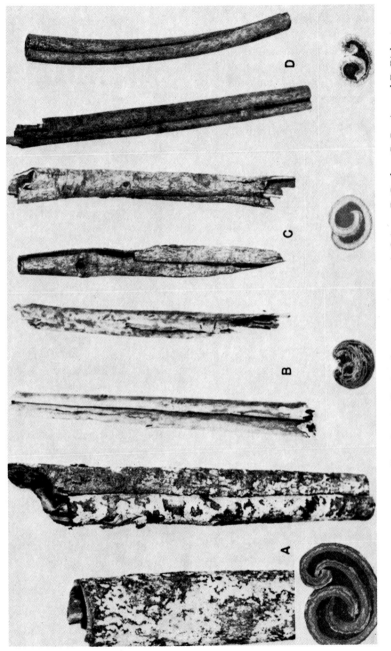

Fig. 5–10. Cinnamon bark quills in longitudinal and transverse views: A, Saigon; B, Ceylon; C, Cassia; and D, Djakarta.

months old. The leaves, branches, and stem tips are distilled with steam for the volatile oil. The bark is cut transversely and longitudinally and peeled. In Sri Lanka and Indonesia, the bark is scraped while fresh to remove epidermis and cork; in China, it is planed to remove partially the cork. In Sri Lanka, many layers of the thin inner bark are rolled into one quill; in Indonesia, several layers may be quilled together; and in China and Vietnam, each layer is quilled separately or only 2 or 3 layers are quilled together.

Saigon cinnamon yields from 2 to 6% of volatile oil; cassia cinnamon, 0.5 to 1.5%; and Ceylon cinnamon, 0.5 to 1%. Other constituents are mannitol, which causes the sweetness of the bark, and tannin, which is abundant in cassia cinnamon.

Uses. Saigon, Ceylon, and cassia cinnamon are carminatives and flavors.

The powdered cinnamon found in the grocery trade is frequently a blend of several kinds of cinnamon. The blending is done either to improve the aromatic quality or to cheapen the product.

Cinnamon oil is the volatile oil distilled with steam from the leaves and twigs of *Cinnamonum cassia* (Nees) Nees ex Blume (Fam. Lauraceae) and rectified by distillation. It is also known as **cassia oil.**

Cinnamon oil is a yellowish to brownish liquid that becomes darker and thicker by age or by exposure to air and possesses the characteristic odor and taste of cassia cinnamon.

The principal constituent of the oil is cinnamic aldehyde, 80 to 95%; the remainder consists of terpenes, such as cineole, p-cymene, (−)-linalool and β-caryophyllene, and other compounds, such as eugenol.

Uses and Dose. Cinnamon oil is used as a flavoring agent; it is also a carminative and pungent aromatic. It has antiseptic properties.

Cinnamaldehyde, cinnamic aldehyde, or cinnamyl aldehyde contains not less than 98% of C_8H_7CHO.

Cinnamaldehyde is obtained naturally from cassia oil or synthetically from a mixture of benzaldehyde and acetaldehyde by the action of sodium hydroxide.

It should be stored in well-filled, tight, light-resistant containers protected from excessive heat.

LEMON PEEL

Lemon is the fruit of *Citrus limon* (Linné) Burmann filius (Fam. Rutaceae).

Lemon peel is the outer yellow rind of the fresh ripe fruit of *C. limon*. *Limon* is from *limun*, the name of the fruit. The plant is a small evergreen tree with shining leaves and is indigenous to northern India but cultivated to a considerable extent in such subtropical regions as southern Spain, southern Italy, Sicily, southern California, Florida, Jamaica, and Australia. The history of the lemon parallels that of the orange; it has been known since the beginning of the written history of India, its native land.

The cultivation of lemon trees and the picking, selecting, and storing of lemon fruits constitute an important industry.

The outer, lemon-yellow or dark yellow layer (peel) is removed by grating or paring. It has a highly fragrant, distinctive odor and an aromatic taste.

Lemon peel contains a volatile oil, a small quantity of hesperidin, bitter principles, a principle resembling tannin, and calcium oxalate.

Uses. Lemon peel is a flavoring agent, a stimulant, and a stomachic. It is employed chiefly in combination with other drugs.

Lemon oil is the volatile oil obtained by expression, without the aid of heat, from the fresh peel of the fruit of *C. limon*, with or without the previous separation of the pulp and the peel. Six processes are utilized in the recovery of oil of lemon; five of these processes yield an oil meeting pharmaceutic requirements.

1. The outer portion of the rind, which contains the volatile oil, is removed by grating; the resultant raspings are placed in canvas bags and subjected to pressure. The resultant turbid oil is allowed to stand until the sediment separates, after which the oil is decanted.

2. The sponge process is employed to a considerable extent in Sicily and along the Riviera. The lemon is peeled and pieces of the peel are pressed flat so that they flex and rupture the oil cells. The oil is absorbed by the sponge which, when it becomes saturated, is squeezed out, and the process is repeated.

3. The entire fruit is rotated in a saucer-shaped container that has several rows of sharp metal pins and is called an *écuellé a piquer*. The pins rupture the oil cells, and the exuding oil collects in a long narrow depression in the bottom of the saucer, which also serves as the handle. This method is now used in the West Indies.

4. During the machine process used in Italy, the oil is separated mechanically using a principle similar to that of the *écuellé a piquer*. Only the peel is subjected to this method.

5. Cold-pressed California oil is obtained by the application of extremely high pressure to the lemons and the rapid removal of the juice and oil. The juice-and-oil mixture is then separated by high-speed centrifugal separation at the lowest feasible temperature and in the shortest possible time.

6. Some lemon oil is obtained by distillation. Such oil is not comparable with the expressed oil and does not conform to pharmaceutic standards. Distilled oil is usually used for the preparation of terpeneless oil of lemon.

Lemon oil contains about 90% of terpenes consisting chiefly of (+)-limonene, the main hydrocarbon present in a range of 70 to 80%, and other monoterpene hydrocarbons, especially β-pinene and γ-terpinene (approximately 8 to 10% of each). The most important contributors to lemon-oil flavor are neral and geranial (together called citral). Some lemon oils contain up to 13% of citral, but a range of 2 to 4% is optimum for a high-quality oil. The primary esters in lemon oil are neryl and geranyl acetates, and they are believed to be important in providing a full-bodied lemon flavor.

Lemon oil that has a terebinthinate odor must not be used or dispensed; such an odor indicates decomposed terpenes or added turpentine oil.

UsES. Lemon oil is a flavoring agent. It has stimulant, carminative, and stomachic properties. It is a valuable commodity used not only in food flavorings but also in cosmetics and liquid cleansers because the aroma and flavor are widely accepted by consumers. In 1967, the dollar value of lemon oil consumed in the United States was $11 million, making it the number one volatile oil in dollar value and representing 2.5 million pounds of oil.

Turpentine oil was formerly used as an adulterant, but has been replaced by terpenes obtained in the preparation of terpeneless oils. California-type lemon oil should contain between 2.2 and 3.8% of total aldehydes (principally citral) and Italian-type lemon oil between 3.0 and 5.5%. Yet, even such a citral content is no criterion of purity because citral from a cheaper source (lemongrass oil obtained from *Cymbopogon citratus* [D.C.] Staph. [Fam. Gramineae], which contains about 80% citral) may be added. Only a careful check of the physical and chemical constants of the oil can determine its purity.

Terpeneless oils. Lemon oil and orange

oil, by virtue of their high terpene content, often develop a terebinthinate odor during storage. A considerable amount of these terpenes may be removed by distillation under reduced pressure. A terpeneless lemon oil with a citral content of 40 to 50% may be prepared. In terpeneless orange oil, about 95% of the terpenes have been removed. Such oils are not subject to deterioration and may be employed in smaller quantities to obtain the same organoleptic effect. They are, however, considerably higher in price than are the natural oils.

KETONE VOLATILE OILS

Ketones occurring in volatile oils may be divided into (1) monocyclic terpene ketones, including menthone, carvone, piperitone, pulegone (see Fig. 5–9), and diosphenol (a crystalline ketone in buchu); and (2) dicyclic ketones including camphor, fenchone, and thujone.

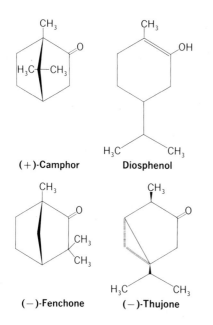

(+)-Camphor   Diosphenol

(−)-Fenchone   (−)-Thujone

The more important drugs of this category are camphor, spearmint, and caraway (Table 5–4).

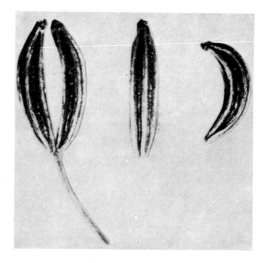

Fig. 5–11.   Caraway fruits, magnified 6 times.

CAMPHOR

Camphor is a ketone obtained from *Cinnamomum camphora* (Linné) Nees et Ebermaier (Fam. Lauraceae) (natural camphor) or produced synthetically (synthetic camphor). *Camphora* is from the Arabic *kafur*, meaning chalk. The plant is a large evergreen tree indigenous to eastern Asia but naturalized in the Mediterranean region, Sri Lanka, Egypt, South Africa, Brazil, Jamaica, Florida, and California. Early references to camphor do not refer to the laurel camphor but rather to the Borneo camphor (borneol, see page 113), which reached Arabia in the sixth century and Europe in the twelfth. Laurel camphor appeared in Europe in the seventeenth century. When Japan annexed Taiwan, a government monopoly was created (1900). From that time until World War II, about 80% of the world's supply of natural camphor (about 4 million kg per year) was produced in Taiwan where the tree occurs naturally in abundance and is also extensively cultivated; the remaining 20% was produced largely in Japan and southern China. Since 1945, the production of syn-

Table 5–4. Ketone Volatile Oil Drugs

Name	Botanical Origin	Part Used	Geographic Origin	Important Constituents	Use
Caraway (Fig. 5–11)	the biennial herb, *Carum carvi* (Umbelliferae)	the dried, ripe fruit	northern Europe, United States	5–7% volatile oil	flavor
Caraway oil	the biennial herb, *Carum carvi* (Umbelliferae)	volatile oil distilled with steam from the dried, ripe fruit	northern Europe, United States	50–60% (+)-carvone, 40–50% (+)-limonene	flavor, carminative
Buchu	the low shrub, *Barosma betulina, B. crenulata,* or *B. serratifolia* (Rutaceae)	the dried leaf	South Africa	volatile oil containing about 30% diosphenol	diuretic in OTC drugs for menstrual problems, De-witt's Flowaway Water®, Fluidex®, Odrinil®
Wormwood oil (absinthe oil)	A shrubby perennial herb, *Artemisia absinthium* (Compositae)	volatile oil distilled with steam from the dried leaves and flowering tops	United States, southern Europe, northern Africa	(+)-thujone, camphene, phellandrene, β-caryophyllene	counterirritant in OTC drugs, Absorbant Rub®, Absorbine Jr.®
Cedar leaf oil	the tree, *Thuja occidentalis* (Cupressaceae)	volatile oil distilled with steam from the fresh leaves	eastern United States, Canada	(+)-thujone, (−)-fenchone, α-pinene	counterirritant in OTC drug, Vicks Vaporub®

thetic camphor has gradually lessened the demand for the natural product; nevertheless, Japanese and Taiwan camphor still occur on the market.

Natural camphor occurs as a crystalline product in clefts in the woody stems and roots and, to a greater extent, dissolved in the volatile oil. The wood is chipped and distilled with steam, and 1 pound of crude camphor is obtained from 20 to 40 pounds of chips. The crude camphor is then freed of oil by centrifugation and pressing and finally resublimed and pressed into the familiar cakes.

Before World War II, about 6.5 million kg of synthetic camphor were produced annually in Europe and the United States. During the war, the production of synthetic camphor practically replaced the natural derivative. Since the war, production of natural camphor has been resumed, but it will never assume its former prominence.

Synthetic camphor is made from pinene, the principal constituent of turpentine oil. The starting point is the stumps of felled pine trees previously used in turpentining. A number of complex methods have been used for producing synthetic camphor, but all are based on: (1) converting pinene into bornyl esters, which are (2) hydrolyzed to isoborneol, and (3) finally oxidized to camphor.

The specific rotation of natural camphor is between +41° and +43°. Synthetic camphor is the optically inactive racemic form.

Uses. Camphor is a topical antipruritic, rubefacient, and anti-infective employed as 1 to 3% in preparations for use on the skin. Commercially it is used in the manufacture of certain plastics.

Nonprescription Products. Camphor is used as an antipruritic in Hist-A-Balm Medicated Lotion®, Rhuli Cream®, and Noxzema Medicated Cream® and as a rubefacient in external analgesic preparations, such as Heet®, Mentholatum®, Minit-Rub®, Sloan's Liniment®, and Vicks Vaporub®. It is also an ingredient of Campho-Phenique® for athlete's foot and Blistex® for cold sores.

Note. Camphor must be labeled to indicate whether it is obtained from natural sources or is prepared synthetically.

SPEARMINT

Spearmint consists of the dried leaf and flowering top of Mentha spicata Linné (M. viridis Linné) (common spearmint) or of M. cardiaca Gerard ex Baker (Scotch spearmint) (Fam. Labiatae). Spicata is from the Latin spica, meaning a spike, and refers to the arrangement of the flowers. The plant is a perennial herb that closely resembles peppermint, is indigenous to Europe, and is naturalized and cultivated in various parts of North America. Spearmint is extensively cultivated in Washington, Idaho, Wisconsin, Michigan, and Indiana. More than 25,000 acres are presently devoted to spearmint cultivation in the state of Washington, and the average yield is 83 pounds per acre. Total production of spearmint oil amounts to about 3 million pounds annually. The plant appears in many of the old herbals, and its mention in early medieval lists demonstrates that it was cultivated in the convent gardens of the ninth century.

Spearmint closely resembles peppermint, but the stems are usually more purple. The leaves are sessile or nearly so, inflorescence is either in slender, interrupted cylindric spikes or crowded lanceolate spikes, and the bracts are 7 to 10 mm in length (Fig. 5–12). Odor and taste are aromatic and characteristic; the taste is not followed by a cooling sensation.

Spearmint is comprised of resin, tannin, and a volatile oil (about 0.5%) that contains carvone.

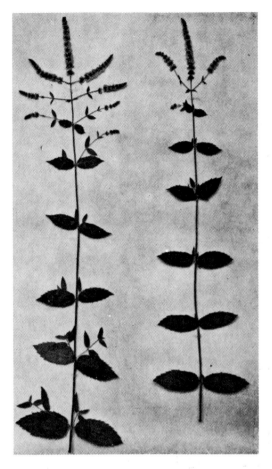

Fig. 5–12. *Mentha spicata* (spearmint) showing opposite, sessile leaves and interrupted terminal inflorescences. (Photo, courtesy of A. M. Todd Company, Kalamazoo, Michigan.)

Uses. Spearmint is classed as a flavor. It possesses carminative properties.

Spearmint oil is distilled with steam from the fresh, overground parts of the flowering plant of *Mentha spicata* or of *M. cardiaca*. It contains not less than 55%, by volume, of carvone ($C_{10}H_{14}O$). Most of the supply of spearmint oil is produced in the same area as is peppermint oil.

Spearmint oil is a colorless, yellow or greenish yellow liquid that has the characteristic odor and taste of spearmint.

Spearmint oil contains from 45 to 60% of (−)-carvone, 6 to 20% of alcohols, and 4 to 20% of esters and terpenes, chiefly (−)-limonene, cineole, and (−)-pinene. The carvone is optically isomeric with the (+)-carvone found in oil of caraway and oil of dill.

Uses. Spearmint oil is a flavor. It possesses carminative properties and is used to a considerable extent in the chewing gum industry. A 1972 government survey showed that the estimated domestic use of spearmint oil was 50% toothpaste and mouthwash, 47% chewing gum, and 3% other.

PHENOL VOLATILE OILS

Two kinds of phenols occur in volatile oils: those that are present naturally and those that are produced as the result of destructive distillation of certain plant products.

Eugenol (see Fig. 5–3), thymol, and carvacrol are the most important phenols occurring in volatile oils. Eugenol occurs in clove oil, myrcia oil, and other oils; thymol and carvacrol occur in thyme oil and others; and creosol and guaiacol occur in creosote and pine tar.

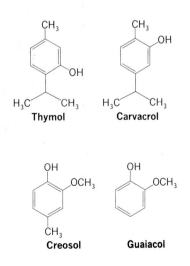

Thymol

Carvacrol

Creosol

Guaiacol

Table 5–5. Phenol Volatile Oil Drugs

Name	Part Used	Botanical Origin	Geographic Origin	Important Constituents	Use
Thyme oil	volatile oil distilled with steam from the flowering plant	an evergreen herbaceous shrub, *Thymus vulgaris, T. zygis* and its variety *gracilis* (Labiatae)	Spain, Italy, France, Germany, England, United States	thymol, carvacrol, *p*-cymene, (−)-α-pinene, myrcene, (−)-linalool	antiseptic in the OTC drugs, Unguentine Cream®, Dewitt's Oil for Ear Use®
Myrcia oil (bay oil)	volatile oil distilled with steam from the leaves	the tree, *Pimenta racemosa* (Myrtaceae)	West Indies	55–65% eugenol, (−)-α-phellandrene, (±)-limonene, isoeugenol, γ-terpinene	perfume
Creosote (beechwood creosote)	mixture of phenols obtained from wood tar produced by destructive distillation of wood	the tree, *Fagus grandiflora* (Fagaceae) and other trees	United States	guaiacol, creosol	disinfectant in the OTC drug, Dewitt's Toothache Drops®; expectorant in the OTC drugs, Creomulsin®, Creo-Terpin®

The more important drugs containing phenol volatile oils are thyme, clove, myrcia oil, creosote, pine tar, and juniper tar (Table 5–5).

Thymol is a phenol having the formula $C_{10}H_{14}O$.

Thymol may be obtained from thyme oil (*Thymus vulgaris* Linné), from horsemint oil (*Monarda punctata* Linné), from *Monarda didyma* Linné oil, from ajowan oil (*Carum copticum* Bentham et Hooker), or it may be prepared synthetically from m-cresol or p-cymene. The oil may be treated in 2 ways to obtain thymol crystals: (1) it may be subjected to freezing temperatures causing the thymol to crystallize, or (2) it may be treated with sodium hydroxide solution, the aqueous solution of sodium thymol being separated and decomposed with acid, thus liberating the thymol, which is subsequently purified.

Thymol occurs as large colorless crystals or as a white crystalline powder. It has an aromatic thymelike odor and a pungent taste. Thymol may be readily microsublimed.

USES AND DOSE. Thymol is an antifungal and antibacterial agent. It is employed topically in lotions, creams, and ointments in concentrations ranging from 0.1 to 1%.

NONPRESCRIPTION PRODUCTS. Thymol is used in the feminine hygiene products Bo-Car-Al®, PMC Douche Powder®, Stomaseptine®, and Zonite®; in the otic products Auro Ear Drops® and Stall Otic Drops®; in the external analgesics Vicks Vaporub® and Zemo Liquid®; and in Listerine® mouthwash.

CLOVE

Clove or cloves is the dried flower bud of *Eugenia caryophyllus* (Sprengel) Bullock et Harrison (*E. caryophyllata* Thunberg) (Fam. Myrtaceae) (Fig. 5–13). *Eugenia*, which is Latin, and *caryophyllus*, which is Greek, mean "nut-leaf," and refer to the

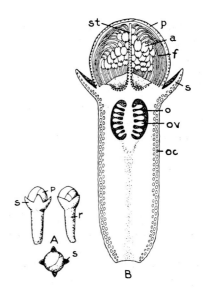

Fig. 5–13. *Eugenia caryophyllus: A*, Entire flower buds in side and upper views showing the cylindric receptacle (*r*), the 4 calyx teeth (*s*), and the globular closed corolla consisting of 4 petals (*p*). *B*, Longitudinal section through the flower bud showing petals (*p*), anthers (*a*), filaments (*f*), style (*st*), ovary (*o*), ovules (*ov*), and oil cells (*oc*).

nutlike flower buds; "clove" is from the Latin *clavus*, meaning a nail, and refers to the shape of the whole spice.

The plant is a tree that grows to 15 meters in height and is indigenous to the Molucca Islands but cultivated on the islands of Penang, Ambon, Pemba, Zanzibar, Sumatra, Madagascar, and Mauritius as well as in the Seychelles and the West Indies. The buds are gathered when they change from green to crimson and are carefully dried in the sun.

The average yield of dried cloves per tree approximates 7 pounds, although a large tree in a favorable year may produce as much as 40 pounds.

Buds are separated from their individual stems by hand and spread out on coconut mats to dry. In sunny weather, drying requires 4 or 5 days; in cloudy weather, a longer time is required. When rain threatens, the buds must be covered and protected. During proper drying, the buds lose about two thirds of their original weight.

The best cloves come from Pemba, but four fifths of the world's supply comes from Zanzibar. Clove was known to the Chinese before 266 B.C. The Dutch, who won possession of the Spice Islands in 1605, endeavored to create a monopoly and destroyed all the trees except those on the islands of Ambon and Ternate. In 1770, however, the French succeeded in introducing the tree onto Mauritius and Réunion. From there, its cultivation spread to other clove-growing areas. Almost 65% of the world's supply of cloves is ground and mixed with tobacco in cigarettes and consequently smoked. The largest consumer is Indonesia, which imports more than half of Tanzania's cloves each year.

Clove contains a volatile oil, 14 to 20%; gallotannic acid, 10 to 13%; oleanolic acid; vanillin; and the chromone, eugenin.

Uses. Clove is a carminative and a flavor.

Clove oil is the volatile oil distilled with steam from the dried flower buds of *Eugenia caryophyllus*. It contains not less than 85%, by volume, of total phenolic substances, chiefly eugenol ($C_{10}H_{12}O_2$).

Clove oil is a colorless or pale yellow liquid that becomes darker and thicker by age or exposure to air and has the characteristic odor and taste of clove.

The oil contains free eugenol (70 to 90%), eugenol acetate, and β-caryophyllene. Together these constituents comprise about 99% of the oil, but they do not account for the characteristic, fresh, fruity note of clove oil. This is owing to several minor constituents, especially methyl-n-amyl ketone.

Uses. Clove oil is classed as a flavor. It is commonly employed as a toothache remedy that is applied topically to dental cavities as required. Clove oil also possesses antiseptic, counterirritant, and carminative properties. Oils with a particu-

larly high content of eugenol are used in the commercial production of vanillin (see page 75).

Approximately 1 million pounds of clove oil are imported into the United States annually.

NONPRESCRIPTION PRODUCTS. Clove oil is used in Noxzema Medicated Cream®, Dr. Hands' Teething Lotion®, and Lavoris® mouthwash.

Eugenol or 4-allyl-2-methoxyphenol is a phenol, $C_{10}H_{12}O_2$, obtained from clove oil and from other sources. It is usually prepared from clove oil by shaking with a 10% solution of sodium hydroxide to form sodium eugenolate. The mixture is washed with ether, and the sodium eugenolate is then decomposed with sulfuric acid. The eugenol is separated by steam distillation. It is a colorless or pale yellow, thin liquid that has a strongly aromatic odor of clove and a pungent spicy taste.

Uses. Eugenol is classed as a dental analgesic. It is applied topically to dental cavities and is incorporated in dental protectives.

NONPRESCRIPTION PRODUCTS. Eugenol is an ingredient in the toothache preparations Benzodent®, Jiffy Toothache Drops®, and Numzident®.

PINE TAR

Pine tar, pix pini, or pix liquida is the product obtained by the destructive distillation of the wood of *Pinus palustris* Miller or of other species of *Pinus* Linné (Fam. Pinaceae).

Pine tar is a viscid, blackish brown liquid. It is noncrystalline, translucent in thin layers, and becomes granular or crystalline (owing to the separation of pyrocatechin) and opaque with age. Pine tar's odor is peculiar, empyreumatic, and aromatic; its taste is pungent.

Pine tar consists of a resinous substance admixed with a small quantity of turpentine, acetic acid, methyl alcohol, and various volatile empyreumatic substances. On distillation, 4 distinct classes of products are obtained: (1) an aqueous distillate, from 10 to 20%, consisting chiefly of acetic acid, methyl alcohol, and acetone; (2) a light oily distillate, from 10 to 15%, distilling under 150° C, and consisting of mesitylene, toluene, xylene, cumene, and benzene, products that are used as solvents for varnishes and similar substances; (3) a heavy oily distillate, about 15%, distilling over between 150° and 250° C and consisting of the creosote oils, i.e., phenol, creosol, paraffin, naphthalene, pyrene, chrysene, retene, and other substances; and (4) a black resinous mass, called **pitch** (50 to 65%), which has the odor of tar.

USES. Pine tar is a local irritant and an antibacterial agent. It also possesses expectorant properties.

NONPRESCRIPTION PRODUCTS. Pine tar is used in the eczema and psoriasis preparations, Packer's Pine Tar® and Polytar®.

Rectified tar oil is the volatile oil from pine tar that is rectified by steam distillation. It is a thin liquid, at first colorless, but eventually reddish brown. It has a strong empyreumatic odor and taste, but does not form a tarry deposit. It consists largely of hydrocarbons, such as pinene, some phenol compounds, and acetic and other acids.

USES AND DOSE. It is used as an expectorant and in ointments or lotions as a parasiticide and an irritant. Usual dose is 0.2 ml.

NONPRESCRIPTION PRODUCT. Pinex® cough syrup.

JUNIPER TAR

Juniper tar, cade oil, oleum juniperi empyreumaticum, or pix juniperi is the empyreumatic volatile oil obtained from the woody portions of *Juniperus oxycedrus* Linné (Fam. Cupressaceae).

The heartwood of the shrub, which is known as prickly cedar and is indigenous to southern France and other countries bordering the Mediterranean, is cut into shavings. These are packed tightly in retorts or kilns that have a drain and are then heated for several hours or days. The distillate separates into an upper oily layer, which constitutes the official product, a middle aqueous layer, and a lower layer of pitch.

Juniper tar is a viscid, clear, dark brown liquid with a tarry odor and a faintly aromatic, bitter taste. It contains the sesquiterpene, cadinene, associated with some phenolic and empyreumatic compounds.

USES. Juniper tar is a local antieczematic. Topically it is employed as a 1 to 5% ointment. It is also used as a parasiticide.

NONPRESCRIPTION PRODUCT. Polytar®.

PHENOLIC ETHER VOLATILE OILS

A number of phenolic ethers occur in volatile oils. The following are the more important examples: anethole (see Fig. 5-3) from anise and fennel (Table 5-6), safrole from sassafras (see page 495), nutmeg, and Japanese star anise.

Derivatives of safrole are also often found in volatile oils. Notable among these

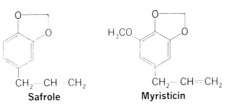

Safrole

Myristicin

Table 5–6.   Phenolic Ether Volatile Oil Drug

Name	Part Used	Botanical Origin	Geographic Origin	Important Constituents	Use
Fennel oil	volatile oil distilled with steam from the dried, ripe fruit	the perennial herb, *Foeniculum vulgare* (Umbelliferae)	central and eastern Europe, India, Japan	50–60% anethole, (+)-fenchone, (+)-α-pinene	flavor, carminative

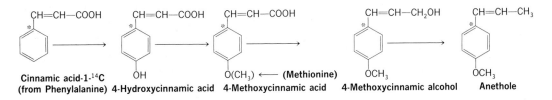

Fig. 5—14. Biosynthesis of anethole.

is myristicin (methoxysafrole) from nutmeg.

Biosynthesis of Phenolic Ethers. Studies of anethole biosynthesis in *Foeniculum vulgare* have revealed that formation takes place from phenylalanine (shikimic acid-phenylpropanoid pathway, see Fig. 5—5) via a number of intermediates (Fig. 5—14). A cell-free enzyme system capable of effecting the conversion has been prepared. Methionine serves as a methyl donor for the methoxylation reaction. Other structurally related phenolic ethers are presumably formed by similar pathways.

Some of the drugs containing phenolic ether volatile oil are anise, fennel, and myristica.

ANISE OIL

Anise or aniseed is the dried, ripe fruit of *Pimpinella anisum* Linné (Fam. Umbelliferae). *Pimpinella* is Latin and means two winged, referring to the bipinnate leaves; *anisum* is the old Arabic name for anise.

The plant is an annual herb indigenous to Asia Minor, Egypt, and Greece and cultivated in South America, Germany, Spain, Italy, and southern Russia (Fig. 5—15). The drug is derived from cultivated plants; Spanish anise is preferred.

Anise is one of the oldest known medicines and spices. It was mentioned by Theophrastus, Dioscorides, and Pliny and was one of the plants cultivated on the imperial farms of Charlemagne in the ninth century.

Anise contains volatile oil (1 to 3%), consisting of about 80 to 90% of anethole; fixed oil, up to 30%; proteins; and sugars.

Uses. Anise is a flavor and a carminative. The fruits are used as a flavor in certain types of bakery products.

Adulterants. Italian anise may be admixed with conium, which is distinguished by the absence of hairs and vittae and the presence of coniine. Coniine is determined by the development of the characteristic mouselike odor when rubbing up the powder with alkalies or placing it in a solution of potassium or sodium hydroxide.

Anise oil is the volatile oil distilled with steam from the dried fruit of *Pimpinella anisum* Linné (Fam. Umbelliferae), or from the dried, ripe fruit of *Illicium verum* Hooker filius (Fam. Magnoliaceae). The oil from the latter source is known as Chinese star anise oil.

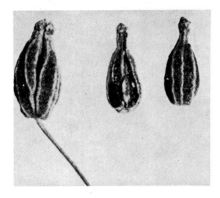

Fig. 5—15. Italian anise, magnified 6 times.

Anise oil is obtained largely from Spain, the southern Soviet Union, and Bulgaria, whereas star anise oil is distilled in southern China. The oils are much alike in constituents and physical properties. Anise oil is a colorless or pale yellow, strongly refractive liquid that has the characteristic odor and taste of anise.

The oil contains 80 to 90% of anethole plus small amounts of methyl chavicol, (+)-α-pinene, linalool, and anisaldehyde.

If solid matter separates, carefully warm the anise oil at a low temperature until it is completely liquefied and mix thoroughly before using. Anise oil should be preserved in well-filled, tight containers; exposure to excessive heat should be avoided.

Uses. Anise oil is a flavoring agent; however, it has carminative properties.

Anethole is (E)-p-propenylanisole. It is obtained from anise oil and other sources or is prepared synthetically. Anethole is a colorless or faintly yellow liquid at or above 23°C. At about 21°C, it solidifies to a crystalline mass that melts at 22 to 23°C. It has a sweet taste and the aromatic odor of anise. Because it is affected by light, anethole should be preserved in tight, light-resistant containers.

Uses. Anethole is a flavoring agent. It has carminative properties also.

Chinese anise or star anise is the dried, ripe fruit of *Illicium verum* Hooker filius (not *I. anisatum* Linné) (Fam. Magnoliaceae), a tree indigenous to southeastern Asia and cultivated in southern China, Vietnam, Japan, the Philippines, and Jamaica. However, the fruits have not been readily available in the United States for several years.

Illicium yields a volatile oil (anise oil) consisting chiefly of anethole (5 to 6% from the pericarp and 1.7 to 2.7% from the seed). Illicium was used as a stimulant and carminative.

Japanese star anise, shikimmi, or skimmi, the fruit of *I. religiosum* Siebold et Zuccarini (also known as *I. anisatum* Linné), is **very poisonous.** It is obtained from trees that are extensively cultivated in Japan, especially in groves of Buddhist temples. The fruits may be dangerous because of their resemblance to Chinese star anise, but the 2 kinds are seldomly mixed. The carpels (Fig. 5–16) are somewhat smaller than Chinese anise and the summit is acuminate and terminated by a short curved beak. Their odor is different from anise and resembles oil of sassafras or

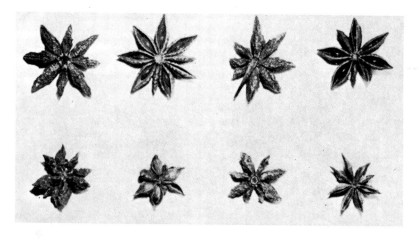

Fig. 5–16. Chinese star anise (top) and Japanese star anise (bottom).

laurel. The taste is intensely pungent and becomes aromatic, somewhat bitter, and camphorlike.

The Japanese star anise yields about 1% of a volatile oil with an unpleasant odor, quite unlike that of Chinese star anise. It is not produced commercially. The toxicity of the fruit is attributed to a principle designated hananomin.

NUTMEG

Nutmeg or myristica is the dried, ripe seed of *Myristica fragrans* Houttuyn (Fam. Myristicaceae) deprived of its seed coat and arillode and with or without a thin coating of lime (Fig. 5–17). The tree is indigenous to the Molucca and neighboring islands and is now extensively cultivated in other tropical regions, including the West Indies. The botanic name, *Myristica fragrans*, refers to the fragrance of the nutmeg. The commercial supply is largely derived from the Malay Archipelago. The trees bear continuously. Two or three crops are collected yearly. First the fleshy pericarp is removed and then the arillode, which constitutes mace when dried, is removed. The seeds are dried, requiring from 3 to 6 weeks, and then the brittle testa is cracked off.

With the exceptions of those from Penang, nutmegs are partially coated with lime to protect them from attack by insects. Over 5 million pounds of whole nutmegs are imported into the United States annually; over 80% of this amount comes from Indonesia.

Nutmegs were introduced into Europe by the Arabs about the middle of the twelfth century but were not a prevailing article of commerce until the sea routes to the Indies were opened in the sixteenth century. They played an important part in the Dutch spice monopoly until the tree began to be cultivated in other parts of the world (1800).

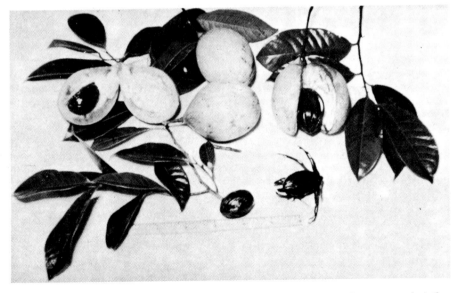

Fig. 5–17. Nutmeg *(Myristica fragrans)* showing the one-seeded fruits (called nutmeg apples), the exposed seeds which are partially covered by the arillode (mace), and the characteristic leaves. The arillode has been partly peeled from a nutmeg seed (right center) to show how it can be removed. (Photo, courtesy of Dr. Julia F. Morton, Director, Morton Collectanea, University of Miami.)

Nutmeg contains fixed oil, 25 to 40%, that is solid at ordinary temperatures, sometimes occurs in prismatic crystals, and is known as "nutmeg butter"; volatile oil, 8 to 15%, that contains myristicin and safrole; proteins in considerable amounts; and starch.

Uses. Myristica is a flavor and a condiment. Recently, it has attracted attention as a useful agent for controlling diarrhea associated with certain carcinomas.

In recent years, nutmeg has gained a reputation, especially among prison inmates, as a hallucinogenic agent. However, the relatively large amount (up to 15 g) that must be ingested to cause the desired intoxication also produces flushing of the skin, tachycardia, absence of salivation, and other undesirable side effects. The active principle(s) responsible for the effects on the central nervous system have not been identified with certainty, but elemicin and myristicin are believed to be involved. Some theories involve the in vivo biotransformation of these nutmeg constituents into amphetaminelike, nitrogen-containing metabolites.

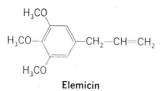

Elemicin

Nutmeg oil or myristica oil is the volatile oil distilled with steam from the dried kernels of the ripe seeds of *Myristica fragrans*. The oil is a colorless or pale yellow liquid that has the characteristic odor and taste of nutmeg.

East Indian nutmeg oil possesses different properties than those of West Indian nutmeg oil. The label of the container must indicate whether the oil is of East Indian or West Indian origin.

The oil contains *safrole* and *myristicin* (methoxysafrole), the chief constituents; methoxyeugenol; 60 to 80% of (+)-camphene; β-terpineol; α- and β-pinene; myrcene; (±)-limonene; and cineole.

Uses. Nutmeg oil is a flavoring agent. It possesses carminative properties.

OXIDE VOLATILE OILS

Cineole (eucalyptol) is found in eucalyptus and several other volatile-oil-yielding drugs. It is also called cajuputol because it occurs in cajuput. Coumarin (see page 76), the lactone of coumarinic acid (o-hydroxycinnamic acid), occurs widely throughout the legume family. It is discussed in the glycosidal drugs.

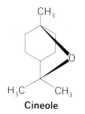

Cineole

EUCALYPTUS OIL

Eucalyptus is the dried, scythe-shaped leaf of *Eucalyptus globulus* Labillardière or of other species of *Eucalyptus* (Fam. Myrtaceae) (Fig. 5–18). This tree is indigenous to eastern Australia and Tasmania and is cultivated in southern Europe and in California. *Eucalyptus* is Greek and means well-covered, alluding to the lidlike cover of the buds, and *globulus* is Latin and refers to the form of the fruit. The commercial supply of the drug is largely from southern France, Spain, Portugal, Angola, and South Africa. The tree requires much water and has been used to dry up marsh land.

Eucalyptus contains volatile oil, 3 to 6%; several resins; and tannic acid.

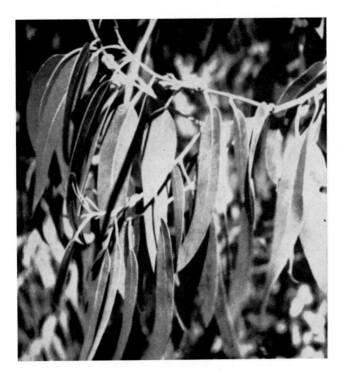

Fig. 5–18. Branch of eucalyptus tree showing fruits and scythe-shaped leaves.

Eucalyptus oil is the volatile oil distilled with steam from the fresh leaf of *E. globulus* or from other species of *Eucalyptus*. The oil is a colorless or pale yellow liquid that has a characteristic, aromatic, somewhat camphoraceous odor and a pungent, spicy, cooling taste.

Eucalyptus oil contains not less than 70% of cineole ($C_{10}H_{18}O$). Eucalyptus oil must be free from eucalyptus oils containing large amounts of phellandrene.

More than 300 species of *Eucalyptus* are recognized by botanists and several different chemical races of a single species may exist. For this reason, the chemistry of the various eucalyptus oils is an extremely complex subject.

Eucalyptus oils intended for medicinal use contain about 70 to 85% cineole, plus lesser amounts of volatile aldehydes, terpenes, sesquiterpenes, aromatic aldehydes and alcohols, and phenols. Many of these minor components have irritant properties and are removed by redistillation of the oil. Oils intended for industrial purposes have piperitone and/or phellandrene as their principal components. Other eucalyptus oils used in perfumery are rich in geraniol and its esters and citronellal.

Over 450,000 pounds of eucalyptus oil are imported into the United States annually.

USES. Eucalyptus oil is classed as a flavor. It is frequently used as an antiseptic, diaphoretic, and expectorant.

Cineole or eucalyptol is obtained from eucalyptus oil and from other sources. It is a colorless liquid that has a characteristic, aromatic, camphoraceous odor and a pungent, cooling, spicy taste. Cineole may be obtained (1) from eucalyptus oils by fractional distillation and subsequent freezing of the distillate or by treating eucalyptus oil with phosphoric acid and subsequently

Table 5–7. Ester Volatile Oil Drugs

Name	Part Used	Botanical Origin	Geographic Origin	Important Constituents	Use
Lavender oil	volatile oil distilled with steam from the fresh flowering tops	the dwarf shrub, *Lavandula angustifolia* (Labiatae)	Europe, United States, Northern Africa	30–60% (−)-linalyl acetate, (−)-linalool, cineol, γ-terpinene	perfume
Pine needle oil (dwarf pine needle oil)	volatile oil distilled with steam from the fresh leaf	the tree, *Pinus mugo* and its variety *pumilio* (Pinaceae)	central Europe	3–10% bornyl acetate, α-pinene, β-pinene, (−)-limonene	perfume, flavor
Mustard oil (allyl isothiocyanate)	volatile oil obtained by maceration with water of the dried, ripe seed with subsequent steam distillation	the annual herb, *Brassica nigra* or *B. juncea* (Cruciferae)	temperate climates worldwide	not less than 93% allyl isothiocyanate	rubefacient in the OTC drug, Musterole®

decomposing the cineole-phosphoric acid with water, or (2) from terpin hydrate as a dehydration product on treatment with acids.

USE. Cineole is classed as a flavor. It has properties similar to those of eucalyptus oil.

NONPRESCRIPTION PRODUCTS. Cineole and eucalyptus oil are employed in a wide variety of products, such as nasal inhalers and sprays, Dristan®, Sine-Off Once-A-Day®, Vicks Sinex®; feminine hygiene products, Bo-Car-Al® and Stomaseptine®; external analgesics, Antiphlogistine®, Mentholatum Deep Heating®, Minit-Rub®, and Vicks Vaporub®; and mouthwashes, Chlorazine®, Listerine®, and Odara®.

RELATED SUBSTANCE. A somewhat similar oil is **cajuput oil,** the volatile oil distilled from the fresh leaves and twigs of several varieties of *Melaleuca leucadendron* Linné (Fam. Myrtaceae) and rectified by steam distillation. Cajuput oil contains from 50 to 65% of cineole (cajuputol) terpineol, and various terpenes. It is used externally as a parasiticide and internally as a carminative, stimulant, and diaphoretic.

ESTER VOLATILE OILS

A wide variety of esters occurs in volatile oils. The most common are the acetates of terpineol, borneol, and geraniol. It is common practice to age perfumes to permit esterification, thus improving bouquet. Other examples of esters in volatile oils are allyl isothiocyanate in mustard oil and methyl salicylate in wintergreen oil (Table 5–7).

Biosynthesis of Esters. Terpene esters are generally formed from the respective alcohols by reaction with aliphatic acid moieties (commonly acetic acid), as was indicated for menthyl acetate. Formation of aromatic esters, at least in the case of methyl salicylate, involves the reverse process; that is, the aromatic acid reacts with an aliphatic alcohol (commonly methanol) to form the ester.

Labeled cinnamic acid has been incorporated into methyl salicylate by *Gaultheria procumbens*. The reactive form of cinnamic acid is presumably an ester of coenzyme A. The biosynthetic pathway (Fig. 5–19) involves o-hydroxylation of the

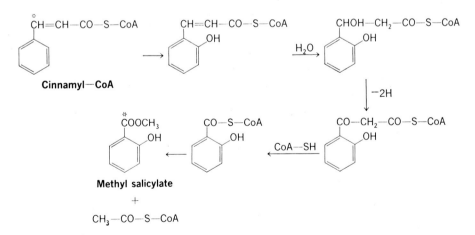

Fig. 5–19. Proposed biosynthetic pathway leading to methyl salicylate.

cinnamic acid and subsequent side-chain degradation.

Among the drugs in this section are lavender oil, dwarf pine needle oil, mustard oil, and gaultheria oil.

GAULTHERIA OIL

Gaultheria, wintergreen, teaberry, and checkerberry consists of the dried leaves of *Gaultheria procumbens* Linné (fam. Ericaceae), a low shrublike perennial with slender creeping or subterranean stems and branches that ascend from 5 to 15 cm in height. The leaves are alternate and evergreen, the flowers are white and axillary, and the fruit is a bright red, globular, aromatic berry. The plant is common in coniferous woods throughout the eastern United States and Canada. The leaves are coriaceous, the upper surface is dark green and shining, and the under surface is pale green. The odor is distinct and aromatic, and the taste is aromatic and astringent.

Methyl salicylate (see Fig. 5–3) is produced synthetically or is obtained by maceration and subsequent distillation with steam from the leaves of *G. procumbens* Linné (Fam. Ericaceae) or from the bark of *Betula lenta* Linné (Fam. Betulaceae). It contains not less than 98% of $C_8H_8O_3$. The product must be labeled to indicate whether it was made synthetically or was distilled from either of the plants mentioned. This oil is also known as **gaultheria oil, wintergreen oil, betula oil, or sweet birch oil.**

In several eastern states the oil is obtained by distilling wintergreen plants that have been chopped into small pieces and allowed to stand in water for about 12 hours. The oil may be purified by rectification with steam. When the oil is distilled from birch bark, the process is much the same. Methyl salicylate is made synthetically by distilling a mixture of salicylic acid and methyl alcohol.

Methyl salicylate is a colorless, yellow or red liquid that has the characteristic odor and taste of wintergreen. Synthetic oil and that obtained from *Betula* are optically inactive, but the oil obtained from *Gaultheria* is slightly levorotatory.

Methyl salicylate, the chief constituent of this oil, is formed when the glycoside, gaultherin, is hydrolyzed by the naturally occurring enzyme, gaultherase, in the presence of water.

Wintergreen oil contains, in addition to methyl salicylate, an ester that splits into enanthic alcohol and an acid. Enanthic alcohol and its ester possess the characteristic odor that distinguishes natural wintergreen oil from synthetic methyl salicylate.

USES AND DOSE. Methyl salicylate is a pharmaceutic aid (flavor) for aromatic cascara sagrada fluidextract. In addition, it has local irritant, antiseptic, and antirheumatic properties. For topical use, 10 to 25% concentrations in lotions and solutions are employed. Wintergreen oil has been used as a flavor for many years; however, large doses of this drug have produced toxic symptoms. Ingestion of 10 ml by children has caused death. Symptoms of poisoning include nausea, vomiting, pulmonary edema, and convulsions.

The principal adulterant of natural wintergreen oil is synthetic methyl salicylate.

READING REFERENCES

Amoore, J. E.: *Molecular Basis of Odor*, Springfield, Illinois, Charles C Thomas, Publisher, 1970.

Billot, M., and Wells, F. V.: *Perfumery Technology*, Chichester, England, Ellis Horwood Limited, 1975.

Charlwood, B. V., and Banthorpe, D. V.: The Biosynthesis of Monoterpenes, In *Progress in Phytochemistry*, Vol. 5, Reinhold, L., Harborne, J. B., and Swain, T., eds., Oxford, Pergamon Press Ltd., 1978.

Chemical Technology, Vol. V, *Natural Organic Materials and Related Synthetic Products*, New York, Barnes & Noble Books, 1972.

Croteau, R., and Loomis, W. D.: Biosynthesis and Metabolism of Monoterpenes, Flavours, 6(5):292, 1975.

Dorland, W. E., and Rogers, J. A., Jr.: *The Fragrance and Flavor Industry*, Mendham, New Jersey, Wayne E. Dorland Co., 1977.

Erickson, R. E.: The Industrial Importance of Monoterpenes and Essential Oils, Lloydia, 39(1):8, 1976.

Friedrich, H.: Phenylpropanoid Constituents of Essential Oils, Lloydia, 39(1):1, 1976.

Furia, T. E., and Bellanca, N., eds.: *Fenaroli's Handbook of Flavor Ingredients*, 2nd ed., Vol. 1, Cleveland, Ohio, CRC Press, Inc., 1975.

Green, R. J.: Peppermint and Spearmint Production in the United States—Progress and Problems, Flavors, 6(4):246, 1975.

Guenther, E.: *The Essential Oils*, Vols. I–VI, New York, D. Van Nostrand Co., Inc., 1949–1952.

Haslam, E. C.: *The Shikimate Pathway*, London, Butterworth & Co. (Publishers) Ltd., 1974.

Hefendehl, F. W., and Murray, M. J.: Genetic Aspects of the Biosynthesis of Natural Odors, Lloydia, 39(1):39, 1976.

Kalbhen, D. A., and Braun, U.: Evidence for the Biogenic Formation of Amphetamine Derivatives from Components of Nutmeg, Pharmacology, 9:312, 1973.

Lawrence, B. M.: Commercial Production of Noncitrus Essential Oils in North America, Perfumer & Flavorist, 3(6):21, 1979.

Masada, Y.: *Analysis of Essential Oils by Gas Chromatography and Mass Spectrometry*, New York, John Wiley & Sons, Inc., 1976.

Nes, W. R., and McKean, M. L.: *Biochemistry of Steroids and Other Isopentenoids*, Baltimore, University Park Press, 1977.

Newman, A. A.: *Chemistry of Terpenes and Terpenoids*, London, Academic Press Inc., Ltd., 1972.

Poucher, W. A.: *Perfumes, Cosmetics and Soaps*, 7th ed., Vols. I–II, Revised by Howard, G. M., London, Chapman and Hall Ltd., 1974.

Shaw, P. E.: Citrus Essential Oils, Perfumer & Flavorist, 3(6):35, 1979.

Theimer, E. T., and McDaniel, M. R.: Odor and Optical Activity, J. Soc. Cosmet. Chem., 22(1):15, 1971.

Weil, A. T.: Nutmeg as a Narcotic, Economic Botany, 19(3):194, 1965.

Chapter 6

Resins and Resin Combinations

Resins are amorphous products with a complex chemical nature. They are usually formed in schizogenous or in schizolysigenous ducts or cavities and are end products of metabolism. Physically, resins are usually hard, transparent, or translucent and, when heated, soften and finally melt. Chemically, they are complex mixtures of resin acids, resin alcohols, resinotannols, esters, and resenes. They are insoluble in water, and some investigators believe resins are oxidation products of the terpenes. Several resins are used in pharmacy and in the arts, among which rosin, guaiac, and mastic are typical examples.

Resins often occur in more or less homogeneous mixtures with volatile oils; the mixtures are known as **oleoresins.** Natural oleoresins are exemplified by turpentine and copaiba; pharmaceutic oleoresins are derived from ginger and capsicum. Oleoresins also occur in mixtures with gums; these mixtures are called **oleo-gum-resins.** Because gums are water-soluble carbohydrate derivatives, they can be separated from oleoresins rather easily. Oleo-gum-resins include asafetida and myrrh. The nomenclature of these resinous combinations is, at best, artificial because small amounts of volatile oil are often present in resins, and small amounts of gum are often present in oleoresins.

Balsams are resinous mixtures that contain cinnamic acid, benzoic acid, or both, or esters of these acids. Benzoin, Peru balsam, Tolu balsam, and styrax are typical balsams. The term "balsam" has been erroneously applied to some oleoresins, e.g., balsam of copaiba. This error has occasionally led to some confusion.

In a few cases, resins are found in glycosidal combinations; such combinations are called **glucoresins** or, more properly, **glycoresins.** Such glycoresins are found in jalap and podophyllum.

RESINS

When resins are separated and purified, they are usually brittle, amorphous solids that fuse readily when heated, after passing through a preliminary stage of softening. They are insoluble in water, but dissolve in alcohol or other organic solvents. These solutions on evaporation deposit the resin as a varnishlike film. Resins burn with a characteristic, smoky flame.

Resins may be the final products in destructive metabolism. Many are believed to be oxidation products of the terpenes. They are usually more or less complex mixtures and their principal constituents may be classified as follows:

Resin Acids. These contain a large proportion of oxyacids, usually combining the properties of carboxylic acids and phenols. They occur both in the free state and as esters. They are soluble in aqueous solutions of the alkalies, usually forming soaplike solutions or colloidal suspensions. Their metallic salts are known as resinates, and some of these resinates are used extensively in the manufacture of cheap soaps and varnishes. Examples of resin acids are abietic acid in rosin or colophony, copaivic and oxycopaivic acid in copaiba, and commiphoric acid in myrrh.

Resin Alcohols. Complex alcohols of high molecular weight, known as **resinotannols,** give a tannin reaction with iron salts. **Resinols** do not give such a reaction. The resin alcohols occur in the free state and as esters in combination with simple aromatic acids (benzoic, salicylic, cinnamic, and umbellic). The following

resinotannols have been isolated: aloeresinotannol from aloe, peruresinotannol from balsam of Peru, siaresinotannol and sumaresinotannol from benzoin, and toluresinotannol from balsam of Tolu. The following are examples of resinols: benzoresinol from benzoin and storesinol from storax.

Resenes. Complex neutral substances devoid of characteristic chemical properties are called resenes. They do not form salts or esters and are insoluble in and resist hydrolysis by alkalies.

Glycoresins. These are complex mixtures yielding sugars and complex resin acids on hydrolysis, as the resin of jalap.

Pharmaceutic Resins. Pharmaceutic resins are usually obtained (1) by extracting the drug with alcohol and precipitating the resin in water, as with resins of jalap and podophyllum; (2) by separating the oil from oleoresin by distillation, as rosin from turpentine and copaivic resin from copaiba; or (3) by collecting the natural product that has exuded as oleoresin from the plant through natural or artificial punctures and from which the natural oil has partially evaporated into the atmosphere, as mastic.

Biosynthesis of Resin Components. The exact chemical identity of most constituents of resin mixtures is unknown; thus, detailed information on the biosynthesis of these plant constituents is lacking. Many resin components are consid-

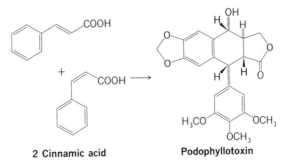

2 Cinnamic acid   Podophyllotoxin

Fig. 6–1. Proposed biosynthetic origin of podophyllotoxin.

ered to arise by oxidation of polymerized terpenoid metabolites. Acetate and mevalonate are incorporated into some resins, and a surprisingly rapid rate of "resin acid" turnover in pine has been suggested by studies with $^{14}CO_2$.

The aromatic acids in balsams are undoubtedly formed via the shikimic acid-phenylpropanoid pathway. Phenylpropanoid precursors are also believed to be involved in the formation of more complex resin components. The lignan, podophyllotoxin, which presumably arises via an oxidative coupling of 2 cinnamic acid residues (Fig. 6–1), is an example of this type of resin component. This belief is supported by the observed 1.4% incorporation of radioactivity into podophyllotoxin during preliminary feeding studies using phenylalanine-U-^{14}C and *Podophyllum emodi*.

ROSIN

Rosin or colophony is a solid resin obtained from *Pinus palustris* Miller and other species of *Pinus* Linné (Fam. Pinaceae).

The commercial grades of rosin vary in color from light amber (the finest or "water-white" grade) to almost black (and very dirty); the latter is used principally for destructive distillation and the production of "rosin oils." Rosin has a great variety of technical uses. Only the light-colored transparent rosins are used medicinally.

Rosin usually occurs as shiny, sharp, angular fragments that are translucent, amber-colored, and often covered with a yellowish dust. Rosin is hard, brittle, and easily pulverized. Its fracture is shallow-conchoidal; its odor and taste are faintly terebinthinate. Rosin is soluble in alcohol, ether, benzol, carbon disulfide, acetic acid, fixed and volatile oils, and in solutions of potassium or sodium hydroxide.

The alcoholic solution of rosin becomes milky white when added to water. When fragments of rosin are heated in water, they melt, flow together, and form a sticky mass.

Rosin contains from 80 to 90% of the anhydrides of abietic acid (which, on treatment with alcohol, are changed into crystalline abietic acid); sylvic acid, which is probably a decomposition product of abietic acid; sapinic acid; pimaric acid and other acids; and resene, a hydrocarbon.

Uses. Rosin is used as a stiffening agent in cerates, plasters, and ointments. It is employed in veterinary medicine as a diuretic. Commercially, rosin is used in the manufacture of varnishes, varnish and paint dryers, printing inks, soap, sealing wax, floor coverings, and numerous other products. Rosin is frequently used as an adulterant of other resinous products.

PODOPHYLLUM

Podophyllum consists of the dried rhizome and roots of *Podophyllum peltatum* Linné (Fam. Berberidaceae) (Fig. 6–2). It is also known as **mayapple** or **mandrake.**

The generic name is Greek and means footlike leaf; *peltatum* means shieldlike. The plant is a perennial herb that has a long, jointed, and branching rhizome. The rhizomes are dug either early in the spring or in the autumn after the aerial parts have died down. Most of the commercial supplies come from the central United States and from Virginia and North Carolina. The drug was known to the Indians, who introduced it to the early settlers. The drug should not be confused with mandragora, referred to as mandrake by the ancient Greeks and Asiatics (see page 209).

Mayapple is an important American botanic drug; the annual production is several hundred tons and supplies both domestic and export demands.

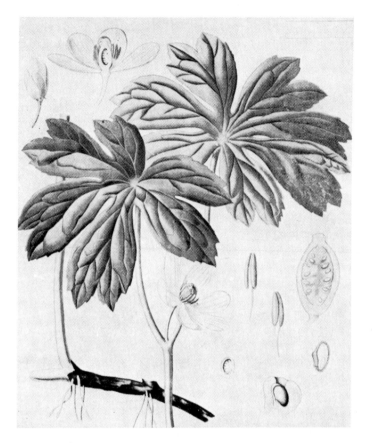

Fig. 6–2. *Podophyllum peltatum:* A portion of the long, horizontal, branched, nearly cylindric, dark brown rhizome, with internodes 2 to 10 cm in length, roots from the underside of the nodes, and a stem-scar, aerial stem, or bud from the upper side; the 2 large, peltate, deeply lobed leaves arising from the top of the stem with the large, white-petaled flower between them; the bud and the flower in median longitudinal section (upper left corner); the stamens, the ovary in cross-section, the fruit in longitudinal section, the ovule and the seed in longitudinal section (lower right corner).

Podophyllum contains 3.5 to 6% of a resin whose active principles are lignans. These include podophyllotoxin (20%), α-peltatin (10%), and β-peltatin (5%). A number of lignan glycosides are in the plant, but because of their water solubility, they are lost during the normal preparation of the resin.

The antimitotic and purgative properties of these compounds depend on a lactone ring in the *trans* configuration. Treatment with mild alkali produces epimerization with formation of the stable *cis* isomers, which are physiologically inactive. Picropodophyllin is an inactive *cis* isomer produced in this way from the active *trans* podophyllotoxin.

Podophyllum yields not less than 5% of podophyllum resin.

USES. Podophyllum possesses drastic purgative properties; however, it is employed in the form of podophyllum resin as an antimitotic and caustic.

ALLIED PLANTS. Indian podophyllum, the rhizome of *Podophyllum emodi* Wallich, a plant growing on the lower slopes of the

Himalayas, is larger and yields 11.4 to 12% of resin that contains about twice as much podophyllotoxin as the resin obtained from *P. peltatum*.

Podophyllum resin is also known as **podophyllin** and is the powdered mixture of resins removed from podophyllum by percolation with alcohol and by subsequent precipitation from the concentrated percolate when added to acidified water.

The precipitated resin is washed twice with water, and is dried and powdered. It is an amorphous powder that varies in color from light brown to greenish yellow and turns darker when subjected to temperatures exceeding 25° C or when exposed to light. It has a slight, peculiar, bitter taste and is highly irritating to the eye and to mucous membranes in general.

USES AND DOSE. Podophyllum resin is a caustic for certain papillomas. It is applied topically as a 25% dispersion in compound benzoin tincture or in a 70 to 96% solution of alcohol. Podophyllum resin has also been used as a drastic purgative and as a hydragogue cathartic. The dose employed was 10 mg.

A number of lignans with lactone rings in the *trans* configuration are the tumor-inhibiting constituents of podophyllum resin. Such compounds include podophyllotoxin, several podophyllotoxin derivatives, and α- and β-peltatin. The peltatins are responsible for most of the purgative effects of the drug.

PROPRIETARY PRODUCT. Podoben®.

ERIODICTYON

Eriodictyon or yerba santa is the dried leaf of *Eriodictyon californicum* (Hooker et Arnott) Torrey (Fam. Hydrophyllaceae). *Eriodictyon* is Greek and means woolly, referring to the hairy leaves. The plant is an evergreen shrub indigenous to the mountains of California and northern Mexico.

The drug has been employed by the Indians of California for many years.

Eriodictyon contains a resin, eriodictyol (the aglycone of eriodictin), xanthoeriodictyol, chrysoeriodictyol, homoeriodictyol, eriodictyonic acid, formic acid, butyric acid, volatile oil, and tannin.

USES AND DOSE. Eriodictyon is a flavor used to disguise the bitterness of certain preparations, such as those containing quinine. It has also been used as a stimulating expectorant in doses of 1 g.

JALAP

Jalap or jalap root is the dried, tuberous root of *Exogonium purga* (Wendoroth) Bentham (Fam. Convulvulaceae). Jalap yields not less than 9% of resins. *Exogonium* is Greek and means "outside" and "offspring," referring to the exserted stamens and pistils; Jalapa is the name of the city in Mexico from which the drug was first obtained. The plant is a perennial, twining herb indigenous to the mountains of Mexico and cultivated in Mexico, India, and, to some extent, in the West Indies. The plant possesses thin, horizontal, underground runners. The tuberous roots arise from the nodes of the runners. The roots are usually dug in the fall, placed in nets, and dried over open fires. This latter process accounts for their empyreumatic odor. Our nation's supply comes entirely from Vera Cruz.

Jalap contains resin, 8 to 12%; volatile oil; starch; gum; and sugar. The resin contains a number of glycosides, such as ipurganol, a phytosterol glycoside (also found in certain *Ipomoea* species) and jalapin, a mixture of acidic glycosides. It also contains β-methyl esculetin and palmitic and stearic acids.

USE AND DOSE. Jalap is a cathartic and is generally considered a hydragogue and a drastic purgative. Usual dose is 1 g.

Jalap resin is prepared by extracting powdered jalap with an alcohol-water mixture. The percolate is concentrated to one-fourth the weight of drug used and is then slowly poured into water and constantly stirred. The precipitated resin is washed with hot water, collected, and dried.

Jalap resin occurs as yellowish brown masses or powder. It is a cathartic possessing hydragogue activity. Usual dose is 125 mg.

MASTIC

Mastic, mastiche, or mastich is the concrete resinous exudate from *Pistacia lentiscus* Linné (Fam. Anacardiaceae). Mastic is Greek and means to chew; *Pistacia* is from the Persian *pistah*, the name of the pistachio tree; *lentiscus* refers to the lenticular cavities into which the resin is secreted. The plant is a shrub or small tree indigenous to the Mediterranean region and cultivated in the Grecian archipelago, especially on the island of Chios. The resinous juice collects in cavities in the inner bark. Long incisions are made in the trunk and in larger branches through which the resin exudes. The resin finally collects in small tears on the outside. The origin of the use of mastic is lost in antiquity; it is mentioned by both Theophrastus and Pliny. Mastic has long been chewed by Oriental women as a breath sweetener and is a common article in Oriental bazaars. Its employment in medicine dates back to about the thirteenth century.

Mastic contains about 90% of a resin, consisting of α-resin (mastichic acid), which is soluble in alcohol, and β-resin (masticin), which is insoluble in alcohol, and a volatile oil, 1 to 2.5%, which has the balsamic odor of the drug and consists chiefly of (+)-pinene. A bitter principle is also present.

Use. Mastic is used in the form of a dental varnish to seal cavities.

KAVA

Kava or kava-kava is the dried rhizome and roots of *Piper methysticum* Forster (Fam. Piperaceae). The plant is a large shrub widely cultivated in Oceania; its underground parts have been extensively used by the natives of these islands in the preparation of an intoxicating beverage.

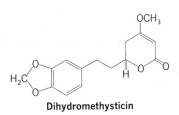

Dihydromethysticin

The drug contains, in addition to large quantities of starch, about 5 to 10% of a resin from which 6 different, closely related styrylpyrones have been isolated in pure form: yangonin, desmethoxyyangonin, kawain, dihydrokawain, methysticin, and dihydromethysticin. Pharmacologic studies have shown that all of the kava pyrones are more or less potent, centrally acting skeletal muscle relaxants. In addition to inducing changes in motor function and reflex irritability, they possess antipyretic and local anesthetic properties. Differences in action are largely quantitative. The central nervous and peripheral activities of the kava pyrones are sufficient to account for the native use of the drug.

CANNABIS

Cannabis, Indian hemp, marihuana, or pot consists of the dried flowering tops of the pistillate plants of *Cannabis sativa* Linné (Fam. Moraceae).

The plant is an annual herb indigenous to central and western Asia and is culti-

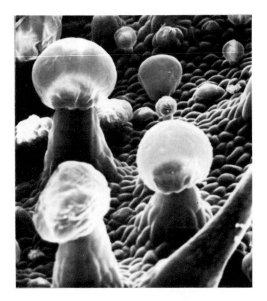

Fig. 6-3. Scanning electron micrograph of stalked and sessile glandular trichomes on the bract of a female plant of *Cannabis sativa*. The glands contain resin. Magnification 390 ×. (Photo, courtesy of Dr. Charles T. Hammond, Department of Biology, Wabash College.)

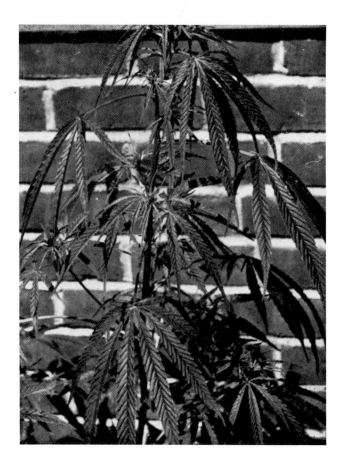

Fig. 6-4. American cannabis.

vated in India and other tropical and temperate regions for the fiber and seed. *Cannabis* is the ancient Greek name for hemp.

Cannabis was used in China and India, spread slowly through Persia to Arabia where the resin was known as **hashish,** and probably was introduced into European and American materia medica about the time of Napoleon.

Through long years of selective cultivation, 2 genetic types of cannabis have evolved. One, designated the drug type, is rich in THC. The other, referred to as the hemp type, contains little active principle (cannabidiol is the predominant cannabinoid) but has the elongated bast fibers desired in the manufacture of rope.

The amount of resin found in the pistil-

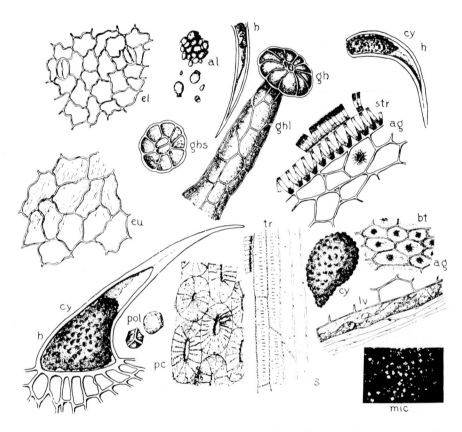

Fig. 6–5. Powdered cannabis. *el*, Epidermis from lower surface of leaves with sinuate vertical walls and numerous oval stomata, and *eu*, from upper surface, with straight walls and no stomata; *h*, nonglandular hairs, numerous, unicellular, rigid, curved, with a slender pointed apex and an enlarged base, usually containing a cystolith *(cy)*, but frequently broken, and the cystolith freed; glandular hairs of 2 kinds, 1 with a short 1-celled stalk *(ghs)* and the other with a long multicellular stalk *(ghl)*, the head *(gh)* in both kinds being globular and consisting of 8 to 16 cells; *bt*, fragments of bracts and leaves showing yellowish brown laticiferous vessels *(lv)*, numerous rosette aggregates *(ag)* of calcium oxalate, 5 to 30 μ in diameter, strands of spiral *(str)* or reticulate *(tr)* vessels, and phloem; *(pc)*, fragments of fruits with palisadelike, nonlignified cells with yellowish brown, finely porous walls; tissues of embryo and endosperm with numerous oil globules and aleurone grains *(al)*, the latter 5 to 10 μ in diameter and displaying crystalloids and globoids; *pol*, pollen grains; *mic*, photomicrograph of leaf fragment showing a rosette aggregate of calcium oxalate crystals in nearly every cell. (Drawings by Paul D. Carpenter.)

late flowering tops of *C. sativa* markedly decreases when the plants are grown in the more temperate climates (Fig. 6–3). Thus, Indian cannabis yields 20% or more of resin; Mexican cannabis 15% or less; Kentucky hemp 8% or less; Wisconsin hemp 6% or less. The active principles are found in the resin in about the same or in even smaller ratios than those just indicated. The hemp leaves contain a small amount of the resin.

Indian cannabis is prepared rather carefully from the pistillate flower heads only and contains relatively few leaves. Mexican and American cannabis consist of the whole upper portion of the stalk of the pistillate plant. Indian cannabis may have an activity many times greater than that of a poor quality of American cannabis. (Figure 6–4 shows the American cannabis plant; Figure 6–5 shows the structural elements in powdered cannabis.)

The unusual sensations induced in man by the uncontrolled use of cannabis are obtained more promptly and with less drug by inhaling the smoke of burning cannabis than by oral dosage. The importation into the United States of rather crude **Mexican cannabis (marihuana)** cigarettes began several decades ago. As the demand for these cigarettes **(reefers)** increased and the habit of smoking them spread to school children, federal and state narcotic agents started a campaign to stamp out their sale. The importation of Indian cannabis was prohibited and even large areas of naturally growing American hemp were destroyed. This campaign continues. The substitution of a poor quality drug for the high quality Indian cannabis and the marihuana campaign resulted in discontinued medicinal use of cannabis in the United States.

Indian cannabis yields 15 to 20% of a resin that contains the major active euphoric principle $(-)$-Δ^9-*trans*-tetrahydrocannabinol, commonly referred to as

Δ^9-THC. This compound was isolated almost simultaneously by 2 teams of investigators. One team viewed the compound as a dibenzopyran derivative and assigned the aforementioned name. The other group applied a monoterpene nomenclature, resulting in the designation Δ^1-*trans*-tetrahydrocannabinol. Both names are commonly found in the literature, but the dibenzopyran nomenclature is now more widely used in this country.

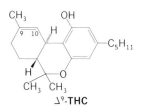

Δ^9-**THC**

Other constituents isolated from cannabis resin include cannabinol, cannabidiol, cannabidiolic acid, cannabichromene, cannabigerol, and Δ^8-*trans*-tetrahydrocannabinol. Tetrahydrocannabinols (Δ^8- and Δ^9-THC) possess euphoric activity, cannabinol is weakly active, and cannabichromene and cannabidiolic acid are sedative principles. Δ^9-THC has been synthesized and the pure compound utilized for physiologic studies in human beings. It was found to be more potent when smoked than when taken orally.

Cannabis is cultivated to a considerable extent for its bast fibers, **hemp,** and for its fruits, **hempseed;** the latter contain about 20% of a fixed oil that is expressed and used in the manufacture of paints and soap; the cake meal is used as cattle food.

OLEORESINS

Oleoresins are homogeneous mixtures of resins and volatile oils.

There is no sharp line of demarcation between these various types of resinous substances, and classification is some-times difficult. Small proportions of vol-atile oils are present in many resins. De-pending on the relative amount of volatile oil in the mixture, oleoresins may be liq-uid, semisolid, or solid. Usually, there is a small amount of "natural" exudate from oleoresin-containing trees owing to insect stings, broken branches, and other in-juries, but the commercial supplies are generally obtained by artificial incision through the bark and even into the wood.

TURPENTINE

Turpentine, gum turpentine, or gum thus is the concrete oleoresin obtained from *Pinus palustris* Miller and from other species of *Pinus* (Fam. Pinaceae).

"Gum" turpentine or "gum" is a com-mon name among the collectors and deal-ers of turpentine, but is a misnomer from the scientific standpoint. Turpentine is not related to the true gums and mucilages of carbohydrate origin.

Turpentine is collected from the longleaf pine (*P. palustris* Miller) and from the slash pine (*P. elliottii* Engelmann var. *elliottii*) that grow in North and South Carolina, Georgia, and northern Florida. The trees form vast forests and present a characteristic appearance owing to the "face" of the cut surface (Fig. 6–6). Tur-pentine yields depend on the treatment

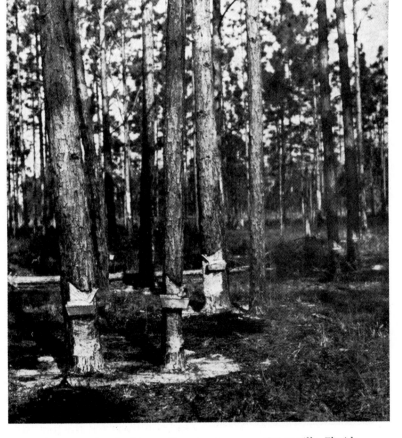

Fig. 6–6. Stand of turpentine pine trees near Gainesville, Florida.

and the size of the tree. Large trees measuring 45 to 50 cm in diameter are preferred although smaller trees may be turpentined also. If skillfully worked, trees yield for 15 to 20 years.

The oleoresin is secreted in ducts located directly beneath the cambium in the sapwood. During the spring of the year, bark is chipped from the tree by using a "bark hack," a long-handled cutting blade (Fig. 6–7). Following removal of the rounded chip, a spray of 50% solution of sulfuric acid is applied to the freshly cut surface. As the sap (oleoresin) flows, it is guided by metal gutters into containers attached directly to the tree trunk; the thick

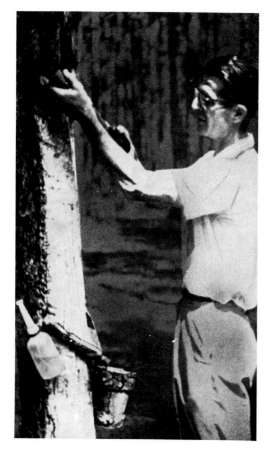

Fig. 6–7. Demonstration of method of cutting turpentine pine trees. Note the acid bottle.

liquid that collects is removed periodically and taken to the turpentine still.

The older method of chipping "deep and often" into the wood does not produce as much flow, requires more man-hours of labor per tree, and, because of the flat surface of the face, deteriorates the value of the butt log for lumbering purposes. Another method of collecting, i.e., making a "box" in the trunk to collect the sap, is no longer used.

The acid treatment collapses the thin-walled parenchyma cells that line the resin ducts. This allows the duct channels to become larger, providing a more rapid flow of oleoresin and reducing the chances of hardened secretions blocking the outlets. The acid does not stimulate greater production of oleoresin by the tree, but it enables more oleoresin from the ducts to escape, thus prolonging the flow. If applied properly, acid treatment does not injure the tree. This method has been much more successful than the fungous culture method used several years ago.

The usual turpentining season lasts about 32 weeks. The product of the first year's cutting is superior and is known as "virgin" turpentine. On steam distillation, it yields from 15 to 30% of volatile oil (turpentine oil, see page 114), whereas the product of the second or third year may yield not more than 10% of oil. The hot filtered residue left after distillation constitutes rosin (see page 146).

The United States is the world's largest producer of rosin and turpentine, accounting for about 70% of the supply. This industry is often referred to as "naval stores" trade because the wooden sailing vessels of the seventeenth century used enormous quantities of tar and pitch obtained from the coniferous forests of Europe. Since then, the trade has followed the location of the pine forests, moving from New England southward as the trees were depleted or became inaccessible.

Turpentine occurs as yellowish, opaque

masses that are lighter internally, more or less glossy, sticky when warm, and brittle in the cold. Its odor and taste are characteristic. It is freely soluble in alcohol, ether, chloroform, and glacial acetic acid.

The drug constituents are volatile oil and resin. It contains not more than 2% of foreign organic matter.

USE. It is employed externally as a counterirritant.

CAPSICUM

Capsicum or cayenne pepper is the dried, ripe fruit of *Capsicum frutescens* Linné, known in commerce as African chillies, of *C. annuum* Linné var. *conoides* Irish, known in commerce as tabasco pepper, of *C. annuum* var. *longum* Sendt, known in commerce as Louisiana long pepper, or of a hybrid between the Honka variety of Japanese capsicum and the old Louisiana sport capsicum, known in commerce as Louisiana sport pepper (Fam. Solanaceae). Capsicum must be labeled to indicate which variety is contained in the package.

Capsicum is from the Latin *capsa*, meaning a box, and refers to the partially hollow, boxlike fruit; *frutescens* is Latin and refers to the shrubby character of the plant; and *annuum* is Latin and refers to the annual character of the plant.

C. frutescens is a small spreading shrub, reaching 1 meter in height and is indigenous to tropical America and cultivated in tropical localities in Africa, India, America, and Japan. Apparently, the more tropical the climate, the more pungent the fruit. *C. annuum* is an herbaceous, annual form cultivated in mildly temperate to semitropical localities in central and southern Europe, Mexico, United States, and other countries. It is cultivated under the names of garden pepper, paprika, pimiento, Mexican chillies, Tabasco pepper, and others. All of these are less pungent than African chillies, but are desirable as condiments. The medicinal value of capsicum as a rubefacient depends on its pungency.

African cayenne comes chiefly from Kenya and Tanzania in East Africa and Sierra Leone in West Africa and is usually designated in the trade by the port from which it is shipped. Japanese chillies, usually exported from Kobe, are somewhat less pungent than African capsicum, but more pungent than Madras or Bombay chillies from India. Of the millions of pounds annually imported into the United States, about one half comes from India, one third from Japan, and one sixth from Africa.

Capsicum was first mentioned in 1494 by Chauca, a physician who accompanied Columbus on his second voyage to the West Indies. Plants were introduced into India by the Portuguese at an early date and later into Africa.

Tabasco peppers are about twice the size and Louisiana peppers up to 10 times the size of African capsicum. The outer epidermis of the pericarp of these peppers consists of irregular (not quadrangular) cells with thickened and strongly beaded, lignified, radial walls. They also possess a hypodermis of elongated cells with thickened, strongly beaded radial walls of cellulose or cuticularized cellulose. These features readily distinguish these peppers, in whole or powdered form, from genuine African capsicum.

Capsicum contains capsaicin (about 0.02%), an extremely pungent principle, in the dissepiments of the fruit. Capsaicin is a phenol having the formula:

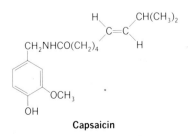

Capsaicin

It imparts a distinctly pungent taste to water, even when diluted to 1 part in 11 million parts of water. Capsicum also contains about 1.5% of a volatile oil, a fixed oil, carotenoids, and up to 0.2% of ascorbic acid (vitamin C).

USES AND DOSE. Capsicum is an irritant and a carminative; it is used as a rubefacient and also as a stimulant and a condiment. Usual dose is 60 mg. **Capsicum oleoresin** has the same properties. Usual dose is 15 mg.

PROPRIETARY PRODUCTS. Capsicum is an ingredient in a number of external analgesic preparations including Heet®, Infra-Rub®, Omega Oil®, and Sloan's®.

ALLIED DRUGS. Paprika, Hungarian paprika, or Turkish paprika is a large-fruited pepper obtained from varieties of *C. annuum.* It apparently is indigenous to America and was first introduced to Spain and then to Greece, Turkey, and Hungary. The fruits, when fresh, are 5 to 10 cm in length, 5 to 7 cm in diameter, more or less inflated, and bright red.

Spanish paprika or pimiento is paprika grown in Spain. The succulent pericarp is used for stuffing olives, and the dry pod is ground as a spice.

GINGER

Ginger or zingiber is the dried rhizome of *Zingiber officinale* Roscoe (Fam. Zingiberaceae), known in commerce as Jamaica ginger, African ginger, and Cochin ginger (Fig. 6–8). The outer cortical layers are often either partially or completely removed. *Zingiber* is from the Arabic Zindschebil, meaning root of Zindschi (India). The specific name refers to its use as an ingredient of preparations made in drug shops.

The ginger plant is propagated in Jamaica by rhizome cuttings that are planted in March and April. The rhizomes are dug and peeled in December and

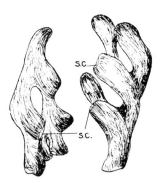

Fig. 6–8. Jamaica ginger: Irregularly branched rhizomes (4 to 16 cm long and 4 to 20 mm thick) from which the cork has been removed, showing depressed stem scars *(sc)* at the ends of the branches; the rhizomes are longitudinally striate, somewhat yellowish to light brown in color, break with a short-fibrous, starchy-resinous fracture, and have an aromatic odor and a pungent, aromatic taste.

January. As soon as they are peeled, the rhizomes are washed in water for hours, then dried in the sun for 5 to 6 days. They are covered at night and during rainy weather.

Ginger was known in China as early as the fourth century B.C. It was used as a spice by the Greeks and Romans. From the eleventh to the thirteenth centuries, ginger was a common import from the East. Marco Polo observed it in China and India from 1280 to 1290. Ginger was introduced into Jamaica and other islands of the West Indies by the Spaniards, and drug exports from the West Indies to Spain were made in considerable quantities as early as 1547. Exports from Jamaica to all parts of the world amount to more than 2 million pounds annually.

Ginger owes its characteristic aroma to about 1 to 3% of a volatile oil, the principal constituents of which are 3 sesquiterpenes: bisabolene, zingiberene, and zingiberol. The characteristic pungency of the drug is attributed to ginger oleoresin from which 2 aromatic ketones, zingerone and shogaol, have been isolated. In addition, ginger contains more than 50% of starch.

USES AND DOSE. Ginger is classed as a flavor; it is used as a condiment, an aromatic stimulant, and a carminative. The dose is 0.6 g. **Ginger oleoresin** has the same properties. Much of the ginger consumed in the present-day market is used in the manufacture of ginger ale.

WHITE PINE

White pine or white pine bark is the dried inner bark of *Pinus strobus* Linné (Fam. Pinaceae). The white or Weymouth Pine is the principal timber pine of the northern United States and Canada. The outer corky layer of the bark is removed before the inner portion is dried.

Pinus is the ancient Latin name, probably akin to *pinna*, and means a feather, referring to the somewhat featherlike foliage of many of the species. The specific name, *strobus*, pertains to the cones or strobiles.

The alcoholic extract forms about 30% of the drug and contains tannic acid and an oleoresin. The bark contains considerable mucilage and a small quantity of coniferin; the latter is usually present in the cambial layer of all of the species of *Pinus* as well as in other genera of the Pinaceae.

USE AND DOSE. White pine has expectorant properties. The usual dose is 2 g.

PROPRIETARY PRODUCTS. Cheracol®, Creomulsion®, and Prunicodeine®.

COPAIBA

Copaiba or balsam copaiba is an oleoresin derived from South American species of *Copaifera (Copaiba)* (Fam. Leguminosae). The oleoresin is formed in schizolysigenous cavities in the wood and seems to be a metamorphosed product of the cell walls; these cavities sometimes contain several liters of the oleoresin. The trees are tapped or boxed (see turpentine, page 153) to the center of the tree and the oleoresin conducted directly to containers. A tree frequently yields 20 to 24 liters.

It should be noted that the term *balsam* is erroneously applied. Copaiba is an oleoresin and contains neither benzoic nor cinnamic acid. It consists of a volatile oil, resin acids, and a small quantity of a bitter principle.

USES AND DOSE. Copaiba was used as a genitourinary disinfectant. It has diuretic, stimulant, expectorant, and laxative properties. The dose is 1 ml.

OLEO-GUM-RESINS

Oleo-gum-resins are mixtures of resin, gum, volatile oil, and, frequently, small quantities of other substances. The principal oleo-gum-resins are myrrh and asafetida.

MYRRH

Myrrh or gum myrrh is an oleo-gum-resin obtained from *Commiphora molmol* Engler, from *C. abyssinica* (Berg) Engler, or from other species of *Commiphora* Jacquin (Fam. Burseraceae). The name myrrh is from the Arabic *murr*, meaning bitter; *Commiphora* is Greek and means gum bearing; *molmol* is the native Somali name; and *abyssinica* refers to the habitat of the plants. The plants are small trees that sometimes attain the height of 10 meters and are found growing on the Arabian peninsula and in Ethiopia and Somalia.

The oleo-gum-resin exudes naturally or from incisions made in the bark; it is at first a yellowish color, but soon hardens in the intense heat of these countries, becomes darker, and is then collected. There are 2 principal commercial varieties of myrrh: **Africa or Somali myrrh** and **Arabian or Yemen myrrh.** The former is considered the better of the two. Practically all of the commercial supply comes from Somalia.

There are numerous references to myrrh in the Old Testament, but it is highly possible that the product thus designated was bdellium. Myrrh was an ingredient of the embalming material of the Egyptians. Its use in incense and perfumes in ceremonial religious life since the days of remote antiquity is well known. Theophrastus, Pliny, and other early writers mention myrrh, and from early times it has been valued in domestic medicine for its aromatic qualities.

Myrrh contains a yellow or yellowish green, rather thick, volatile oil, 2.5 to 8%, that has the characteristic odor of myrrh; resin, 25 to 40%, composed of several constituents, among which are resin acids (α-, β-, and γ-commiphoric acids), resenes, and phenolic compounds, one of which yields protocatechuic acid and pyrocatechin; gum, about 60%, consisting of soluble and insoluble portions and forming a mucilage that does not readily ferment (being of the acacia type) and yielding arabinose as one of the products of hydrolysis; and a bitter principle, sparingly soluble in water but soluble in alcohol.

USES. Myrrh is a protective; it has also been employed as a stimulant and a stomachic. It is used in mouthwashes as an astringent.

PROPRIETARY PRODUCTS. Astring-O-Sol® and Odara®.

ASAFETIDA

Asafetida or gum asafetida is the oleogum-resin obtained by incising the living rhizomes and roots of *Ferula assafoetida* Linné, *F. rubricaulis* Boissier, *F. foetida* (Bunge) Regel, and probably of other species of *Ferula* (Fam. Umbelliferae). *Assafoetida* is from the Latin *asa*, meaning gum, or from the Arabic *aza*, meaning healing. The Latin *foetida* refers to the ill-smelling, offensive odor of the drug.

Asafetida is sometimes referred to as devil's dung.

The plants are perennial branching herbs that reach up to 3 meters in height and are indigenous to eastern Iran and western Afghanistan. A substance supposed to be asafetida has been used under the name of *Laser* in Iran and India since time immemorial. It appears in Sanskrit works under the name of *Hingu*. It has long been employed by the Arabs, who no doubt introduced it into Europe during the Middle Ages.

Asafetida occurs as a soft, sometimes almost semiliquid mass, as irregular masses of agglutinated tears, or as separate ovoid tears that range from 1 to 4 cm in diameter and which, when fresh, are tough, yellowish white and translucent. These tears change in color gradually to pinkish, violet-streaked, and finally reddish brown. They are hard and brittle when dry. Internally, the tears are milky-white and opaque, odor is persistently alliaceous, and taste is bitter, alliaceous, and acrid. Asafetida should be kept in tightly closed bottles.

The drug contains from 4 to nearly 20% of a volatile oil, 40 to 65% of resin, and about 25% of gum. The main constituent of the oil is isobutylpropanyl disulfide that is accompanied by a number of related organic disulfides. Some terpenes are apparently also present. The resin consists of asaresinotannol, both free and combined with ferulic acid. Umbelliferone is also present in combined form.

USES AND DOSE. Asafetida has been used as a carminative, an expectorant, an antispasmodic, and a laxative. The dose is 400 mg. Asafetida tincture is commercially available.

BALSAMS

Balsams are resinous mixtures that contain large proportions of benzoic acid, cinnamic acid, or both, or esters of these acids.

Benzoin is sometimes referred to as a balsamic resin. The medicinal balsams include Tolu balsam, Peru balsam, styrax (Levant and American), and benzoin (Siam and Sumatra).

STORAX

Storax is a balsam obtained from the trunk of *Liquidambar orientalis* Miller, known in commerce as Levant storax, or of *L. styraciflua* Linné, known in commerce as American storax (Fam. Hammamelidaceae). Storax is also known as **liquid storax** or **styrax.**

The term *styrax* is from the Arabian *assitirax*, meaning a sweet-smelling exudation; *Liquidambar* is from the Latin *liquidus*, meaning fluid, and from the Arabian *ambar*, meaning amber; *orientalis* means pertaining to the Orient; and *styraciflua* means to flow storax.

L. orientalis is a tree that attains a height of about 15 meters and grows in Asia Minor. *L. styraciflua* is a tree that attains a height of up to 40 meters and grows in southern North America, Central America, and northern South America. Levant storax is a pathologic product; its formation is induced by bruising or puncturing the bark of the tree in early summer, thereby causing the cambium to produce new wood with balsam-secreting ducts. In autumn, the bark, which is more or less saturated with balsam, is peeled off and the balsam is recovered by pressing. The bark is then boiled in hot water and pressed again. The balsam is poured into casks or cans and is usually exported via Smyrna.

Most of the American storax is produced in Central America where large forests of *L. styraciflua* are found. The balsam exudes into natural pockets between the bark and the wood and may be located by excrescences on the outside of the bark. These pockets, which contain up to 4 kg of the balsam, are tapped with gutters and the balsam is led into containers. The balsam is exported in tin cans. A large quantity is also produced in the United States but is used mostly in the tobacco industry for flavoring cigarettes.

The early Arabian physicians were acquainted with storax, and it is mentioned as early as the twelfth century. Most of the styrax used in pharmacy comes from Turkey and Honduras.

Levant storax occurs as a viscid, grayish to grayish brown, more or less opaque, semiliquid mass that deposits a heavier, dark brown, oleoresinous stratum on standing. American storax is a nearly clear, yellowish brown semiliquid that becomes hard, opaque, and darker colored. Storax is transparent in thin layers; its odor is agreeable and its taste is balsamic. Storax is insoluble in water, but almost completely soluble in warm alcohol.

Levant storax consists of about 50% of 2 resin alcohols, α-storesin and β-storesin, which are partly free and partly in combination with cinnamic acid. α-Storesin is amorphous, but forms a crystalline compound with potassium. β-Storesin occurs as white flakes that do not form a crystalline compound with potassium. Storax also contains storesin cinnamate, 10 to 20%; styracin or cinnamyl cinnamate, 5 to 10%, in needle-crystals that are colorless, odorless, and tasteless; phenylpropyl cinnamate, 10%, a liquid with the odor and taste of styrax; volatile oil, 0.5 to 1%; a trace of vanillin; free cinnamic acid, from 2 to 5%; and small amounts of several other substances. Free cinnamic acid may be obtained from storax by microsublimation with a yield of up to 20%.

American storax contains related storesins and other principles of levant storax: it yields 7% of volatile oil by steam distillation and contains about 28% of cinnamic acid, 23% of cinnamein, 35% of resin esters, and 2% of resin acids.

USES AND DOSE. Storax is a pharmaceutic aid for compound benzoin tincture. It has been used as a stimulant, an expectorant, and an antiseptic. When used internally, the dose is 1 g.

PERUVIAN BALSAM

Peruvian balsam, Peru balsam, or balsam of Peru is obtained from *Myroxylon pereirae* (Royle) Klostzsch (Fam. Leguminosae). *Myroxylon* is from the Greek *myron*, meaning ointment, and *xylon*, meaning wood; *pereirae* is in honor of Jonathan Pereira (1804 to 1853), an English pharmacognosist. "Peru" refers to the early importation of the balsam into Spain via Lima, Peru.

The balsam trees attain a height of about 25 meters and are especially abundant along the coast of El Salvador in Central America. The tree has been naturalized in Florida and in Sri Lanka. It was frequently referred to by writers who described the conquest of Guatemala in 1524. In the seventeenth century, the drug appeared in German pharmacy, after which its use became universal.

The balsam is a pathologic product and is formed by injury to the trees. The tree is beaten on 4 sides and then scorched with a torch to cause the bark to separate from the trunk. Four intermediate strips are left uninjured so as not to kill the tree. Within a week, the bark drops from the trunk and the balsam begins to exude freely from the exposed wood. The areas are then wrapped with rags that are removed from time to time when they become saturated with balsam. The rags are then boiled with water and, as the water cools, the balsam settles out, is recovered, strained, and packed, usually in tin cans. Most of the commercial supply comes from El Salvador, although some is produced in Honduras.

Peruvian balsam occurs as a dark brown, viscid liquid that appears reddish brown and transparent in thin layers. It is free from stringiness or stickiness and has an empyreumatic, aromatic, vanillalike odor and a bitter, acrid, persistent taste.

The drug contains cinnamein, about 60%, which is a volatile oil consisting chiefly of benzyl cinnamate and a lesser amount of benzyl benzoate; resin esters, 30 to 38%, which are composed mostly of peruresinotannol cinnamate and benzoate; vanillin; free cinnamic acid; peruviol; and other substances in small amounts.

Uses. Peru balsam is a local protectant and rubefacient; it also is a parasiticide in certain skin diseases. It is an antiseptic and vulnerary and is applied externally, either alone, in alcoholic solution, or in the form of an ointment.

Proprietary Products. The drug is employed for its astringent properties in various preparations used to treat hemorrhoids. These include Anusol® and Eudicaine® suppositories and Wyanoid® ointment and suppositories.

TOLU BALSAM

Tolu balsam is a balsam obtained from *Myroxylon balsamum* (Linné) Harms (Fam. Leguminosae). Tolu balsam is sometimes called balsam of Tolu.

The balsam trees grow abundantly along the lower Magdalena River in Colombia. Tolu is a district near Cartagena, where the balsam was once extensively produced.

Balsam of Tolu is usually considered to be a pathologic product similar to balsam of Peru or coniferous oleoresins. V-shaped incisions are made through the bark and sap wood, and calabash cups receive the flow of balsam. Similar cuts are made higher on the trees; sometimes as many as 20 incisions are made on a tree. The balsam is collected from the cups and transferred to tin containers in which it is shipped.

Some balsam of Tolu is also produced in Venezuela, and trees are now being cultivated in the West Indies. Tolu balsam was used by the natives in Colombia and Venezuela. Monardes (1574) described its collection, stating that the drug was much esteemed by the Indians and later by the Spanish, who introduced it into Europe.

Much of the balsam of Tolu entering the United States comes from Great Britain, where a certain amount of the volatile oil has been removed. Sufficient oil remains, however, so that the balsam meets the official requirements.

Tolu balsam occurs as a plastic solid that gradually hardens, becoming brown or yellowish brown. It is transparent in thin layers; brittle when old, dried, or exposed to cold, and shows numerous crystals of cinnamic acid. Its odor is agreeably aromatic, resembling that of vanilla, and its taste is aromatic and slightly pungent.

The drug contains resin esters, 75 to 80%, chiefly toluresinotannol cinnamate with a small quantity of the benzoate; volatile oil, 7 to 8%, chiefly benzyl benzoate; free cinnamic acid, 12 to 15%; free benzoic acid, 2 to 8%; vanillin; and other constituents in small quantities.

Uses. Tolu balsam is a pharmaceutic aid for compound benzoin tincture. It is sometimes used as an expectorant and is extensively used as a pleasant flavoring in medicinal syrups, confectionery, chewing gum, and perfumery.

BENZOIN

Benzoin is the balsamic resin obtained from *Styrax benzoin* Dryander, *S. paralleloneurus* Perkins, known in commerce as Sumatra benzoin, *S. tonkinensis* (Pièrre) Craib ex Hartwich, or other species of the Section *Anthostyrax* of the genus *Styrax*, known in commerce as Siam benzoin (Fam. Styraceae). *Styrax* is the ancient Greek name of storax, the name applied to a sweet-scented gum and to the tree producing it; *benzoin* is from the Arabic *ben*, meaning fragrant, or the Hebrew *ben*, meaning a branch, and *zoa*, an exudation,

meaning the juice of the branch; *tonkinensis* is named after Tonkin, the northern region of Vietnam.

The plants are trees of medium height that grow in southeastern Asia and the East Indies. *S. benzoin* is cultivated throughout Sumatra; *S. tonkinensis* in Thailand, Vietnam and Laos. Benzoin is a pathologic product developed by incising the bark. After about 2 months, the exuding balsamic resin becomes less sticky and firm enough to collect.

The first tapping of *S. benzoin* yields the so-called almond tears. The second tapping yields a more fluid substance. The almond tears and the fluid substance are imported into Singapore and are admixed (possibly with adulterants) to produce block benzoin.

In Thailand, the separate tears are scraped from the trees. New incisions are continually made until the trees die. The tree contains no secretory cells, nor does it contain the constituents of the balsamic resin until it is incised. The bark of the normal tree contains considerable tannin. The resinotannols in benzoin are probably produced from this tannin. Benzoin was unknown to the Greeks and Romans. It was first mentioned by Ibn Batuta, who visited Sumatra in the fourteenth century. In the fifteenth century, it still appeared as a precious balsam, but in the sixteenth century it was an article of Venetian commerce.

The use of Siam benzoin is confined almost entirely to perfumery. The tears of Siam benzoin are graded according to size and color; the smaller tears and siftings are darker in color. In pharmacy, only the Sumatra benzoin is used. Before World War II, Sumatra benzoin was obtained directly from Sumatra; today almost all Sumatra benzoin is imported from Singapore.

Sumatra benzoin occurs as blocks or irregular masses composed of tears of variable size imbedded in a translucent or opaque matrix. It is brittle and the tears internally are milky white, becoming soft when warmed and gritty when chewed. The matrix is reddish or grayish brown; the odor is agreeable, balsamic, and resembles that of styrax; the taste is aromatic and resinous.

Siam benzoin occurs mostly in separate concavo-convex tears that are yellowish brown to rusty brown externally and milky white on the freshly broken surface. The tears are brittle but become soft when warmed and plastic when chewed. It has a vanillalike odor.

Siam benzoin consists principally of coniferyl benzoate (60 to 70%), plus smaller amounts of free benzoic acid (10%), the triterpene, siaresinol, (6%), and a trace of vanillin.

Sumatra benzoin contains free balsamic acids, chiefly cinnamic (10%) and benzoic (6%), as well as esters derived from them. Triterpene acids, especially 19-hydroxyoleanolic and 6-hydroxyoleanolic, and traces of vanillin, phenylpropyl cinnamate, cinnamyl cinnamate, and phenylethylene are also present.

Sumatra benzoin yields not less than 75% of alcohol-soluble extractive; Siam benzoin yields not less than 90% of alcohol-soluble extractive.

Uses. Benzoin possesses antiseptic, stimulant, expectorant, and diuretic properties.

Compound benzoin tincture is employed as a topical protectant and is applied as required. It contains benzoin, aloe, storax, and Tolu balsam and is valuable as an expectorant when vaporized.

Benzoic acid (C_6H_5COOH) is now a synthetic product but was first obtained by sublimation from Sumatra benzoin.

It occurs as white crystals, usually in the form of scales or needles. It has a slight odor of benzoin and is volatile at moderate temperatures, freely so in steam.

Benzoic acid and its sodium salt are extensively used as a preservative of foods, drinks, fats, pharmaceutic preparations, and other substances. Medicinally, it is used primarily as an antifungal agent. It is an ingredient in benzoic and salicylic acids ointment (Whitfield's ointment), which is effective in the treatment of athlete's foot and, to a lesser extent, ringworm.

READING REFERENCES

Balbaa, S. I., Karawya, M. S., and Girgis, A. N.: The Capsaicin Content of Capsicum Fruits at Different Stages of Maturity, Lloydia, *31* (3):272, 1968.

Bernfeld, P., ed.: *Biogenesis of Natural Compounds*, 2nd ed., New York, Pergamon Press, Inc., 1967.

Efron, D., ed.: *Ethnopharmacologic Search for Psychoactive Drugs*, Public Health Service Publication No. 1645, Washington, D.C., U.S. Government Printing Office, 1967.

Emmenegger, H., Stähelin, H., Rutschmann, J., Renz, J., and von Wartburg, A.: Zur Chemie und Pharmakologie der *Podophyllum*-Glucoside und ihrer Derivate, Arzneim. Forsch., *11* (4,5):327, 459, 1961.

Guenther, E.: Ginger in Jamaica, Coffee and Tea Ind., *82*(1):169, 1959.

Howes, F. N.: *Vegetable Gums and Resins*, Waltham, Massachusetts, Chronica Botanica Co., 1949.

Mantell, C. L., Kopf, C. W., Curtis, J. L., and Rogers, E. M.: *The Technology of Natural Resins*, New York, John Wiley & Sons, Inc., 1942.

Nahas, G. G.: *Marihuana—Deceptive Weed*, New York, Raven Press, Publishers, 1975.

Pravatoroff, N.: Ginger—The Properties and Chemistry of Some Natural Spicy Compounds, Mfg. Chemist, *38*(3):40, 1967.

Schroeder, H. A.: The p-Hydroxycinnamyl Compounds of Siam Benzoin Gum, Phytochemistry *7*(1):57, 1968.

Walker, G. T.: Balsam of Peru, Perfumery Essent. Oil Record, *59*(10):705, 1968.

Waller, C. W., Johnson, J. J., Buelke, J., and Turner, C. E.: *Marihuana: An Annotated Bibliography*, New York, Macmillan Information, 1976.

Chapter 7

Steroids

Steroids comprise a natural product class of compounds that is widely distributed throughout nature. The diversity of biologic activities of steroids includes the development and control of the reproductive tract in man, (estradiol, progesterone, testosterone), the molting of insects (ecdysone), and the induction of sexual reproduction in aquatic fungi (antheridiol). In addition, steroids contribute to a wide range of therapeutic applications, such as cardiotonics (digitoxin), vitamin D precursors (ergosterol), oral contraceptive agents (semisynthetic estrogens and progestins), anti-inflammatory agents (corticosteroids), and anabolic agents (androgens).

NOMENCLATURE

A steroid is any compound that contains a cyclopentanoperhydrophenanthrene nucleus. The chemical nomenclature of steroids is based on this fundamental carbocycle with adjacent side-chain carbon atoms. Each parent tetracyclic hydrocarbon bears a specific stem name, and some of the principal hydrocarbons are shown in Figure 7–1. Steroids are numbered and

rings are lettered as indicated in the structural formula for cholesterol. If one or more of the carbon atoms shown in the structure of cholesterol is not present, the numbering of the remainder is undisturbed.

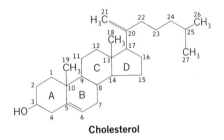

Cholesterol

When the rings of a steroid are denoted as projections onto the plane of the paper, an atom or group attached to a ring is termed α (alpha) if it lies below the plane of the paper or β (beta) if it lies above the plane of the paper. In formulas, bonds to atoms or groups attached in an α configuration are shown as broken (〰〰〰) lines, and bonds to atoms or groups attached in a β configuration are shown as solid lines.

163

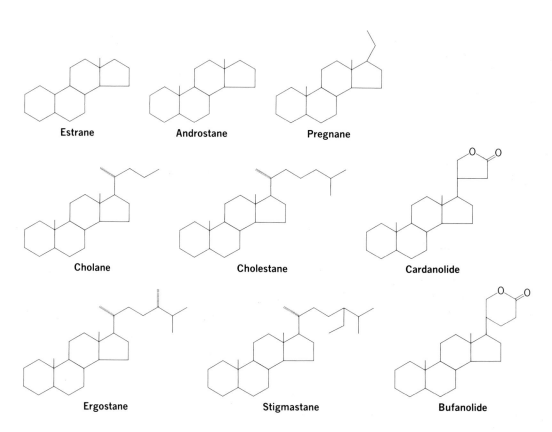

Fig. 7–1. Principal steroid stereoparent hydrocarbons.

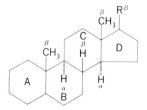

Fig. 7–2. Orientation of steroid substituents.

The use of a steroid stem name implies that atoms or groups attached at the ring-junction positions 8, 9, 10, 13, and 14 are oriented as shown in Figure 7–2 (8β, 9α, 10β, 13β, 14α), and a carbon chain (R) attached to position 17 is assumed to be β oriented. The configuration of hydrogen or

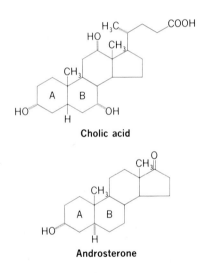

Cholic acid

Androsterone

a substituent at the ring-junction position 5 is always designated by adding α or β after the numeral 5. This numeral and letter are placed immediately before the stem name. The implication of these conventions of nomenclature is that, in most steroids, rings B and C and rings C and D are fused *trans*, whereas rings A and B may be fused either *cis* or *trans*. For example, the bile acid, cholic acid, has a *cis*-fused A/B ring junction. The chemical name of cholic

acid is 3α, 7α, 12α-trihydroxy-5β-cholan-24-oic acid. The sex hormone androsterone, chemical name 3α-hydroxy-5α-androstan-17-one, has a *trans*-fused A/B ring junction.

BIOSYNTHESIS

Steroids are formed biosynthetically from isopentenyl pyrophosphate (active isoprene) and involve the same sequence of reactions as does terpenoid biosynthesis. In fact, the triterpenoid squalene is an intermediate in steroid biosynthesis. Most knowledge of the biosynthesis of steroids has been derived from studies of cholesterol production. Although this compound is not necessarily a direct precursor of all other steroids, its formation may be considered as a general mechanism of steroid biosynthesis. The familiar acetate $\rightarrow\rightarrow$ mevalonate $\rightarrow\rightarrow$ isopentenyl pyrophosphate $\rightarrow\rightarrow$ squalene $\rightarrow\rightarrow$ cholesterol pathway is outlined in Figure 7–3.

In plants and animals, squalene is converted to the 2,3-epoxide, and the cyclization might be concerted because no intermediates have been isolated between oxidosqualene and cycloartenol or lanosterol. As shown in Figure 7–3, a proton initiates the cyclization by attacking the epoxide bond, which then sets off a succession of electron migrations from the 5,10-, 8,9-, 13,14-, and 17,20-double bonds. The resulting carbonium ion, which has a positive charge at C-20, is stabilized by rearrangements involving 2 hydride shifts (17$\rightarrow$20, 13$\rightarrow$17) and 2 methyl shifts (14$\rightarrow$13, 8$\rightarrow$14). These shifts result in the migration of the positive charge to C-8 and, with the loss of a proton from C-9, either the 9,10,19-cyclopropane ring of cycloartenol or the 8,9-double bond of lanosterol may be formed. The conversion of the C_{30} compound, lanosterol, to the C_{27} steroid, cholesterol, involves the loss of 3 methyl groups, the shift of a double bond,

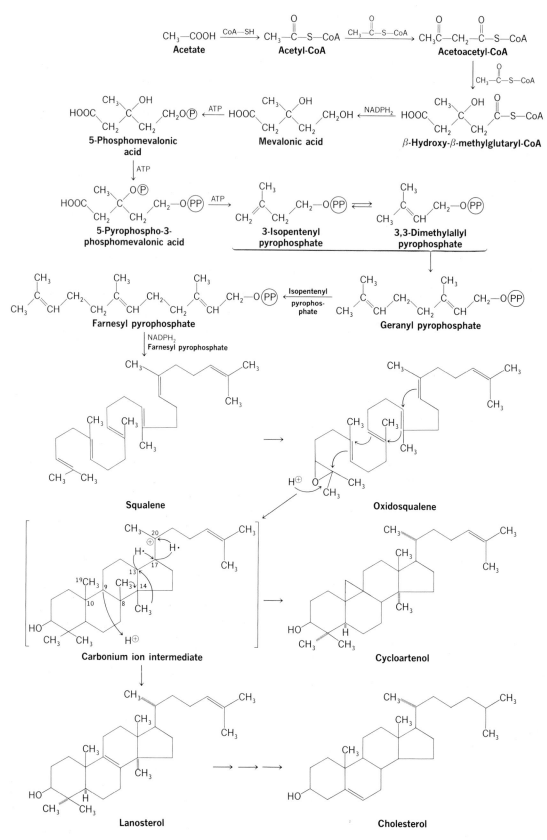

Fig. 7–3. Biosynthesis of cholesterol.

and a reduction of a double bond. The sequence in which these reactions take place may vary depending on the organism. Consequently, numerous intermediates, including zymosterol, have been isolated that represent various stages in this transformation.

STEROLS

The first steroids isolated from nature were a series of C_{27}-C_{29} alcohols that were found in the lipid fractions of many tissues. These compounds were solids and therefore named **sterols** from the Greek

stereos, meaning solid (Fig. 7–4). The most widely occurring sterol is cholesterol. It was first isolated from human gallstones and, because it is a constituent of animal cell membranes, it has been found in all animal tissue. It is one of the chief constituents of lanolin and therefore is found in many drug products. Until recently, cholesterol was thought to be restricted to the animal kingdom; however, it has now been identified in algae, fungi, actinomycetes, bacteria, ferns, and higher plants.

Much has been written about cholesterol and human health. Cholesterol is present in atherosclerotic plaques, and feeding of

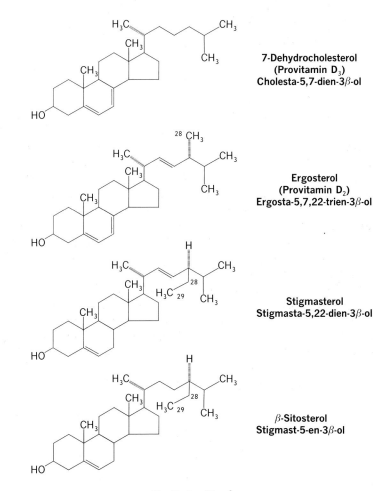

**7-Dehydrocholesterol
(Provitamin D₃)
Cholesta-5,7-dien-3β-ol**

**Ergosterol
(Provitamin D₂)
Ergosta-5,7,22-trien-3β-ol**

**Stigmasterol
Stigmasta-5,22-dien-3β-ol**

**β-Sitosterol
Stigmast-5-en-3β-ol**

Fig. 7–4. Sterols.

cholesterol to susceptible animals has induced atherosclerosis. In man, atherosclerosis is frequently associated with conditions in which the blood cholesterol is elevated. However, at the present time, the evidence of a causal relationship between cholesterol and atherosclerosis is still indirect.

The principal sterol in fungi is ergosterol. This C_{28} sterol arises biosynthetically through a transmethylation reaction of the cholestane side chain involving S-adenosyl methionine. Ergosterol is also known as provitamin D_2 because, upon ultraviolet irradiation, a series of isomerizations with the subsequent opening of ring B results in the formation of vitamin D_2. Vitamin D_3 is formed in the same manner from 7-dehydrocholesterol. This compound occurs in small amounts with cholesterol in animal tissue, including the skin of man, where irradiation from the sun catalyzes the formation of vitamin D_3. The vitamin D compounds are discussed in the chapter on vitamins.

The most common sterol in plants is β-sitosterol, a C_{29} compound. It has been shown that a second transmethylation from methionine accounts for the C-29 atom. The drug **sitosterols** is a mixture of β-sitosterol (stigmast-5-en-3β-ol) ($C_{29}H_{50}O$) and certain saturated sterols. It contains not less than 95% of total sterols and not less than 85% of unsaturated sterols calculated as β-sitosterol. It occurs as a white, essentially odorless, tasteless powder that is practically insoluble in water. In general, sitosterols are widely distributed throughout the plant kingdom and may be obtained from wheat germ oil, rye germ oil, corn oil, cottonseed oil, and other seed oils.

Sitosterols is a hypocholesterolemic agent used in the treatment of atherosclerosis. The sitosterols are poorly absorbed and compete with cholesterol for absorption sites in the intestine. Reduced cholesterol absorption may result in a decreased blood level of *beta* lipoproteins which, in turn, may prevent the deposition of atherosclerotic plaques in the blood vessels. The usual dose is 3 g, 3 times a day before meals. Sitosterols suspension (Cytellin®) is a hydroalcoholic suspension of β-sitosterol and a small amount of dihydro-β-sitosterol (stigmast-3β-ol).

Closely related to β-sitosterol is the sterol, stigmasterol, which was first isolated from calabar beans but is also found in soybean oil. The double bond at position 22 of stigmasterol allows it to be more readily converted into the pregnane-type steroid hormones than can β-sitosterol; consequently, the extraction of stigmasterol from soybean oil is an important commercial process.

BILE ACIDS

In the liver of man and other animals, the side chain of cholesterol is degraded to C_{24} steroids, which possess a C-24 carboxyl. These steroids are collected in the bile; therefore, they are referred to as the bile acids (Fig. 7–5). The primary bile acids formed in the liver of man are cholic acid and chenodesoxycholic acid. Desoxycholic acid and lithocholic acid are also found in substantial amounts in mammalian bile; however, they are not formed in the liver. They are produced in the intestinal tract by the action of microorganisms on cholic acid to form desoxycholic acid and on chenodesoxycholic acid to form lithocholic acid. Their presence in the bile is attributed to enterohepatic circulation. Generally, the bile acids do not exist in the free state, but are conjugated through a peptide bond to either glycine or taurine (Fig. 7–6). The conjugated bile acids are discharged into the duodenum where they act as emulsifying agents to aid in the intestinal absorption of fat. Bile salts are the sodium salts of the

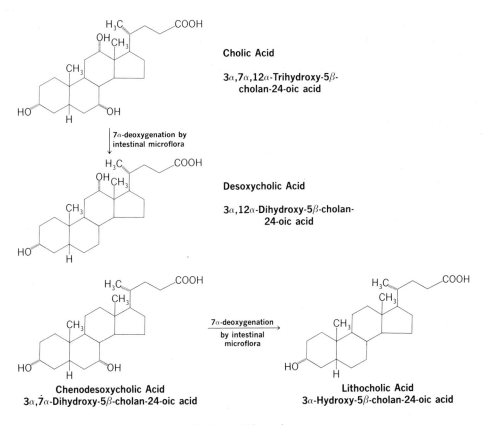

Fig. 7–5. Bile acids.

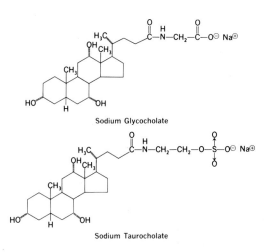

Fig. 7–6. Conjugated bile acids.

conjugated acids and are the principal constituents of ox bile extract, which is used therapeutically as a choleretic. It is usually given in a dose of 300 mg when biliary secretion seems deficient.

Ox bile extract is prepared by partial evaporation of fresh ox bile, precipitation of the mucus and albuminous matter with alcohol, filtering, washing, and evaporating the combined filtrates to dryness at a temperature not exceeding 80° C. It contains an amount of the sodium salts of glycocholic acid and taurocholic acid equivalent to not less than 45% of cholic acid.

Nonprescription Product. Bilron Pulvules®.

Although still in investigational stages, the use of **chenodesoxycholic acid** to dissolve gallstones promises to be a significant advance in drug therapy. This bile acid decreases the hepatic synthesis of cholesterol which, in turn, reduces the output of cholesterol into the bile and therefore permits the dissolution of cholesterol stones. The most frequently used dose is 10 to 15 mg/kg/day. Small stones may dissolve in 3 to 12 months; however, dissolution of larger stones may require up to 3 years. Lifetime therapy may be necessary because stones may recur when therapy is discontinued.

CARDIAC GLYCOSIDES

Some steroids present in nature are characterized by the highly specific and powerful action that they exert on the cardiac muscle. These steroids occur as glycosides with sugars attached at the 3-position of the steroid nucleus. Because of their action on the heart muscle, they are named cardiac glycosides (Fig. 7–7). The

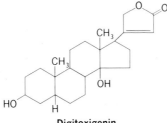

Digitoxigenin
3β,14-dihydroxy-5β,14β-card-20(22)-enolide

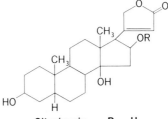

Gitoxigenin   R = H
3β,14,16β-trihydroxy-5β,14β-card-
20(22)-enolide

Gitaloxigenin   R = CHO
16β-formyloxy-3β,14-dihydroxy-
5β,14β-card-20(22)-enolide

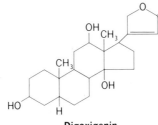

Digoxigenin
3β,12β,14-trihydroxy-5β,14β-card-20(22)-enolide

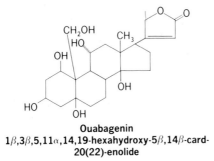

Ouabagenin
1β,3β,5,11α,14,19-hexahydroxy-5β,14β-card-
20(22)-enolide

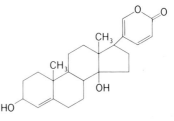

Scillarenin A
3β,14-dihydroxy-14β-bufa-4,20,22-
trienolide

Fig. 7–7. Structural formulas of several aglycones of cardiac glycosides.

steroid aglycones or genins are of 2 types: a cardenolide or a bufadienolide. The more prevalent in nature are the cardenolides, which are C_{23} steroids that have as a 17β side chain an α,β-unsaturated 5-membered lactone ring. The bufadienolides are C_{24} homologs of the cardenolides and carry a doubly unsaturated 6-membered lactone ring at the 17-position. The bufadienolides derive their name from the generic name for the toad, *Bufo* (the prototype compound bufalin was isolated from the skin of toads). An unusual aspect of the chemistry of both cardenolides and bufadienolides is that the C/D ring junction has the *cis*-configuration. To obtain optimum cardiac activity, the aglycone should possess an α,β unsaturated lactone ring that is attached β at the 17-position of the steroid nucleus and the A/B and C/D ring junctions should have the *cis*-configuration. Metabolic reduction of the double bond in the lactone ring of digoxin to form dihydrodigoxin may explain why certain individuals are refractory to digoxin therapy. If the glycoside is cleaved, the aglycone retains cardiac activity; however, the sugar portion of the glycoside confers on the molecule solubility properties important in its absorption and distribution in the body. Oxygen substitution on the steroid nucleus also influences the distribution and metabolism of glycosides. In general, the more hydroxy groups on the molecule, the more rapid the onset of action and the subsequent dissipation from the body.

The use of the cardiac glycosides in therapeutics stems from the ability of these compounds to increase the force of systolic contraction. An increase in contractility in the failing heart results in a more complete emptying of the ventricle and a shortening in the length of systole. Thus, the heart has more time to rest between contractions. As the myocardium recovers owing to increased cardiac output and circulation, the heart rate is decreased through a reflex vagal effect. In addition, the improved circulation tends to improve renal secretion, which relieves the edema often associated with heart failure.

In the use of cardiac glycosides to treat congestive heart failure, the patient is given an initial loading dose of the drug in order to bring the heart under the influence of the drug. Because the amount required varies with the patient and the drug used, the preparation is given in divided doses while titrating the dose against signs of improvement. The patient is usually maintained indefinitely after the loading dose by administering a daily maintenance dose that replaces the amount of drug that is metabolized and excreted. In toxic concentrations, the glycosides may increase cardiac automaticity and lead to ectopic tachyarrhythmia. Ventricular extrasystoles are the most frequent effect. With all the glycosides, the therapeutic level appears to be approximately 50 to 60% of the toxic dose. This finding explains why careful dosage must be determined experimentally for each patient.

Despite numerous experimental investigations, the mechanism of action of the cardiac glycosides is still not completely known; however, observations have implicated Na^+, K^+-ATPase as the receptor enzyme. This enzyme catalyzes the active transport of Na^+ out of the cell and the subsequent transport of K^+ into the cell. Inhibition of Na^+, K^+-ATPase by the cardiac glycoside possibly affects cation fluxes in and out of the myocardial cell. The end result is an increase in Na^+ and a decrease in K^+ within the cell which, in turn, results in an increase in Ca^{++}. When the level of free Ca^{++} reaches a certain value, it antagonizes the inhibitory action of troponin. This antagonism permits the formation of actomyosin, which results in the contraction of the myocardium.

Drug Interactions. This postulated mechanism implicating intracellular cation levels explains the development of toxicity symptoms in patients with certain plasma-electrolyte imbalances who receive cardiac glycoside therapy. Potassium depletion increases the susceptibility to cardiac glycoside toxicity; therefore, patients on concomitant therapy with such potassium-depleting drugs as thiazide diuretics and corticosteroids with mineral corticoid activity may require potassium supplementation or a reduced dosage of cardiac glycosides. Conversely, patients treated with cardiac glycosides should not commence the excessive ingestion of any product containing absorbable calcium,

e.g., milk, calcium gluconate, and dibasic and tribasic calcium phosphate. Also, such patients should not be given parenteral calcium because hypercalcemia can potentiate the cardiac effect.

DIGITALIS

Digitalis or foxglove is the dried leaf of *Digitalis purpurea* Linné (Fam. Scrophulariaceae) (Fig. 7–8). Its potency is such that, when assayed as directed, 100 mg are equivalent to not less than 1 USP digitalis unit (100 mg of the USP Digitalis Reference Standard). *When digitalis is*

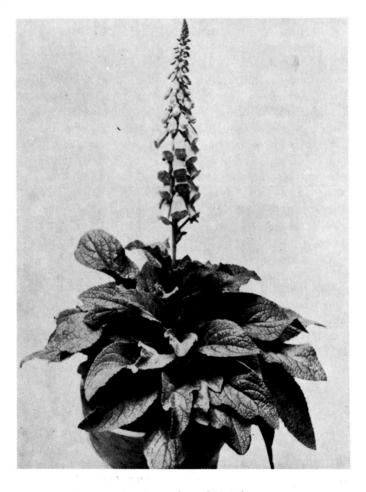

Fig. 7–8. Specimen plant of *Digitalis purpurea.*

prescribed, powdered digitalis is to be dispensed.

Powdered digitalis is digitalis dried at a temperature not exceeding 60° C, reduced to a fine or a very fine powder, and adjusted, if necessary, to conform to the official potency by admixture with sufficient lactose, starch, exhausted marc of digitalis, or with a powdered digitalis that has either a lower or a higher potency.

Digitalis is from the Latin *digitus*, meaning a finger, and refers to the finger-shaped corolla, so named by Tragus in 1539; *purpurea* is Latin and refers to the purple color of the flower. The plant is a biennial herb, probably indigenous to central and southern Europe and naturalized in various parts of Europe and in the northern and western United States and Canada.

Digitalis seems to have been used externally by the Welsh. Parkinson recommended it in 1640, but its internal use was not in vogue until its recommendation by Withering in 1776. It is an important drug and has been official in most pharmacopeias of the world since the eighteenth century.

Digitalis lanata or Grecian foxglove is the dried leaves of *Digitalis lanata* Ehrhart, a plant indigenous to southern and central Europe. It is the source of several official glycosides.

The leaves of other *Digitalis* species, *D. dubia, D. ferruginea, D. grandiflora, D. lutea, D. mertonensis, D. nervosa, D. subalpina,* and *D. thapsi,* also show the presence of cardiac glycosides.

CULTIVATION OF DIGITALIS. Until recently, digitalis was cultivated in Pennsylvania by the S. B. Penick Company. At present, however, digitalis and the digitalis glycosides used in the U.S. are obtained principally from England and Germany. In Germany, *D. purpurea* and *D. lanata* seeds, which have been developed through strain selection to yield plants with maximum drug potency and with resistance to plant

diseases, are sown in greenhouses in March. From the middle of May until the beginning of June, the young plants are planted outside in relatively small plots (1 to 10 acres). The areas of cultivation are centered around a commercial drying unit for medicinal plants at a distance of not more than 20 km. To insure potency, the leaves must be rapidly and gently dried at 50 to 60° C as soon as the plants are harvested. This procedure must be followed because the leaf contains hydrolytic enzymes which, if not rapidly inactivated, cleave the glycosidic linkages, thereby giving rise to the less active genins. Also, excess heat may split off water from the tertiary hydroxy group at position 14 of the steroid nucleus, thereby forming the inactive anhydro compound.

The annual crop is harvested from the middle of September to the end of October. The weight of a fresh plant ranges from 200 to 500 g. The yield per acre, depending on the quality of the soil and the effort and skill of the farmer, may vary from 2.5 to 5.5 tons fresh weight/acre, which corresponds to approximately 0.6 to 1.4 tons dry weight/acre.

The harvested crop utilizes only the first year's leaves (Fig. 7–9), which develop as a dense rosette. Some of the plants remain undisturbed to permit development of the flowering stalk during the second season. These flowering stems are the source of seeds for future use. With the exception of the plants used for seed production, all other plants are harvested; consequently, fresh cultivation of young plants is begun each year.

CONSTITUENTS. The drug contains a large number of glycosides, of which the most important from a medicinal viewpoint are digitoxin, gitoxin, and gitaloxin. The total concentration of these 3 glycosides varies appreciably with the plant source and the conditions of growth. Also, because all are secondary glycosides derived by hydroly-

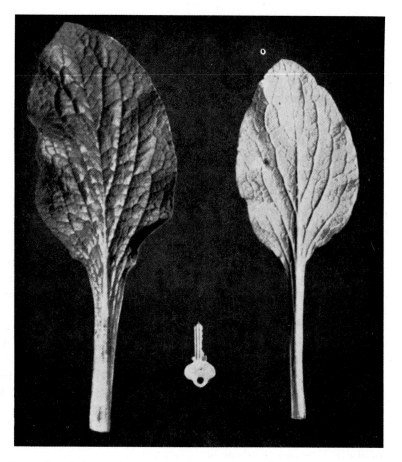

Fig. 7–9.   Mature digitalis leaves showing the prominent veins of the dorsal and ventral surfaces. Note the winged petiole.

sis of some of the sugars from the primary or parent glycosides occurring in the leaf, their concentration depends on the manner of treatment of the plant material following harvesting. Careful experiments have revealed that the secondary glycoside content in the leaf is about 10 to 20% of the primary glycoside concentration. Reported total concentrations of digitoxin, gitoxin, and gitaloxin range from 0.09% in a poor-quality Spanish sample to 0.225% in a superior Japanese leaf; the average concentration approximates 0.16%.

Nearly 30 other glycosides have been identified in the drug. The major

glycosides, in terms of concentration, include: purpurea glycoside A, purpurea glycoside B, glucogitaloxin, glucodigitoxigenin-bis-digitoxiside, glucogitaloxigenin-bis-digitoxiside, glucoevatromonoside, glucogitoroside, glucolanadoxin, digitalinum verum, glucoverodoxin, stropeside, and verodoxin (see Table 7–1).

Assay. Digitalis and its preparations must be assayed biologically to insure their potency; however, because the crystalline glycosides are definite chemical entities, they are assayed chemically. A number of test animals have been used in

Table 7-1. Composition of the Principal Glycosides of *Digitalis purpurea*

Glycoside	Sugars
Derivatives of Digitoxigenin	
Purpurea glycoside A	3 digitoxose, 1 glucose
Digitoxin	3 digitoxose
Gluco-digitoxigenin-bis-digitoxoside	2 digitoxose, 1 glucose
Gluco-evatromonoside	1 digitoxose, 1 glucose
Derivatives of Gitoxigenin	
Purpurea glycoside B	3 digitoxose, 1 glucose
Gitoxin	3 digitoxose
Gluco-gitoroside	1 digitoxose, 1 glucose
Digitalinum verum	1 digitalose, 1 glucose
Stropeside	1 digitalose
Derivatives of Gitaloxigenin	
Gluco-gitaloxin	3 digitoxose, 1 glucose
Gitaloxin	3 digitoxose
Gluco-gitaloxigenin-bis-digitoxoside	2 digitoxose, 1 glucose
Gluco-lanadoxin	1 digitoxose, 1 glucose
Gluco-verodoxin	1 digitalose, 1 glucose
Verodoxin	1 digitalose

the past: guinea pigs, frogs, and cats. The animal now employed in the assay procedure is the pigeon.

Standardization is determined by comparison of the effect of a known dilution of the drug with that of a similar dilution of the USP Digitalis Reference Standard. Adult pigeons are anesthetized lightly with ether, immobilized, and their alar vein is exposed and cannulated. Definite volumes of the diluted preparation are introduced at 5-minute intervals until the pigeon dies from cardiac arrest.

The bioassay of digitalis leaf can be criticized because of the inability of the method to predict oral potency of the drug. For example, gitoxin in the leaf would contribute to the intravenous assay potency but, because it is poorly absorbed from the GI tract, it would not contribute significantly to the cardiac effect. This observation assumes additional significance when one considers that the amount of gitoxin present in the leaf may vary greatly depending on the genetics of the plant or the manner in which the drug is harvested and prepared for market. As a precautionary measure, care should be taken to maintain patients on one brand of digitalis tablets. This precaution decreases the chances of dispensing a preparation with an oral potency that is either reduced or greater than that obtained by the patient in a prior prescription.

USES AND DOSE. Digitalis is used in the form of tablets or capsules to treat congestive heart failure, supraventricular tachycardia, atrial flutter, and atrial fibrillation. Usual initial dose is 1.5 g divided over 24 to 48 hours; maintenance is 100 mg daily. Usual initial dose range is 1 to 2 g; maintenance is 100 to 200 mg daily. Dose must be reduced by 25 to 50% for the elderly, for patients with lean body mass, and for patients with metabolic or electrolyte disorders. The onset of action is 2 to 4 hours, and maximal effect occurs in 12 to 14 hours. Complete dissipation of the drug from the body takes 2 to 3 weeks.

PRESCRIPTION PRODUCTS. Pil-Digis® and Digifortis® represent the whole leaf of D. purpurea; Digiglusin® contains the products from the specially prepared leaf of D. purpurea.

DIGITOXIN

Digitoxin is a cardiotonic glycoside obtained from D. purpurea, D. lanata, and other suitable species of Digitalis. It is a highly potent drug and should be handled with exceptional care. Digitoxin occurs as a white or pale buff, odorless, microcrystalline powder. It is a bitter substance that is practically insoluble in water and slightly soluble in alcohol. Digitoxin is the most toxic of the active constituents of the leaves and is cumulative in action.

USE AND DOSE. Digitoxin is a cardiotonic that increases the tone of cardiac muscle and thus causes the heart to empty more effectively. Usual initial dose for rapid digitalization, orally or intravenously, is 800 μg, followed by 200 μg at 6- to 8-hour intervals for 2 to 3 doses. For slower digitalization, the dose is 100 to 200 μg 1 to 3 times daily to a total of 1.2 to 1.8 mg; maintenance is 50 to 200 μg once a day. The same precautions of use and duration of drug action that apply to digitalis also apply to digitoxin.

PRESCRIPTION PRODUCTS. Digitoxin is represented by Crystodigin® and Purodigin®.

Gitalin, more properly referred to as gitalin fraction or gitalin (amorphous), is an amorphous mixture of glycosides obtained from the leaf of D. purpurea. It was first derived from a cold-water extract of digitalis leaves. The mixture is composed of gitaloxin (13 to 19%), its decomposition product, gitoxin (13 to 19%), and digitoxin (14 to 20%). Minor components include stropeside, verodoxin, gitoxigenin, and digitoxigenin. Gitalin is a yellowish white,

bitter, amorphous powder that is soluble in alcohol, in chloroform, and in about 800 parts of water. In the dried state, gitalin is quite stable, retaining its action without any change in potency or quality for periods of as long as 2 years. It is rapidly absorbed following oral administration and has the same action and uses as digitalis.

USE AND DOSE. Gitalin is employed in the treatment of congestive heart failure. Some clinicians believe it has a greater margin of safety than other digitalis preparations, but others report no essential difference. It may remain effective when adequate doses of other digitalis preparations cannot be tolerated. Usual dose, maintenance, is 0.5 mg daily (equivalent to 100 mg of the leaf). Usual dose range, maintenance, is 250 μg to 1.25 mg daily. The same precautions of use and duration of drug action that apply to digitalis also apply to gitalin.

PRESCRIPTION PRODUCT. Gitaligin®.

DIGITONIN

Digitonin is a crystalline saponin found in the leaves and seeds of D. purpurea. On hydrolysis, digitonin yields 1 molecule of digitogenin, 2 of glucose, 2 of galactose, and 1 of xylose. The commercial product contains between 70 and 80% of digitonin; the remainder consists of related saponins of minor importance. It is practically insoluble in water, but forms a soapy suspension.

USE. Digitonin forms an insoluble complex with cholesterol and has been used in the determination of cholesterol in blood plasma, bile, and tissue. It is not employed internally; however, it is available for reagent purposes.

DIGITALIS LANATA

Nearly 70 different glycosides have been detected in the leaves of D. lanata. The composition of 18 of the most important of

Table 7–2. Composition of the Principal Glycosides of *Digitalis lanata*

Glycoside	Sugars
Derivatives of Digitoxigenin	
Lanatoside A	3 digitoxose, 1 acetyl group, 1 glucose
Acetyldigitoxin (α and β forms)	3 digitoxose, 1 acetyl group
Gluco-evatromonoside	1 digitoxose, 1 glucose
Gluco-digitoxigenin-glucomethyloside	1 glucomethylose, 1 glucose
Gluco-digifucoside	1 fucose, 1 glucose
Neo-gluco-digifucoside	1 fucose, 1 glucose
Derivatives of Gitoxigenin	
Lanatoside B	3 digitoxose, 1 acetyl group, 1 glucose
Gluco-gitoroside	1 digitoxose, 1 glucose
Digitalinum verum	1 digitalose, 1 glucose
Derivatives of Gitaloxigenin	
Lanatoside E	3 digitoxose, 1 acetyl group, 1 glucose
Gluco-lanadoxin	1 digitoxose, 1 glucose
Gluco-verodoxin	1 digitalose, 1 glucose
Derivatives of Digoxigenin	
Lanatoside C	3 digitoxose, 1 acetyl group, 1 glucose
Desacetyllanatoside C	3 digitoxose, 1 glucose
Acetyldigoxin (α, β, and γ forms)	3 digitoxose, 1 acetyl group
Digoxin	3 digitoxose
Gluco-digoxigenin-bis-digitoxoside	2 digitoxose, 1 glucose
Derivatives of Diginatigenin	
Lanatoside D	3 digitoxose, 1 acetyl group, 1 glucose

these is listed in Table 7–2. All are derivatives of 5 different aglycones, 3 of which (digitoxigenin, gitoxigenin, and gitaloxigenin) also occur in *D. purpurea*. The other 2 types of glycosides derived from digoxigenin and diginatigenin occur in *D. lanata* but not in *D. purpurea*. As noted in the table, the 5 types of primary glycosides are designated lanatosides A through E, according to the identity of the aglycone. The lanatosides are sometimes referred to as digilanids, especially in the older literature.

None of the primary glycosides of *D. lanata* is identical to those found in *D. purpurea*. Even those that have the same aglycone differ by the presence of an acetyl group attached to the third digitoxose residue. Removal of the acetyl group and sugar residues by selective hydrolysis results in secondary glycosides, some of which, e.g., digitoxin, occur in both species. NOTE: Glycosides derived from aglycones of the C and D series may be obtained only from *D. lanata*.

DIGOXIN

Digoxin is a cardiotonic glycoside obtained from the leaves of *D. lanata*. It is a highly potent drug and should be handled with exceptional care. Digoxin occurs as colorless or white crystals or as a white, crystalline powder. Variable bioequivalence among different brands of digoxin tablets has been demonstrated. Because of the low therapeutic index of the drug, it is recommended that, in the absence of good comparative bioavailability data, a patient should not be changed from one brand to another after a reasonable therapeutic effect has been achieved with one preparation. Otherwise, either a toxic or nontherapeutic effect may result owing to a change in the bioavailability of the drug.

USE AND DOSE. Digoxin is used in the treatment of congestive heart failure and cardiac tachyarrhythmia. It is a prompt-acting glycoside when given orally and has an onset of action of from 1 to 2 hours and a maximal effect in 6 to 8 hours. The drug is eliminated in 3 to 6 days. It is also administered parenterally for a more rapid effect. Usual dose ranges are: for rapid digitalization, initially, 500 to 750 μg orally, followed by 250 to 500 μg every 6 to 8 hours until full digitalization; or, initially, 250 to 500 μg intravenously, followed by 250 μg at 4- to 6-hour intervals, if needed, to a total dose of 1 mg. The usual oral maintenance dose range and the dose for slow digitalization is 125 to 500 μg daily. The same precautions of use that apply to digitalis also apply to digoxin.

PRESCRIPTION PRODUCT. Lanoxin®.

LANATOSIDE C

Lanatoside C is a glycoside obtained from the leaves of *D. lanata. It is extremely poisonous.* Lanatoside C occurs as colorless or white crystals or as a white, crystalline powder.

It is easily soluble in methyl or ethyl alcohol. Although only slightly soluble in water, this solubility suffices for its therapeutic use. On enzymatic and alkaline hydrolysis, the glucose and acetyl radicals are liberated and leave the glycoside digoxin. Further acid hydrolysis splits off 3 molecules of digitoxose leaving the aglycone, digoxigenin. Lanatoside C is a stable, easily absorbed, and promptly effective preparation that can serve as a potent therapeutic agent.

USE AND DOSE. Lanatoside C is employed in the treatment of congestive heart failure. Usual initial dose range, orally, is 5 to 10 mg; maintenance is 0.5 to 1.5 mg.

PRESCRIPTION PRODUCT. Cedilanid®.

DESLANOSIDE

Deslanoside is desacetyllanatoside C. Deslanoside occurs as white crystals or as a white, crystalline powder. It is hygroscopic, absorbing about 7% of moisture when exposed to air, and is highly potent.

USE AND DOSE. Deslanoside is a cardiotonic and is frequently used to attain rapid initial loading by parenteral administration. Onset of action is 10 to 30 minutes; maximal effects occur in 2 to 3 hours with dissipation in 3 to 6 days. Usual dose range, intramuscularly or intravenously for digitalization, is, initially, 0.8 mg, then 0.4 mg every 2 to 4 hours to a maximum of 2 mg. Because deslanoside is more soluble than lanatoside C, it provides a more efficient preparation for intravenous administration. The same precautions of use that apply to digitalis also apply to deslanoside.

PRESCRIPTION PRODUCT. Cedilanid D®.

OUABAIN

Ouabain is a glycoside of ouabagenin and rhamnose. It may be obtained from the seeds of *Strophanthus gratus* (Wall et Hook.) Baillon or from the wood of *Acokanthera schimperi* (A. DC.) Schwf. (Fam. Apocynaceae). *It is extremely poisonous.* Ouabain is also known as G-strophanthin.

Strophanthus seeds have long been used by the native Africans in the preparation of arrow poisons. These poisons were first observed in western Africa by Hendelot and in East Africa by Livingstone. Early specimens sent to Europe established the powerful cardiac properties of the seeds.

Ouabain is assayed by spectrophotometry rather than by bioassay. Because of its well-defined physical characteristics and crystalline structure, ouabain has been used as a reference standard for the assay of the cardiac glycosides; however, the availability of pure digitoxin and digoxin for assay purposes has obviated the use of ouabain as a reference standard for these glycosides.

USE AND DOSE. Ouabain is the most rapidly acting cardiac glycoside available. It is administered intravenously for the treatment of acute cardiac failure, 250 to 500 μg initially, then 100 μg repeated every hour, if necessary, to a total of 1 mg divided over 24 hours. The onset of action is 3 to 10 minutes, maximal effect is 30 to 60 minutes, and dissipation from the body is 24 to 48 hours.

SQUILL

Squill or squill bulb consists of the cut and dried, fleshy inner scales of the bulb of the white variety of *Urginea maritima* (Linné) Baker, known in commerce as white or Mediterranean squill; or of *U. indica* Kunth, known in commerce as Indian squill (Fam. Liliaceae). The central portion of the bulb is excluded during its processing.

Scilla is from the Greek *skilla*, meaning to split, and refers to the separating scales; *Urginea* may be from the Latin *urgere*, meaning to press, and refers to the compressed seed; *maritima* is Latin and refers to the habitat of the plant on the Mediterranean coasts of Spain, France, Italy, Greece, Algeria, and Morocco. The bulbs, which grow half immersed in the sandy soil near the sea, are gathered late in August, and, after removal of the membranous outer scales and the central portion, the fleshy scales are cut into transverse pieces and dried. The best commercial variety of white squill comes from Italy, but because

of high labor costs, relatively small quantities are now obtained from that country. India is now the major producer of squill.

Squill contains about a dozen cardioactive glycosides of which the principal one, scillaren A, comprises about two thirds of the total glycoside fraction. On hydrolysis, it yields the aglycone scillarenin, a bufadienolide, plus rhamnose and glucose. Other minor glycosides include glucoscillaren A (scillarenin + rhamnose + glucose + glucose) and proscillaridin A (scillarenin + rhamnose).

USES AND DOSE. Squill is an expectorant, but it also possesses emetic, cardiotonic, and diuretic properties. The usual dose is 100 mg.

NONPRESCRIPTION PRODUCT. Sedatussin® contains squill.

Red squill consists of the bulb or bulb scales of the red variety of *U. maritima*, which is imported for use as a rat poison. It should not be present in the medicinal squill and may be detected by the presence of red, pink, or purple epidermal or parenchymal tissues.

Most of the squill imported into the United States is of the red variety. Each year, a considerable tonnage is used as a rodenticide. Rodents lack the vomiting reflex, which makes red squill particularly lethal to these animals. The inadvertent ingestion by human beings of plant materials that contain cardiac glycosides induces the vomiting reflex and reduces the life-threatening aspects of the toxic manifestations.

OTHER CARDIOACTIVE DRUGS

A number of plants contain cardioactive glycosides, and some of them have been employed for many years as cardiac stimulants and diuretics. Several are more potent than digitalis, but they are less reliable because their dosage cannot be controlled properly. Although most of these drugs were recognized officially for years and were considered efficacious, they have been superseded by digitalis and its derivatives. A few are currently under reinvestigation.

Convallaria or lily-of-the-valley root is the dried rhizome and roots of *Convallaria majalis* Linné (Fam. Liliaceae). More than 20 cardioactive glycosides have been isolated from this drug. Principal among these is convallatoxin, a monoglycoside composed of the genin of K-strophanthin (strophanthidin) and the sugar of G-strophanthin (rhamnose). Other minor glycosides include convallatoxol and convalloside.

Apocynum, black Indian hemp, dog bane, or Canadian hemp consists of the dried rhizome and roots of *Apocynum cannabinum* Linné or *A. androsaemifolium* Linné (Fam. Apocynaceae). The chief constituent is cymarin, although apocannoside and cyanocannoside have also been isolated from *A. cannabinum.*

Adonis or pheasant's eye is the dried overground portion of *Adonis vernalis* Linné (Fam. Ranunculaceae). Cardioactive glycosides identified in the drug include adonitoxin, cymarin, and K-strophanthin.

Cactus grandiflorus or night-blooming cereus consists of the fresh, succulent stem of wild-growing *Selenicereus grandiflorus* (Linné) Britton et Rose (Fam. Cactaceae).

Black hellebore or Christmas rose is the dried rhizome and roots of *Helleborus niger* Linné (Fam. Ranunculaceae). The chief constituent is hellebrin. Black hellebore possesses cardiac stimulant properties in contrast to green hellebore (see veratrum viride), which is a cardiac depressant.

Another plant that contains a cardiac glycoside is *Nerium oleander* Linné (Fam. Apocynaceae). The leaves have been used to treat cardiac insufficiency. The chief constituent is oleandrin, a 3-glycosido-16-acetyl derivative of gitoxigenin.

Strophanthus is the dried, ripe seed of *Strophanthus kombe* Oliver, or of *S. hispidus* DeCandolle (Fam. Apocynaceae), that is deprived of the awns and possesses a potency, per gram, equivalent to not less than 55 mg of USP Reference Ouabain when assayed biologically in cats.

K-strophanthoside, also known as strophoside, is the principal primary glycoside in both *S. kombe* and *S. hispidus.* It is composed of the genin, strophanthidin, coupled to a trisaccharide consisting of cymarose, β-glucose, and α-glucose. α-Glucosidase removes the terminal α-glucose to yield K-strophanthin-β, and the enzyme, strophanthobiase, contained in the seed converts this to cymarin plus glucose. A mixture of these glycosides, existing in the seed in concentrations of up to 5%, was formerly designated strophanthin or K-strophanthin. Recent studies have revealed additional glycosides as minor constituents.

Whereas digitalis is the drug of choice in the United States, strophanthus and its derivatives are frequently preferred in Europe. Strophanthus belongs to the cardiotonic series of drugs and has an action similar to that of digitalis.

STEROID HORMONES

The steroid hormones can be divided into 2 classes, the **sex hormones** and the **adrenocortical hormones.** The former are produced primarily in the gonads and mediate the growth, development, maintenance, and function of the reproductive tract and the accessory sex organs. These hormones fall into 3 chemically and physiologically distinct categories: the **estrogens** and **progestins,** which regulate various functions of the female reproductive tract, and the **androgens,** which stimulate the development of the male reproductive organs. The adrenocortical hormones are produced by the outer cortical portion of the adrenal glands, and they are divided into 2 classes, depending on their biologic activity. The hormones that principally affect the excretion of fluid and electrolytes, with a subsequent sodium retention, are called mineralocorticoids; those that affect intermediary metabolism are termed glucocorticoids.

The production of steroid hormones in the body is initiated by the releasing factors of the hypothalamus, which travel to the anterior lobe of the pituitary gland where they induce the release of tropic hormones into the blood. When stimulated by the appropriate tropic hormone, steroids are synthesized at the target site, either the adrenal cortex or the gonads. Steroid level in the blood is held in balance by a mechanism of feedback regulation that is mediated through the hypothalamus. When excess active steroid is in the blood that reaches the hypothalamus, the production of the hypothalamic releasing factors is stopped (Fig. 7–10).

This phenomenon of feedback regulation can cause problems in drug therapy with steroid hormones. For example, prolonged therapy with corticosteroids may

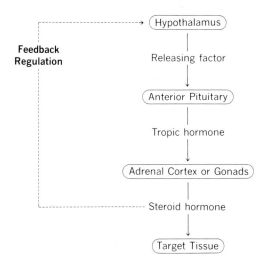

Fig. 7–10. Regulation of steroid hormone production.

cause irreversible atrophy of the adrenal cortex. A high corticosteroid level in the body suppresses the hypothalamus from secreting the corticotropin-releasing factor which, in turn, suppresses release of corticotropin. The lack of stimulatory impact of this anterior pituitary hormone results in atrophy of the adrenal cortex.

Biosynthesis of Steroid Hormones. Biosynthesis of the numerous steroid hormones of the adrenal cortex, gonads, and placenta is an extremely complex specialty field. Only the briefest essentials can be presented here. When one realizes that more than 70 different steroids have been isolated from the adrenal gland alone, one can easily understand why the biosynthetic relationships are complex.

Like other steroids of biologic origin, these hormones are derived from the well-known acetate-mevalonic acid pathway which, in this case, leads first to cholesterol (see Fig. 7–3 for details). Partial side-chain degradation of cholesterol leads to pregnenolone and then to progesterone, both of which serve as precursors of the other steroid hormones.

The conversion of cholesterol to pregnenolone is catalyzed by a mixed-function oxidase enzyme complex that involves a desmolase and requires O_2 and NADPH. This conversion appears to be the rate-limiting step in steroid hormone biosynthesis and is under the influence of the tropic hormones of the anterior pituitary. In the case of ACTH stimulation of steroidogenesis, ACTH activates adrenal cortical adenyl cyclase, which causes a rise in cyclic AMP and a subsequent activation of glycogen phosphorylase. This enzyme breaks down glycogen to produce glucose-6-phosphate, which then is oxidized via the hexose monophosphate shunt pathway, yielding NADPH. An increase in the availability of this coenzyme increases the activity of the desmolase and the hydroxylase reactions.

Enzymes in the adrenals and the gonads remove the side chain and hydroxylate the steroid nucleus in the 17α-position to form the androgens. After loss of the angular 19-methyl group, androgens are aromatized to estrogens. The adrenals also hydroxylate progesterone in positions 21, 11, and/or 17 to produce the classic adrenocortical hormones. Production of aldosterone involves 18-hydroxylation and dehydrogenation reactions.

Some of the principal conversions are illustrated in the simplified scheme shown in Figure 7–11.

The steroid hormones are bound to proteins, primarily albumins, for transport in the blood. These steroid-protein complexes per se are physiologically inert and protect the steroid from metabolic inactivation. The strength of binding varies and can be generalized by classification as follows: the corticosteroids tend to be weakly bound, the estrogens are more strongly bound, and progesterone and testosterone are intermediate between the 2 extremes.

Reductive processes are normally involved in the metabolism of steroid hormones. The di-, tetra-, and hexahydric metabolites may be formed and usually entail progressive reduction of the 4-ene, 3-keto, and 20-keto functions. The reduced forms are usually excreted as the more soluble uronides or sulfate esters involving the 3-oxygen function. In the case of the metabolism of estradiol and testosterone, the initial metabolic reaction is oxidative,

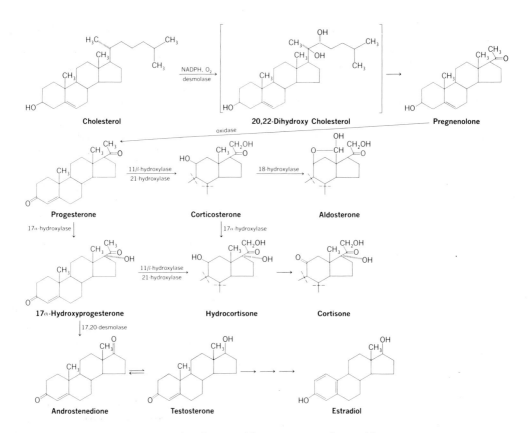

Fig. 7–11. Biosynthesis and bioconversion of steroid hormones.

involving the 17-hydroxyl function, but subsequent metabolic steps are reductive with eventual conjugation.

Mechanism of Action. The steroid hormones have diverse actions, and several specific receptor proteins, varying with the particular target tissue, have been isolated for each action. Structural changes of the hormone may affect the affinity or activity on one receptor and have little or no effect on other receptors. For example, changes in the chemical structure of testosterone allow for the separation of the androgenic activity from the anabolic activity of this hormone. The same applies when separating the glucocorticoid/mineralocorticoid activity of corticosteroids. Also, steroid hormones do not act through an increase in cyclic AMP, but rather through a stimulation of protein synthesis. A possible explanation of this mechanism is that the steroid binds with the specific receptor protein in the cytoplasm of the target cell. This complex enters the nucleus, where it is bound to the chromosome through a specific acceptor protein associated with chromatin. The interaction of steroid, of cytoplasm receptor protein, and of the chromosomal receptor protein may lead to a derepression of a segment of chromosome, which would result in the increased production of a particular enzyme protein. For example, mineralocorticoids produce an increase in the synthesis of enzymes that are necessary for active transport of Na^+, which leads directly to increased Na^+ reabsorption in the renal tubules.

Commercial Production of Steroids. The steroid hormones and their semi-synthetic analogs represent a multi-million-dollar annual business for the American drug industry. When one considers the social, political, and economic implications associated with the use of oral contraceptive drugs, the importance of steroids to mankind cannot be ques-

tioned. At the present time, the principal source of the steroid chemical nucleus used in the drug industry is the plant kingdom; however, in the not too distant past, the source of steroid hormones was from the gonads and adrenal glands of animals that were used as food by man. The amount of hormone present in these glands was extremely small and large quantities of glands were required to isolate milligram quantities of hormone; consequently, it was not practical to use the pure hormone in therapy. For example, in 1934, Schering Laboratories, Berlin, needed 625 kg of ovaries from 50,000 sows in order to obtain 20 mg of pure crystalline progesterone.

Today, the steroid industry represents the culmination of efforts by many scientists; however, a few can be singled out for their pioneering work in steroid chemistry. One of these men is Russell E. Marker. Marker is responsible for the discovery of a commercially feasible conversion of steroidal sapogenins to progesterone. His early work involved the search for plant species that were rich in steroidal sapogenins. When he found that Mexican yams, various species of *Dioscorea*, were rich in these compounds, he moved to Mexico City in 1943 where he isolated diosgenin from *D. macrostachy (D. mexicana)*, known in Mexico as *cabeza de negro*. From diosgenin, employing the chemical degradation illustrated in Figure 7–12, he managed to prepare more than 3 kg of progesterone (at the time valued at $8 a gram). This hormone and the process used to prepare it were the foundation stones for the Syntex Company.

During the 1930s, several scientists, including E. C. Kendall, a chemist at the Mayo Clinic, and T. Reichstein, a chemist at the Federal Institute of Technology, Zurich, Switzerland, almost simultaneously and independently isolated steroids from the adrenal cortex of cattle. Stimulated by the potential therapeutic

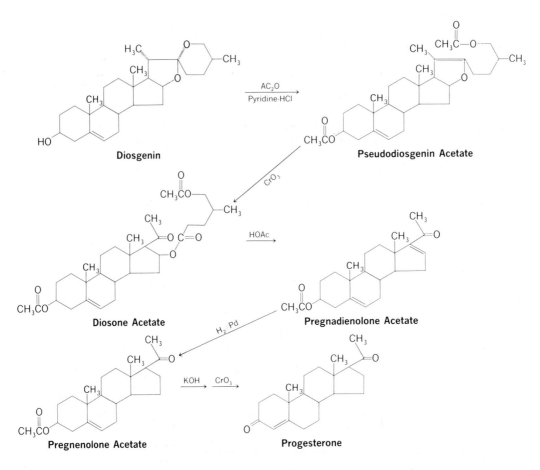

Fig. 7–12.   The Marker degradation.

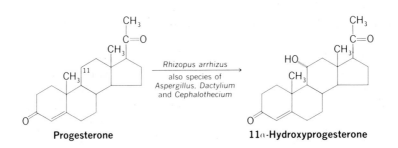

Fig. 7–13.   Introduction of oxygen function into the 11-position of the steroid nucleus.

importance of these compounds, the Merck Company in 1944 successfully produced 15 mg of cortisone from 1 kg of desoxycholic acid utilizing 36 separate chemical steps. However, in 1949 when P. S. Hench of the Mayo Clinic announced cortisone's dramatic effectiveness in treating rheumatoid arthritis, the increased demand for cortisone required a more readily available and inexpensive source. The problem was solved in 1952 when scientists at the Upjohn Company found a microorganism, *Rhizopus arrhizus*, that could convert progesterone, a readily available starting material because of the Marker degradation, to 11α-hydroxyprogesterone in an 80 to 90% yield. The extremely difficult problem of introducing an oxygen function in the 11-position of the steroid nucleus by using chemical methods was therefore solved (Fig. 7–13).

A vast amount of research resulted in extension and improvement of this basic procedure with other precursors and numerous microorganisms. Relatively inexpensive starting materials, such as stigmasterol from soybeans, hecogenin from the sisal industry, or diosgenin from *Dioscorea* species, are now employed.

Stigmasterol may be converted chemically to progesterone, which is, in turn, incubated in large fermentors with suitable microorganisms under specified conditions to yield 11α-hydroxyprogesterone, which may then be converted chemically to cortisone. Similarly, cortexolone (Richstein's substance S) is prepared chemically from diosgenin and is then converted by *Streptomyces fradiae* or *Cunninghamella blakesleeana* to cortisol (hydrocortisone).

Cortisone or cortisol is dehydrogenated in the Δ^1-position by *Corynebacterium simplex* or by *Fusarium* species to yield prednisone or prednisolone, respectively.

Certain microorganisms also can hydroxylate synthetically prepared fluoro-

steroids in the 16α-position to produce triamcinolone (Fig. 7–14).

ADRENAL CORTEX

The adrenal cortex is essential to life. Removal of about 85% of cortical tissue is lethal in a few days. In animals so treated, life may be maintained by the administration of extracts or homones of the adrenal cortex.

Cortical deficiency in animals is marked by a loss of appetite and weight, vomiting and diarrhea, weakness, and a fall in temperature, metabolism, and blood pressure. There is a loss of blood fluid, with resulting concentration of blood, and a fall in serum sodium, with a rise in serum glucose and potassium. Kidney damage is frequently present. These developments can be prevented or restored to normal by the administration of cortical extracts and frequently by the simple use of a high sodium, low potassium intake.

The human counterpart of this deficiency picture is seen in the clinical development of Addison's disease (chronic adrenocortical insufficiency), usually owing to tuberculosis or tumor of the adrenal cortex. Associated with this disease are degeneration of the gonads, a marked increase in capillary permeability, and an increased sensitivity to insulin. Sodium loss with potassium retention may be the outstanding condition of the disease. If untreated, Addison's disease terminates fatally in 1 to 3 years, usually owing to hypoglycemia, dehydration, nutritional disturbances, or secondary infection.

Excessive adrenal cortical activity, as in tumors or because of the presence of accessory cortical tissue, results in profound growth abnormalities, especially seen in the external genitalia and in the secondary sex characteristics. In young children, there is precocious sexual development

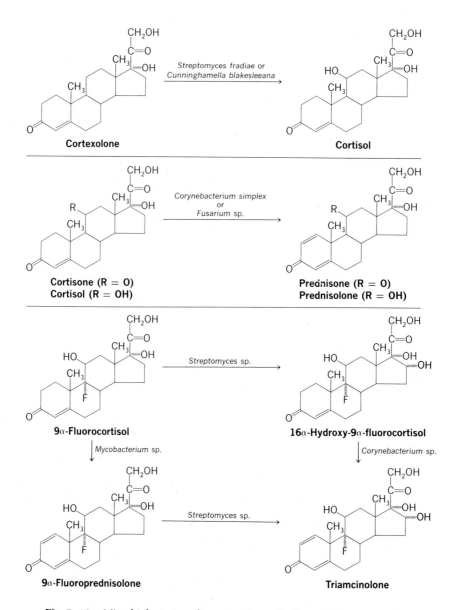

Fig. 7–14. Microbiologic transformation in production of glucocorticoids.

and desire and obesity or unusual muscular development. In adult females, virilism usually develops, associated with a masculine appearance, often with homosexuality. The bearded lady of the circus frequently falls into this category. Treatment of cortical hyperactivity is principally surgical.

Some 70 or more steroids have been isolated from cortical extracts. These exhibit in some degree the action of adrenal cortex. Some, in addition, manifest estrogenic, androgenic, and progesteronelike activity, further indicating the close relationship between the adrenal cortex and the gonads.

Adrenocortical steroids include cortisone, hydrocortisone, desoxycorticosterone, and aldosterone. Cortisone and hydrocortisone comprise the majority of the hormones that regulate protein and carbohydrate metabolism. They have been referred to as the glucocorticoids. Aldosterone and desoxycorticosterone have been referred to as mineralocorticoids. Aldosterone is the principal adrenal steroid that regulates sodium, potassium, and water balance in the organism; however, it is not available for therapeutic use. Also, many agents that are considered primarily as glucocorticoids possess variable mineralocorticoid activity as well.

Preparations of the adrenal cortex are used most effectively in replacement therapy for such conditions as Addison's disease or surgically caused adrenal cortex deficiency. An injection containing a mixture of hormonal substances from the adrenal cortex has been used in replacement therapy. Presumably, use of such a crude mixture offers the advantage of administering all of the active glandular hormones rather than only individual hormones that have been recognized and are available in pure form. However, controlling responses with undefined preparations is difficult, and the subtle responses potentially elicited by the mixed extracts are not easily recognized; thus, the trend in replacement therapy favors the use of pure hormonal substances.

The glucocorticoids are also used for their anti-inflammatory activity; therapy based on this pharmacologic response is an effective palliative approach in rheumatoid arthritis and a number of other conditions involving the inflammatory response. However, caution must be used in balancing the advantages and disadvantages of prolonged durations of corticosteroid therapy, such as may be involved in arthritic conditions. Exogenous sources of corticosteroids may cause a disruption in the physiologic balance among the biosynthetically related steroid hormones; toxic manifestations in such situations often involve changes that are normally considered to be dominated by gonadal hormones. As was discussed earlier, another potential problem of serious consequence is irreversible atrophy of the adrenal cortex.

Glucocorticoid therapy provides palliative treatment of symptoms in many allergic disorders, such as bronchial asthma, and is lifesaving for patients in anaphylactic shock. These compounds are used as immunosuppressive agents in organ transplants and autoimmune disorders and as antitumor agents in the treatment of malignancies, especially in certain leukemias and lymphomas.

Drug Interactions. Barbiturates and diphenylhydantoin can induce the hepatic drug-metabolizing enzymes, such as hydrocortisone hydroxylase, which results in an increased degradation of corticosteroids. Therefore, concomitant therapy with one of these drugs may require an increase in the dose of the corticosteroid.

Because of an increase in hepatic gluconeogenesis during glucocorticoid therapy, the dose of hypoglycemic agents may have to be adjusted upward in diabetic patients receiving corticosteroids.

Desoxycorticosterone or desoxycortone is 21-hydroxypregn-4-ene-3,20-dione, a steroid hormone that was identified by Reichstein and his associates in 1938. Later, it was synthesized from stigmasterol. Present drug supplies are obtained by synthetic means.

This hormone is classified as a mineralocorticoid. Desoxycorticosterone functions primarily to restore a balance of sodium and potassium in body fluids and to restore kidney function in cortical deficiency. Death from hypoglycemia may occur when Addison's disease is treated with desoxycorticosterone alone; such cases also require the use of a glucocorticoid.

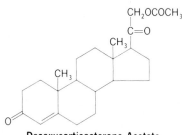
Desoxycorticosterone Acetate

The hydroxyl function at C-21 of desoxycorticosterone is esterified, normally with acetic acid, in pharmaceutic formulations. It is effective when administered buccally, but better and more uniform results follow intramuscular injection. Pellets can be successfully implanted in the subcutaneous tissues for even more prolonged action. Usual dose of desoxycorticosterone acetate, intramuscularly or subcutaneously, is 1 to 6 mg daily.

PRESCRIPTION SPECIALTIES. Doca Acetate®, Percorten Acetate®, Percorten Pivalate® (the trimethylacetate ester).

Cortisone or 17,21-dihydroxypregn-4-ene-3,11,20-trione is one of the glucocorticoid substances of the adrenal cortex. The acetate ester of this hormone is used intramuscularly, orally, and topically to treat a wide variety of situations, such as rheumatoid arthritis, other collagen diseases, Addison's disease, and certain allergic and asthmatic conditions. An appreciable sodium-retaining property can be a major problem with the systemic use of cortisone. Usual dose, orally, is 25 to 300 mg a day; intramuscularly, 20 to 300 mg a day.

PRESCRIPTION SPECIALTY. Cortone® Acetate.

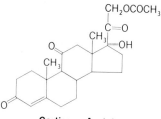
Cortisone Acetate

Cortisol or Hydrocortisone (Kendall's compound F) is $11\beta,17,21$-trihydroxypregn-4-ene-3,20-dione. It is considered the principal glucocorticoid substance of the adrenal cortex. This hormone and its acetate ester are used intramuscularly, orally, and topically for the same purposes as is cortisone acetate. Intra-articular administration of cortisol always involves the acetate ester. Hydrocortisone sodium phosphate and hydrocortisone sodium succinate are water soluble and are used in parenteral formulations when intravenous administration is indicated.

There are indications that cortisol is slightly more potent in some patients than cortisone and gives slightly better overall effects. However, it may exhibit the same disadvantages of sodium retention that were noted with cortisone.

The usual oral dose of hydrocortisone is 5 to 60 mg, 3 or 4 times a day. Topically, it is applied as a 0.5 to 2.5% cream or ointment. Hydrocortisone acetate is usually administered intra-articularly, 5 to 75 mg at each site, repeated at 2- to 3-week intervals. Both hydrocortisone sodium phosphate and hydrocortisone sodium succinate are employed intravenously or intramuscularly in usual doses equivalent to 15 to 240 mg of hydrocortisone a day for the hydrocortisone sodium phosphate and the equivalent of 100 to 500 mg of hydrocortisone, repeated at 1- to 10-hour intervals for hydrocortisone sodium succinate.

PRESCRIPTION SPECIALTIES. Cortef®, Cortef® Acetate, Solu-Cortef®, Hydrocortone®, Hydrocortone® Phosphate.

The potential therapeutic utility of the glucocorticoids has promoted intensive efforts to discover modifications of the naturally occurring hormones that will be more potent and more specific in their activity. The best success has been achieved with desired increases in potency. Prednisone (Deltasone®, Meticorten®, Paracort®) and prednisolone (Deltra-Cortef®, Hydeltrasol®, Meticortelone®, Sterane®) represent early achievements in these efforts. Elimination of any mineralocorticoid activity has been a major objective; a degree of success has been attained with such compounds as betamethasone (Celestrone®), dexamethasone (Decadron®, Dexameth®. Hexadrol®), fluprednisolone (Alphadrol®), methylprednisolone (Medrol®), paramethasone (Haldrone®), meprednisone (Betapar®) and triamcinolone (Aristocort®, Kenacort®), but the ideal of total separation of mineralocorticoid activity from glucocorticoid substances has not yet been achieved. It is interesting to note that successful modifications in the basic steroid molecule fall into 4 categories:

1. Δ^1-dehydrogenation
2. 16α-hydroxylation
3. 6α- or 9α-fluorination
4. 6α-, 16α-, or 16β-methylation.

GONADS

The ovaries and testes are exocrine (ova, sperm) as well as endocrine (hormonal) in function. They develop under the influence of anterior pituitary hormones, particularly:

1. The follicle-stimulating hormone (FSH) leads to the development of the ovarian follicles, to their formation of ova and of estrogen, and to the development of the testes and the maturation of the spermatozoa.

2. The luteinizing hormone (LH) is necessary to the development of the corpora lutea in the ovarian follicles after ovulation, to the formation of progesterone by the corpora lutea, and to the production of androgen in the matured testis.

Androgens (male hormones) and estrogens (female follicular hormones) act to:

1. Develop and maintain the secondary characters of sex.

2. Depress anterior pituitary function, leading in turn to the depression of the testis or the ovary.

Progesterone (corpus luteum hormone) similarly depresses anterior pituitary function and presents a mixed antagonism-synergism with estrogenic activity, as will be indicated later.

Gonadal hyperactivity or excessive therapy may thus result in a picture of precocious or excessive sexual development, with the generalized effects of anterior pituitary depression. Gonadal hypoactivity, as occurs in the natural menopause or following surgical removal of the gonads, results in a mixed picture of sexual regression and enhanced anterior pituitary activity with psychic disturbance and the involvement of other endocrine glands, particularly the thyroid.

TESTES

Following castration in the male, the sex organs atrophy, and sexual desire and activity are diminished. These functions are restored by the administration of testis hormone. Hypogonadism (eunuchoidism) is inadequate development of the testes, owing to pituitary disorder, infection, or other disease. Therapy of this condition is still in the experimental stages.

Hypergonadism is most frequently seen in young males, owing to testis tumors; this results in precocious development of sex organs and male characteristics. Therapy is usually surgical.

Testosterone is believed to be the true testis hormone, although it has been identified only in the bull's testis. It was synthesized by Ruzicka from cholesterol in 1936. Androsterone and dehydroandrosterone are urinary excretion products, relatively inactive in man.

Testes hormone preparations have been valuable in the replacement therapy of male castrates and eunuchoid states and in the treatment of certain female ovarian dysfunctions. Much of this therapy is still in the experimental stages. Testosterone is not an aphrodisiac and its use may produce the general effects of anterior pituitary depression. It may produce virilism in the female, and skin reactions similar to acne vulgaris may frequently develop.

Anabolic effects, especially with regard to protein synthesis and nitrogen retention in the body, have been noted with androgens. This action is potentially useful as supportive therapy in a number of debilitating conditions. Attempts have been made to prepare steroid compounds that separate anabolic effects from other androgenic activities, and the ultimate limitations on this therapeutic approach are keyed to the success of these efforts. The ideal separation has not been achieved with such compounds as methylandros-tenediol, methandrostenolone, and other anabolic substances that are currently available.

Testosterone or 17β-hydroxyandrost-4-en-3-one is the active male hormone. The quantities used for drug purposes are prepared synthetically. The 17-hydroxyl function of testosterone is readily oxidized and metabolized to the much less physiologically active keto compound. Thus, testosterone is not administered orally. The hormone may be used buccally, implanted subcutaneously, or injected intramuscularly. However, many formulations for these purposes utilize derivatives of the hormone, such as the cypionate, ethanthate, and propionate esters of the 17-hydroxyl group, which are characterized by delayed absorption and destruction. Usual dose of testosterone, intramuscularly, is 25 mg as needed; implantation, 300 mg.

Prescription Specialties. Delatestryl®, Oreton®, Oreton® Propionate.

The introduction of a methyl substituent at C-17 is another manipulation that has been used to circumvent the chemical and metabolic instability of testosterone. Preparations of methyltestosterone (Android®, Metandren®, Oreton® Methyl) are used buccally and orally for androgenic purposes.

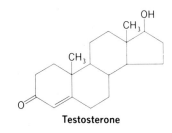

Testosterone

OVARY

The human ovaries are paired organs. One is situated on each lateral pelvic wall in the posterior layer of the broad ligament, behind and below the lateral extremity of each Fallopian tube (oviduct). Each is about the size and shape of an unshelled almond and weighs about 4 to 8 g.

Ova develop within primitive ovarian follicles (Graafian follicles) under the influence of the follicle-stimulating hormone of anterior pituitary. Ovulation with the extrusion of one ovum from a ripened follicle normally occurs each month during the childbearing period. The ruptured follicle undergoes cellular change to become the corpus luteum under the influence of the luteinizing hormone of anterior pituitary. The ovary elaborates 2 types of hormones; namely, the estrogens, elaborated in the developing Graafian follicle and probably also in the placenta during pregnancy; and the progestins, normally elaborated by the corpus luteum and, in the later half of pregnancy, by the placenta.

Estrogens. Deficiency in estrogenic activity is most frequently experienced in the normal menopause or following surgical removal of the ovaries. Local changes in the tissues of the vagina and vulva may result from estrogenic deficiency of any cause. The estrogens are necessary to:

1. Develop and maintain secondary female sex characters.

2. Develop and maintain the uterus and the vagina.

3. Aid in the presecretory development of the mammary glands.

4. Act as a growth hormone for uterine smooth muscle cells during pregnancy.

Estrogens act further to excite or sensitize the uterine muscle and to depress the anterior pituitary function. Preparations of estrogenic substances are employed in the management of:

1. Symptoms of the natural or surgical menopause.

2. Local atrophic and degenerative changes in the adult vagina and vulva, resulting from estrogen deficiency.

3. Gonorrheal vaginitis in the young female child, by inducing an adult type of vaginal epithelium resistant to the gonococcus.

4. Suppression of lactation in engorged, painful mammary glands, presumably by a direct action in the breast.

5. Prostatic cancer in the male, presumably by balancing an excessive persistence of androgen—the principle of "biochemical castration."

The natural ovarian hormones are steroids. The 3 major estrogenic hormones are estradiol and its oxidation products, estriol, and estrone. These hormones can be isolated from pregnancy urine and can be prepared synthetically. Other estrogenic substances occur naturally, and amorphous mixtures of some of these steroids obtained from a pregnant mare's urine are used in therapy under the designations of conjugated and esterified estrogens.

Estrogens may be administered orally, parenterally, by implantation, or by inunction for systemic activity. Orally administered natural estrogens are destroyed in greater part. Estriol is the best of the pure, naturally occurring estrogens for oral use; oral efficiency of estriol is about one-fifth that achieved by parenteral administration. Conjugated and esterified estrogens are also used orally, and the introduction of an ethinyl substituent at C-17 of estradiol gives a potent, orally effective compound; the usual dose of ethinyl estradiol (Estinyl®, Feminone®) is 50 μg, 1 to 3 times a day.

As much as 90% of parenterally administered natural estrogens may be destroyed. This factor, in addition to rapid absorption, tends to diminish their efficiency and the effective period of therapy. Pharmaceutic manipulations, which have proved useful in achieving a prolonged action, include the use of esters, such as cypionate or valerate, and of formulations involving sterile vegetable oils. These manipulations slow absorption and destruction of the hormones; they also lessen the side effects of nausea and vomiting.

Implantation of the estrogens or their esters provides an even longer duration of action than do preparations administered intramuscularly. Suppositories containing estrogenic substances provide local treatment of changes in the vagina or vulva, or treatment of gonorrheal vaginitis in female children, with a minimum of systemic effect.

The natural estrogens exhibit carcinogenic properties, upon prolonged administration, to animal strains having hereditary susceptibility to mammary cancer. On this basis, some people feel that estrogens should be contraindicated in women who have a personal or family history of mammary or genital cancer.

Estradiol. Estradiol or estra-1,3,5(10)-triene-3,17β-diol is used orally, injected intramuscularly, and implanted subcutaneously. Usual dose, orally, 1 to 2 mg daily; implantation, 25 mg, as necessary.

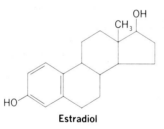

Estradiol

The usual intramuscular maintenance doses of the estradiol esters are 1 to 5 mg every 2 to 3 weeks for the cypionate (Depo-Estradiol®) and 10 to 40 mg every 1 to 4 weeks for the valerate (Delestrogen®).

Estrone. Estrone or estra-1,3,5(10)-trien-3-ol-17-one is used intramuscularly. The usual dose is 100 μg to 2 mg per week for menopausal symptoms.

PRESCRIPTION SPECIALTY. Theelin®.

The designation **conjugated estrogens** refers to a mixture of the sodium salts of the sulfate esters of the estrogenic substances that are of the type excreted by pregnant mares. This mixture of estrogenic substances must contain not less than 50% and not more than 65% of sodium estrone sulfate and not less than 20% and not more than 35% of sodium equilin sulfate. Equilin is estra-1,3,5(10),7-tetraen-3-ol-17-one and is one of the estrogens that appears in pregnant mare's urine in increasing quantities as the stage of pregnancy advances; equilin is only slightly less potent than estradiol. Conjugated estrogens may be administered orally or parenterally. Usual dose for menopausal symptoms, orally, 300 μg to 1.25 mg, daily, cyclically, and a progestin may be added the last 7 to 10 days.

PRESCRIPTION SPECIALTIES. Menotabs®, Premarin®.

The designation **esterified estrogens** also refers to a mixture of the sodium salts of the sulfate esters of the estrogenic substances that are of the type excreted by pregnant mares. This mixture differs from conjugated estrogens because it has more estrone and less equilin metabolites. It must contain not less than 75% and not more than 85% of sodium estrone sulfate and not less than 6.5% and not more than 15% of sodium equilin sulfate. It is used orally for the same purposes and in the same dosage range as are preparations of conjugated estrogens.

PRESCRIPTION SPECIALTIES. Amnestrogen®, Menest®, Evex®.

A number of stilbene derivatives, as well as various other compounds, have estrogenic activity. These synthetic substances are active orally and have been used in some instances as therapeutic substitutes for the estrogenic steroids. These stilbene derivatives are absorbed rapidly, destroyed slowly, and active for a prolonged period. However, the side effects of nausea and vomiting also tend to be enhanced. Diethylstilbestrol is probably the best known of these substances, but other useful derivatives include chlorotrianisene (Tace®) and dienestrol.

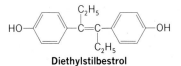

Diethylstilbestrol

Corpus Luteum—Progestin. The corpus luteum is essential to the maintenance of human pregnancy during the first half of the term. Its principal hormonal functions are:

1. Preparation of the uterine mucosa to receive the fertilized ovum.

2. Development of the maternal placenta.

3. Continuation of the development of the mammary glands in preparation for lactogenic action of anterior pituitary.

4. Suppression of ovulation for the duration of pregnancy.

5. Antagonism of the stimulating effect of estrogens on the uterine muscle to produce a relaxation of the uterus.

The active hormone of the corpus luteum is progesterone. It can be prepared synthetically from a number of steroidal substances. Progesterone is relatively inactive on oral administration, and it is given buccally or parenterally. This hormone is used in the treatment of amenorrhea, dysmenorrhea, endometriosis, functional uterine bleeding, premenstrual tension, and threatened or habitual abortion.

Progesterone. Progesterone is pregn-4-ene-3,20-dione. Usual dose, intramuscularly, is 5 to 100 mg.

PRESCRIPTION SPECIALTIES. Progelan in Oil®, and Profac-O®.

A number of synthetic progestins have been developed that have such advantages over progesterone as fewer side effects when administered over prolonged periods, oral efficacy, and greater potency. Such compounds as hydroxyprogesterone caproate in oil (Delalutin®), methoxyprogesterone acetate (Provera®), and norethindrone (Norlutin®) may be used as therapeutic substitutes for the natural hormone.

One of the normal physiologic functions of progesterone is to suppress ovulation during pregnancy. This hormone is not formed during the first half of a normal menstrual cycle, but administration of it or of some other progestational agent during this part of the menstrual period offers an effective means of birth control. When progestins are used as oral contraceptives, some estrogenic substance is frequently added, either by combined formulation or sequential administration, to the therapeutic approach to reduce side effects.

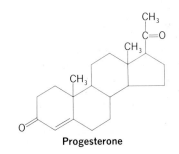

Progesterone

Progesterone is also available in an intrauterine device (IUD). The hormone is dissolved in silicone oil, and the flexible polymer of the IUD acts as a membrane to allow for the slow release of progesterone (65 μg daily) into the uterine cavity. The IUD contains enough progesterone to last 1 year, and the failure rate is about 2%. The failure rate of the same device without progesterone is approximately 18%. The product is called Progestasert®.

READING REFERENCES

IUPAC-IUB Revised Tentative Rules for Nomenclature of Steroids, J. Org. Chem., 34(6):1517, 1969.

Beher, W. T.: Bile Acids. In *Monographs on Atherosclerosis*, Vol. VI, Kritchevsky, D., Pollack, O. J., and Simms, H. S., eds., Basel, S. Karger AG, 1976.

Bodem, G., and Dengler, H. J., eds.: *Cardiac Glycosides*, Berlin, Springer-Verlag, 1978.

Briggs, M. H., and Brotherton, J.: *Steroid Biochemistry and Pharmacology*, New York, Academic Press, Inc., 1970.

Charney, W., and Herzog, H. L.: *Microbial Transformations of Steroids*, New York, Academic Press, Inc., 1967.

Cope, C. L.: *Adrenal Steroids and Disease*, Philadelphia, J. B. Lippincott Co., 1972.

Fisch, C., and Surawicz, B.: *Digitalis*, New York, Grune and Stratton, 1969.

Freedman, M. A., and Freedman, S. N.: *Introduction to Steroid Biochemistry and Its Clinical Application*, New York, Harper & Row, 1970.

Frieden, E., and Lipner, H.: *Biochemical Endocrinology of the Vertebrates*, Englewood Cliffs, New Jersey, Prentice-Hall, Inc., 1971.

Goodwin, T. W.: *Aspects of Terpenoid Chemistry and Biochemistry*, New York, Academic Press, Inc., 1971.

Greene, R.: *Human Hormones*, New York, McGraw-Hill Book Co., 1970.

Heftman, E.: *Steroid Biochemistry*, New York, Academic Press, Inc., 1970.

Iizuka, H., and Naito, A.: *Microbial Transformation of Steroids and Alkaloids*, State College, Pennsylvania, University Park Press, 1967.

James, V. H. T., ed.: *Hormonal Steroids*, Amsterdam, Excerpta Medica, 1971.

Johns, W. F., ed.: *MTP International Review of Science: Steroids*, Organic Chemistry, Series 1, Vol. VIII, Baltimore, University Park Press, 1973.

Johns, W. F., ed.: *International Review of Science: Steroids*, Organic Chemistry, Series 2, Vol. VIII, London, Butterworth & Co. (Publishers) Ltd., 1976.

Lehmann, F., P. A., Bolivar, G., A., and Quintero, R., R.: Russell E. Marker, Pioneer of the Mexican Steroid Industry, J. Chem. Educ., *50*(3):195, 1973.

McCann, S. M., ed.: *Endocrine Physiology*, Baltimore, University Park Press, 1974.

Makin, H. L. J., ed.: *Biochemistry of Steroid Hormones*, Oxford, Blackwell Scientific Publications, 1975.

Marks, B. H., and Weissler, A. M., eds.: *Basic and Clinical Pharmacology of Digitalis*, Springfield, Illinois, Charles C Thomas, 1972.

Miller, L. P., ed.: *Phytochemistry, Organic Metabolites*, Vol. II, New York, Van Nostrand Reinhold Co., 1973.

Moss, A. J., and Patton, R. D.: *Antiarrhythmic Agents*, Springfield, Illinois, Charles C Thomas, 1973.

Nair, P. P., and Kritchevsky, D., eds.: *The Bile Acids; Chemistry, Physiology, and Metabolism*, Vols. I and II, New York, Plenum Press, 1971, 1973.

Nes, W. R., and McKean, M. L.: *Biochemistry of Steroids and Other Isopentenoids*, Baltimore, University Park Press, 1977.

Newman, A. A.: *Chemistry of Terpenes and Terpenoids*, London, Academic Press, Inc. Ltd., 1972.

Pasqualini, J. R., ed.: *Receptors and Mechanism of Action of Steroid Hormones*, Parts I and II, New York, Marcel Dekker, Inc., 1976, 1977.

Rickenberg, H. V., ed.: *MTP International Review of Science: Biochemistry of Hormones*, Biochemistry Series 1, Vol. VIII, Baltimore, University Park Press, 1974.

Sanders, H. J.: Arthritis Drugs, Chem. Eng. News, Aug. 12, 46, 1968.

Schulster, D., Burstein, S., and Cooke, B. A.: *Molecular Endocrinology of the Steroid Hormones*, London, John Wiley & Sons, Ltd., 1976.

Singh, B., and Rastogi, R. P.: Review Article: Cardenolides—Glycosides and Genins, Phytochemistry, *9*(2):315, 1970.

Tepperman, J.: *Metabolic and Endocrine Physiology*, Chicago, Year Book Medical Publishers, Inc., 1973.

Thomas, J. A., and Mawhinney, M. G.: *Synopsis of Endocrine Pharmacology*, Baltimore, University Park Press, 1973.

Thomas J. A., and Singhal, R. L., eds.: *Molecular Mechanisms of Gonadal Hormone Action*, Baltimore, University Park Press, 1975.

Thomas, R., Boutagy, J., and Gelbart, A.: Synthesis and Biological Activity of Semisynthetic Digitalis Analogs, J. Pharm. Sci., *63*(11):1649, 1974.

Chapter **8**

Alkaloids

Alkaloids are extremely difficult to define because they do not represent a homogeneous group of compounds from either the chemical, biochemical, or physiologic viewpoint. Consequently, except for the fact that they are all organic nitrogenous compounds, reservations must be appended to any general definition. All alkaloids occur in plants, but some are found in animals, and practically all have been reproduced in the laboratory by chemical synthesis. Most possess basic properties, owing to the presence of an amino nitrogen, and many, especially those pertinent to pharmacy and medicine, possess marked physiologic activity. In spite of the difficulties attending a precise definition, the term alkaloid is extremely useful and is commonly applied to basic nitrogenous compounds of plant origin that are physiologically active.

The alkaloids appear to have a restricted distribution in the plant kingdom. This observation is based on the incomplete investigations of plants up to the present time; considerable research must be accomplished before definite statements concerning the occurrence of alkaloids can be made. Among the angiosperms, the Leguminosae, Papaveraceae, Ranunculaceae, Rubiaceae, Solanaceae, and Berberidaceae are outstanding alkaloid-yielding plants. The Labiatae and Rosaceae are almost free of alkaloids; the gymnosperms only rarely contain them (Taxaceae). Although it has been claimed that the monocotyledons do not generally produce alkaloids, investigations indicate that the Amaryllidaceae and Liliaceae are 2 of the most promising families (of a list of 11) in which to search for alkaloid-yielding plants.

Specific alkaloids of complex structures are ordinarily confined to specific plant families (hyoscyamine in Solanaceae, colchicine in Liliaceae). Nicotine, which is found in a number of widely scattered plant families, is not an exception to this rule because of the biosynthetic simplicity of its structure. However, the occurrence of ergot alkaloids in the fungus *Claviceps purpurea* and certain *Ipomoea* species (Convolvulaceae) is a definite exception and may be attributed to either parallel or convergent evolution of certain complex biochemical pathways. Alkaloids may

195

occur in various parts of the plant: in seeds (physostigma, areca), in fruits (conium), in leaves (belladonna, coca), in underground stems (sanguinaria), in roots (belladonna root), in rhizomes and roots (ipecac, hydrastis), and in barks (cinchona). They are also found in the fungi (ergot, *Amanita citrina*).

The names of the alkaloids are obtained in various ways: (1) from the generic name of the plant yielding them (hydrastine, atropine), (2) from the specific name of the plant yielding them (cocaine, belladonnine), (3) from the common name of the drug yielding them (ergotamine), (4) from their physiologic activity (emetine, morphine), and (5) occasionally from the discoverer (pelletierine).

Sometimes a prefix or suffix is added to the name of a principal alkaloid to designate another alkaloid from the same source (quinine, quinidine, hydroquinine). By agreement, chemical rules designate that the names of all alkaloids should end in "ine."[*]

Alkaloids usually contain 1 nitrogen atom, although some, like ergotamine, may contain up to 5. The nitrogen may exist as a primary amine (RNH_2), as a secondary amine (R_2NH), or as a tertiary amine (R_3N).

Because the nitrogen atom bears an unshared pair of electrons, such compounds are basic and resemble ammonia's chemical properties. The degree of basicity varies greatly, depending on the structure of the molecule and the presence and location of other functional groups. Like ammonia, the alkaloids are converted into their salts by aqueous mineral acids, and when the salt of an alkaloid is treated with hydroxide ion, nitrogen gives up a hydrogen ion and the free amine is liberated. Quaternary ammonium compounds [$R_4N^+X^-$], such as tubocurarine chloride or berberine chloride, have 4 organic groups covalently bonded to nitrogen, and the positive charge of this ion is balanced by some negative ion. The quaternary ammonium ion, having no proton to give up, is not affected by hydroxide ion; consequently, quaternary ammonium compounds have chemical properties quite different from those of the amines.

In spite of the difficulty in precisely characterizing alkaloids by definition, they do have in common a surprising number of physical and chemical properties. For the most part, the alkaloids are insoluble or sparingly so in water, but the salts formed on reaction with acids are usually freely soluble. The free alkaloids are usually soluble in ether, chloroform, or other relatively nonpolar, immiscible solvents in which, however, the alkaloidal salts are insoluble. This permits a ready means for the isolation and purification of the alkaloids as well as for their quantitative estimation. Most of the alkaloids are crystalline solids, although a few are amorphous. An additional few, coniine, nicotine, and sparteine, which lack oxygen in their molecules, are liquids. Alkaloidal salts are crystalline, and their crystal form and habit are often a useful means of rapid microscopic identification.

Alkaloids are usually classified according to the nature of the basic chemical structures from which they derive. A number of these structures are shown in Figure 8–1. Arecoline, lobeline, and nicotine are derivatives of **pyridine** and **piperidine;** atropine, hyoscyamine, and hyoscine are derived from **tropane,** a condensation product of pyrrolidine and piperidine; the cinchona alkaloids, quinine, quinidine, cinchonine, and cinchonidine, contain **quinoline** as the principal nucleus; hydrastine, (+)-tubocurarine, emetine, and the opium alkaloids are characterized by the **isoquinoline** nucleus. Other types include ergonovine, reserpine, and strychnine, which derive from the **indole** ring; pilocarpine, which

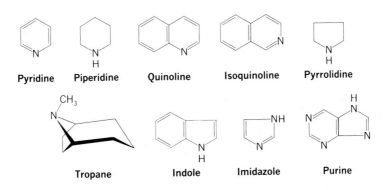

Fig. 8–1. Important nitrogen-containing ring structures present in alkaloidal drugs.

has the **imidazole** ring; caffeine and theobromine, which are **purine** bases, and protoveratrine, which contains a **steroidal** structure.

The alkaloids, like other amines, form double salts with compounds of mercury, gold, platinum, and other heavy metals. These double salts are usually obtained as precipitates, and many of them are microcrystallographically characteristic. The common alkaloidal reagents include Wagner's (iodine in potassium iodide), Mayer's (potassium mercuric iodide), Dragendorff's (potassium bismuth iodide), and many others. The alkaloids usually possess a bitter taste.

Much has been written about the possible function of alkaloids in plants and about the reasons why they occur there. Some of the possibilities that have been discussed include their functions as (1) poisonous agents protecting the plant against insects and herbivores, (2) end products of detoxification reactions representing a metabolic locking-up of compounds otherwise harmful to the plant, (3) regulatory growth factors, or (4) reserve substances capable of supplying nitrogen or other elements necessary to the plant's economy.

Although certain exceptions exist because of the diverse nature of alkaloids, the evidence for any result of alkaloid formation useful to the existence of the plant is slight. Perhaps the best example of such a result is found in the wild plants of certain arid regions, where overgrazing by domestic animals has taken place for centuries. An extremely high percentage of such plants contains alkaloids that, because of their bitter taste or toxic properties, apparently confer survival value on the species producing them. Plants lacking such distasteful substances were long ago exterminated. However, to avoid being teleologic, we must emphasize that protection, like the other postulated functions, is a consequence of, not a reason for, alkaloid formation.

Perhaps alkaloids should be viewed as products of metabolic experimentation that reflect the intermediary evolutionary stages now attained by plants. Alkaloid formation is probably best regarded as a metabolic act involving longer or shorter reaction sequences that begin with substances normal and essential in plant metabolism and end with compounds not necessarily serving such a purpose. Because the process is genetically controlled, an alkaloid-producing plant is merely a plant in which this additional metabolic reaction has evolved through mutation of one or more genes. Proof that such changes occur irrespective of the utility of ultimate products is given by the thousands of pigments, tannins, polysaccharides, glycosides, volatile oils, and resins to which no essential role in plant metabolism can be ascribed.

Like many of these other secondary constituents, the alkaloids may be thought of as resulting from a "metabolic error," which will probably be eliminated when plants approach a stage of ultimate adaptation and eliminate all redundant features and processes. They are thus a kind of waste product retained within the organism that produces them. It must be emphasized that, unlike many such substances with which we are familiar, the alkaloids are structurally complex end products of energy-requiring reaction sequences.

The pharmacologic action of alkaloids varies widely: some (morphine, codeine) are analgesics and narcotics whereas others (strychnine, brucine) are central stimulants. Some (atropine) are mydriatics whereas others (physostigmine, pilocarpine) are myotics. Some (ephedrine) cause a rise in blood pressure, but others (reserpine) produce a fall in excessive hypertension. In fact, the alkaloids are capable of extensive physiologic activity.

Various schemes for the classification of alkaloids have been suggested. The following plan is based on the ring structure or nucleus of the chief alkaloid group in the plant drug: (1) pyridine-piperidine combined, (2) tropane, (3) quinoline, (4) isoquinoline, (5) indole, (6) imidazole, (7) steroid, (8) alkaloidal amine, and (9) purine.

The biosynthesis of many alkaloidal structures can be rationalized through simple chemical reactions that involve amino acids. The amino acids that most often serve as alkaloidal precursors include phenylalanine, tyrosine, tryptophan, histidine, anthranilic acid, lysine, and ornithine. Some of the general reactions of particular importance include the decarboxylation and transamination of the amino acids to yield a corresponding amine or aldehyde. These can react to form a Schiff base which, in turn, can react with a carbanion in a Mannich-type condensation. These general reactions are illustrated in Figure 8–2. Specific examples of alkaloid biosynthesis are discussed under the various structural groups of alkaloids.

PYRIDINE-PIPERIDINE ALKALOIDS

Upon reduction, the tertiary base, pyridine, is converted into the secondary base, piperidine. These 2 nuclei form the basis of this group.

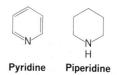

Pyridine   Piperidine

This group is sometimes divided into 3 subgroups: (1) derivatives of piperidine,

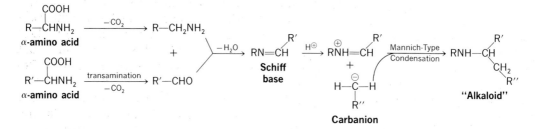

Fig. 8–2. General reactions in alkaloid biosynthesis.

including lobeline from lobelia; (2) derivatives of nicotinic acid, including arecoline from areca; and (3) derivatives of both pyridine and pyrrolidine, including nicotine from tobacco. The important alkaloidal drugs and their alkaloids that are classified in this group are areca, arecoline hydrobromide, lobelia, lobeline, and nicotine.

BIOSYNTHESIS OF PYRIDINE-PIPERIDINE ALKALOIDS

Nicotine. More than 65 years ago, the Swiss chemist Trier proposed that nicotine was biosynthesized from nicotinic acid and proline. If proline is considered a representative of the ornithine-proline-glutamic acid group, this remarkable hypothesis may be considered correct. However, numerous experiments conducted principally during the last 2 decades still have not clarified completely all of the reactions involved in the production of nicotine in *Nicotiana* species. The biosynthetic pathways leading to this compound are summarized in Figure 8–3.

Tracer studies have shown that ornithine is incorporated into nicotine by tobacco plants. This incorporation results in

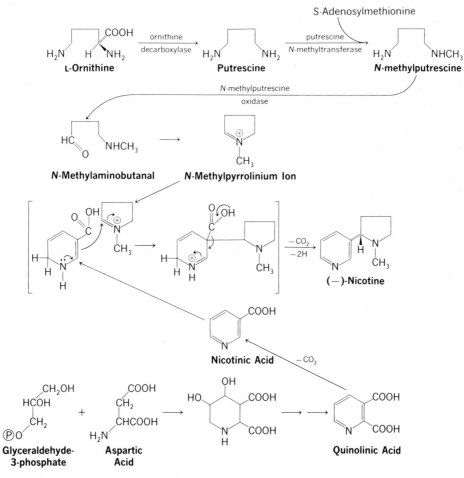

Fig. 8–3. Biosynthesis of nicotine.

a symmetric labeling pattern of nicotine. Putrescine, N-methylputrescine, and N-methylaminobutanal are all incorporated, and the key intermediate is thought to be the N-methylpyrrolinium ion which, through electrophilic aromatic substitution, attaches to C-3 of the pyridine ring of nicotinic acid. Nicotinic acid is formed in higher plants and certain microorganisms via quinolinic acid by the condensation of glyceraldehyde-3-phosphate and aspartic acid.

Nicotine is primarily a product of root metabolism, but the formation of small amounts, as well as subsequent reactions such as the demethylation of nicotine, can occur in the leaves of plants.

ARECA

Areca, areca nut, or betel nut is the dried, ripe seed of *Areca catechu* Linné (Fam. Palmae). *Areca* is the Spanish and Portuguese term for the betel nut. *Catechu* is the East Indian name for an astringent extract or juice. *Areca catechu* is a beautiful tall palm extensively cultivated in India, southeastern Asia, the East Indies, and to some extent East Africa. The fruit is a nut that contains a single seed with a thin seed coat and a large ruminate endosperm. The seeds are removed from the fruits, boiled in water containing lime, and dried. India is a major producer of areca, but its production is mostly consumed domestically. The United States imports the drug from Sri Lanka. Sri Lanka also exports to India when areca is in short supply.

Areca is mixed with lime, the leaves of *Piper betle* Linné, and occasionally gambir. The mixture is used as a stimulant masticatory in India and the East Indies. In India, the mixture is known as "pun-supari." Betel chewing has been practiced since early times. The natives chew fresh betel nuts; dried betel nuts are used for pharmaceutic purposes. The value of areca

as a taenicide apparently has been known in the East for a long time but was not known to western civilization until 1863.

Areca contains several alkaloids that are reduced pyridine derivatives. Among them are arecoline (arecaidine methyl ester), arecaidine (N-methyl guvacine), guvacine (tetrahydronicotinic acid), and guvacoline (guvacine methyl ester). The total alkaloid content can reach 0.45%. Arecoline, the most abundant and physiologically most active alkaloid, is a liquid occurring to the extent of about 0.2%. Areca also contains tannin (about 15%), lipids, volatile oils, and gum.

USE AND DOSE. Areca is classified as an anthelmintic in veterinary practice and is employed as a vermicide and taenifuge. Usual dose in dogs is 2 to 4 g; in sheep, 4 to 8 g, based on the weight of the animal.

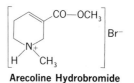

Arecoline Hydrobromide

LOBELIA

Lobelia or Indian tobacco consists of the dried leaves and tops of *Lobelia inflata* Linné (Fam. Lobeliaceae). *Lobelia* was named in honor of Matthias de L'Obel, a Flemish botanist (1538 to 1616); *inflata* refers to the fruit, which is hollow and distended. The plant is an annual herb indigenous to the eastern and central United States and to Canada.

Commercial supplies come from collecting stations in North Carolina, Virginia, and Tennessee. It should be collected after a portion of the capsules has become inflated; then it should be carefully dried and preserved. Lobelia was employed by the Indians, when necessity required, as a substitute for tobacco. Its emetic properties were first observed in 1785, and the drug was introduced into medicine in 1807.

The drug contains 14 alkaloids, of which lobeline is the major and most important, a pungent volatile oil, resin, lipids, and gum.

Lobeline, (−)-lobeline, or *alpha* lobeline (to distinguish it from a mixture of the lobelia alkaloids formerly designated as lobeline) occurs as colorless crystals that are slightly soluble in water but readily soluble in hot alcohol.

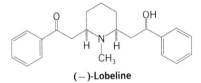

(−)-Lobeline

Uses and Dose. Galenic preparations of lobelia were formerly used for expectorant purposes. Lobeline is a respiratory stimulant, but its action is somewhat unreliable and its duration is brief. Other effects resemble those of nicotine. For this reason, 0.5- to 1.5-mg doses of lobeline sulfate are incorporated in tablets or lozenges that are intended to aid in breaking the tobacco habit (smoking deterrents). The effectiveness of such treatment requires scientific verification.

TROPANE ALKALOIDS

Tropane is a dicyclic compound formed by the condensation of a pyrrolidine precursor (ornithine) with 3 acetate-derived carbon atoms. Both pyrrolidine and piperidine ring systems can be discerned in the molecule.

The 3-hydroxy derivative of tropane is known as tropine. Its esterification with (−)-tropic acid yields hyoscyamine (tropine tropate), which may be racemized to form atropine.

BIOSYNTHESIS OF TROPANE ALKALOIDS

Because of the commercial importance of hyoscyamine and scopolamine, investigation of their biosynthesis has been extensive, especially in *Datura* species. Feeding studies with labeled ornithine have revealed that this amino acid is incorporated stereospecifically to form the pyrrolidine ring of tropine. The remaining 3 carbon atoms are derived from acetate and thus complete the piperidine moiety. Methylation results via transmethylation from S-adenosylmethionine to complete the tropine nucleus.

Phenylalanine is the precursor of tropic acid. Tracer studies have shown that the side chain of the amino acid undergoes a novel type of intramolecular rearrangement during the conversion. Esterification of tropic acid with tropine produces hyoscyamine. These reactions are summarized in Figure 8–4.

The important drugs and alkaloids in this group are belladonna leaf, hyoscyamus, stramonium, atropine, hyoscyamine, scopolamine, coca, and cocaine.

BELLADONNA

Belladonna leaf, belladonna herb, or deadly nightshade leaf consists of the dried leaf and flowering or fruiting top of *Atropa belladonna* Linné or of its variety *acuminata* Royle ex Lindley (Fam. Solanaceae) (Fig. 8–5). Belladonna leaf yields not less than 0.35% of alkaloids.

Atropa is from *Atropos,* meaning inflexible, the name of the Greek Fate who cuts the thread of life, and probably alludes to the poisonous character of the drug. Belladonna is from the Italian *bella,* meaning beautiful, and *donna,* meaning lady. (The juice of the berry, when placed in the eyes,

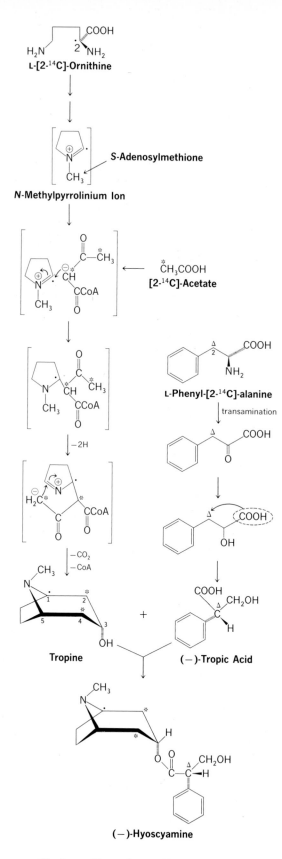

Fig. 8-4. Biosynthesis of hyoscyamine.

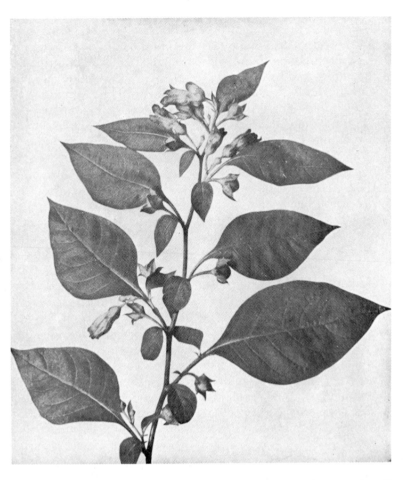

Fig. 8–5. *Atropa belladonna* showing the alternate, petiolate, ovate, entire leaves, in the axils of which are the solitary fruits or flowers with large, leafy bracts.

causes dilation of the pupils. thus giving a striking appearance.)

The plant is a perennial herb that grows to a meter in height. It is indigenous to central and southern Europe and to Asia Minor and is cultivated in sunny locations in England, Germany, India, and the United States. At present, the chief source of supply is the Balkans.

Belladonna was probably known to the ancients, but the first authentic notice appeared in 1504. The poisonous character of the plant has been known for many years, particularly in its indigenous localities. It was the subject of many treatises during the eighteenth century. Its mydriatic properties were first recorded in 1802, but its analgesic properties were not recognized until 1860. The leaves were used earlier than the root, whose use did not occur until about 1860.

The stems are cut about halfway down when the fruits begin to form and the alkaloids are most abundant. After rains or irrigation, the plant produces a second crop of leaves and flowers, which are gathered in the fall. Most of the herb crop is dried or partially dried and extracted with acidified water to obtain the alkaloids. A fine grade of leaf is obtained by hand picking the leaves and drying them rapidly at rather low temperatures and in the shade.

The leaf yields alkaloids in concentrations ranging up to more than 1%. About three fourths of the isolated alkaloid mixture is (−)-hyoscyamine; the remainder is atropine. The latter compound exists, at most, only in traces in fresh plant material. Atropine is formed by racemization during the extraction process. Small but varying amounts of other bases are found in the root, but not in the leaf. These include apoatropine, belladonnine, cuscohygrine, and scopolamine.

The yield of alkaloids averages as follows: roots, 0.6%; stems, 0.05%; leaves, 0.4%; unripe berries, 0.19%; ripe berries, 0.21%; seeds, 0.33%.

USES AND DOSE. Belladonna acts as a parasympathetic depressant, which accounts for its use as a spasmolytic agent. It possesses anticholinergic properties and is used to control excess motor activity of the gastrointestinal tract and spasm of the urinary tract.

Belladonna leaf is commonly administered in the form of belladonna tincture. The usual dose of the tincture is 0.6 to 1 ml, 3 or 4 times a day.

PRESCRIPTION PRODUCTS. Belladonna alkaloids: Bellafoline®. Belladonna extract: Belap SE®. Among the preparations containing mixtures of the belladonna alkaloids in combination with barbiturates or other ingredients are Belladenal®, Bellergal®, Butibel®, and Donnatal®.

NONPRESCRIPTION PRODUCTS. Belladonna is used in the following cold and allergy preparations that have drying effects on mucus secretions: Spantac®, Spen-Cold®, Supres®, Extendac®, Nazac®, Spandecon®. For antidiarrheal preparations in which belladonna is used in combination with either opium alkaloids, kaolin, and/or pectin, see page 228.

Practically no alkaloids are isolated from belladonna on a commercial scale although a total alkaloid fraction of belladonna is available. One must ascertain that this product represents the true, total alkaloids of belladonna rather than an admixture of alkaloids of other solanaceous drugs. Belladonna, hyoscyamus, and stramonium are seldom used in any form other than as the powdered extract, fluidextract, or tincture.

Most of the alkaloids are derived from Egyptian henbane (*Hyoscyamus muticus* Linné). Another important source is *Duboisia*, particularly *Duboisia myoporoides* R. Brown and *D. leichardtii* F. Moeller. The relative percentages of scopolamine and hyoscyamine occurring in *Duboisia* depend on the species used, the area in which the plants are collected, and the season of the year. After *Duboisia* was developed as a source of solanaceous alkaloids (during World War II), T. Smith and H. Smith of Edinburgh, Scotland, developed a purely synthetic process for the formation of atropine starting with tropine. Although this process was successful, it was not economical; at present, atropine and the related alkaloids are still produced from *Duboisia* (see page 209) and from *Hyoscyamus muticus* (see page 207).

SOLANACEOUS ALKALOIDS

The principal alkaloids of this group are (−)-hyoscyamine; atropine [(±)-hyoscyamine]; scopolamine (also known as hyoscine); and the anhydride of atropine (apoatropine) and its stereoisomer, belladonnine. These are tropine derivatives and esters.

Hyoscyamine, $C_{17}H_{23}NO_3$, is the tropine ester of (−)-tropic acid and is readily hydrolyzed by boiling in dilute acids or alkalies to form these compounds (see Fig. 8–4).

The carbon atom α to the carboxyl group

of tropic acid is asymmetric and accounts for the natural occurrence of the optical isomer. When (−)-hyoscyamine is extracted from the plants in which it occurs, it usually is racemized during the process and thus converted into the (±)-compound, which is atropine. The piperidine ring system of tropine can exist in 2 principal conformations. The chair form has the lowest energy requirement. In addition, 2 stereoisomeric forms can exist because of the rigidity imparted to the molecule through the ethane chain across positions 1 and 5. Pharmacologically, the most active isomer results when the esteratic group is substituted axial at position 3, as in the case of (−)-hyoscyamine and atropine.

Use and Dose. Hyoscyamine is an anticholinergic. Usual dose is 300 μg, 4 times a day.

Hyoscyamine sulfate is the sulfate of an alkaloid usually obtained from species of Hyoscyamus Linné or other genera of Solanaceae. *It is extremely poisonous.* Hyoscyamine sulfate occurs as white, odorless crystals or as a crystalline powder; it is deliquescent and is affected by light.

Use and Dose. Hyoscyamine sulfate is an anticholinergic. Usual dose is 125 to 250 μg, 3 or 4 times a day.

Prescription Product. Levsin®, Anaspaz®, Levamine®, Cystospaz®.

Hyoscyamine hydrobromide resembles the sulfate in appearance and, although it is affected by light, it is not deliquescent. It is an anticholinergic. Usual dose is 250 μg to 1 mg.

Atropine, $C_{17}H_{23}NO_3$, is an alkaloid obtained from botanic sources [usually from *Atropa belladonna* Linné, from species of *Datura* Linné, and from *Hyoscyamus* Linné (Fam. Solanaceae)] or produced synthetically. *It is extremely poisonous.* Synthetic production of atropine is more costly than extraction from natural sources and cannot compete in price. Formerly,

Hyoscyamus muticus represented the chief natural source; however, atropine is now also obtained from species of *Duboisia* (see page 209). It pre-exists in the solanaceous plants only in traces and is formed from hyoscyamine during the process of extraction.

Atropine occurs as colorless, needlelike crystals or as a white, crystalline powder; it is optically inactive, but usually contains some levorotatory hyoscyamine, the limit of which produces an angular rotation not to exceed −0.70°.

Use and Dose. Atropine is an anticholinergic. Usual dose is 250 μg, 3 times a day.

Atropine sulfate occurs as colorless crystals or as a white, crystalline powder. *It is extremely poisonous.* It effloresces in dry air, is slowly affected by light, and is an anticholinergic. Usual dose, tablets, is 300 to 600 μg, 3 or 4 times a day; injection, 400 to 600 μg, 4 to 6 times a day, and as an antidote to cholinesterase inhibitors, intravenously, 2 to 4 mg initially, followed by intramuscularly, 2 mg repeated every 5 to 10 minutes until muscarinic symptoms disappear or signs of atropine toxicity appear. Topically to the conjunctiva, 0.1 ml of a 0.5 to 4% solution, 3 times a day.

Scopolamine or hyoscine is an alkaloid that is particularly abundant in *Datura fastuosa* var. *alba* and in *D. metel*. It is an ester that, upon hydrolysis, yields tropic acid and scopoline, a base resembling tropine.

It occurs as an almost colorless, syrupy liquid from its chloroformic solution and as colorless crystals from its ether solution. It is levorotatory.

Scopolamine hydrobromide or hyoscine hydrobromide ($C_{17}H_{21}NO_4 \cdot HBr \cdot 3H_2O$) occurs as colorless or white crystals or as a white, granular powder that is odorless and slightly efflorescent in dry air. *It is extremely poisonous.*

Use and Dose. Scopolamine hydrobromide is classified as an anticholinergic.

The usual dose, both orally and parenterally, is 320 μg to 1.1 mg as a single dose and topically to the conjunctiva, 0.05 to 0.1 ml of a 0.2 to 0.5% solution, 1 or more times a day.

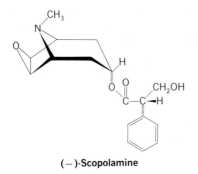

(−)-Scopolamine

Atropine and scopolamine are competitive with acetylcholine at the postganglionic synapse (muscarinic site) of the parasympathetic nervous system. Clinically useful effects obtained from blocking the muscarinic activity of acetylcholine are an antispasmodic effect used principally to relieve spasms of the bowel in the treatment of spastic colitis, gastroenteritis, and peptic ulcer; an antisecretory effect used to reduce respiratory secretions in anesthesia (antisialogogue), gastric secretions in peptic ulcer therapy, and nasal and sinus secretions in common cold and allergy medications; and a mydriatic and cycloplegic effect used to prevent adhesions between the iris and lens of the eye in cases of iritis.

Atropine is an antidote in cases of poisoning caused by cholinesterase inhibitors such as physostigmine and organophosphate insecticides.

Scopolamine has a depressant activity on the central nervous system and has been used to treat motion sickness and, in combination with morphine as "twilight sleep," was extensively used in the past as a sedative and preanesthetic medication during labor (amnesic analgesic). Because of the dangers involved, the use of this product has been abandoned.

Toxicity symptoms that can occur during the therapeutic use of atropine, scopolamine, and belladonna tincture are skin rash, skin flushing, mouth dryness, difficult urination, eye pain, blurred vision, and light sensitivity. The patient should also be advised that such antacids as alumina gels may interfere with absorption of these drugs when taken simultaneously.

HYOSCYAMUS

Hyoscyamus or henbane is the dried leaf, with or without the stem and flowering or fruiting top, of *Hyoscyamus niger* Linné (Fam. Solanaceae) and contains not less than 0.04% of the alkaloids of hyoscyamus. *Hyoscyamus* is the ancient Greek and Latin name formed from 2 Greek words meaning hog and bean. The plant is poisonous to swine.

The plant is an annual or biennial herb (Fig. 8–6) indigenous to Europe, western Asia, and northern Africa and is cultivated in the Soviet Union, the Balkans, Belgium, England, and Germany, and, to some extent, the United States and Canada. The biennial form is most generally cultivated in England; the annual form is cultivated on the Continent. The leaves should be gathered when the plant is in full flower and should be carefully dried immediately. Dioscorides mentioned the plant, and under the name of henbane, it has been employed in European domestic medicine from the remotest times. It is mentioned in Anglo-Saxon works on medicine written in the eleventh century and in the *Arabian Nights*. After the Middle Ages the drug fell into disuse, but was reintroduced into European medicine about 1760, largely through the efforts of Störck.

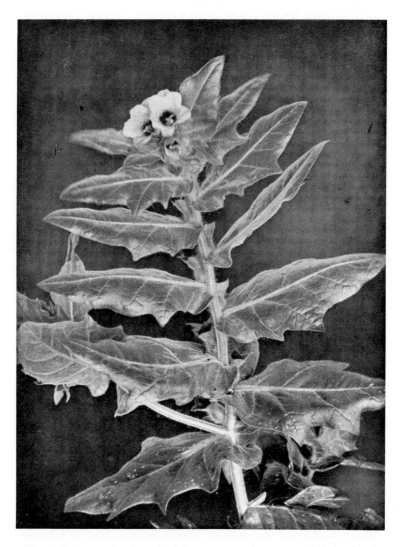

Fig. 8–6.   Flowering branch of *Hyoscyamus niger* var. *agrestis* K. showing sessile, acutely lobed leaves and two of the funnel-form flowers.

The alkaloids, hyoscyamine and scopolamine, 0.05 to 0.15%, of which three-fourths is hyoscyamine, are the active principles.

USE. Hyoscyamus is a parasympatholytic, but the crude drug is rarely employed in medicine today.

Egyptian henbane, the dried leaves and flowering tops of *Hyoscyamus muticus,* yields about 1.5% of total alkaloid, consisting largely of hyoscyamine. The plant is indigenous to and cultivated in Egypt. It is also cultivated in irrigated soils of southern California. The drug is used, perhaps entirely, for the extraction of its alkaloids.

STRAMONIUM

Stramonium, jimson weed, or Jamestown weed consists of the dried leaf and

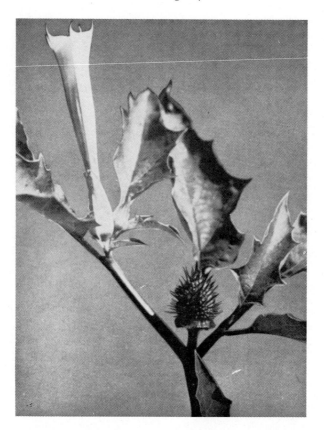

Fig. 8–7. *Datura stramonium* leaves, flower, and fruit.

flowering or fruiting tops with branches of *Datura stramonium* Linné or of its variety *tatula* (Linné) Torrey (Fam. Solanaceae). It yields not less than 0.25% of alkaloids. The name *Datura* is derived from the Sanskrit, *dhattura* and from the Arabic *tatura* or *tatula*, the native name; *stramonium* is from the French *stramoine*, meaning stinkweed. The plant is an annual herb that attains the height of about 2 meters. It is indigenous to the region of the Caspian Sea, naturalized in waste places in Europe and North America, and cultivated in central Europe and South America. The leaves and tops (Fig. 8–7) are collected when the plant is in flower and are carefully dried and preserved. A few years ago, most of the commercial supply was obtained from plants cultivated in Argentina. At present, Europe is again supplying reasonable quantities of the drug. The purple stramonium (*Datura stramonium* var. *tatula*), which is naturalized in the United States from tropical America, is similar to *D. stramonium*, but the stems and flowers are purplish. The active constituents in the 2 plants are alike. Stramonium was grown in England in about the sixteenth century from seeds obtained from Constantinople. The early settlers near Jamestown, Virginia, used it as a "pot herb" with fatal results, thus establishing its common name of Jamestown weed, which was subsequently modified in some areas to jimson weed. It can serve as a source of atropine.

The drug contains hyoscyamine and scopolamine; the former is most abundant.

Use. Stramonium is an anticholinergic and has an action like that of belladonna.

Powdered stramonium is an ingredient in preparations that are intended to burn. The resultant vapor is inhaled for the relief of asthma. These so-called asthma powders were widely sold on an over-the-counter basis until thrillseekers began to ingest them in order to become intoxicated. In 1968, the Food and Drug Administration placed stramonium-containing asthma powders in the prescription-drug category.

Stramonium seed is the ripe seed of *D. stramonium*. The ripening capsules are gathered and dried until the seeds shake out. The seeds are reniform, flattened, 3 to 4 mm in length, bluish black, and minutely reticulate.

Stramonium seed contains about 0.4% of alkaloids, principally hyoscyamine with a small proportion of scopolamine and traces of atropine.

Stramonium is generally regarded as a noxious weed and has frequently caused poisoning in children when seeds were ingested. The chief toxic symptoms are those of atropine poisoning: dilated pupils, impaired vision, dryness of the skin and secretions, extreme thirst, hallucinations, and loss of consciousness. Although newspaper items often describe the circumstances, such cases are also reported in the medical literature. Because the plant is rather widespread, pharmacists may be asked to help in identifying the plant and in applying emergency measures pending arrival of the physician.

OTHER SOLANACEOUS DRUGS

Withania is the dried root of *Withania somnifera* Dunal (Fam. Solanaceae), a plant that grows within a broad range from southern Europe to India, and in Africa. It is cultivated in India, where it has been employed as a sedative since antiquity.

Studies have shown that withania, which is closely related botanically to belladonna and hyoscyamus, contains about a dozen biochemically heterogeneous alkaloids. Tropine and pseudotropine are accompanied by hygrine (pyrrolidine derivative), isopelletierine (piperidine derivative), cuscohygrine (2 pyrrolidine moieties), anaferine (2 piperidine moieties), and anahygrine (1 pyrrolidine moiety and 1 piperidine moiety). The principle responsible for the sedative action of the drug has not yet been determined, but the study of the alkaloids of this drug has advanced our knowledge of the chemical-taxonomic relationships of solanaceous plants.

Duboisia consists of the dried leaves of *Duboisia myoporoides* R. Brown (Fam. Solanaceae), a large shrub indigenous to Australia. The drug contains (−)-hyoscyamine, scopolamine, and a number of related alkaloids, in addition to small amounts of nicotine and nornicotine. Duboisia currently is a chief source of atropine, the racemic mixture of the isomers of hyoscyamine, which is formed during the extraction process. The leaves of *D. leichardtii* F. von Mueller, of Australia, also contain a relatively large percentage of similar alkaloids.

Pituri or Australian tobacco is the leaf of *D. hopwoodii* F. von Mueller and is used in Australia like tobacco. It contains nicotine and nornicotine.

Mandragora or European mandrake is the root of *Mandragora officinarum* Linné and contains hyoscyamine, scopolamine, and mandragorine. This drug and its method of collection are the subjects of many superstitions and folklore tales. It should not be confused with the resin-containing American mandrake (podophyllum), see page 146.

COCAINE

Coca or coca leaves has been described as the dried leaves of *Erythroxylum coca* Lamarck, known commercially as Huanuco coca, or of *E. truxillense* Rusby, known commercially as Truxillo coca (Fam. Erythroxylaceae). The plants are shrubs or small trees that attain a height of about 2 meters and are indigenous to certain areas of South America. They have been cultivated there for centuries, but were later introduced as crops on the islands of Java and Ceylon. *Erythroxylum* is from 2 Greek words meaning red and wood, alluding to the color of the plants; *coca* is the Spanish name for the tree; and *truxillense* is from Truxillo, a coastal city in Peru.

Modern studies have revealed that many of the old concepts regarding this drug were inaccurate. It is now generally recognized that all of these plants characterized by relatively high concentrations of ecgonine bases belong to one polymorphic species, *Erythroxylum coca* Lamarck. Three varieties yielding the commercial drug may be distinguished:

1. var. *coca* (= *E. coca* Lamarck *sensu stricto)* yields Huanuco (Bolivian) coca. The leaves of commerce are large, dark green, and coriaceous with an acute or obtuse apex.
2. var. *spruceanum* Bruck (= *E. truxillense* Rusby) yields both Truxillo (Peruvian) coca and Java coca. In commerce, these leaves are smaller, narrower, thinner, and lighter green than those of the var. *coca.*
3. var. *novogranatense* (Morris) Hieron. yields a type of Truxillo coca from Colombia. It rarely occurs in commerce, but may be distinguished from the previous varieties by its obtuse to emarginate apex.

Most of the present-day supply of the drug is obtained from cultivated plants grown at an altitude of 500 to 2000 meters in Peru and Bolivia. Nearly 100,000 kg of coca leaves are imported into the United States annually. The leaves are collected from twigs that are cut off in the spring, pruned again in June, and pruned for a third time in the fall. Only a small portion of the drug is exported because most of it is chewed by the natives or is used for the manufacture of cocaine. Peru exports a considerable quantity of crude cocaine.

Cocaine was first isolated in 1860, but until 1884, coca was considered as only an inferior substitute for tea. In that year, Koller discovered its local anesthetic properties.

Coca leaves contain 3 basic types of alkaloids: derivatives of ecgonine (cocaine, cinnamylcocaine, α- and β-truxilline), tropine (tropacocaine, valerine), and hygrine (hygroline, cuscohygrine). Only the ecgonine derivatives are commercially important. The composition of the alkaloid mixture in the leaf varies qualitatively and quantitatively according to the variety of the plant and, to some extent, to the stage of development of the leaves when collected.

Huanuco coca contains 0.5 to 1% of ester alkaloids, derivatives of tropine and ecgonine, of which cocaine constitutes the major part. Cuscohygrine is the principal nonester alkaloid in the leaf.

Java coca has a somewhat higher average concentration of ester alkaloids, 1 to 2%, but less than one third of this total is ordinarily represented by cocaine. Cinnamylcocaine makes up most of the remainder of this fraction.

Truxillo coca from Peru, although derived from the same botanic source as Java coca, has a somewhat lower content of ester alkaloids, but a much higher percentage (up to 75%) of this quantity is cocaine. This difference is attributed to the different degrees of maturity of the 2 products. Java leaves are picked in an early stage of de-

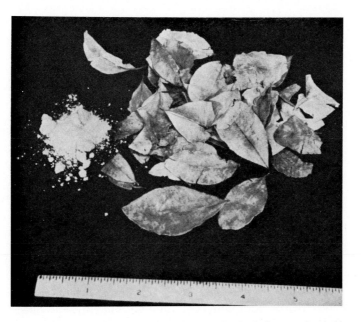

Fig. 8–8. Dried coca leaves *(Erythroxylum coca)* and lime with which they are chewed by Peruvian natives. (Photo, courtesy of Dr. Julia F. Morton, Director, Morton Collectanea, University of Miami.)

velopment when they are rich in total alkaloids. All South American types represent fully developed leaves that contain less total alkaloids, but greater percentages of cocaine. Because the total ecgonine bases are utilizable in the semisynthesis of cocaine, the Java product is quite suitable for this purpose.

Coca leaves were highly valued by the natives long before the Spanish conquest; the shrub was known as "The Divine Plant of the Incas." Monardes published an extensive article on the drug in 1569. The natives chew the leaf, either as such or mixed with lime (Fig. 8–8), and are thus able to travel great distances without experiencing fatigue and without any but the most meager food rations.

At present, coca chewing is an integral part of the native culture pattern in many isolated highland areas of Colombia and in most of the mountainous sections of Peru, Bolivia, and the northwestern part of Argentina. Its use has spread from these areas to the lowlands and is prevalent in most parts of the northwestern Amazon valley in Colombia and Peru.

Much has been written about the effect this habit has on its practitioners. Dr. R. E. Schultes, the well-known ethnobotanist at Harvard University, expressed the following opinion:

"What is very commonly overlooked or even purposely ignored in many governmental and sociologic circles is the fact that coca as chewed by the native is not of necessity physically, socially, and morally dangerous. It has nothing in common with cocaine addiction, and coca chewing does not lead to addiction. . . . Unwise legal prohibitions in certain Andean areas aimed at extirpation of the coca custom have invariably driven the Indian, deprived in his inhospitable cold altitudes of the euphoric coca, to the dangerously poisonous local distilled drinks with an attendant rapid rise in crime."

Cocaine is an alkaloid obtained from the leaves of *Erythroxylum coca* and its varieties. As explained subsequently, much of the alkaloid is actually prepared by semisynthesis, from plant-derived ecgonine.

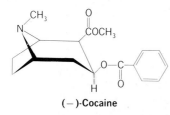

(−)-Cocaine

Cocaine is the methyl ester of benzoylecgonine. When hydrolyzed, it splits into ecgonine, benzoic acid, and methyl alcohol. Cinnamylcocaine splits into ecgonine, methyl alcohol, and cinnamic acid whereas α- and β-truxilline split into ecgonine, methyl alcohol, and α- and β-truxillic acids. (The truxillic acids are isomeric dicinnamic acids.)

The production of cocaine is ordinarily conducted on a large scale by a number of methods that are similar but not identical. Many of the important steps are protected by patents. Ordinarily, the total bases are extracted, the ester alkaloids are converted to (−)-ecgonine by acid hydrolysis, and cocaine is synthesized from it by esterification first with methanol and then with benzoic acid. When this procedure is utilized, only the total content of ecgonine derivatives in the leaf is commercially significant.

USE. Cocaine is a local anesthetic. It is applied topically to mucous membrane as a 1% solution.

Cocaine hydrochloride is the hydrochloride of the alkaloid cocaine. It occurs as colorless crystals or as a white, crystalline powder.

USE. Cocaine hydrochloride is a local anesthetic. It is applied topically to mucous membrane as a 2 to 4% solution.

Cocaine hydrochloride is an ingredient in Brompton's cocktail, which is widely used to control severe pain associated with terminal cancer. Because of its CNS stimulant properties, cocaine counteracts the narcotic-induced sedation and respiratory depression associated with the narcotic analgesic ingredient (morphine or methadone) used in the cocktail. It also potentiates the analgesic effect.

Cocaine and cocaine hydrochloride, as agents of abuse, are generally inhaled or sniffed and are rapidly absorbed across the pharyngeal mucosa, resulting in cerebral stimulation and euphoria. Repeated use results in psychic dependence and tolerance; therefore, cocaine is classified as a Schedule II drug under the Controlled Substances Act.

Cocaine served as the model for a large number of synthetic local anesthetics that have been produced to increase the stability and reduce the toxicity of the natural product. Some of them are vasodilators and are often employed in conjunction with epinephrine. Such compounds are considered in detail in the standard textbooks of medicinal chemistry.

QUINOLINE ALKALOIDS

Alkaloids containing quinoline as their basic nucleus include those obtained from cinchona (quinine, quinidine, cinchonine and cinchonidine) and acronycine from *Acronychia baueri*.

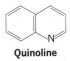

Quinoline

Cinchona and its alkaloids are the only members of this group that are therapeutically important at present. Cinchonine, which is isomeric with cinchonidine, is the parent alkaloid of the quinine series.

Quinine and its isomer, quinidine, represent 6-methoxycinchonine.

BIOSYNTHESIS OF QUINOLINE ALKALOIDS

Alkaloid Precursors. Tryptophan is a precursor of quinine in cinchona. Because quinine is the first secondary compound derived from the amino acid to be considered, it is convenient to review the biosynthesis of tryptophan here.

The biosynthetic pathway leading to tryptophan in higher plants is unknown; however, it has been elucidated in microorganisms using auxotrophic mutants of *Escherichia coli* and *Enterobacter aerogenes* that required tryptophan for growth. In the pathway, shikimic acid, through a series of phosphorylated intermediates, yields chorismic acid, which is an important branch-point intermediate. One branch leads to prephenic acid and the aromatic amino acids, phenylalanine and tyrosine (see page 112). The other leads to anthranilic acid and then to tryptophan. Chorismic acid is converted to anthranilic acid by aromatization and transfer of the amide nitrogen of glutamine. The anthranilic acid then reacts with 5-phosphoribosyl-1-pyrophosphate to

form, via an intermediate, 1(o-carboxyphenylamino)-1-deoxyribulose 5-phosphate, which undergoes ring closure to produce indole-3-glycerol phosphate. The final step in the reaction sequence involves replacement of the glycerol phosphate side chain with serine, thereby yielding tryptophan (Fig. 8–9).

Quinoline Derivatives. Studies with labeled geraniol and tryptophan-2-^{14}C indicate that quinine is metabolically derived from the monoterpenoid-tryptophan pathway that leads to the *Corynanthe*-type indole alkaloids (see page 231). The most distinctive feature of quinine biosynthesis appears to be cleavage of the benzopyrrole ring of the tryptophan moiety and rearrangement to form the quinuclidine nucleus and then the quinoline nucleus. Details of the biosynthetic processes are lacking, but a presumed biogenetic origin involving strictosidine and corynantheal as intermediates is illustrated in Figure 8–10. Both of these compounds are precursors.

CINCHONA

Cinchona, cinchona bark, or Peruvian bark is the dried bark of the stem or of the root of *Cinchona succirubra* Pavon et

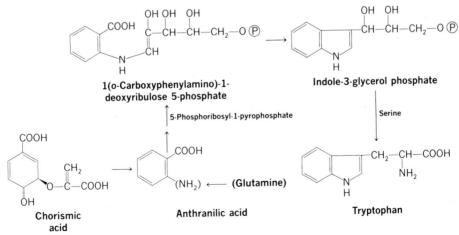

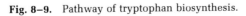

Fig. 8–9. Pathway of tryptophan biosynthesis.

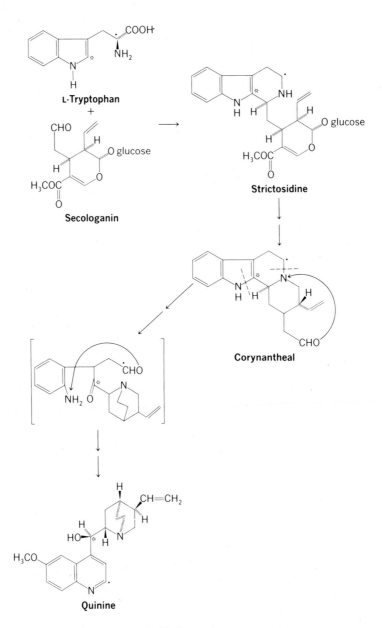

Fig. 8–10. Probable biosynthetic origin of quinine.

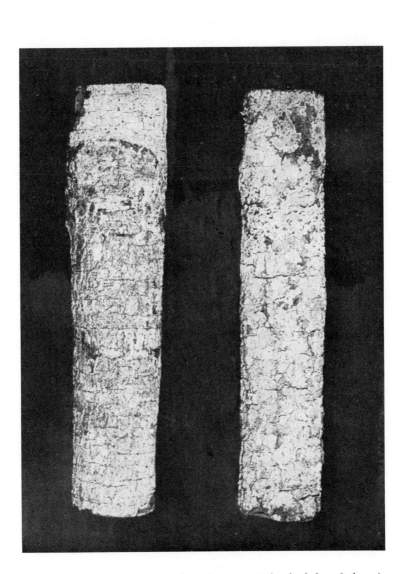

Fig. 8–11. Typical specimens of *Cinchona succirubra* bark from Indonesia.

Klotzsch (Fig. 8–11), or its hybrids, known in commerce as red cinchona; or of *C. ledgeriana* (Howard) Moens et Trimen, *C. calisaya* Weddell, or hybrids of these with other species of *Cinchona*, known in commerce as calisaya bark or yellow cinchona (Fam. Rubiaceae).

Cinchona was named in honor of the Countess of Chinchon, wife of the Viceroy of Peru; *succirubra* is Latin and means red juice; *calisaya* is the Spanish and Indian name in Peru for the bark of a tree; *ledgeriana* is named in honor of Charles Ledger, who introduced *Cinchona* into the East Indies. The plants are trees indigenous to the Andes of Ecuador and Peru. They grow at an elevation of 1000 to 3000 meters and are cultivated in Indonesia and India. There are over 36 known species and hybrids of *Cinchona*.

Just before World War II, Java (Indonesia) supplied over 90% of the world consumption of this important drug. When the Japanese cut off this supply from the world, several synthetic antimalarials (chloroquine, quinacrine, and primacrine) were developed to replace cinchona. Cultivation of cinchona trees was also undertaken in several countries in Central and South America (where it originally occurred). Alkaloid production from these trees during the early months of World War II was a deciding factor in preventing further advances by the Japanese in the Pacific area. Extraction techniques were improved in such a manner as to utilize all of the important alkaloids in any type of cinchona bark that could be obtained from any source.

The Dutch have now resumed the manufacture of cinchona alkaloids using bark obtained from Indonesia. A certain amount of alkaloids is produced in Germany; owing to economic factors, practically none is produced in the United States.

Cultivation gives the opportunity to select seeds from plants producing high-quality bark and to hybridize one choice strain with another. Thus, hybrids of *Cinchona ledgeriana-Cinchona calisaya* produce a higher yield of alkaloids than do either of the parent species. Selected seeds planted in seed beds develop into young plants that can be transplanted within 2 years. The stems tend to grow tall, the lower branches tend to die and drop off, and the tree crowns grow closely, thus shading the trunks. Shade is favorable to the production of quinine. Trees that are 6 to 9 years old possess the maximum amount of alkaloids in the bark. They can easily be uprooted with tractors and the fresh bark of both trunk and roots can then be removed by hand. When young bark is dried, it may have an alkaloidal content 3 times as great as that in bark from an old tree. A considerable amount of cinchona bark enters into the manufacture of vermouth and certain bitter liqueurs.

A number of fantastic tales have been told about the origin of the medicinal use of cinchona. One of these tales states that an Indian in Peru was overcome with fever and was forced to drink stagnant water from a pond into which several cinchona trees had fallen. Enough alkaloids had been extracted by the prolonged maceration that, within hours of drinking the solution, the Indian's fever had abated and he eventually recovered.

A Jesuit missionary learned of the use of the drug from the Indians. He taught others, among them Canizares, the corregidor of Loxa. Canizares sent the bark to Juan de Vega, who at that time was treating the Countess Ana de Osorio, wife of the Count of Chinchon and Viceroy of Peru, for tertian fever. The Countess recovered and shortly thereafter introduced the bark into Europe. The use of cinchona was further spread through the efforts of the Jesuit Order. For the next half century or more, Europe seethed with a controversy over cinchona. The drug was both widely condemned and widely praised. Early names for the drug were Countess bark, Jesuit's bark, and Peruvian bark. It is interesting to note that Linnaeus, when naming the genus, desired to honor the Countess, but omitted the second letter in the name, Chinchon. This error has continued to the present day. The tree yielding cinchona bark was unknown until 1737. In 1854, the Dutch began its introduction into Java, and in 1860, the English introduced it into India.

The alkaloids are chiefly formed in the parenchyma cells of the middle layers of the bark. Cinchona contains some 25 closely related alkaloids, of which the most important are quinine, quinidine, cinchonine, and cinchonidine, and the average yield is 6 to 7%, of which from one-half to two-thirds is quinine in the yellow barks. In the red barks, cinchonidine exists in greater proportion; specimen pieces have yielded as high as 18% of total alkaloids. Another constituent of cinchona is cinchotannic acid, from 2 to 4%, which decomposes into the nearly insoluble cinchona red, occurring in red barks to the extent of 10%. The red color in cinchona bark is caused by an oxidase similar to the oxidase that causes fruits to darken when cut. If the fresh bark is heated in boiling water for 30 minutes and then dried, it does not become red.

In commerce, cinchona bark is priced on the basis of its total alkaloid content and frequently on its quinine content.

USES AND DOSE. Cinchona and its alkaloids have been used in the treatment of malaria fever for many years. Quinine continues to be used for malaria in many parts of the world, but in the United States this alkaloid is utilized primarily in the preparation of effervescent tonic water. Quinidine is now the principal cinchona alkaloid employed therapeutically.

Overdoses of cinchona products result in temporary loss of hearing and in im-paired sight. Ringing in the ears is a toxic symptom. When these symptoms are produced as the result of continuous use of cinchona or of quinine, the condition has been called **cinchonism.** Cinchona was formerly given in doses of 1 g.

Cuprea bark is obtained from *Remijia purdieana* Triana and *R. pedunculata* Flückiger (Fam. Rubiaceae), of central and southern Colombia. It has a copper-red color, is hard, compact and heavy, and contains numerous transversely elongated stone cells and 2 to 6% of alkaloids, of which one-third may be quinine. Cuprea bark is a commercial source of quinidine.

CINCHONA ALKALOIDS

Quinidine, $C_{20}H_{24}N_2O_2$, is a stereo-isomer of quinine and is present in cinchona barks to the extent of 0.25 to 1.25%.

Quinidine sulfate is the sulfate of an alkaloid obtained from various species of *Cinchona* and their hybrids and from *Remijia pedunculata*, or prepared from quinine. It occurs as fine, needlelike, white crystals that frequently cohere in masses. It is odorless, has a bitter taste, and darkens when exposed to light. It is readily soluble in water, alcohol, methanol, and chloroform.

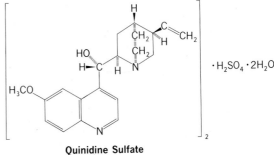

Quinidine Sulfate

USE AND DOSE. Quinidine sulfate is a cardiac depressant and is used particularly to inhibit auricular fibrillation. Usual dose, initially, is 200 to 800 mg repeated at 2- or

3-hour intervals for 5 doses a day; for maintenance, 100 to 300 mg, 3 to 6 times a day. The patient should be instructed to notify the physician if skin rash, fever, unusual bleeding or bruising, ringing in ears, or visual disturbance occurs.

PRESCRIPTION PRODUCTS. Cin-Quin®, Quinidex®, and Quinora®.

Quinidine gluconate occurs as a white powder that is odorless and has a bitter taste. It is used similarly to quinidine sulfate as a cardiac depressant (antiarrhythmic). Usual dose, intramuscularly, is 600 mg, then 400 mg repeated up to 12 times a day, as necessary; intravenous infusion, 800 mg in 40 ml of 5% dextrose injection at the rate of 1 ml per minute.

PRESCRIPTION PRODUCT. Quinaglute®.

Quinidine polygalacturonate affords controlled and more uniform absorption through the intestinal mucosa than does quinidine sulfate. In addition, it produces a lower incidence of gastrointestinal irritation.

PRESCRIPTION PRODUCT. Cardioquin®.

Quinine, $C_{20}H_{24}N_2O_2 \cdot 3H_2O$, is the diastereoisomer of quinidine. It occurs as white, odorless, bulky, bitter crystals or as a crystalline powder. It darkens when exposed to light and effloresces in dry air. It is freely soluble in alcohol, ether, and chloroform, but slightly soluble in water. A large number of its salts are commercially available.

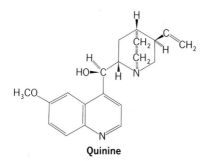

Quinine

Quinine sulfate is the sulfate of an alkaloid obtained from the bark of *Cinchona*

species. It occurs as white, odorless, bitter, fine, needlelike crystals that are usually lusterless. It becomes brownish when exposed to light. It is not readily soluble in water, alcohol, chloroform, or ether.

The drug is an antimalarial. It suppresses but does not cure vivax malaria and was once almost abandoned in this country in favor of chloroquine or other newer synthetic antimalarials. Recently, it has regained considerable importance in the treatment of chloroquine-resistant falciparum malaria. Usual dose is 200 mg to 1 g 3 times a day for 6 to 12 days. The patient should be instructed to notify the physician if ringing in ears or visual disturbance occurs. Daily doses of 0.2 to 0.4 g as a tonic or as an analgesic in the treatment of colds were used extensively in the past; at present, quinine salts are ingredients in certain proprietary cold remedies.

Over 1.5 million avoirdupois ounces of quinine and over 1.1 million ounces of quinidine are imported annually into the United States.

ACRONYCHIA

Acronychia consists of the bark of *Acronychia baueri* Schott (Fam. Rutaceae), an evergreen tree that attains a height of 15 to 20 meters. It is native to New South Wales and Queensland where it is commonly called the scrub ash or scrub yellowwood.

The bark contains a number of quinoline alkaloids, one of which, acronycine, exhibits an extremely broad antitumor spectrum in laboratory animals. Acronycine is an N-methyl acridone and is structurally unrelated to other known antitumor al-

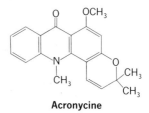

Acronycine

kaloids. Scientific investigations of its activity are in progress.

ISOQUINOLINE ALKALOIDS

The isoquinoline structure occurs in a considerable number of alkaloids in widely separated plant families.

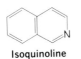

Isoquinoline

Although the more important opium alkaloids (morphine, codeine, thebaine) exhibit a phenanthrene nucleus, the majority of its alkaloids have the isoquinoline ring structure. These phenanthrene alkaloids are derived biosynthetically from benzylisoquinoline intermediates. For this reason, opium is included in this group. Sanguinaria, another member of the Papaveraceae, also contains isoquinoline alkaloids.

The important drugs and their alkaloids of this group are ipecac, emetine, hydrastis, hydrastine, sanguinaria, curare, tubocurarine, berberine, opium and its alkaloids.

BIOSYNTHESIS OF ISOQUINOLINE ALKALOIDS

Although the isoquinoline alkaloids possess relatively complex structures, the basic biosynthetic reactions that account for their formation in plants are relatively simple. These compounds result from the condensation of a phenylethylamine derivative with a phenylacetaldehyde derivative. Both of these moieties are derived from phenylalanine or tyrosine. Administration of tyrosine-2-^{14}C to *Papaver somniferum* resulted in the formation of papaverine labeled in corresponding positions. Norlaudanosoline is an intermediate in this reaction (Fig. 8–12).

Morphine is also formed from 2 molecules of tyrosine, and its biosynthesis is related to the biosynthesis of papaverine. Norlaudanosoline serves as a key intermediate. This medicinally important alkaloid is derived from a benzylisoquinoline metabolite. The biosynthesis of morphine and related alkaloids has been studied extensively, and these experiments provide some of the most complete and detailed observations available for any secondary plant constituent. The biosynthetic pathway leading to morphine is shown in Figure 8–12. A key feature of this pathway is the enzymatically controlled methylation pattern that gives rise to (−)-reticuline, thus facilitating formation of the dienone, salutaridine, which is the first intermediate with a phenanthrene nucleus. Another interesting aspect of this pathway is the biosynthetic relationship of thebaine, codeine, and morphine; stepwise demethylation of the therapeutically unimportant thebaine leads first to the relatively mild analgesic codeine and then to the potent narcotic morphine.

P. somniferum has a highly evolved and useful secondary metabolism that culminates, at least from the therapeutic viewpoint, in morphine. *P. bracteatum* Lindley, a thebaine-producing poppy, appears to lack any significant demethylation capability; this feature is not only useful for biosynthetic studies, but has recently become commercially significant. Because thebaine can be converted to codeine semisynthetically, a source of the latter alkaloid is assured without concomitant production of morphine, which is more subject to abuse by drug addicts. These 2 species emphasize the subtle metabolic difference that frequently separates useful plants from those of only scientific interest.

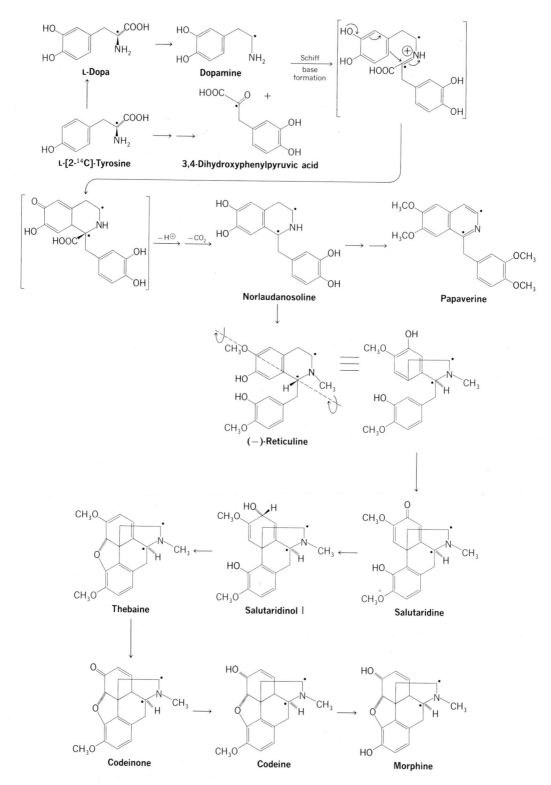

Fig. 8–12. Biosynthesis of papaverine and morphine.

Presumably, morphine and other opium alkaloids are formed primarily in various cells of the poppy plant and are excreted into the laticiferous ducts. However, isolated latex is capable of alkaloid biosynthesis in the presence of suitable precursors and cofactors. The latex is also capable of metabolic destruction of morphine, and diurnal variations in alkaloid composition of the latex have been recorded. These observations, which establish a metabolic function for the latex, are fundamentally significant and undoubtedly contribute to the normal variability in alkaloid composition of crude opium samples.

IPECAC

Ipecac consists of the dried rhizome and roots of *Cephaelis ipecacuanha* (Brotero) A. Richard, known in commerce as Rio or Brazilian ipecac (Fig. 8–13), or of *Cephaelis acuminata* Karsten, known in commerce as Cartagena, Nicaragua, or Panama ipecac (Fam. Rubiaceae). Ipecac yields not less than 2% of the ether-soluble alkaloids of ipecac.

Cephaelis is from 2 Greek words, meaning head and to collect or roll up, and refers to the inflorescence; *ipecacuanha* is Portuguese from the Brazilian Indian *ipekaa-*

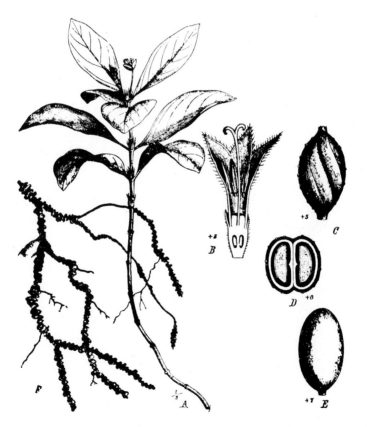

Fig. 8–13. Ipecac plant *(Cephaelis ipecacuanha)*: *A*, flowering shoot; *B*, flower in longitudinal section; *C*, fruit; *D*, fruit in transverse section; *E*, seed; *F*, annulate root.

guene, meaning a creeping plant that causes vomiting; *acuminata* refers to the acute apex of the leaf.

The plants are low, straggling shrubs with slender rhizomes bearing annulated wiry roots. *C. ipecacuanha* is indigenous to Brazil, which furnishes most of the present supply. It has been cultivated to a limited extent in Malaysia and in India. The drug is gathered during the dry season and dried rapidly in the sun for 2 or 3 days. *C. acuminata* is indigenous to the northern portions of Colombia and extends into Panama and Nicaragua; it is exported from Cartagena and Savanilla. Apparently, ipecac was used by the South American Indians. The drug was first mentioned by a Jesuit friar in 1601. It was introduced into Europe by Le Gras in 1672 and by 1690 was well known in medicine.

Ipecac contains 5 alkaloids (2 to 2.5%). The 3 principal alkaloids are emetine, cephaeline, and psychotrine, contained chiefly in the bark, which makes up about 90% of the drug. About 40% of starch is present.

In Rio (Brazilian) ipecac, the total alkaloid content reaches slightly over 2%, about one-third cephaeline and two-thirds emetine. At the present time, the plants are becoming rather scarce despite the laws of most South American countries that require a portion of the root to be planted when collections are made. Roots that are collected are usually immature, and the total alkaloid content barely reaches the minimum percentage.

In Cartagena (Colombia) ipecac and in Panama ipecac, the total alkaloid content reaches 2.2%. The rhizomes and roots from Nicaragua and Costa Rica yield more than 2.5% of total alkaloids. In these 4 varieties, the ratio of emetine to cephaeline is somewhat constant and is composed of about one-third emetine to two-thirds cephaeline.

USES AND DOSE. Ipecac, in the form of a syrup, is an emetic; usual dose is 15 ml and may be repeated once in 20 minutes if emesis does not occur. The dosage should be recovered by gastric lavage if emesis does not occur after the second dose. Ipecac syrup should not be confused with ipecac fluidextract, which is 14 times stronger. Ipecac mixed with opium (as Dover's powder) acts as a diaphoretic. Ipecac syrup is included in poison antidote kits because of its emetic properties (see page 450).

Emetine or methylcephaeline, $C_{29}H_{40}N_2O_4$, is an alkaloid obtained from ipecac or prepared synthetically by methylation of cephaeline. It was discovered by Pelletier and Magendie in 1817.

Emetine hydrochloride is a hydrated hydrochloride of emetine. It occurs as a white, odorless, crystalline powder that becomes yellowish when exposed to light. It is freely soluble in water and alcohol.

USES AND DOSE. Emetine hydrochloride is an anti-amebic. The usual dose is, intramuscularly or subcutaneously, 1 mg per kg of body weight, but not exceeding 60 mg daily, for not more than 5 days. Emetine hydrochloride has been used extensively as an antiprotozoan, particularly in the treatment of amebic dysentery, pyorrhea alveolaris, and other amebic diseases. It possesses expectorant and emetic properties.

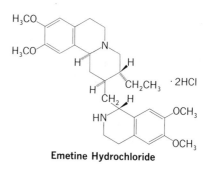

Emetine Hydrochloride

PRESCRIPTION AND NONPRESCRIPTION PRODUCTS. A number of expectorant mixtures include ipecac in their formulas: Cetro-Cirose®, Ipsatol®, Cerose®, Creomulsion®, Quelidrine®, and Sorbutuss®.

HYDRASTIS

Hydrastis or goldenseal consists of the dried rhizome and roots of *Hydrastis canadensis* Linné (Fam. Ranunculaceae).

Hydrastis is Greek and means to accomplish or act with water; the specific name refers to the habitat. The plant is a perennial herb with a short horizontal rhizome that bears numerous long, slender roots. Internally, the rhizome and roots show a golden yellow color. Goldenseal was plentiful in the forests of the eastern United States and Canada; in recent years, it has become almost extinct because of ruthless collection. Its market price is relatively high and, at times, has reached $16 per pound. Goldenseal has been cultivated in Oregon, Washington, North Carolina, Tennessee, Michigan, Wisconsin, and other localities; most of the commercial supply now comes from Arkansas and from the Blue Ridge Mountain area. The plants, propagated from rhizome buds, require 3 to 4 years to produce marketable drug. It is gathered in autumn, the terminal buds are replanted, and the drug is carefully dried. Hydrastis was known to the Cherokee Indians who used it as a dye and an internal remedy. These Indians introduced its use to the early American settlers.

Three alkaloids have been isolated from hydrastis: hydrastine, berberine, and canadine. Of these, hydrastine (1.5 to 4%) is the most important. Hydrastis yields not less than 2.5% of the anhydrous ether-soluble alkaloids of hydrastis.

USE. The hydrastis alkaloids, hydrastine and berberine, are used as astringents in inflammation of the mucous membranes.

Hydrastine is readily soluble in chloroform, alcohol, and ether, but almost insoluble in water. It crystallizes in prisms, melting at 131 to 132° C.

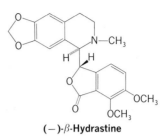

(−)-β-**Hydrastine**

Hydrastine hydrochloride occurs as a white or creamy white powder that is odorless, bitter, and hygroscopic.

Berberine is readily soluble in water, but almost insoluble in ether. The salts of berberine form bright yellow crystals.

SANGUINARIA

Sanguinaria or bloodroot is the dried rhizome of *Sanguinaria candensis* Linné (Fam. Papaveraceae). The generic name is from *sanguinarius*, meaning bloody, and refers to the color of the juice; *canadensis* refers to the plant habitat in Canada. The plant is a low perennial herb (Fig. 8–14) with a horizontal branching rhizome that bears slender roots and contains an orange-red latex. The rhizomes are dug during the early summer, deprived of their roots, and carefully dried. It grows in rich open woodlands in North America east of the Mississippi. Most of the collection takes place in the eastern states. Bloodroot was used by the Indians to stain their faces and was also used as an acrid emetic. Its use in homemade cough remedies seems to have been adopted by the early settlers.

Sanguinaria contains alkaloids of the protopine series, including sanguinarine (about 1%), chelerythrine, protopine, and allocryptopine. These alkaloids are colorless but tend to form colored salts. Sanguinarine yields reddish salts with nitric

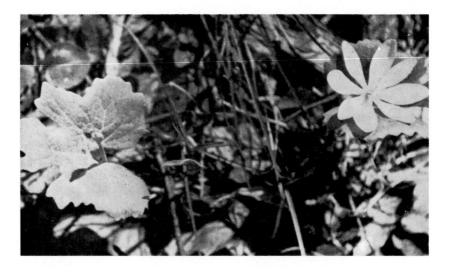

Fig. 8–14. *Sanguinaria canadensis* showing (left) seed pod and characteristic leaf and (right) showy, white flower.

or sulfuric acids; yellowish salts are formed with chelerythrine.

All alkaloids of sanguinaria are found in other members of the Papaveraceae and, like berberine and hydrastine, are isoquinoline derivatives. Species of the families Ranunculaceae, Berberidaceae, Menispermaceae, and Papaveraceae contain alkaloids of this type.

Sanguinaria of good quality contains not more than 5% of the roots of the plant. Shriveled rhizomes that are gray and free from starch should be rejected.

Uses and Dose. Sanguinaria has stimulating expectorant and emetic properties. The usual dose is 125 mg.

Prescription Products. Sedatussin® and Prunicodeine®.

TUBOCURARINE CHLORIDE

Curare or South American arrow poison is a crude dried extract from the bark and stems of *Strychnos castelnaei* Weddell, *S. toxifera* Bentham, *S. crevauxii* G. Planchon (Fam. Loganiaceae) and from *Chondodendron tomentosum* Ruiz et Pavon (Fam. Menispermaceae). The term "curare" is derived from *woorari* or *urari*, Indian words for poison. Curare varies in composition among the Indian tribes. Each tribe modifies the formula in accordance with tribal custom.

The young bark is scraped off the plants, mixed with other substances, and boiled in water and strained or extracted by crude percolation with water. It is evaporated to a paste over a fire or in the sun. The earliest available preparations were named according to the containers in which the drug was packaged: **calabash** (gourd), **tube** (bamboo), or **pot** (clay pot) **curare.** Curare is obtained from the Orinoco basin, the upper Amazon regions, and the eastern Ecuadorian plateau. It is a brownish or black, shiny, resinoid mass with a bitter taste. It is readily soluble in cold water and in dilute alcohol.

Any given sample of the drug contains at least several of a large possible number of alkaloids and quaternary compounds, but the specific composition varies according to the identity of the plant material from which it was prepared. (+)-Tubocurarine, the most important constituent, is a quaternary compound that contains a *bis*-benzylisoquinoline structure. The crude extract exhibits a paralyzing effect on voluntary muscle (curariform effect), but also produces a toxic action on blood vessels as well as a histaminelike effect.

Curare was brought to England by Sir Walter Raleigh in 1595, but it has only recently come into prominence in medical circles. Claude Bernard, Kolliker, Langley, and other investigators studied the effect of curare on mechanisms of neuromuscular activity; however, its heterogeneous nature, its variability, and its uncertain supply limited its use in therapeutics.

Tubocurarine chloride or (+)-tubocurarine chloride is a white or yellowish white to grayish white, odorless, crystalline powder. It is derived from tube curare and was first isolated by Boehm in 1898 and later by King in 1947. King obtained it from *Chondodendron tomentosum* and confirmed the structure as a quaternary ammonium compound. It is soluble in water and in alcohol but is insoluble in acetone, chloroform, and ether.

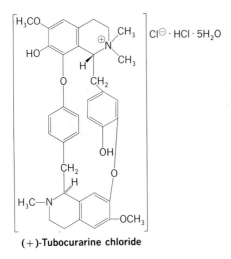

(+)-Tubocurarine chloride

Tubocurarine chloride is standardized by the "head-drop" crossover test in rabbits in which groups of animals for testing

and for control are used on alternate days (crossover). The standard "head-drop" dose is the least amount of the drug capable of producing muscle relaxation so that the head of the animal drops in a characteristic manner.

USES AND DOSE. Tubocurarine chloride is employed as a skeletal muscle relaxant to secure muscle relaxation in surgical procedures without deep anesthesia. It is also used to control convulsions of strychnine poisoning and of tetanus; it is an adjunct to shock therapy in neuropsychiatry and a diagnostic aid in myasthenia gravis. Usual initial dose, intramuscularly or intravenously, is 200 to 400 μg per kg of body weight, not exceeding 27 mg, then 40 to 200 μg per kg, repeated as necessary.

PRESCRIPTION PRODUCT. Metubine Iodide® is a modified tubocurarine product.

OPIUM

Opium or gum opium is the air-dried milky exudate obtained by incising the unripe capsules of *Papaver somniferum* Linné or its variety *album* DeCandolle (Fam. Papaveraceae). The term *opium* is from the Greek *opion*, meaning poppy juice; *Papaver* is the Latin name for the poppy; *somniferum* is Latin and means to produce sleep.

The opium poppy is an annual herb with large, showy, solitary flowers that vary in color from white to pink or purple. The color of its seeds is also variable, ranging from blue-black or gray to yellow-white or rose-brown. Plants that produce the lighter-colored seeds have been classified as variety *album*, but this designation is not employed in modern taxonomic writings. Because of its long history as a cultivated plant, numerous varieties of *P. somniferum* exist, and their taxonomy is extremely complicated.

The plant was first cultivated somewhere in the northeastern corner of the

Mediterranean region, where opium was first produced. Opium was then introduced into India (the date is uncertain). Some scholars credit the introduction to Alexander the Great (327 B.C.), others to the Arabs who invaded the Province of Sind in the eighth century. The first recorded cultivation of the opium poppy in India dates from the fifteenth century, and cultivation began in Macedonia and Persia (Iran) about the middle of the nineteenth century. Opium is commercially produced now in many countries throughout the world, but production is concentrated in a zone that extends from the Turkish Anatolian Plain to the northern border of Laos. The discovery of the medicinal qualities of opium is lost in antiquity. Theophrastus (third century B.C.) mentioned it, and Dioscorides (77 A.D.) distinguished between the juice of the poppy and an extract of the entire plant. In 1806, Sertürner first isolated the alkaloid morphine from opium.

CULTIVATION, COLLECTION, AND COMMERCE. The cultivation of the opium poppy is controlled internationally by the International Narcotics Control Board of the United Nations. At the present time, licit production takes place primarily in India, Turkey, the Soviet Union, and the People's Republic of China, where it is carried out under strict governmental control. Most of the opium destined for the illicit trade originates in Turkey; in remote border areas of Burma, Thailand, and Laos, commonly referred to as the "Golden Triangle"; and in India, Pakistan, and Afghanistan. In a relatively large number of countries, morphine is extracted from poppy straw prepared by cutting and drying the entire overground plant at a suitable stage of development.

For the production of opium, the poppy seeds are sown in October in well-cultivated soil. The seeds germinate in the fall, and the seedlings may be 2 to 3 cm high when snow falls; this protects them

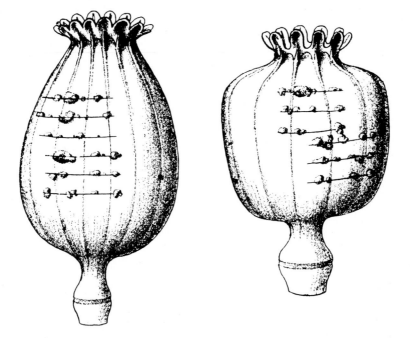

Fig. 8–15. Poppy capsules showing the milky juice exuding from transverse incisions and forming irregular globular masses on the surface. The hardened milky juice forms opium.

from freezing. In the spring, when the plants have attained the height of 15 cm, the fields are cultivated, and the plants are thinned to stand about 60 cm apart. The poppy blossoms in April or May, and the capsules mature in June or July. Each plant bears from 5 to 8 capsules (see Fig. 8–15).

The ripening capsules, about 4 cm in diameter, change from bluish green to yellowish in color. This time is critical for latex collection. The capsules are incised with a knife, which is usually 3-bladed, and the incision is made around the circumference of the capsule. The latex tubes open into one another; therefore, it is not necessary to incise them all. Great skill, however, is required so that the endocarp is not cut. When the endocarp is broken, the latex flows into the interior of the capsule and is lost. The latex, which is at first white, rapidly coagulates and turns brown. This latex is removed early the following morning (scraped off with a knife) and is transferred to a poppy leaf. When sufficient latex is collected, it is kneaded into balls that are wrapped in poppy leaves and dried in the shade. The opium is then inspected and usually packed with the brown-winged fruits of a *Rumex*, which prevents cohering.

Turkish opium reaches the American market in the form of molded or pressed cakes that resemble large bricks. They each weigh about 2 kg and yield about 12 to 14% of anhydrous morphine. The cakes are quite hard and dry on the outside because they are dusted with exhausted materials and then wrapped. In recent years, Indian opium has been packed in pliofilm bags, which are placed in canvas sacks or into wooden cases. The style of packaging of Indian opium depends on the particular orders of the individual purchaser in each country to which it is sent.

Opium occurs in more or less rounded, somewhat flattened masses that are usually about 8 to 15 cm in diameter and weigh from 300 g to 2 kg each. Externally, opium is pale olive-brown or olive-gray and is covered with fragments of poppy leaves and, at times, with fruits of a species of *Rumex* that adheres from the packing. It is more or less plastic when fresh and becomes hard and brittle or tough when kept. Internally, it is coarsely granular or nearly smooth, reddish brown, frequently interspersed with lighter areas, and somewhat lustrous. Its odor is characteristic and its taste is bitter and characteristic.

The principal commercial varieties are:

1. **Turkish opium** most closely conforms to the official description and is the variety generally used for pharmaceutic purposes. It is produced in 12 provinces and certain adjacent districts of Turkey; the principal ports of export are Istanbul and Izmir. The term "druggists' opium" is often applied to Turkish opium from the western provinces, which contains from 10 to 20% of moisture. The name "soft opium" is applied to Turkish opium from the northern and southern provinces, which has a pasty consistency and contains about 30% of moisture. The product from the northern provinces has a high morphine content (10 to 21%). It is imported for alkaloid manufacture and never appears on the market for pharmaceutic purposes.

2. **Indian opium** is produced at Ghazipur and is consumed in India or exported for the American and British trades. It is presently our main source of opium. It usually occurs in soft cakes that weigh about 5 kg each. These cakes are shipped in plastic bags. Indian opium yields about 10% of anhydrous morphine.

3. **Chinese opium,** once of considerable commercial importance, has not been available in this country since the Communist government came to power in China more than 30 years ago. Although the People's Republic of China has not reported to the International Narcotics Con-

trol Board during this period, the domestic production and use of narcotic drugs are strictly controlled. Chinese opium occurs as flat globular cakes usually wrapped in paper and contains from 4 to 11% of morphine.

Approximately 285,000 kg of opium, with a market value in excess of $5 million, are imported into the United States annually.

More than 30 different alkaloids have been obtained from opium and its extracts, some of which are alteration products of the alkaloids occurring naturally in the drug. The most important of these are **morphine,** which exists to the extent of 4 to 21%; **codeine,** 0.8 to 2.5%; **noscapine** (formerly **narcotine**), 4 to 8%; **papaverine,** 0.5 to 2.5%; and **thebaine,** 0.5 to 2%. Other alkaloids include narceine, protopine, laudanine, codamine, cryptopine, lanthopine, and meconidine.

Opium also contains from 3 to 5% of meconic acid, which exists free or in combination with morphine, codeine, and other alkaloids. It forms rhombic prisms that are soluble in water and alcohol and give a red color in solutions of ferric chloride. The color is not altered when diluted hydrochloric acid is added. Because meconic acid is found only in opium, this test may be used for the detection of opium. The total ash yield of opium is from 4 to 8%, with about 0.55% of acid-insoluble ash.

Opium in its normal, air-dried condition yields not less than 9.5% of anhydrous morphine.

USES AND DOSE. Opium is a pharmaceutic necessity for powdered opium. It acts chiefly on the central nervous system; its action first stimulates and then depresses nerve response. It serves as an analgesic, a hypnotic, and a narcotic and checks excessive peristalsis and contracts the pupil of the eye. A dose of 60 mg was formerly listed for opium and powdered opium.

ADULTERANTS. Fragments of the capsules, the pulp of figs and other fruits, tragacanth, beeswax, powdered cumin seed, starch, and such inorganic substances as clay, sand, stone, lead piping, and lead bullets have been found in opium. Starch is not usually admixed with Turkish opium.

Powdered opium yields not less than 10% and not more than 10.5% of anhydrous morphine. Powdered opium of a higher-percentage morphine may be reduced to the official standard by admixture with powdered opium of a lower percentage or with any of the diluents, except starch, permitted for powdered extracts. The diluents may be colored with caramel to simulate the color of the drug.

Powdered opium is used in making Dover's powder and camphorated opium tincture and is combined with other agents in antidiarrheal preparations.

PRESCRIPTION PRODUCTS. Diabismul®, Ekrised®, KBP/O®, Kapinal®.

Paregoric or camphorated opium tincture is classed as an antiperistaltic. The usual dose of paregoric is 5 to 10 ml, 1 to 4 times a day, and it may be mixed before taking with a small amount of water to form a milky solution. It is used in combination with belladonna alkaloids, kaolin, pectin, and/or other ingredients for the symptomatic treatment of diarrhea. Many of these preparations are Schedule V drugs under the Controlled Substances Act.

NONPRESCRIPTION PRODUCTS. Pabizol with Paregoric®, Kenpectin-P®, Parepectolin®, Pecto-Kalin®, Parelixir®, Donnagel-PG®.

Laudanum, opium tincture, or deodorized opium tincture was formerly used similarly to paregoric. Its dose is 0.6 ml, 4 times a day.

Poppy seed or maw seed is the dried seed of *Papaver somniferum* variety *nigrum* DeCandolle. The seeds are bluish black or yellowish white, reniform, from 0.5 to 1 mm in diameter, and reticulate.

They have a yellowish hilum scar, a white oily endosperm, and a curved embryo. Their taste is slight and oily. Poppy seeds are used in baking (poppy seed rolls). They contain about 50% of a fixed oil **(poppy seed oil),** which is used in some parenteral formulations, by artists as a drying oil, and also for food and salad dressings. **Poppy seed oil cake** is used as a cattle food. Poppy seed contains no significant quantity of alkaloids.

ALKALOIDS OF OPIUM

Morphine is the most important of the opium alkaloids. Morphine and the related alkaloids are phenanthrene derivatives. The molecule contains a phenolic and an alcoholic hydroxyl group.

The alkaloid and its salts occur as white, silky crystals, sometimes in cubic masses, or as a fine crystalline powder. It is stable in air, odorless, and bitter-tasting.

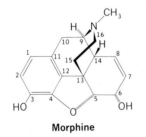

Morphine

Morphine and its salts are classed as narcotic analgesics; they are strongly hypnotic and narcotic. Their use tends to induce nausea, vomiting, constipation, and habit formation. Usual dose of morphine sulfate, parenterally, is 10 mg, 6 times a day, as necessary.

Centrally acting analgesics, in most cases, have certain structural features in common. They are: (1) a central carbon atom with no hydrogen substitution (quaternary), (2) a phenyl group or isostere attached to this carbon atom, (3) a tertiary nitrogen atom, and (4) a 2-carbon bridge separating the tertiary nitrogen atom and the central carbon atom.

Morphine and the related opium alkaloids that have analgesic activity possess these structural features. In the case of morphine, the central carbon atom is C-13; the phenyl ring attached to C-13 is comprised of carbon atoms 1 to 4 and 11 and 12; and the tertiary nitrogen atom is linked via a 2-carbon bridge (C-15, C-16) to the central carbon atom.

Codeine is the most widely used opium alkaloid. It may be either obtained from opium (0.2 to 0.7%) or prepared from morphine by methylation or from thebaine by appropriate reduction and demethylation. Codeine is methylmorphine in which the methyl group replaces the hydrogen of the phenolic hydroxyl group. Codeine and its salts occur as fine needles or as white crystalline powders that effloresce in air.

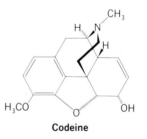

Codeine

Codeine and its salts are narcotic analgesics and antitussives; they are used as sedatives, especially in allaying coughs. Although the action is similar to that of morphine, codeine is considerably less toxic and involves much less danger from habit formation. Usual dose of codeine, codeine phosphate, and codeine sulfate: analgesic is 15 to 60 mg every 4 hours as needed; antitussive, 10 to 20 mg every 4 to 6 hours as needed.

Diacetylmorphine or heroin is formed by the acetylation of morphine; the hydrogen atoms of both the phenolic and alcoholic hydroxyl groups are replaced by acetyl groups. Heroin's action is similar but more pronounced than morphine's action. Because of its potency and the danger from habit formation, its manufacture in the United States is forbidden by law, and its use in medicine has been discontinued.

Apomorphine hydrochloride is formed when morphine is treated with hydrochloric acid in a sealed tube, and one molecule of water is lost. The compound decomposes readily and must be rejected if an emerald green color is produced when it is shaken with distilled water (1 to 100).

Apomorphine is an emetic and is particularly valuable in cases of poisoning because it may be administered subcutaneously. Usual dose, emetic, subcutaneously, is 100 μg per kg of body weight (maximum, 6 mg).

Papaverine occurs naturally in opium to the extent of about 1%, but it may also be produced synthetically. **Papaverine hydrochloride** occurs as white crystals or as a white crystalline powder. It is odorless, but has a slightly bitter taste.

Papaverine hydrochloride is a smooth muscle relaxant. Usual dose, orally, is 150 mg; intramuscularly, 30 mg. Papaverine hydrochloride is represented by Pavabid® and Pavadyl®. It is also used in combination with codeine sulfate (Copavin®). The dose of each is 15 mg.

Hydromorphone hydrochloride or dihydromorphinone hydrochloride differs from morphine hydrochloride because one of the hydroxyl groups of morphine is replaced by a ketone group, and the adjacent double bond is removed. It is prepared by

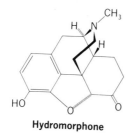

Hydromorphone

reducing morphine in hydrochloric acid solution with hydrogen in the presence of a catalyst.

The drug is a powerful narcotic analgesic and tends to depress strongly the respiratory mechanism. Its dosage is smaller than that of morphine, it causes nausea and constipation less frequently than does morphine, and perhaps is less habit-forming. Usual dose, orally and subcutaneously, 2 mg every 4 hours, as necessary. Dihydromorphinone hydrochloride is represented by the product Dilaudid® Hydrochloride. It is the chief ingredient in Dilocol®.

Hydrocodone bitartrate or dihydrocodeinone bitartrate bears the same relation to codeine as dihydromorphinone does to morphine—a ketone group replaces one of the hydroxyl groups and the adjacent double bond is saturated. It is classed as an antitussive and is an excellent aid in treating a troublesome cough. Usual dose is 5 to 10 mg, 3 to 4 times a day, as necessary. Dihydrocodeinone bitartrate is represented by the products Dicodid® and Codone®.

Noscapine (commonly called **narcotine**) exists in opium as a free base (1.3 to 10%). It possesses no narcotic properties and is therefore sometimes called anarcotine. To eliminate misunderstanding and wrong connotation, the name noscapine is employed in pharmaceutic literature, but narcotine remains as the common chemical designation of this alkaloid.

Noscapine is an antitussive. Usual dose is 15 mg, up to 4 times a day. It is available in syrup and chewable tablets as Tusscapine® and is the chief ingredient in Conar® and Theo-Nar®.

Noscapine hydrochloride or 1-narcotine hydrochloride is a potent cough suppressant and is classified as an antitussive. Usual dose is 15 to 30 mg, 3 to 4 times a day.

A long-standing prescription product

composed of the hydrochlorides of the alkaloids of opium in the same proportion in which they occur in the natural product is Pantopon®. This drug has been freed from inert or irritating gums, waxes, and resins, and it may be administered parenterally as well as orally.

The term **"opioid"** has been devised to refer to the synthetic morphinelike compounds. Many of these substances offer the same narcotic and pain-relieving properties as does morphine, but they are not as habit-forming. Others possess the cough-relieving activity of codeine, but are not addictive.

INDOLE ALKALOIDS

A number of important alkaloids possess an indole ring as part of their structure. Strychnine and brucine (dimethoxystrychnine) from nux vomica and physostigmine from physostigma belong to this group. However, strychnine and brucine also contain a quinoline nucleus, and some authors classify them in the quinoline group.

The important drugs and their alkaloids of the indole group are rauwolfia, reserpine, catharanthus (vinca), vinblastine, vincristine, nux vomica, strychnine, brucine, physostigma, physostigmine, ergot, ergotamine, and ergonovine.

BIOSYNTHESIS OF INDOLE ALKALOIDS

Many of the therapeutically useful indole alkaloids are rather complex multicyclic molecules. Incorporation of a tryptamine moiety into this type of alkaloid was established at a fairly early stage in the study of alkaloid biosynthesis. The origin of the balance of the molecules proved more elusive. However, it is now established that the nontryptophan portions of the molecules are derived from monoterpenoid precursors. Three general monoterpenoid skeletons give rise to most of the complex indole alkaloids; these skeletons are designated as the *Aspidosperma*, *Corynanthe*, and *Iboga* types, taking the names of genera that are rich in alkaloids with the respective monoterpenoid nuclei (Fig. 8–16).

The reactive form of the terpene presumably involves an aldehyde group, and the loss of one carbon atom during the biosynthetic process to give a C_9 unit appears to be fairly common. Most of the details on the sequence of biosynthetic reactions and various rearrangements remain to be clarified. It is suspected that the *Corynanthe* type of monoterpenoid moiety is metabolically the most primitive. Studies on the formation of therapeutically unimportant monomeric alkaloids in *Catharanthus roseus* have demonstrated that the glucoside, secologanin, provides the terpenoid unit. Evidence suggests that secologanin reacts initially with tryptamine to form strictosidine (see Fig. 8–10) and that the glycosidic linkage is cleaved during subsequent metabolic steps.

The *Rauvolfia* alkaloids, ajmaline, reserpine, and serpentine, are derived from a *Corynanthe*-type monoterpenoid precursor. They can be used to illustrate some of

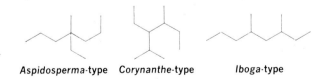

Aspidosperma-type   Corynanthe-type   Iboga-type

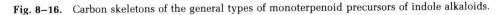

Fig. 8–16. Carbon skeletons of the general types of monoterpenoid precursors of indole alkaloids.

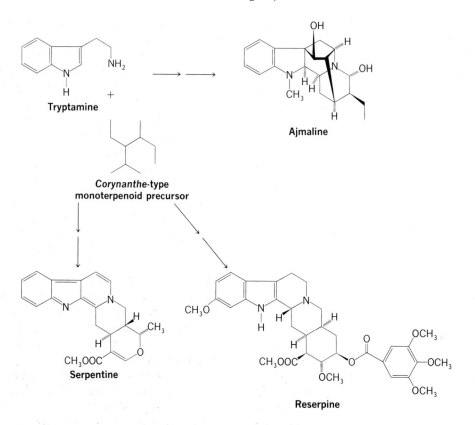

Fig. 8–17. Biosynthesis of *Rauvolfia* alkaloids.

the multicyclic structures that arise during tertiary cyclization and rearrangement steps in biosynthesis (Fig. 8–17).

Ergot Alkaloids. The alkaloids of ergot are also derived from a combination of tryptophan and acetate metabolism. Studies with various physiologic strains of *Claviceps* species, including some significant stereospecific experiments, have clarified many of the key steps leading to the biosynthesis of the lysergic acid nucleus. Dimethylallyl pyrophosphate condenses at the 4-position of tryptophan as an initial step in the pathway (Fig. 8–18). Recent evidence indicates that the next intermediate arises from the N-methylation of dimethylallyltryptophan to give N_{α}-methyldimethylallyltryptophan. The next

anticipated step would be decarboxylation with a subsequent formation of chanoclavine-I. The number of intermediates and enzymatic conversions in these events is still unknown. Concerning the biosynthetic mechanism of alkaloid formation, there is evidence that 2 *cis-trans* isomerizations in the isoprenoid moiety take place in the course of forming the tetracyclic ring system. If the *trans* methyl group of dimethylallylpyrophosphate is radioactively labeled, the *cis* methyl group of chanoclavine-I will be labeled indicating one *cis-trans* isomerization, and the *trans* methyl group of the isoprenoid moiety of agroclavine will be labeled indicating a second isomerization. Agroclavine undergoes stepwise oxidation to elymo-

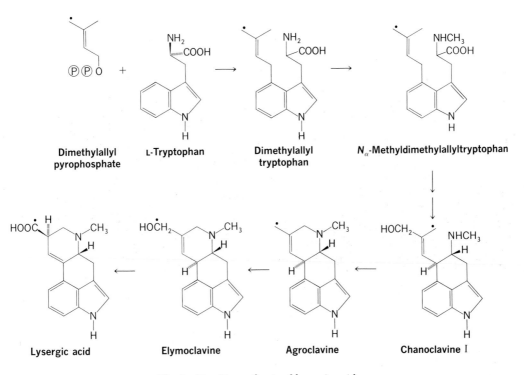

Fig. 8–18. Biosynthesis of lysergic acid.

clavine and eventually to lysergic acid. The carboxyl group of lysergic acid forms a peptide linkage with an amino group of a variety of amino acids or peptide residues to yield the therapeutically useful ergot alkaloids.

Synthesis of lysergic acid derivatives and clavine alkaloids in higher plants (*Ipomoea* species) apparently takes place from the same precursors.

RAUWOLFIA SERPENTINA

Rauwolfia serpentina is the dried root of *Rauvolfia serpentina* (Linné) Bentham ex Kurz (Fam. Apocynaceae). Sometimes fragments of rhizome and aerial stem bases are attached (Fig. 8–19). When assayed as directed, it contains not less than 0.15% of reserpine-rescinnamine group alkaloids, calculated as reserpine. The genus name was selected in honor of Dr. Leonhard

Rauwolf, a noted sixteenth century German botanist, physician, and explorer; *serpentina* refers to the long, tapering, snakelike roots of the plant. It must be emphasized that the name of the drug and the name of the genus of plants from which it derives are spelled differently. For technical reasons, the genus must be spelled with a *v* instead of a *w*. The plant *Rauvolfia serpentina* is thus the correct botanic origin of the drug rauwolfia serpentina (rauwolfia).

For centuries *Rauvolfia serpentina* was used by the medicine men of India to treat a variety of maladies, ranging from snakebite to insanity. In 1563, Garcia de Orta mentioned the plant and its uses in his book on the drugs of India, but European physicians were skeptical of its properties. Consequently, it was not until 1952, when Müller succeeded in isolating the alkaloid, reserpine, that this plant was conceded to

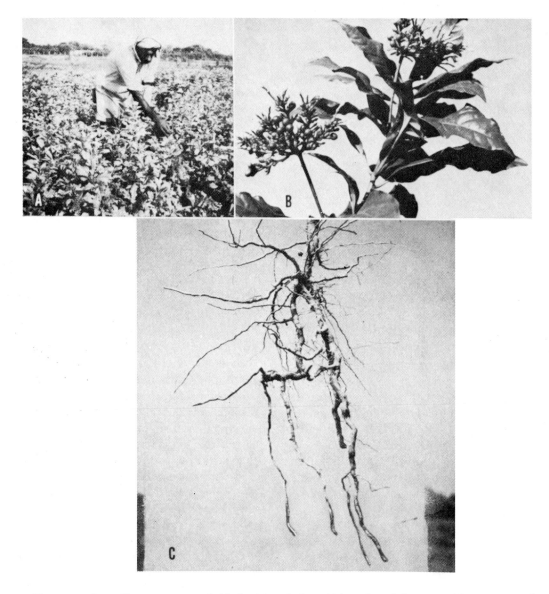

Fig. 8–19. *Rauvolfia serpentina: A*, field of cultivated plants; *B*, branch with flowers and fruits; *C*, typical root system of a 2-year-old plant. (Photo, courtesy of Dr. P. K. Dutta, Regional Research Laboratory, Jammu & Kashmir, India.)

be valuable. In the form of the powdered root, the alkaloidal extract, and purified alkaloids, rauwolfia serpentina has become an exceedingly important therapeutic aid in the treatment and control of hypertension.

The plant is referred to as *sarpagandha* in Sanskrit, *chota-chand* or *chandrika* in Hindi, *pagla-ka-dawa* (insanity cure) in the dialect of Bihar, and also by such other names as *patala-gandhi*, *dhanburua*, and *covanamilpori*. A native plant of India, Burma, Sri Lanka, Vietnam, Malaysia, Indonesia, and the Philippines, rauwolfia occurs in hot moist regions. Practically all commercial supplies at the present time come from India and Thailand. Three varieties of R. serpentina roots have been sold on the Indian markets: Bihar, Dehra Dun, and Assam.

R. serpentina is an erect shrub that reaches 1 meter in height and has cylindric stems. These stems bear pale bark and exhibit a light-colored viscous latex when ruptured. It has leaves that may be simple and opposite or, more commonly, arranged in whorls of 3 to 5. The white or pale rose flowers are arranged in terminal and axillary cymes. The fruit is a single, 2-lobed drupe that turns purplish black when mature.

Three series of alkaloids have been reported: (1) weakly basic indole alkaloids, (2) indoline alkaloids of intermediate basicity, and (3) strong anhydronium bases. The principal alkaloids, reserpine, rescinnamine, and deserpidine, are tertiary indole alkaloids that have a carbocyclic structure in ring E. Other tertiary indole alkaloids exhibit a heterocyclic structure in ring E: δ-yohimbine (identical with ajmalicine), tetrahydroreserpine, raubasine, and reserpinine. Ajmaline, isoajmaline, rauwolfinine, and others are listed as tertiary indoline alkaloids; however, these bases do not have a tranquilizing action. Serpentine, serpentinine, and alstonine are classed as strongly basic anhydronium alkaloids. The latter type is not considered of practical therapeutic importance. From the 25 or more species of *Rauvolfia* investigated, at least 50 alkaloids have been reported.

Powdered rauwolfia serpentina is R. serpentina root reduced to a fine or very fine powder that is adjusted, if necessary, to conform to the official requirements for reserpine-rescinnamine group alkaloids by admixture with lactose or starch or with a powdered rauwolfia serpentina containing a higher or lower content of these alkaloids. It contains not less than 0.15% and not more than 0.20% of reserpine-rescinnamine group alkaloids, calculated as reserpine.

PACKAGING AND STORAGE. Seasonal variation, genetic differences, geographic location, improper handling, improper drying, and other factors account for percentage differences in alkaloid amount. Certain alkaloids hydrolyze easily, and proper storage of the roots, the powdered drug, and the compressed tablets must be observed. Rauwolfia serpentina should be packaged and stored in well-closed containers in a cool, dry place that is secure against insect attack.

USES AND DOSE. Rauwolfia serpentina is a hypotensive. (Reserpine is the chief alkaloid and has strong hypotensive and sedative activity.) A total alkaloidal determination is not indicative of activity unless the proportion of alkaloids is known.

Because at least 50 alkaloids have been isolated, it is easy to understand the claim that the whole root exhibits a medicinal action that is different from that of reserpine. A definite lowering of blood pressure in hypertensive states, a slowing of the pulse, and a general sense of euphoria follow administration. In mild anxiety conditions, the drug has a tranquilizing effect. (The alkaloid has been described as a phenotropic drug because it influences the function of the mind and the affective be-havior). The usual dose of rauwolfia ser-pentina is, initially, 200 mg daily for 1 to 3 weeks; maintenance, 50 to 300 mg daily.

PRESCRIPTION PRODUCTS. Powdered whole root in tablet form is represented by Raudixin®, Rauval®, Wolfina®, and others.

Alseroxylon fraction is a basic pow-dered alkaloidal extract of rauwolfia ser-pentina and is claimed to possess a lack of toxicity over long-range administration. It is given in doses of 2 mg, twice daily.

PRESCRIPTION PRODUCTS. Rautensin® and Rauwiloid®.

Reserpine is a white or pale buff to slightly yellow, odorless, crystalline pow-der that darkens slowly when exposed to light and rapidly when in solution. The structural formula is shown in Figure 8–17.

USES AND DOSE. Reserpine is an antihyper-tensive and tranquilizer. Usual oral dose of reserpine is, initially, 250 µg once a day; maintenance, 100 to 250 µg once a day. The patient should be advised to notify his physician if a change in mood occurs. The intramuscular dose is 500 µg to 1 mg, fol-lowed by 2 to 4 mg, 8 times a day, as neces-sary.

PRESCRIPTION PRODUCTS. Rau-Sed®, Raurine®, Reserpoid®, Sandril®, Serpasil®, and other products.

Reserpine has been obtained in com-mercial quantities from 4 different species of *Rauvolfia*: *R. serpentina, R. micrantha* Hooker filius, *R. tetraphylla* Linné, and *R. vomitoria* Afzelius. Several of these pre-sent problems in the separation of the al-kaloids. In *R. serpentina*, reserpine and re-scinnamine both respond to the extraction procedures, and the end result of the assay procedure is a mixture of both. In *R. tetra-phylla*, reserpine and deserpidine (raunormine) are extracted together; in *R. vomitoria*, reserpine must be separated from the resins.

Laboratory investigators in France have developed a method of synthesizing reser-pine on a commercial scale. However, the natural alkaloid is much less expensive than the synthetic, and, with large quan-tities of *R. vomitoria* available from the Congo, the commercial supplies appear to be sufficient to provide adequate amounts of reserpine and related alkaloids for many years to come. In addition, other species of plants are being studied to ascertain their alkaloidal composition. Because the fam-ily Apocynaceae consists of many addi-tional species, it is probable that untapped sources of reserpine and other valuable al-kaloids may be discovered by pharmacog-nosists and plant chemists.

Rescinnamine is an alkaloid that occurs in several species of *Rauvolfia*. Its appear-ance, properties, and solubility are some-what similar to those of reserpine. Chemi-cally, it is the methyl reserpate ester of 3,4,5-trimethoxy cinnamic acid; its struc-tural formula is:

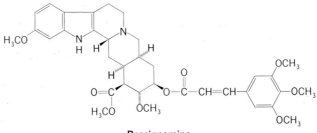

Rescinnamine

Use and Dose. The usual antihypertensive dose of rescinnamine is, initially, 500 μg, 2 times a day and increase dosage gradually, if necessary; maintenance is 250 μg daily. Higher doses should be used cautiously because serious mental depression may be increased considerably.

Prescription Product. Moderil®.

Deserpidine (canescine, recanescine) is an alkaloid obtained from the root of *Rauvolfia canescens* L. Chemically, it is 11-desmethoxyreserpine. It is a wide-range tranquilizer and antihypertensive and is relatively free from the incidence and severity of the side effects that accompany other forms of rauwolfia therapy. It is usually administered orally in doses of 250 μg daily for mild essential hypertension and 500 μg daily for psychiatric disorders.

Prescription Product. Harmonyl®.

Authorities are not in complete agreement as to the relative efficacy or safety of rauwolfia therapy as achieved by administration of the powdered whole root, a total alkaloidal extract, a partial alkaloidal extract, a mixture of the alkaloids, or certain individual alkaloids. In general, 100 mg daily of the standardized alkaloidal extract, or 500 μg to 1 mg of reserpine daily, is an adequate dosage.

In mild or moderate hypertension, rauwolfia or its derivatives may be the sole therapy, but in more severe hypertension, rauwolfia acts synergistically with more potent hypotensive agents. Products are available that utilize combinations of rauwolfia or reserpine with thiazide diuretics and/or other antihypertensive agents.

Prescription Products. Diupres®, Serpasil-Esidrix®, Hydropres®, Salutensin®, Rauzide®, Rautrax-N®, Ser-Ap-Es® and Serpasil-Apresoline®.

Allied Plants. Roots of *Rauvolfia canescens* L. (which are used in India similarly to *R. serpentina*), *R. densiflora*, *R. mi-*crantha, *R. perakensis*, and 2 additional unidentified species of *Rauvolfia* are frequently found as adulterants. The genuine *R. serpentina* roots may be differentiated from roots of the other species by the absence of sclerenchyma tissue in the cortex and secondary phloem and by the shorter and nonfibrous fracture of its thicker pieces. The former restrictions placed on exports of *R. serpentina* roots from India have resulted in the use of other species, particularly for the extraction of reserpine. Root of *R. tetraphylla* Linné obtained from plants growing in Mexico and Guatemala are a source of the alkaloid.

CATHARANTHUS

Catharanthus or vinca is the dried whole plant of *Catharanthus roseus* G. Don (Fam. Apocynaceae), formerly designated *Vinca rosea* Linné. The plant is an erect, everblooming pubescent herb or subshrub that is woody at the base and stands 40 to 80 cm high. It probably originated in Madagascar but is now cosmopolitan in the tropics and is widely cultivated as an ornamental. The flowers are normally violet, rose, or white; ocellate forms are found in cultivated varieties. Botanically, it is closely related to *Vinca minor* Linné, the common periwinkle (Fig. 8–20).

During the course of a modern scientific investigation prompted by the folklore reputation of this plant as an oral hypoglycemic agent, the ability of certain fractions to produce peripheral granulocytopenia and bone marrow depression in rats was observed by the Canadian group of Noble, Beer, and Cutts. Continued study led to the isolation of an alkaloid, vinblastine, which produced severe leukopenia in rats.

Recognizing the anticancer potential of this plant, G. H. Svoboda and coworkers at Eli Lilly and Company isolated an extremely large number of alkaloids from the

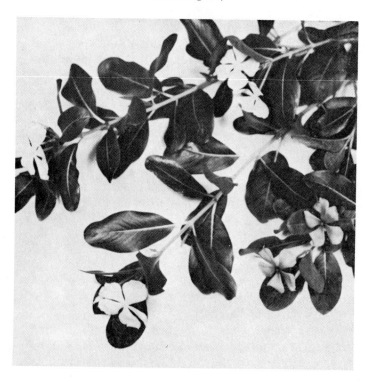

Fig. 8–20. Periwinkle (*Catharanthus roseus*, also known as *Vinca rosea*) showing both white-flowered and pink-flowered varieties. This plant grows abundantly in southern Florida. (Photo courtesy of Dr. Julia F. Morton, Director, Morton Collectanea, University of Miami.)

plant. Of these, 4 dimeric indole-indoline compounds, vinblastine, vinleurosine, vinrosidine, and vincristine, possess demonstrable oncolytic activity. An extremely confusing situation regarding the nomenclature of these alkaloids exists in the scientific literature. The names just mentioned are the United States Adopted Drug Names, but are not the names assigned by the original discoverers who, by tradition, are accorded the privilege of selecting the scientific name for a new chemical compound of complex structure. Equivalent names of these alkaloids are:

U.S. Adopted Drug Names	Scientific Names
Vinblastine	= Vincaleukoblastine (VLB)
Vinleurosine	= Leurosine
Vinrosidine	= Leurosidine
Vincristine	= Leurocristine (LC)

Because the active alkaloids exist in the crude drug in relatively small amounts, enormous quantities of the latter are required for commercial production. Nearly 500 kg of catharanthus are utilized to produce 1 g of vincristine. To satisfy the demand, the plant is collected from both natural and cultivated sources in Madagascar, Australia, South Africa, South America, the West Indies, Europe, India, and the southern United States.

CATHARANTHUS ALKALOIDS

More than 55 different alkaloids have been isolated from catharanthus. They are generally indole and dihydroindole derivatives, some of which occur in other members of the Apocynaceae. These include ajmalicine, tetrahydroalstonine, serpentine, and lochnerine. The alkaloids with antineoplastic activity belong to a new class of dimeric indole-dihydroindole derivatives. Two of them are presently available as prescription drugs.

Vinblastine sulfate is the salt of an alkaloid extracted from catharanthus. It is unstable and is available in sealed ampoules, which should be stored in a refrigerator to insure extended stability. The alkaloid is being used experimentally for the treatment of a wide variety of neoplasms and is recommended for generalized Hodgkin's disease and choriocarcinoma resistant to other therapy. It is administered intravenously or orally in doses regulated by the patient's age, body weight, and white-blood-cell count. Usual dose, intravenously, is 100 μg per kg of body weight initially, each succeeding dose is increased by 50 μg per kg once a week, until a maximum dose is reached as determined by a white-blood-cell count.

PRESCRIPTION SPECIALTY. Velban®.

Vincristine sulfate is also obtained from catharanthus. The structure of this alkaloid is quite similar to that of vinblastine, differing only in the substitution of an N-formyl group for the N-methyl group of vinblastine. Despite the structural similarities, there are differences in the antitumor spectra of the 2 compounds, and no cross-resistance has been observed. Because vincristine sulfate is unstable, refrigerated storage in sealed ampoules is essential. It is recommended for the treatment of acute leukemia and in combination therapy in Hodgkin's disease. Usual dose, intravenously, is 10 to 30 μg per kg of body weight initially, each succeeding dose is increased by 25 μg per kg once a week, not to exceed 2 mg in adults, until optimal therapeutic benefit is seen.

PRESCRIPTION SPECIALITY. Oncovin®.

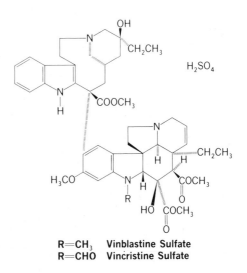

R=CH₃   Vinblastine Sulfate
R=CHO   Vincristine Sulfate

NUX VOMICA

Nux vomica is the dried, ripe seed of *Strychnos nux-vomica* Linné (Fam. Loganiaceae). *Strychnos* is the Greek name for a number of poisonous plants; *nux-vomica* is from 2 Latin words and means a nut that causes vomiting.

The plant is a small tree, about 12 meters tall, that is native to the East Indies and is also found in the forests of Sri Lanka, on the Malabar Coast, and in northern Australia. The fruit is a berry with from 3 to 5 seeds (Fig. 8–21) that are freed from the bitter pulp by washing before exportation. Most of the commercial supply comes from Cambodia and Sri Lanka. The drug was introduced into Europe about the sixteenth century, although it was used mainly for poisoning animals. Its use in medicine began about 1640. The natives of India apparently had no knowledge of its medicinal value.

Nux vomica contains alkaloids, 1.5 to 5%, consisting chiefly of **strychnine** and **brucine,** the former comprising from one third to one half of the total amount. Studies have shown that these alkaloids occur in the large, thick-walled cells of the endosperm, but strychnine is concentrated

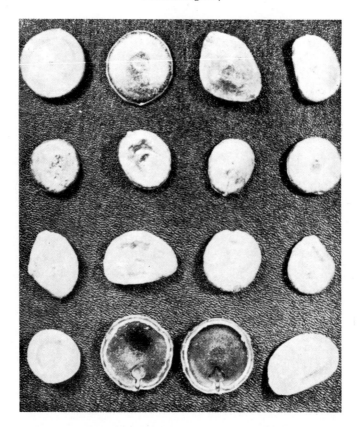

Fig. 8–21.   Nux Vomica: orbicular, compressed, concavo-convex, sometimes irregularly bent, margin acute or rounded, 10 to 30 mm in diameter, 3 to 5 mm in thickness; externally grayish yellow or grayish green, covered with appressed hairs giving the seed a satiny luster, sometimes with adhering dark brown fragments of the fruit pulp; hilum, near the center of one side and a more or less distinct ridge resembling a raphe extending from it to the micropyle; very hard when dry, tough when damp; internally whitish, horny; endosperm in two more or less regular concavo-convex halves; embryo small, situated near the micropyle, and with two heart-shaped cotyledons; inodorous; taste intensely and persistently bitter. The two halves of the seed at the middle of the bottom row show the two cotyledons and the caulicle of the embryo lying against the endosperm.

in the cells near the center of the seed and brucine in the outer cells near the epidermis.

Use. Nux vomica and the seeds of the closely related *Strychnos ignatii* Bergius **(ignatia** or **St. Ignatius bean)** serve as a commercial source of strychnine and brucine. The former alkaloid is commonly marketed as strychnine sulfate or strychnine phosphate.

Strychnine and brucine (dimethoxy-strychnine) are obtained from nux vomica or ignatia by extraction with dilute sulfuric acid. The solution is concentrated. The alkaloids are precipitated with lime, separated by means of solvent, and purified by recrystallization. Brucine is far more soluble in water and in alcohol than is strychnine; however, strychnine sulfate is somewhat more soluble in these 2 solvents than is brucine sulfate.

Strychnine is interesting pharmacologically and is a valuable tool in physiologic and neuroanatomic research. It is extremely toxic, functioning as a central stimulant. Fatal poisoning in human beings ordinarily results from doses of 60 to 90 mg. The drug is seldom employed in modern medical practice, but is utilized as a vermin killer. Brucine, which is less toxic than strychnine, is used commercially as an alcohol denaturant.

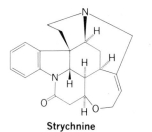

Strychnine

PHYSOSTIGMINE

Physostigma, Calabar bean, or ordeal bean is the dried, ripe seed of *Physostigma venenosum* Balfour (Fam. Leguminosae) yielding not less than 0.15% of the alkaloids of physostigma.

The name *Physostigma* is Greek and means an inflated or bladderlike stigma (Fig. 8–22); *venenosum* is Latin and means full of poison. The plant is a perennial, woody climber that grows on the banks of streams in West Africa, particularly in the vicinity of the Gulf of Guinea. In 1846, Daniell described the use of the seed, known as *esere* by the natives of old Calabar, to prove the innocence or guilt of persons accused of crime.

Calabar bean contains several alkaloids, physostigmine (eserine), eseramine, geneserine, and physovenine. Physostigmine is the major alkaloid and is present in the cotyledons to the extent of 0.04 to 0.3%.

Physostigmine or eserine is an alkaloid usually obtained from the dried, ripe seed of *P. venenosum*. It occurs as a white, odorless, microcrystalline powder that may acquire a red tint when exposed to heat, light, air, or contact with traces of metals. Therefore, physostigmine should be preserved in tight, light-resistant containers in quantities not exceeding 1 g.

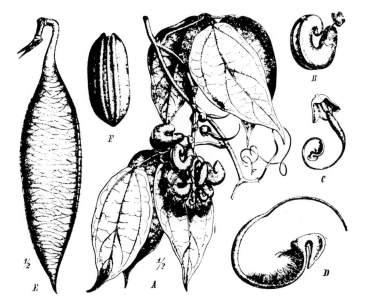

Fig. 8–22. *Physostigma venenosum: A*, flowering branch; *B*, a single flower; *C*, flower showing ovary and part of the calyx; *D*, enlarged view of style and stigma; *E*, legume; *F*, seed. (After Bentley and Trimen.)

USE AND DOSE. Physostigmine is a reversible inhibitor of the cholinesterases. It is employed in ophthalmology to treat glaucoma, usually in the form of a 0.25% ointment that is applied topically to the conjunctiva up to 4 times a day.

Physostigmine salicylate or eserine salicylate is the salicylate of the alkaloid, physostigmine. It is a white powder that also acquires a red tint when exposed to the conditions described under physostigmine. It also should be preserved in tight, light-resistant containers in quantities not exceeding 1 g.

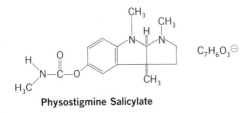

$C_7H_6O_3^{\ominus}$

Physostigmine Salicylate

USES AND DOSE. Physostigmine salicylate is a cholinergic (ophthalmic) and is administered topically, 0.1 ml of a 0.25 to 0.5% solution, to the conjunctiva 1 to 4 times a day. Because it prolongs and exaggerates the effect of acetylcholine, physostigmine salicylate is given by injection as an antidote in poisonings caused by anticholinergic agents.

PRESCRIPTION PRODUCTS. For ophthalmic use, Isopto Eserine®; for poisoning antidote, Antilirium®.

Physostigmine sulfate or eserine sulfate is the sulfate of the alkaloid, physostigmine. This white, microcrystalline powder is deliquescent in moist air and acquires the red tint previously described. Storage requirements are the same as for physostigmine and physostigmine salicylate. It is a cholinergic (ophthalmic) whose dose is, topically, 0.1 ml of a 0.25 to 0.5% solution to the conjunctiva up to 4 times a day.

ERGOT

Ergot, rye ergot, or secale cornutum was formerly defined in the official compendia as the dried sclerotium of *Claviceps purpurea* (Fries) Tulasne (Fam. Hypocreaceae) developed on plants of rye, *Secale cereale* Linné (Fam. Gramineae). Ergot was required to yield not less than 0.15% of the total alkaloids of ergot calculated as ergotoxine and water-soluble alkaloids equivalent to not less than 0.01% of ergonovine.

The generic name, *Claviceps*, refers to the clublike character of the sclerotium; *purpurea* refers to its purple color. Because these sclerotia are long and somewhat pointed, the common name of **spurred rye** has been applied to the drug.

Because galenic preparations of the crude drug are seldomly employed in pharmacy in this country, ergot has been omitted from the official compendia. Nevertheless, its alkaloids continue to enjoy widespread use as extremely important medicinal agents. It therefore appears worthwhile to redefine, in light of modern knowledge, the source of these active compounds.

At present, ergot alkaloids are obtained on a commercial scale from both parasitic and saprophytic sources. The former is the dried sclerotium of *Claviceps purpurea* (Fries) Tulasne (Fam. Clavicipitaceae) developed on rye plants, *Secale cereale*. Some alkaloids are also obtained from the fermentation broth in which the mycelium of selected strains of *Claviceps paspali* Stevens & Hall has been grown saprophytically in submerged culture.

The qualitative and quantitative composition of the alkaloids obtained from either source is influenced by a number of factors, but especially by the identity of the strain (chemical race) of organism involved. At present, both peptide alkaloids and nonpeptide (water-soluble) alkaloids are obtained from parasitically developed ergot sclerotia. Only the latter type is produced commercially in saprophytic culture. However, lysergic acid produced by fermentation is converted on a commercial scale to the peptide alkaloid, ergotamine, by chemical semisynthesis.

In the absence of official standards, the word, ergot, may be used in a variety of ways to describe either one or more species of Claviceps, the mycelium produced by these species in saprophytic culture, or the resting body (sclerotium) of the fungus produced parasitically on rye plants. When the crude drug ergot is referred to in this book, it designates the latter product.

Some knowledge of the rather complex life cycle of the ergot fungus is required to understand the different methods of production of the alkaloids. In nature, the organism is parasitic. In the spring, one of its spores comes into contact with the ovary of a grass, frequently rye, where it germinates, forming hyphal strands that penetrate into the host tissue. The hyphae eventually form a mass of tissue known as a **mycelium,** which supplants the ovary. Some of the hyphal strands produce asexual spores, known as conidiospores, which become suspended in a viscous, sugary liquid, known as honeydew. Honeydew is secreted by the mycelium. Insects are attracted to this honeydew and carry it and the spores to other host plants where the process is repeated. This stage of development of the organism is termed the sexual or **sphacelial stage.**

In the second stage of development, the mycelium eventually replaces the entire ovary, then gradually hardens, becomes dark purple, and forms a resting body, known as a **sclerotium** (Fig. 8–23). The sclerotium, in turn, normally falls to the ground, overwinters, and, in the spring, produces sexual spores or ascospores that repeat the entire cycle. This second phase

of development of the organism is referred to as the sexual or **ascigerous stage.**

When ergot spores are germinated in a suitable nutrient medium in the laboratory (saprophytic growth), hyphae are formed. The hyphae produce mycelium and conidiospores, but no further development occurs. Because the medicinally useful alkaloids are normally produced only during the latter stages of parasitic sclerotial development, the difficulties in producing them in saprophytic mycelial culture are apparent.

Before the introduction of modern agricultural practices, the fungus periodically invaded rye fields in Russia and in eastern European countries, and the ergot sclerotia were harvested with the rye grains. Rye flour made from the contaminated rye grains was subsequently made into rye bread and ingested. Thus, the fungus was responsible for severe outbreaks of a disease, both in man and in cattle, which is today known as ergotism. Two distinct types are recognized. One, common in parts of France, was characterized by the appearance of gangrene in the extremities. The gangrene was caused by the restricted blood flow resulting from the vasoconstrictor action of the ergot alkaloids. The second type, which frequently occurred east of the Rhine in Germany, was characterized by convulsions. Although the factors responsible for the different types of ergotism have not been completely clarified, it is believed that the convulsive variety is associated with a dietary deficiency of vitamin A. Before the causative agent was known, gangrenous ergotism was often referred to as "St. Anthony's fire." As early as 1582, the drug was known to promote uterine contractions.

Originally, the main sources of supply for ergot were Spain, Russia, and the Balkan countries; however, Russia (the Soviet Union) and the Balkans export little ergot

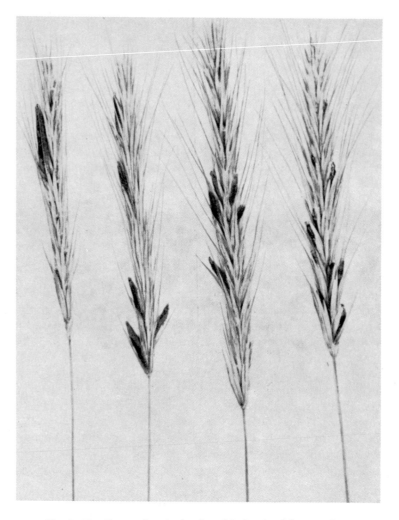

Fig. 8–23. Ergot sclerotia developed in heads of the rye plant.

today. Because of the currency exchange, much of the Spanish ergot is exported through Portugal. Currently, considerable ergot is cultivated in Czechoslovakia, Germany, Hungary, and Switzerland. Entire fields of rye are utilized for this purpose. Prior to fertilization, the flowers of the plants are artificially inoculated with condiospores of *Claviceps purpurea*. Different types of inoculative apparatus are employed. A small (15 cm × 15 cm), hand-operated puncture board studded with eyed or grooved needles that are dipped into a spore suspension before application to the rye inflorescence is the simplest device, but requires an adequate supply of inexpensive labor. The same principle is utilized in motor-driven machines with needle-studded inoculating rollers that are mounted on the front of tractors and are capable of inoculating 5 to 7 acres of rye per day.

Cultured conidiospores are utilized for the inoculum. Much effort has been devoted to the isolation, development, and selection of the best strains of C. *purpurea* for field cultivation. Strains capable of producing about 0.35% of selected alkaloids, principally ergotamine, are now employed.

Approximately 6 weeks after inoculation, the mature sclerotia are harvested. They may be picked by hand or collected by machines developed especially for this purpose in Hungary and Germany. Sclerotia not collected in these ways can be harvested with the grain and separated after threshing by sieving, by specific gravity, or by electrostatic attraction processes. Ergot must be dried immediately after collection and stored properly to prevent deterioration.

The yield of ergot varies considerably, but if the weather has been reasonably favorable and the cultivation has been done well, the yield amounts to 30 to 100 kg or more per acre. If performed by hand, labor involved in collecting and harvesting the ergot amounts to at least 6 hours per kg. This may be reduced appreciably by mechanization, but a substantial investment in machinery is then required. These factors, coupled with the present low price and limited market for the crude drug, have discouraged the field cultivation of ergot in the United States. Although ergot is not cultivated on a commercial scale in this country, the electrostatic attraction process is utilized to separate the naturally occurring drug from quantities of grain. The small domestic supply thus obtained is not uniform in quality or quantity.

Successful saprophytic production of ergot alkaloids dates from the monumental work, first published in 1948, of Matazo Abe of the Takeda Pharmaceutical Industries in Japan. The principal alkaloids produced by Abe's strains and by other strains of the fungus subsequently isolated by A. Stoll and his colleagues at the Sandoz Company in Switzerland were found to be new ergoline derivatives. These compounds, although closely related, proved not to be derivatives of lysergic acid and were designated as clavine alkaloids (see Fig. 8–18). Although their discovery furnished great impetus to the scientific investigation of ergot alkaloid production in saprophytic culture, the clavine alkaloids proved disappointing from the pharmacologic and, consequently, from the commercial viewpoint.

Large-scale production of lysergic acid derivatives in submerged culture was finally achieved in 1960 by A. Tonolo, E. B. Chain, and coworkers of the Istituto Superiore de Sanita in Italy. These investigators utilized an artificially virulented strain of C. *paspali* Stevens & Hall, which produced several simple lysergic acid derivatives, especially (+)-lysergic acid methylcarbinolamide, in stirred fermenters containing a suitable medium. Yields reaching up to 6 mg per ml of nutrient medium have been obtained in 7 to 10 days. A United States patent covering this process was assigned by the investigators to Societa Farmaceutici Italia. The alkaloids obtained can be converted to lysergic acid, which is utilized for the semisynthesis of ergonovine and ergotamine.

CONSTITUENTS. Ergot contains or produces a large number of alkaloids, the most important of which are ergonovine, ergotamine, and a mixture of ergocristine, ergokryptine, and ergocornine that has been marketed for many years under the name, ergotoxine. The alkaloids are often separated into 2 groups based on their solubility in water. Ergonovine is the principal component of the water-soluble fraction. Ergotamine and the ergotoxine group are water-insoluble and are often referred to as peptide alkaloids. Significant semisynthetic alkaloids include methylergonovine, dihydroergotamine, Hydergine®, methysergide, and LSD.

The medicinally useful alkaloids, either

natural or semisynthetic, are all derivatives of (+)-lysergic acid. Because that compound is readily converted to its isomer, (+)-isolysergic acid, the corresponding isolysergic acid derivatives often accompany the (+)-lysergic acid alkaloids in the plant material or are produced during the course of extraction. Isolysergic acid derivatives are practically physiologically inert. They are named by inserting an additional syllable, -in, to the name of the corresponding lysergic acid derivatives, e.g., ergotamine-ergotaminine.

In addition to its characteristic alkaloids, ergot contains a large number of other constituents, including several pigments, a fixed oil (up to 35%), and steroids (ergosterol). Two compounds that contribute to the physiologic activity of the crude drug are histamine and tyramine.

STANDARDS AND ASSAY. Ergot contains not more than 8% of moisture. The use of a cartridge of a nonliquefying, inert, dehydrating agent to maintain low humidity in the container of ergot is desirable. Ergot is assayed for its alkaloid content by colorimetric procedures involving the use of p-dimethylaminobenzaldehyde.

USE. Ergot is used as a source of ergot alkaloids. In the past, galenic preparations were used for their oxytocic properties.

ERGOT ALKALOIDS

Ergonovine maleate or ergometrine maleate occurs as a white or faintly yellow, odorless, microcrystalline powder. It is affected by light and is readily soluble in water, but less soluble in alcohol.

The alkaloid was discovered almost simultaneously in 1935 by 5 independent research groups, and it was assigned 4 different names. To resolve the conflict, a fifth name, ergonovine, was officially adopted in the United States. That title has not been accepted elsewhere. Ergometrine is used

in practically all other countries, except Switzerland where ergobasine is preferred. Establishment of a clear-cut priority is difficult but, based on the first isolation of a pure compound, probably should be awarded to ergobasine. Even in the United States, the accepted chemical name of the isolysergic acid isomer of ergonovine is ergometrinine.

Because of its ready solubility in water, this alkaloid has marked advantages over the other ergot alkaloids (Fig. 8–24). The oxytocic effect of the drug, either orally, subcutaneously, or intramuscularly, is sometimes noted within 5 minutes after giving the dose, and its effect is more marked than that of either ergotoxine or ergotamine. However, the vasoconstrictor action is much less marked.

USE AND DOSE. Ergonovine maleate is an oxytocic and produces much faster stimulation of the uterine muscles than do other ergot alkaloids. It is used for the prevention and treatment of postpartum hemorrhage caused by uterine atony. Usual dose is, orally, 200 to 400 μg, 2 to 4 times a day; intramuscularly or intravenously, 200 μg, repeated after 2 to 4 hours if necessary.

PRESCRIPTION PRODUCT. Ergotrate Maleate®.

Methylergonovine maleate is a semisynthetic homolog of ergonovine prepared from lysergic acid and 2-aminobutanol. It occurs as a white to pinkish tan, microcrystalline powder.

USE AND DOSE. Methylergonovine maleate is an oxytocic reputed to be slightly more active and longer acting than ergonovine. Usual dose is the same as ergonovine.

PRESCRIPTION PRODUCT. Methergine®.

Ergotamine tartrate occurs as colorless crystals or as a white, crystalline powder, sparingly soluble in water or in alcohol. Ergotamine possesses oxytocic properties, but it is not employed for that effect. It is categorized as a specific analgesic in migraine. Usual dose is, orally or sublin-

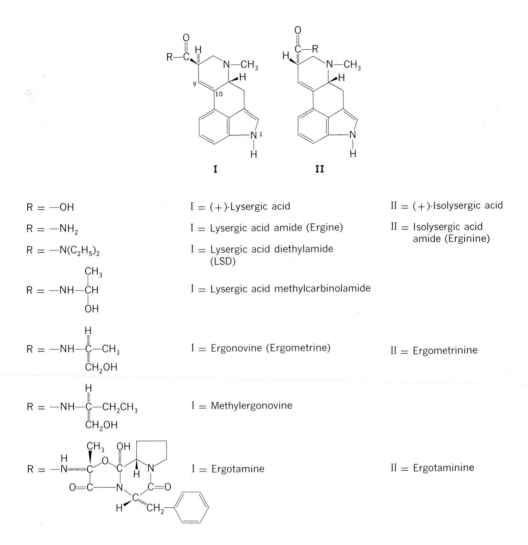

Fig. 8–24. Structural relationships of ergot alkaloids.

gually, 1 to 2 mg, then 1 to 2 mg every 30 minutes, if necessary, to a total of 6 mg per attack; intramuscularly or subcutaneously, 250 to 500 μg, repeated in 40 minutes, if necessary. The patient should be advised to initiate therapy at onset of attack and to lie down in a quiet and darkened room for 2 hours after taking medication.

PRESCRIPTION PRODUCTS. Ergomar®, Ergostat®, Gynergen®, Medihaler Ergotamine®.

Ergotamine tartrate is used with caffeine for the treatment of migraine headache. Both act as cerebral vasoconstrictors; caffeine is believed to enhance the action of ergotamine.

PRESCRIPTION PRODUCTS. Cafergot®, Migral®, Wigraine®.

Dihydroergotamine mesylate is the salt of a semisynthetic alkaloid prepared from ergotamine by hydrogenation of the Δ^9 double bond in the lysergic acid nucleus. Dihydroergotamine is employed in the treatment of migraine because it is more effective and better tolerated than the parent alkaloid. Usual dose is, parenterally, 1 mg, and may be repeated at 1-hour intervals to 3 mg.

PRESCRIPTION PRODUCT. D.H.E. 45®.

Ergotoxine was formerly employed as a reference standard in the form of **ergotoxine ethanesulfonate,** which was discontinued because it was a variable mixture of 3 closely related alkaloids, ergocristine, ergokryptine, and ergocornine. A mixture of equal parts of these component alkaloids is hydrogenated to eliminate the Δ^9 double bond of the lysergic acid nucleus and to yield an equivalent mixture of dihydroergocristine, dihydroergokryptine, and dihydroergocornine. The methanesulfonates (mesylates) of this mixture are marketed for the treatment of selected symptoms in elderly patients. They produce vasorelaxation, increased cerebral blood flow, lowering of systemic blood pressure, and bradycardia. Usual dose is, sublingually, 0.5 mg, 4 to 6 times daily; intramuscularly or intravenously, 0.3 mg, daily or every other day.

PRESCRIPTION PRODUCTS. Circanol®, Hydergine®, Spengine®, Trigot®, Deapril-ST®, Gerigine®, Tri-Ergone®.

Methysergide maleate is the salt of methylergonovine that has an additional methyl group attached to the nitrogen at position 1 of the lysergic acid nucleus. It is prepared by semisynthesis from lysergic acid. Methysergide is a serotonin antagoninst (antiadrenergic) employed in the prophylaxis of vascular headache. Usual dose is, orally, 4 to 6 mg daily in divided doses.

The patient should be advised to take medication with meals and to notify the physician if cold, numb, or painful hands, leg cramps, abdominal or chest pain, or change in skin color occurs.

PRESCRIPTION PRODUCT. Sansert®.

Lysergic acid diethylamide or LSD does not occur in nature, but is prepared by semisynthesis. The compound has a 2-fold action, producing a predominant central sympathetic stimulation that parallels a slight depression. Discovered by A. Hofmann in 1943 during the course of experiments directed toward the synthesis of analeptics, it is the most active and most specific psychotomimetic agent known. The effective oral dose in man is 30 to 50 μg. LSD is of considerable interest and value in experimental psychiatry. Because of widespread misuse, the drug is available, at this writing, only to qualified scientific investigators.

DRUGS RELATED TO ERGOT

The active principles of **ololiuqui,** an ancient Aztec hallucinogenic drug still used in Mexico for magicoreligious purposes, have been identified as ergot alkaloids. Seeds of ololiuqui, *Rivea corymbosa* (Linné) Hallier filius (Fam. Convolvulaceae), as well as certain closely related *Ipomoea* species (commonly known as morning glories) and *Argyreia* species, contain up to about 0.05% of total alkaloids. (+)-Lysergic acid amide (ergine), the principal psychotomimetic compound in these species, is accompanied by (+)-isolysergic acid (erginine), ergonovine, (+)-lysergic acid methylcarbinolamide, and certain clavine alkaloids.

Many of these morning glories are widely cultivated ornamentals. The ready availability of their seeds has led to misuse by thrill-seeking teenagers and adults who ingest the seeds to experience hallucinations. Needless to say, the practice is dangerous because of the extreme potency of the active principles.

Occurrence of the biosynthetically complex ergot alkaloids in both fungi and higher plants is unusual and of considerable chemotaxonomic interest. Aside from *Claviceps* species and the members of the Convolvulaceae, ergot alkaloids have been reported only in 4 other fungi, *Aspergil-*

lus fumigatus Fres., Penicillium chermesinum Biourge, Penicillium roquefortii Thom, and Rhizopus arrhizus Fischer. Only clavine alkaloids were detected in these latter species.

IMIDAZOLE ALKALOIDS

The imidazole (glyoxaline) ring is the principal nucleus in pilocarpine from pilocarpus. Pilocarpine is a monoacidic tertiary base containing a lactone group as well as the imidazole nucleus. Obvious structural similarities suggest that this alkaloid probably is formed from histidine or a metabolic equivalent, but experimental confirmation of such a biosynthetic origin is lacking.

Pilocarpus and pilocarpine are the important drugs of this group.

PILOCARPINE

Pilocarpus or jaborandi consists of the leaflets of Pilocarpus jaborandi Holmes (Pernambuco jaborandi), of P. microphyllus Stapf (Maranham jaborandi), or of P. pinnatifolius Lemaire (Paraguay jaborandi) (Fam. Rutaceae). The plants are shrubs indigenous to Brazil.

All of the commercial kinds of pilocarpus, when freshly dried, yield from 0.5 to 1% of the alkaloid pilocarpine. Isopilocarpine, pilocarpidine, and pilosine are also present in some of the species. Even under ideal storage conditions, the leaves lose at least half of their alkaloidal content in 1 year through deterioration. Leaves that are 2 years old are practically worthless.

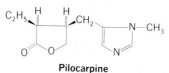

Pilocarpine

Pilocarpine is the lactone of pilocarpic acid, an acid with a glyoxaline nucleus. It is an oily, syrupy liquid, though its salts crystallize easily. It may be obtained by treating the powdered leaves with sodium carbonate, extracting with benzene, and then shaking the benzene extract with dilute hydrochloric or nitric acid. The aqueous solution is then made alkaline and shaken with chloroform; the chloroform solution is then shaken with acid, and the alkaloidal salt is allowed to crystallize.

Pilocarpine hydrochloride is the hydrochloride of an alkaloid obtained from the dried leaflets of Pilocarpus jaborandi or of P. microphyllus. It is hygroscopic.

Pilocarpine nitrate is the nitrate of the alkaloid. It is stable in air, but is affected by light.

Pilocarpine hydrochloride occurs as colorless, translucent, odorless, faintly bitter crystals; pilocarpine nitrate occurs as shiny, white crystals.

Use and Dose. Both pilocarpine hydrochloride and pilocarpine nitrate are cholinergic (ophthalmic) drugs used in the treatment of glaucoma. They are applied topically, 0.05 to 0.1 ml of a 0.25 to 10% solution of pilocarpine hydrochloride or of a 0.5 to 6% solution of pilocarpine nitrate to the conjunctiva, 1 to 6 times a day. The patient should be advised to wash hands immediately after application. Pilocarpine is sometimes administered (5 mg) orally or subcutaneously to stimulate the secretion of saliva, especially in patients undergoing therapy with ganglionic blocking agents.

Prescription Products. Pilocarpine hydrochloride is an ingredient in Pilocel®, Adsorbocarpine®, Pilocar®, Almocarpine®, Pilomiotin®, E-carpine®, and Isopto Carpine®.

STEROIDAL ALKALOIDS

The steroidal alkaloids are characterized by the cyclopentenophenanthrene nucleus. They are apparently either formed from cholesterol, or they and cholesterol have a common precursor. The results of preliminary tracer experiments are consistent with this idea.

The important drugs and their alkaloids of this group are veratrum viride, veratrum album, and protoveratrine.

VERATRUM VIRIDE

Veratrum viride, American or green hellebore consists of the dried rhizome and roots of *Veratrum viride* Aiton (Fam. Liliaceae) (Fig. 8–25).

Veratrum is from the Latin *vere*, meaning truly, and *ater*, meaning black. *Viride* is Latin and means green. The plant grows in wet meadows in the mountainous sections of New England and the eastern United States, North Carolina, Tennessee, and northern Georgia. Most of the commercial drug is collected in New York State and eastern Canada. The rhizomes are dug, cleaned, cut longitudinally, and dried. The drug was known to the Indians, who probably introduced its use to the early settlers.

Different investigators in the past have standardized veratrum viride on the guinea pig, dog, mouse, pigeon, and *Daphnia magna*, a macroscopic water crustacean that possesses a myogenic heart. *D. magna* was the basis for the Craw unit: the amount of veratrum viride that caused cardiac arrest in that organism. At present, dogs are used as the test animals, and the unit is called the Carotid Sinus Reflex Unit (CSR Unit). One unit repre-

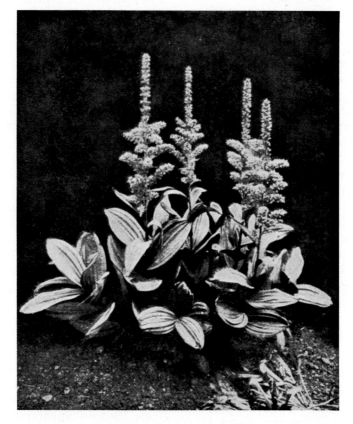

Fig. 8–25. Plants of *Veratrum viride* growing in the Royal Botanic Society's Gardens (London) and showing the parallel-veined leaves with entire margin and the large terminal panicles of flowers.

sents the amount necessary to elicit the carotid sinus blockage in an anesthetized dog; 13 such units equal the activity of 1 Craw unit.

Veratrum viride contains a large number of alkaloids customarily classified in 3 groups on the basis of their chemical constitution. Group I, consisting of esters of the steroidal bases (alkamines) with organic acids, includes cevadine, germidine, germitrine, neogermitrine, neoprotoveratrine, protoveratrine, and veratridine. Group II includes pseudojervine and veratrosine, which are glucosides of the alkamines. The alkamines themselves, germine, jervine, rubijervine, and veratramine, comprise group III. The ester alkaloids, germidine and germitrine, are probably the most important therapeutically. The complexity and relative instability of these constituents account for the problems encountered in the biologic standardization of this drug.

Uses and Dose. Veratrum viride possesses hypotensive, cardiac-depressant, and sedative properties. It is valuable in the treatment of hypertension. Small doses principally affect blood pressure without notably changing respiratory rate or cardiac rate. The drug has its most uniform effects in small doses. The dose is 100 mg.

Veratrum viride, in the form of the tincture, was used for many years by American physicians as a cardiac depressant. This form of medication was abandoned when a study of the alkaloids demonstrated their hypotensive properties.

Prescription Products. A product containing whole powdered veratrum viride is Veralzem®. A mixture of alkaloids known as **"cryptenamine"** (a unique fraction obtained by selective isolation from veratrum viride) is present in Unitensen®. A mixture of the highly purified alkaloids of veratrum viride, **"alkavervir,"** is contained in Veriloid®.

White hellebore or European hellebore is the dried rhizome of Veratrum album, Linné (Fam. Liliaceae). It is similar to V. viride, but is indigenous to central and southern Europe. White hellebore is similar in appearance and structure to green hellebore, but the external color is much lighter.

The drug contains a complex mixture of ester alkaloids, glycoalkaloids, and alkamines similar, and in some cases identical, to those occurring in veratrum viride. Two ester alkaloids, protoveratrine A and protoveratrine B, are the most active.

Uses. White hellebore possesses hypotensive properties, but the crude drug is not used therapeutically. It serves as a source for the isolation of the alkaloids. Both white and green hellebores are also employed as insecticides.

Protoveratrines A and B are the active alkaloids of V. album and represent the

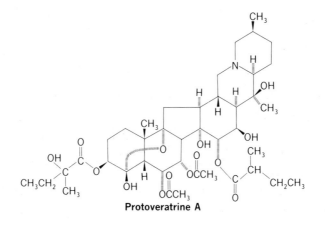

Protoveratrine A

constituents possessing hypotensive activity. On hydrolysis, both yield protoverine, acetic acid, methylbutyric acid, and methylhydroxybutyric acid (A) or methyldihydroxybutyric acid (B). Although they are generally combined for their therapeutic effect, protoveratrine A is sometimes employed separately. Both are free of serious side effects in doses that produce a significant drop in blood pressure. Protoveratrine A is sold as Pro-Amid®.

ALKALOIDAL AMINES

The alkaloids in this group do not contain heterocyclic nitrogen atoms. Many are simple derivatives of phenylethylamine and, as such, are derived from the common amino acids, phenylalanine or tyrosine. Some of the alkaloids in this category whose biosynthesis has been studied utilizing labeled precursors include hordenine in barley *(Hordeum vulgare)*, mescaline in the peyote cactus *(Lophophora williamsii)*, ephedrine in *Ephedra distachya*, cathine [(+)-norpseudoephedrine] in the khat plant *(Catha edulis)*, and colchicine in the autumn crocus *(Colchicum autumnale)*.

Ring A and carbon atoms 5, 6, and 7 of colchicine derive from the phenylalanine-cinnamic acid pathway in *Colchicum*

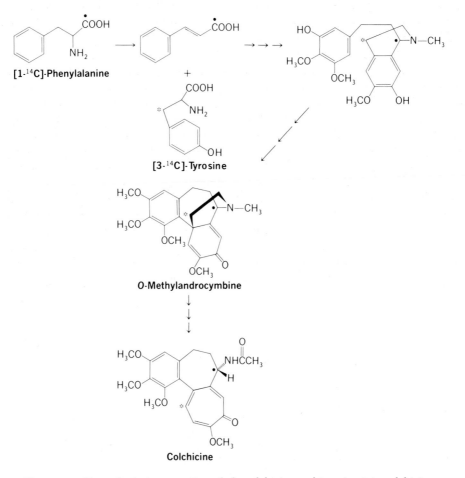

Fig. 8–26. Biosynthetic incorporation of phenylalanine and tyrosine into colchicine.

species (Fig. 8–26). Tyrosine cannot replace phenylalanine as a precursor for this part of the molecule. Radioactivity from tyrosine-3-^{14}C is incorporated into the C-12 position of the tropolone ring. Many of the details of the biosynthetic pathway are unknown; a phenethylisoquinoline intermediate is suspected, and androcymbine also occurs in *Colchicum*. Labeled acetate is readily incorporated into the acetyl group of the molecule, presumably during a terminal phase of biosynthesis.

Other alkaloidal amines are tryptamine derivatives and, as such, are biosynthesized from tryptophan. Examples include gramine in *Hordeum vulgare*, psilocybin in the Mexican hallucinogenic mushroom, *Psilocybe semperviva*, and serotonin and bufotenine in a number of plant and animal species.

The drugs and their alkaloids classified as alkaloidal amines are ephedra, ephedrine, colchicum seed, colchicum corm, colchicine, khat, and peyote.

EPHEDRINE

Ephedra or ma huang is the entire plant or the overground portion of *Ephedra sinica* Stapf (Fam. Gnetaceae). In Chinese characters, "ma" means astringent and "huang" means yellow, probably referring to the taste and color of the drug. It has

been used as a medicine in China for more than 5000 years. Its use in modern medicine began in 1923 with the discovery of the valuable properties of ephedrine. The plant is found near the sea coast in southern China, and this source formerly supplied most of the American market. At the present time, northwestern India and Pakistan represent the areas from which ephedra is obtained.

The plant is a low, dioecious, practically leafless shrub that grows 60 to 90 cm high. The stem is green, slender, erect, small ribbed and channeled. It is 1.5 mm in diameter and usually terminates in a sharp point. At the nodes, which are 4 to 6 cm apart, the leaves appear as whitish, triangular, scarious sheaths. Small blossoms appear in the summer.

Ephedrine or (−)-*erythro*-α-[1-(methylamino) ethyl] benzyl alcohol is an alkaloid produced commercially either by the extraction of plant material (*Ephedra* sp.) or by a chemical procedure involving a reductive condensation between L-1-phenyl-1-acetylcarbinol and methylamine (Fig. 8–27). This yields L-ephedrine essentially free from the D-isomer. The carbinol precursor used in the reaction is produced biosynthetically by the fermentative action of brewer's yeast on benzaldehyde.

Studies indicate that the reaction involves the dismutation of pyruvic acid to lactic acid and acetyl-CoA which, in turn,

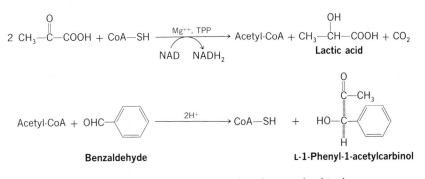

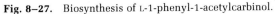
Fig. 8–27. Biosynthesis of L-1-phenyl-1-acetylcarbinol.

condenses with benzaldehyde to yield L-1-phenyl-1-acetylcarbinol.

An undesirable by-product of the fermentation process is benzyl alcohol, which is produced as a result of competition for the benzaldehyde by the carbinol synthesizing system and another enzyme, alcohol dehydrogenase. Addition of structural analogs of nicotinamide to the fermentation medium appreciably reduces benzyl alcohol production. These probably function by competing with NAD for its enzyme site because $NADH_2$ is required as the H^+ donor in the reductive reaction.

Ephedrine occurs as white, rosette or needle crystals, or as an unctuous mass. It is soluble in water, alcohol, chloroform, ether, and in liquid petrolatum. The latter solution is turbid if the ephedrine is not dry. Ephedrine melts between 33 and 40° C, depending on its water content.

USES AND DOSE. Ephedrine is classed as an adrenergic (bronchodilator); it excites the sympathetic nervous system, causes vasoconstriction and cardiac stimulation, and produces effects similar to those of epinephrine. It produces a rather lasting rise of blood pressure, causes mydriasis, and diminishes hyperemia. The alkaloid may be used in 0.5 to 2% oil spray.

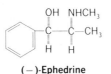

(−)-Ephedrine

Ephedrine sulfate, $(C_{10}H_{15}NO)_2 \cdot H_2SO_4$, is the sulfate of the alkaloid obtained from the natural sources or prepared synthetically. It occurs as fine, white, odorless crystals or as a powder and darkens when exposed to light. Ephedrine sulfate is an adrenergic; usual dose is, orally or parenterally, 25 to 50 mg, 6 to 8 times a day, as necessary. For external use, intranasally,

0.1 to 0.15 ml of a 1 to 3% solution, 2 or 3 times a day.

Ephedrine hydrochloride, $C_{10}H_{15}NO \cdot HCl$, also occurs as fine, white, odorless crystals or as a powder and is affected by light.

It has the same pharmacologic properties as ephedrine and is used as a sympathomimetic. Usual dose is 25 to 50 mg, every 3 or 4 hours. Both of these salts are readily soluble in water and in hot alcohol, but not in ether.

PRESCRIPTION PRODUCTS. The crude drug, ephedra, is contained in Ephedrol® with Codeine. Ephedrine salts are ingredients in the following products: Calcidrine®, Dainite®, Epragen®, I-Sedrin®, Quadrinal®, Tedral®, and many others.

ALLIED PLANTS. In addition to *Ephedra sinica* (the source of ma huang) and *E. equisetina* Bunge (the chief source of the extracted alkaloid), *E. distachya* Linné also yields ephedrine. These plants grow in northern China, India, and Spain in sandy and clay soil. Attempts to grow the plants in the United States, particularly in the Dakotas, were successful, but not economically feasible.

COLCHICINE

Colchicum seed is the dried, ripe seed of *Colchicum autumnale* Linné (Fam. Liliaceae). **Colchicum corm** is the dried corm of the same species.

The genus name is from Colchis on the Black Sea, where the plant flourishes; *autumnale* refers to the season when the plant blooms. The plant is cultivated in England, central and southern Europe, and northern Africa, where it grows in moist meadows. It is also cultivated as an ornamental in the United States. Two to six flowers with long perianth tubes develop from the corm buds in the fall (hence, the name **autumn crocus**). The seed is collected in July and August and the corm in the spring before leaf development. Italy and Yugoslavia produce most of the supply of the seed and the corm.

Dioscorides mentions a *Colchicum*. The Arabs recommended the use of the corm for gout in medieval times, but the drug was abandoned because of its toxicity. It again came into use in Europe about the middle of the seventeenth century.

Colchicum contains the alkaloid colchicine, up to 0.8% in the seed and 0.6% in the corm.

Use. Colchicum is a source of colchicine.

Colchicine, $C_{22}H_{25}NO_6$, is an alkaloid obtained from various species of Colchicum, usually *Colchicum autumnale*. It has also been found in other genera of the lily family. Colchicine has one amido nitrogen atom. The compound lacks pronounced basicity and does not form a well-defined series of salts as do other alkaloids. Nevertheless, it is precipitated by many alkaloid reagents and is conventionally considered an alkaloid. (See Fig. 8–26 for the structural formula.)

Colchicine occurs as pale yellow, amorphous scales or powder that gradually turns darker when exposed to light. It is soluble in water and ether and is freely soluble in alcohol and chloroform.

Use and Dose. Colchicine is used as a suppressant for gout. Usual prophylactic dose is, orally, 500 to 650 μg, 1 to 3 times a day; intravenously, 500 μg to 1 mg, 1 or 2 times a day.

Proprietary Products. Colsalide®. Colchicine is combined with probenecid in the following: ColBENEMID®, Colbeni-Mor®, Proben-C®, Robenecol®.

The use of colchicine to double chromosomes has opened a large field in plant genetics. Any numeric change in chromosome number entails a mutation that becomes evident in a number of the characteristics of the experimental plant. New varieties of plants of economic and pharmacognostic value may result from further

research. The interrelationship between the action of colchicine and mitosis is being investigated in animals; preliminary experiments show that injections of colchicine can effect the dispersal of tumors; thus, it has been employed experimentally in the treatment of various neoplastic diseases.

OTHER ALKALOIDAL AMINE DRUGS

Khat or Abyssinian tea consists of the fresh leaves of *Catha edulis* Forskal (Fam. Celastraceae). The plant is a small tree or shrub native to tropical East Africa. It is cultivated extensively in the Ethiopian highlands near Harar and to a lesser extent in other parts of East Africa, in South Africa, and in Yemen. Fresh leaves are regularly transported by air to areas distant from the centers of cultivation.

The leaves are chewed habitually by many people in East Africa and the Arabian countries to alleviate the sensations of hunger and fatigue. Authorities disagree as to the safety of the practice. The Expert Committee on Addiction-Producing Drugs of the World Health Organization does not classify khat as a drug that produces habituation or addiction, but the French government considers it a narcotic. Regardless, khat-chewing is a theologically accepted and lawful custom in Arabian and African countries today.

Khat contains about 1% of (+)-norpseudoephedrine, on the basis of air-dried material, which occurs without any notable admixture of isomers or related bases. The central stimulant activity of the crude drug is well accounted for by this amount of (+)-norpseudoephedrine.

Peyote or mescal buttons consists of the dried tops of *Lophophora williamsii* (Lemaire) Coulter (Fam. Cactaceae), growing in northern Mexico and the southwestern United States (Fig. 8–28). The main axis of the plant lies beneath the ground,

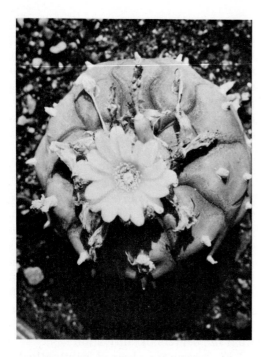

Fig. 8–28. *Lophophora williamsii:* top view of flowering plant. (Photo, courtesy of Dr. J. L. McLaughlin, Department of Medicinal Chemistry and Pharmacognosy, Purdue University.)

and from it arise a number of aerial shoots that are button-shaped or disklike and reach 20 to 50 mm in diameter. In the center of each disk are a tuft of hairs and usually one or more pink flowers.

This plant has been associated with Indian ceremonies for many years. It disturbs normal mental function and effects concomitant hallucinations and euphoria. Ingestion of mescal buttons results in mydriasis accompanied by unusual and bizarre color perception. Flashing lights and vivid configurations characterize the visions at first; later, the colors become dim and the subjects become drowsy; eventually, sleep is produced.

The drug contains several alkaloids, including mescaline (the most active of the peyote constituents), anhalanine, anhalamine, and anhalidine. Mescaline (3,4,5,-

trimethoxy-β-phenylethylamine) also occurs in other cacti, e.g., *Trichocereus* species, or it may be produced synthetically.

Mescaline is regarded as the first of a series of hallucinogens or psychotomimetics. Others are psilocybin (obtained from the mushroom *Psilocybe mexicana* Heim) and lysergic acid diethylamide (LSD). All of these drugs have proved valuable in experimental psychiatry.

PURINE BASES

The purines are derivatives of a heterocyclic nucleus consisting of the 6-membered pyrimidine ring fused to the 5-membered imidazole ring. Purine itself does not occur in nature, but numerous derivatives are biologically significant. The pharmaceutically important bases of this group are all methylated derivatives of 2,6-dioxypurine (xanthine). Caffeine is 1,3,7-trimethylxanthine, theophylline is 1,3-dimethylxanthine, and theobromine is 3,7-dimethylxanthine (see page 259).

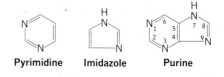

Pyrimidine   Imidazole   Purine

Caffeine is synthesized from the same precursors in *Coffea arabica* as are the purine bases in all other biologic systems that have been investigated. Carbon atoms 2 and 8 derive either from formate or from any compound that can give rise to an active 1-carbon fragment (serine, glycine, formaldehyde, and methanol). These same compounds, as well as methionine, are active precursors of the N-methyl groups of the molecule. Carbon atom 6 is derived from carbon dioxide and carbons 4 and 5, together with the nitrogen at 7, from glycine. The nitrogen atom at position 1 derives from aspartic acid, but those in positions 3 and 9 originate from the amide nitrogen of glutamine.

The drugs of this group are coffee, caffeine, guarana, kola, maté, tea, theophylline, cocoa, and theobromine.

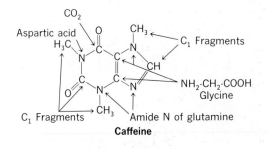

Caffeine

CAFFEINE-CONTAINING DRUGS

Kola, cola, or kolanuts is the dried cotyledon of *Cola nitida* (Ventenat) Schott et Endlicher, or of other species of *Cola* (Fam. Sterculiaceae). It yields not less than 1% of anhydrous caffeine. Kolanut is important because of its caffeine content and its flavor. Its principal use in the United States is in the manufacture of nonalcoholic beverages. In the tropical countries where it grows, the fresh nut is chewed as a stimulant, similar to the betel nut (see page 200). *C. nitida* is a large tree indigenous to West Africa between Sierra Leone and the Congo. It is also cultivated in East Africa, Sri Lanka, Indonesia, Brazil, and the West Indies, particularly in Jamaica. The commercial supplies come chiefly from cultivated plants that grow in West Africa and in the West Indies.

Kolanuts in Jamaica are harvested twice a year when the pods ripen (May and June and again in October and November). The chocolate-colored pods, which range from 5 to 10 cm in length, are shaken from the tree and gathered immediately. The seeds are removed from the pods, and the outer coat is cut off, exposing the bare cotyledons. These cotyledons are then carefully graded because only sound cotyledons do not deteriorate quickly. Fresh kolanuts tend to mold and spoil rather easily; they must be transported to the markets quickly for local consumption. Kolanuts prepared for shipment to the United State are split in half, dried in the sun, and shipped in bags.

Kolanuts contain caffeine, up to 3.5%, and theobromine, less than 1%. In the fresh nuts, these purine derivatives are bound to the tannin, kolacatechin. During the drying process, the complex is split, yielding free caffeine and theobromine and converting the colorless kolacatechin to the red-brown kola red.

USE. Kola possesses the central stimulating action of caffeine. It is an ingredient in several carbonated beverages.

Coffee bean or coffee seed is the dried, ripe seed of *Coffea arabica* Linné or *C. liberica* Hiern (Fam. Rubiacae), deprived of most of the seed coat.

Roasted coffee is coffee roasted until it acquires a dark brown color and develops the characteristic aroma.

The plants are small evergreen trees or shrubs with lanceolate, acuminate, entire, slightly coriaceous, dark green, short-petiolate leaves, which are partly united with the short interpetiolar stipules at the base. The name *Coffea* is from the Turkish *qahveh* or the Arabic *qahuah*, the name of a beverage. The coffee plant is indigenous to Ethiopia and other parts of eastern Africa and is widely cultivated in tropical countries, notably in Indonesia, Sri Lanka, and Central and South America, particularly Brazil. More than 600,000 tons are produced annually in the latter country. The yield from one tree is between 0.5 and 5 kg.

The fruit is a small spheroidal or ellipsoidal drupe with 2 locules, each containing one seed or coffee bean. There are 2 methods of freeing the seeds from the parchmentlike endocarp: (1) the fruits are allowed to dry and are then broken, and (2)

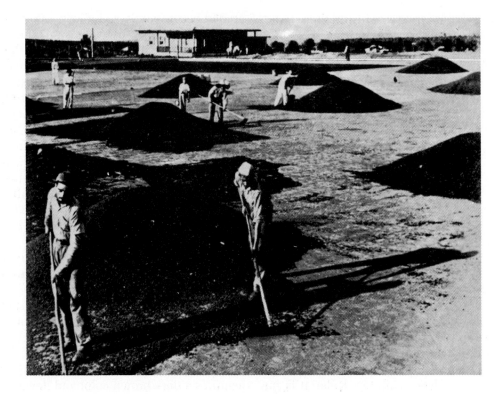

Fig. 8–29. Coffee beans being sun-dried in the state of São Paulo, Brazil. (Photo, courtesy of U.S. Department of Agriculture.)

the wet method in which the sarcocarp is removed by means of a machine, and the 2 seeds with the parchmentlike endocarp are allowed to dry in such a manner as to undergo a fermentation, and after drying, the endocarp is removed (Fig. 8–29). The green seeds are sent into commerce and roasted.

Coffee seeds contain from 1 to 2% of caffeine; about 0.25% of trigonelline (N-methylbetaine of nicotinic acid); from 3 to 5% of tannin; about 15% of glucose and dextrin; 10 to 13% of a fatty oil consisting chiefly of olein and palmitin; and 10 to 13% of proteins. They yield 4 to 7% of total ash, nearly all of which is acid-soluble.

When the coffee is roasted, the seeds swell, change in color to dark brown, and develop the characteristic odor and flavor.

The aroma is caused by an oil known as caffeol, consisting of about 50% furfurol with traces of valerianic acid, phenol, and pyridine. It is produced during the roasting process. At the same time, the caffeine is freed from its combination with chlorogenic acid with which it exists in the unroasted seed. The caffeine may be partially sublimed during this roasting process; much of the caffeine of commerce is collected in condensers attached to coffee roasters.

The action of coffee depends principally on the caffeine, which acts on the central nervous system, the kidneys, the muscles, and the heart. However, chlorogenic acid and caffeol are also physiologically active, and some of the unpleasant side effects connected with coffee consumption, at least in certain persons, have been attributed to these compounds. The usual cup of coffee contains about 100 mg of caffeine, about 1/15 of the estimated maximal daily dose. Although coffee is mainly a dietetic, it is also a stimulant and a diuretic. It is of value in the treatment of poisoning by certain central nervous system depressants.

Decaffeinized coffee is prepared by extracting most of the caffeine from the coffee bean, yet retaining the pleasant characteristic aroma of coffee. Such preparations normally contain up to 0.08% of caffeine. Decaffeinized coffee has an extensive American market and brings a higher price than the ordinary roasted coffee.

Guarana is a dried paste composed chiefly of the crushed seed of *Paullinia cupana* Kunth (Fam. Sapindaceae). The plant is a climbing shrub native to Brazil and Uruguay. The seeds are collected by the Indians and roasted over fires for about half a day; the kernels are ground with water to a pasty mass in crude stone mortars and molded into cylindric sticks that are dried in the sun or over fires.

Guarana enters into the preparation of a stimulating beverage that is used like tea and coffee by the people of Brazil. Guarana was introduced into France from South America in 1817, and caffeine (2.5 to 5%) was discovered as its principal constituent in 1840. The drug also contains 25% of tannin (cathechutannic acid).

In recent times, guarana has been extensively promoted as a stimulating drug. Its action is caused by the caffeine present, but it also possesses astringent properties.

Maté or Paraguay tea consists of the leaves of *Ilex paraguariensis* St. Hil. (Fam. Aquifoliaceae). Maté contains caffeine (up to 2%) and tannin. It is used in large doses as a laxative or purgative; it also has diaphoretic and diuretic properties. It is employed in South America in the preparation of a tealike beverage.

CAFFEINE

Caffeine or 1,3,7-trimethylxanthine occurs in coffee, tea, cacao, guarana, kola and maté. Although caffeine can be produced synthetically, it is usually prepared from tea, tea dust, or tea sweepings, or recovered from coffee roasters. Caffeine is anhydrous or contains one molecule of water of hydration.

Caffeine occurs as a white powder or as white, glistening needles matted together in fleecy masses. It has a bitter taste. Caffeine may be sublimed without decomposition when heated.

The solubility of caffeine in water is markedly increased by the presence of citric acid, benzoates, salicylates, and bromides; medicinal compounds of this class are citrated caffeine and caffeine and

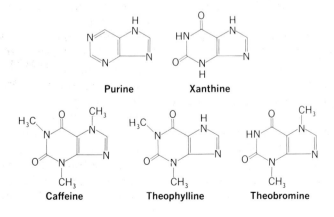

Purine   Xanthine

Caffeine   Theophylline   Theobromine

sodium benzoate. The latter is most suitable for intramuscular injection.

USE AND DOSE. Caffeine and its related compounds are central stimulants. Usual dose of caffeine is 200 mg, of citrated caffeine, 300 mg, of caffeine and sodium benzoate injection, parenterally, 500 mg.

PRESCRIPTION SPECIALTIES. Caffeine is an ingredient in a number of products, including: Empirin® Compound, Fiorinal®, Cafergot®, Wigraine®. In all of these drugs, it is combined with other therapeutic agents.

THEOPHYLLINE

Thea or tea consists of the prepared leaves and leaf buds of *Camellia sinensis* (Linné) O. Kuntze (Fam. Theaceae), a shrub or tree with alternate, evergreen leaves. The tea tree is indigenous to eastern Asia and is now extensively cultivated in China, Japan, India, and Indonesia. The generic name is Greek and means goddess; *sinensis* refers to its Chinese origin.

Green tea is prepared in China and Japan by rapidly drying the freshly picked leaves in copper pans over a mild artificial heat. The leaves are often rolled in the palm of the hand as they dry.

Black tea is prepared in Sri Lanka and India by heaping the fresh leaves until fermentation has begun. They are then rapidly dried artificially with heat.

Tea occurs as more or less crumpled, bright green or blackish green masses. Its odor is agreeable and aromatic; its taste is pleasantly astringent and bitter.

Tea contains 1 to 4% of caffeine (theine) and small amounts of adenine, theobromine, theophylline, and xanthine; about 15% of gallotannic acid; and about 0.75% of a yellow volatile oil that is solid at ordinary temperatures and has a strongly aromatic odor and taste.

The stimulating action of tea is essentially that of the contained caffeine; its astringent properties are owing to the tannin content. It is used mainly as a beverage, containing about 30 to 60 mg of caffeine in a normal cup. Tea leaf waste and tea dust represent important sources for the extraction of caffeine.

Theophylline or 1,3-dimethylxanthine is isomeric with theobromine and was first isolated from tea in 1885. It is prepared synthetically from caffeine or by other means. Theophylline occurs as a white, odorless, bitter cystalline powder that is soluble in about 120 parts of water. It is rendered more soluble when combined with basic compounds. Aminophylline or theophylline ethylenediamine, theophylline monoethanolamine, choline theophyllinate, and theophylline sodium glycinate are commonly employed in medicine.

USES AND DOSE. Theophylline and related compounds are utilized principally as smooth muscle relaxants. In addition, theophylline possesses diuretic properties. Usual dose of theophylline is, orally, the equivalent of 2.4 mg of anhydrous theophylline per kg of body weight every 6 hours initially, adjusted as necessary to control symptoms with a usual optimal dosage of 4.8 mg per kg of body weight every 6 hours. Usual dose of aminophylline is, orally, 3 mg per kg of body weight every 6 hours adjusted as necessary to an optimal dosage of 6 mg per kg every 6 hours and, intravenously, 250 to 500 mg every 6 hours.

Aminophylline is also a valuable diuretic. It exhibits dilating action on the pulmonary vessels in relieving asthma and can lower venous pressure in certain cases of heart failure.

PRESCRIPTION PRODUCTS. Theophylline: Bronkodyl®, Theophyl®, Theospan®, Theolair®, Accurbron®, Sustaire®; Aminophylline: Mini-Lix®, Lixaminol®, Somophyllin®, Phyllocontin®; Theophylline Monoethanolamine: Fleet Brand

Theophylline®; Theophylline Sodium Glycinate: Glynazan®, Synophylate®, Theofort®; Choline Theophyllinate: Choledyl®. Amesec® and Amodrine® contain aminophylline in combination; Tedral® and Bronkotabs® contain theophylline.

THEOBROMINE

Theobromine or 3,7-dimethylxanthine is a compound prepared from the dried, ripe seed of Theobroma cacao Linné (Fam. Sterculiaceae), or is made synthetically. It occurs as a white, crystalline powder with a bitter taste and sublimes at about 260° C.

The base is slightly soluble in cold water or in alcohol, but is readily soluble when mixed with salts that form basic solutions, such as calcium salicylate, sodium acetate, or sodium salicylate.

USES AND DOSE. Theobromine is a diuretic and a smooth muscle relaxant. It has little simulant action on the central nervous system and hence is preferred over caffeine in cardiac edema and in angina pectoris. The usual dose is 200 mg, 3 times daily.

PRESCRIPTION PRODUCTS. Athemol® contains theobromine magnesium oleate.

READING REFERENCES

Bové, F. J.: The Story of Ergot, Basel, S. Karger AG, 1970.

Dalton, D. R.: The Alkaloids, New York, Marcel Dekker, Inc., 1979.

Emboden, W.: Narcotic Plants (revised and enlarged), New York, MacMillan Publishing Co., Inc., 1979.

Fell, K. R., and Ramsden, D.: Colchicum: A Review of Colchicums and the Sources, Chemistry, Biogenesis and Assay of Colchicine and its Congeners, Lloydia 30(2):123, 1967.

Floss, H. G.: Biosynthesis of Ergot Alkaloids and Related Compounds, New York, Pergamon Press Ltd., 1976.

Glasby, J. S.: Encyclopedia of the Alkaloids, Vols. I–III, New York, Plenum Press, 1975 and 1977.

Gröger, D.: Ergot, Microbial Toxins, 8:321, 1972.

Gröger, D.: Ergot Alkaloids—Recent Advances in Chemistry and Biochemistry. In Antibiotics and Other Secondary Metabolites, Hütter, R., Leisinger, T., Nüesch, J., and Wehrli, W., eds., New York, Academic Press, Inc., 1978.

Grundon, M. F., ed.: A Specialist Periodical Report: The Alkaloids, Vols. VI–VIII, London, The Chemical Society, Burlington House, 1976–1978.

Kritikas, P. G., and Papadaki, S. P.: The History of the Poppy and of Opium and Their Expansion in Antiquity in the Eastern Mediterranean Area. Bull. Narcotics, U.N. Dep. Social Affairs, 19(3):17, 1967 and 19(4):5, 1967.

Luckner, M.: Secondary Metabolism in Plants and Animals, New York, Academic Press, Inc., 1972.

Mann, J.: Secondary Metabolism, Oxford, Oxford University Press, 1978.

Manske, R. H. F., ed.: The Alkaloids, Vols. V–XVI, New York, Academic Press, Inc., 1955–1977.

Manske, R. H. F., and Holmes, H. L., eds.: The Alkaloids, Vols. I–IV, New York, Academic Press, Inc., 1950–1954.

Manske, R. H. F., and Rodrigo, R. G. A., eds.: The Aklaloids, Vol. XVII, New York, Academic Press, Inc., 1979.

Miller, L. P., ed.: Phytochemistry: Organic Metabolites, Vol. II, New York, Van Nostrand Reinhold Co., 1973.

Pelletier, S. W., ed.: Chemistry of the Alkaloids, New York, Van Nostrand Reinhold Co., 1970.

Raffauf, R. F.: A Handbook of Alkaloids and Alkaloid-Containing Plants, New York, John Wiley & Sons, Inc., 1970.

Robinson, T.: The Biochemistry of Alkaloids, New York, Springer-Verlag, Inc., 1968.

Saxton, J. E., ed.: A Specialist Periodical Report: The Alkaloids, Vols. I–V, London, The Chemical Society, Burlington House, 1971–1975.

Schultes, R. E., and Hofmann, A.: The Botany and Chemistry of Hallucinogens, Springfield, Illinois, Charles C Thomas, 1973.

Shamma, M.: The Isoquinoline Alkaloids; Chemistry and Pharmacology, New York, Academic Press, Inc., 1972.

Shamma, M., and Moniot, J. L.: Isoquinoline Alkaloids Research 1972–1977, New York, Plenum Press, 1978.

Taylor, W. I., and Farnsworth, N. R., eds.: The Catharanthus Alkaloids, New York, Marcel Dekker, Inc., 1975.

Thomas, K. B.: Curare: Its History and Usage, Philadelphia, J. B. Lippincott Co., 1964.

Wiesner, K., ed.: MTP International Review of Science: Alkaloids, Organic Chemistry, Series 1, Vol. IX, Baltimore, University Park Press, 1973.

Wiesner, K. F., ed.: *International Review of Science: Alkaloids*, Organic Chemistry, Series 2, Vol. IX, London, Butterworth & Co. (Publishers) Ltd, 1976.

Waller, G. R., and Nowacki, E. K.: *Alkaloid Biology and Metabolism in Plants*, New York, Plenum Press, 1978.

Willaman, J. J., and Schubert, B. G.: *Alkaloid-bearing Plants and Their Contained Alkaloids*, Washington, D. C., Agricultural Research Service, U.S.D.A., Technical Bulletin No. 1234, 1961.

Willaman, J. J., and Li, H.-L.: Alkaloid-bearing Plants and Their Contained Alkaloids, 1957–1968, Lloydia, *33* (3A, supplement):1, 1970.

Chapter 9

Peptide Hormones and the Endocrine System

Hormones are mammalian metabolites that are produced by endocrine or ductless glands, are released directly into the blood, and are involved in eliciting responses by specific body organs and tissues. These biologically active metabolites either are steroidal or are derived from amino acids. The latter group of hormones consists primarily of peptides of various sizes, but a few nonpeptide metabolites (epinephrine, thyroxine) are known. Pertinent details about the nonsteroidal hormones and general aspects of endocrine products used as therapeutic agents will be discussed in this chapter. Specific details about the steroid hormones were presented previously (see page 180).

HISTORIC DEVELOPMENT

Present therapeutic use of endocrine products is an outgrowth of the primitive practice of organotherapy. The use by Magnus in the thirteenth century of pow-

dered hog testis in male impotence and of rabbit uterus in female sterility were direct progenitors of present therapy. The basic philosophy for the use of mammalian organs was ably expressed by Vicary in the sixteenth century when he said, "In what part of the body the faculty you would strengthen lies, take the same part of the body of another creature in whom the faculty is strong, as a medicine."

The origin and early development of endocrine therapy was empiric, but most of the present knowledge of endocrine function and therapy is the result of intensive investigations conducted over the past 30 years. Standardized powdered glands and glandular extracts initially provided more reproducible effects and better therapeutic control than did randomly selected glands, and isolated hormonal substances have offered additional advantages in most cases. Modern technology has permitted the ready synthesis of many hormones, including a number of peptides, and the preparation of substances that mimic the actions of natural hormones (e.g., prednisone-cortisone).

Much of the obvious progress in the endocrine area is reflected in the nature of available products. However, a more precise comprehension of their physiologic functions and improved diagnostic procedures have contributed significantly to therapeutic advancement.

GENERAL PHYSIOLOGIC INVOLVEMENT AND THERAPEUTIC PHILOSOPHIES

Hormones function as chemical transmitters of selective stimuli between the various endocrine glands and specific body organs and tissues. Sufficient information is available to permit some generalizations about the modes by which hormones influence the metabolism of target cells and maintain homeostasis. The size and lipophilic character of steroids permit penetration of cell membranes, but many peptide hormones will not enter cells in the absence of a specialized transport system. The latter hormones, in many cases, bind to receptors on the surface of the cell and act in one of two ways: (1) to induce directly changes in membrane permeability for ions, glucose, amino acids, etc., or (2) to induce the production of a secondary messenger such as cyclic AMP, which transmits the signal of the hormone within the cell. Hormones that control membrane permeability, either directly or indirectly, include the estrogens, growth hormone, glucagon, glucocorticoids, insulin, testosterone, and vasopressin. Induction of enzyme formation and modification in the rate of enzymatic reactions are other known mechanisms of hormonal action.

Physiologic control of hormone formation or release to regulate hormone level is a vital aspect of maintaining metabolic homeostasis and integrity of body function. Two general regulatory mechanisms are currently recognized. There is a feedback mechanism that responds to change in concentration of some substance in the blood. The key substance may be a hormone or some other metabolite. For example, an increase in blood glucose in normal persons stimulates the release of insulin, and increased levels of triiodothyronine-thyroxine cause a decrease in thyrotropin secretion owing to an inhibition of the secretion of thyrotropin-releasing factor by the hypothalamus (see page 181). The second mechanism involves external stimuli and is mediated by the hypothalamus; the hypothalamus secretes releasing factors that act on the anterior pituitary to increase the release of specific tropic hormones.

Some manifestations of hormonally controlled processes are rather subtle, and their significance in the normal individual is usually recognized only by people trained in the health sciences. However, the widely recognized influence of the gonadal hormones on the development and function of the reproductive organs and sex characteristics illustrates the general type of fundamental involvement of hormones.

There is appreciable interaction among the functions of the various endocrine glands and a close correlation between the endocrine system and the central and autonomic nervous systems. Thus, a primary disturbance in an endocrine gland or therapy with a hormone may have far-reaching effects. Caution must be exercised in therapeutic management of such complex situations to avoid dangerous or irrational developments.

Disturbance in the function of an endocrine gland may take the form of excessive activity (hyperfunction) or diminished activity (hypofunction), to any degree. The most frequently encountered therapeutic situations involve the hypofunctioning gland. Replacement therapy merely uses endocrine preparations to supplement or totally replace abnormally low levels of endogenous hormone. Early diagnosis and treatment are essential in this type of therapy to avoid irreversible changes that can occur, such as cretinism, giantism, and other comparable conditions. Use of hormones for replacement purposes is usually long-term therapy, and, because these potent substances are normal body metabolites, serious side effects are usually minimal if caution is taken to balance the administered dosage with replacement needs. Insulin utilization provides a good example of this type of approach to a hypofunctioning endocrine system.

Hypofunctioning glands that retain some degree of activity can potentially be stimulated to approach normal activity by the use of drugs that are not hormones per se or by the inhibition of the normal catabolic processes to conserve the limited supply of hormone. There are many variations to this type of therapeutic approach, but they all require metabolic capability in the glandular tissue and a thorough knowledge of biochemical detail. This general approach will probably become more useful in the future when greater knowledge is available.

Hormonal substances are not employed in treatment of hyperfunctioning endocrine glands. Antimetabolites may offer some potential for eliminating the deleterious effects of abnormally high levels of hormones. Alternate approaches to this kind of problem include surgical removal of part of the hyperfunctioning gland or selective destruction of some of the glandular tissues. Various radiation treatments, including the use of ^{131}I in certain thyroid conditions, represent the latter approach.

Sometimes, hormones have therapeutic utility for pharmacologic actions that are not directly related to normal endocrine functions. The use of glucocorticoids for anti-inflammatory and antirheumatic purposes falls into this category (see page 187). The potential danger of serious side effects is considerably greater when hormones are used for specific pharmacologic actions than when they are used for replacement therapy. Prolonged therapeutic use of a hormone, such as cortisone, may cause irreversible atrophy of the endocrine gland that normally produces the hormone or may induce other undesirable secondary responses. The safest use of a hormone as a therapeutic agent involves a short duration of therapy, e.g., the use of oxytocin to induce labor or to control postpartum hemorrhage. This short-term approach avoids problems associated with prolonged upset of the delicate balance among various endocrine systems.

COMMERCIAL PRODUCTION

Many drugs employed in medical practice and generally classified as endocrine products are by-products of the meat-packing industry. Thyroid, pancreas, adrenal, and pituitary glands of bovine and porcine origin are used for such purposes. The active principles obtained from such glands may vary in quantity and quality, depending on species, so that specific manufacturing processes are developed and used with particular species in mind.

Glands used in the manufacture of pharmaceutic products are collected in government-inspected packinghouses and must conform to the regulations of the Meat Inspection Department of the United States Department of Agriculture. Only glands from carcasses that are classified by federal inspectors as edible may be used.

Endocrine glands are technically fresh meat and must be processed in a manner that prevents deterioration. Glands are normally quick-frozen as soon as they are removed from the animal carcasses and maintained in a frozen state until processed. Processing varies with the nature of the ultimate endocrine product. The glands, in many cases, are subjected to extraction and fractionation treatments to yield purified hormones. However, the continued therapeutic acceptance of desiccated thyroid is a pragmatic reminder that satisfactory results sometimes can be achieved without costly isolation of the active principles. Frozen thyroid gland is simply dehydrated, defatted, powdered, standardized, and made into suitable dosage forms.

Chemical synthesis is a logical approach to insuring the ready availability of adequate supplies of any natural metabolite of known structure and therapeutic utility. The feasibility of synthetic procedures is governed to a large degree by the complexity of the molecule and by the technical knowledge relating to the given type of compound. Hormones present no exception to these generalizations. Perhaps the only unusual feature that is applied commercially in the production of certain hormones involves the action of selected biologic systems on foreign substrates. Various microorganisms metabolize certain steroids to give useful compounds. An indication of the significant contribution of microbial biotransformation of steroids is included in the steroid chapter (see page 185).

The Merrifield solid-phase synthesis of peptides is a technologic development of the 1960s of major significance for endocrine therapy. This technique involves basically attaching a carboxy-terminal amino acid to a resin column and synthesizing a polypeptide by passing a programmed sequence of reacting solutions through the column. There is no need to isolate each intermediate, the process can be automated, and commercially feasible synthesis has already been extended to peptides containing 24 to 32 amino acid residues (cosyntropin and calcitonin, respectively). A number of peptide hormones that were previously isolated from glandular materials are now prepared synthetically, and

the prospects for new developments in the area of peptides with hormonal activity are among the best for any group of therapeutic agents.

ADRENAL GLANDS

The **adrenals** (suprarenals) in man comprise a pair of small glands; one is situated over the superior medial aspect of each kidney. Each average gland measures $5 \times 25 \times 50$ mm; together the adrenals weigh 4 to 18 g.

The adrenals were first described by Eustachius in the sixteenth century and were long supposed to function in the inhibition of fetal urination and in the prevention of renal stones in the adult. Knowledge of adrenal function began with Addison in 1849 and is still far from complete.

Each adrenal consists embryologically, histologically, and functionally of 2 distinct glandular entities that are grossly combined into one organ. Cells of the adrenal cortex secrete steroid hormones, which were discussed previously (see page 185).

The adrenal medulla is composed of cells that migrated out from the embryonic neural crest and are analogous to the peripheral sympathetic neurons of the autonomic nervous system. The adrenal medulla secretes epinephrine and norepinephrine (normally in a ratio approximately 17 : 3) and functions as a sympathetic postganglionic structure.

The adrenal medulla is not essential for life, and no diseases of deficiency are known. Therapeutic use of these hormones is based on the pharmacology of sympathomimetic amines and not on the principle of replacement. Epinephrine elicits vasoconstrictor and vasopressor responses, acting in general as a sympathomimetic agent of rapid onset but brief duration of action. Bronchodilation, resulting from epinephrine's beta-receptor adrenergic activity, is particularly useful in acute asthmatic attacks. The labile catechol function precludes oral administration of epinephrine, which must be administered by subcutaneous or intramuscular injection or absorbed through a mucous membrane.

The catecholamine hormones are metabolically inactivated in several ways. A major pathway involves catechol O-methylation, but oxidative deamination with monoamine oxidase is especially significant owing to the therapeutic use of MAO inhibitors.

Biosynthesis of Epinephrine. From the biosynthetic viewpoint, epinephrine may be considered as an alkaloidal amine of the phenylpropanoid type. Its derivation from tyrosine has been demonstrated experimentally. Tyrosine is oxidized to dihydroxyphenylalanine (dopa), which is decarboxylated and oxidized in the side chain. The norepinephrine thus produced is converted to epinephrine by transfer of a methyl group from active methionine (Fig. 9–1). The rate-limiting step appears to be the conversion of tyrosine to dopa.

Epinephrine is (−)-3,4-dihydroxy-α-[(methylamino)methyl] benzyl alcohol. It may be isolated as a hormone from adrenal medulla or may be prepared synthetically. Dextrorotatory epinephrine is almost completely inactive, and optically inactive mixtures have approximately half the activity of natural epinephrine. The specific rotation of epinephrine is not less than

−50° and not more than −53.5°. Epinephrine occurs as a white to nearly white, microcrystalline, odorless powder that gradually darkens when exposed to light and air.

Prescription Product. Adrenalin®.

Epinephrine is incorporated into a variety of pharmaceutic formulations for therapeutic utilization. The hormone is frequently solubilized in aqueous preparations using hydrochloric acid or tartaric acid (bitartrate), and a water-soluble borate complex is sometimes used in ophthalmology. Acidity favors the stability of this labile compound, but no epinephrine-containing solution should be used if a brown color or a precipitate has formed. Formulations for therapeutic use of this hormone include a 1:1000 aqueous solution for topical purposes, a 1:100 aqueous solution for inhalation, a sterile 1:1000 aqueous solution for parenteral administration, a sterile suspension in oil for prolonged systemic action, and several ophthalmic solutions (1:50 to 1:200) for use in open-angle glaucoma.

Levarterenol or (−)-norepinephrine is (−)-α-(aminomethyl)3,4-dihydroxybenzyl alcohol. It is usually used as the bitartrate salt, which is a white or faintly gray, crystalline powder. It slowly darkens when exposed to air and light. Solutions of this hormone should not be used if they are brown in color or contain a precipitate. Levarterenol is a sympathetic stimulant closely related in chemical structure and

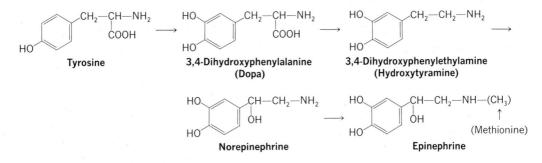

Fig. 9–1. Biosynthesis of epinephrine.

pharmacologic action to epinephrine. Its chief difference in clinical utility lies in its predominantly *alpha*-receptor adrenergic activity. It is a strong peripheral vasoconstrictor and is especially useful in restoration of blood pressure in acute hypotensive situations.

USUAL DOSE. Levarterenol bitartrate is usually administered by intravenous infusion. Usually, the equivalent of 4 mg of levarterenol is placed in 1000 ml of 5% dextrose injection and infused at a rate adjusted to maintain blood pressure.

PRESCRIPTION PRODUCT. Levophed®.

THYROID GLAND

The **thyroid gland** in man consists of 2 lobes that are lateral and inferior to the anterior aspect of the larynx and are connected across the larynx by an isthmus to produce a U-shaped structure averaging 30 g in weight. Galen vaguely described the thyroid in the second century, but its identity as a ductless gland was first described by Holler in 1776. Interestingly, Roger of Palermo used sponges and seaweed, high in iodine content, in the treatment of goiter (thyroid enlargement) in the twelfth century.

Thyroid gland mobilizes dietary iodine, converting it to an organic compound that can accelerate metabolic processes. It is necessary to the development and function of all body cells. The actual molecular form of the thyroid hormone or hormones, exclusive of calcitonin which has a hypocalcemic action that is distinct from the physiologic responses usually associated with this gland, remains unclear. The iodine-containing levorotatory amino acids, thyroxine and triiodothyronine, occur in the gland and are physiologically active upon oral administration. These metabolites also occur in the gland bound with globulin (thyroglobulins), and the exogenously administered amino acids could conceivably bind with serum protein to form physiologically active molecules that are responsible for the ultimate hormonal action. The thyroid gland can store thyroglobulins and other iodometabolites. The release of these thyroid hormones appears to be controlled by thyrotropin, a hormone of the anterior pituitary.

Manifestations of hypothyroidism may be caused by an iodine deficiency and a resulting lack of precursor moieties for the hormonal substances (simple hyperplastic goiter, which is characterized by a compensatory enlargement of the gland), by a deficiency of thyrotropic factors, or by other metabolic irregularities. The first two causes may be corrected by adding iodine to the diet or administering thyrotropin, respectively. Naturally, replacement therapy with thyroid hormones can be used for a deficiency of any origin.

A hypothyroid condition results in some degree of cretinism in infants and of myxedema in adults. Cretinism is characterized by retarded and abnormal growth; arrested sexual development; mental deficiency; thickened, dry skin; thickened tongue; coarsened features; and a fall in the metabolic rate. The features of myxedema include general lethargy; retarded mental processes; increased body fat; susceptibility to cold and fatigue; cardiac dilatation; dry, thickened skin; and coarsened features with a thickened, protruding tongue.

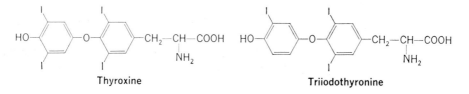

Thyroxine   Triiodothyronine

Thyroid hyperactivity results in thyrotoxicosis characterized by increased heart rate, blood pressure, nervous excitability, and metabolic rate; muscular weakness with tremor; loss of body weight and fat; and an increased tolerance to cold but intolerance to heat. When accompanied by protrusion of the eyeballs (exophthalmos), the condition is known as exophthalmic goiter (Graves' or Basedow's disease). The course is marked by occasional crises or "storms," which may result in abrupt death. These symptoms of thyroid hyperactivity may result from overdosage of thyroid preparations; thus, the rationality of using thyroid preparations in obesity "cures" is questionable. Treatment of organic hyperthyroidism is principally surgical, aided by radioactive iodine and by antimetabolites such as propylthiouracil. Improved manipulation of the latter aids may even supplant surgery in selected cases.

Preparations of thyroid hormones are useful for replacement therapy in cretinism or myxedema. Early diagnosis and treatment are essential in cretinism to avoid irreversible body and mental retardation. These preparations are also employed to prevent myxedema in cases when the thyroid gland must be surgically removed. Preparations from the thyroid gland are sometimes used as pharmacologic agents for their influence on various metabolic processes, but the success of such therapy is difficult to predict.

The responses elicited by exogenous thyroxine and triiodothyronine differ quantitatively. Triiodothyronine exhibits a more rapid onset and a shorter duration of action. This difference appears to be related to the extent of ionization of the 4'-phenolic group in the respective substances at physiologic pH. Thyroxine is approximately 90% ionized and is predominantly protein bound in the blood. The reversible binding to plasma proteins is apparently electrostatic, and the strength of the bond varies among the different plasma proteins. Drugs such as salicylates and diphenylhydantoin disrupt the weaker bonds (potential drug-drug interaction) to increase the physiologic impact of thyroid hormones.

Relative binding and biopharmaceutic properties of thyroxine and triiodothyronine are also illustrated by their normal serum levels. The normal human serum levels of triiodothyronine range from 60 to 160 ng per ml, but the concentration of thyroxine is approximately 60 times higher.

Biosynthesis of Thyroid Hormone. The reactions leading to thyroxine formation in the thyroid gland are still incompletely understood. The first step in the biosynthesis is a peroxidation of iodide to "active iodine," which then reacts with tyrosine to first form 3-monoiodotyrosine and subsequently 3,5-diiodotyrosine. Two molecules of the latter compound react to form thyroxine. Alternatively, a molecule of the diiodotyrosine may react with a molecule of monoiodotyrosine to form triiodothyronine, which is then iodinated to yield thyroxine (Fig. 9–2). Some evidence shows that thyrotropin exerts an influence on the condensation of 2 molecules of the iodoamino acids to yield either thyroxine or triiodothyronine, and some degree of reversibility has been noted

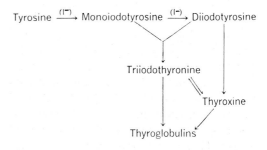

Fig. 9–2. Biosynthesis of thyroid hormones.

for the biosynthetic conversion of triiodothyronine to thyroxine. Triiodothyronine is the most active of the known thyroid metabolites, but the significance of its metabolic relationship with thyroxine relative to biologic control processes is unclear.

Deiodination in various body tissues is the major catabolic pathway for thyroxine and triiodothyronine. However, other metabolic pathways are known, including deamination and oxidation in the kidney to form acetic acid analogs and conjugation in the liver followed by biliary excretion. Some differences have been detected in the latter pathway. The β-glucuronide is the major conjugation product of thyroxine, but the sulfate ester is more common for triiodothyronine. None of the catabolic pathways is especially rapid, and manipulation of these processes offers no significant potential for achievement of therapeutic objectives.

Thyroid is the cleaned, dried, and powdered thyroid gland previously deprived of connective tissue and fat. It is obtained from domesticated animals that are used for food by man. Thyroid contains not less than 0.17% and not more than 0.23% of iodine in thyroid combination and is free from iodine in inorganic or any form of combination other than that peculiar to the thyroid gland. A desiccated thyroid of a higher iodine content may be brought to this standard by admixture with a desiccated thyroid of a lower iodine content or with lactose, sodium chloride, starch, or sucrose.

USE AND DOSE. Thyroid is effective in oral therapy. Usual dose is 15 to 180 mg daily. The effect of a single dose of thyroid orally, or of thyroxine orally or intravenously, is not manifest for some 24 to 48 hours; it reaches a maximum in 8 to 10 days and decreases slowly over a period of several weeks. Hence, accumulation may occur,

and dosage schedules must be adjusted individually to the needs of the patient.

PRESCRIPTION PRODUCTS. Thermoloid®, Thyrar®, Thyro-Teric®, Thyrocrine®, Tuloidin®.

Thyroglobulin is obtained by fractionation of porcine thyroid gland. It contains not less than 0.7% of organically bound iodine, and the ratio of thyroxine and triiodothyronine is approximately 5:2. The source is restricted to Sus scrofa Linné var. domesticus Gray (Fam. Suidae) because the hog accumulates especially high levels of the thyroid hormones and has a higher proportion of triiodothyronine.

USE AND DOSE. Thyroglobulin is used in essentially the same manner as thyroid. The usual daily dose is 16 to 200 mg.

PRESCRIPTION PRODUCT. Proloid®.

Sodium levothyroxine is the sodium salt of the levo isomer of thyroxine, an active physiologic principle obtained from the thyroid gland of domesticated animals used for food by man. It can also be prepared synthetically. It contains not less than 61.6% and not more than 65.5% of iodine.

USES AND DOSE. Sodium levothyroxine is classed as a thyroid hormone. It is used for replacement therapy of reduced or completely absent thyroid function (manifested as myxedema, cretinism, and mild forms of hypothyroidism). It may be valuable in cases of sterility or habitual abortion, chronic arthritis, vascular disturbances of the extremities, skin lesions associated with dryness, and certain other conditions. Usual dose is 25 to 300 μg once a day.

PRESCRIPTION PRODUCTS. Levoid®, Levothroid®, Noroxine®, Synthroid®.

Sodium liothyronine is the sodium salt of the levorotatory isomer of 3,3',5-triiodothyronine. This physiologically active compound is a naturally occurring thyroid hormone, but quantities needed for commercial purposes are provided by chemical synthesis. It contains not less than 53.7% and not more than 57.1% of iodine.

USE AND DOSE. Sodium liothyronine is used for the same purposes as is sodium levothyroxine. Some evidence shows that sodium liothyronine is more readily absorbed upon oral administration than are other thyroid preparations. The usual dose is the equivalent of 5 to 100 μg of liothyronine, once a day.

PRESCRIPTION PRODUCTS. Cytomel®, Cytomine®.

Liotrix is a 4:1 mixture of synthetic sodium levothyroxine and sodium liothyronine. The effects of this mixture are claimed to resemble closely those of endogenous thyroid secretion and to give laboratory protein-bound-iodine test results that are more consistent with clinical response than are the results obtained with other preparations.

PRESCRIPTION PRODUCTS. Euthyroid®, Thyrolar®.

Consensus equivalents for comparison of the various thyroid preparations, based on 65 mg (1 gr) of thyroid are: thyroglobulin, 65 mg; sodium levothyroxine, 100 μg; sodium liothyronine, 25 μg; and liotrix formulation, 50 μg of lexothyroxine and 12.5 μg of liothyronine.

Sodium dextrothyroxine is the salt of the synthetically prepared dextrorotatory isomer of thyroxine. This substance is effective in high dose (up to 8 mg daily) for the treatment of hypothyroidism, but its use for such purposes is usually restricted to patients with cardiac disease who cannot tolerate other thyroid medications.

Dextrothyroxine also reduces β-lipoproteins, and it has been classed as a hypocholesteremic agent. Its greatest therapeutic utility may be in this area, but patients must be monitored carefully for ischemic myocardial changes and other adverse reactions. The hypocholesteremic dosage regimen starts with 1 mg daily for a month; the dosage is increased in 1-mg increments at intervals no shorter than 1 month until a satisfactory lowering of β-lipoprotein has been achieved or until a maximum daily dose of 8 mg is reached.

PRESCRIPTION PRODUCT. Choloxin®.

PITUITARY

The human **pituitary gland or hypophysis** is situated in a small cavity in the sphenoid bone at the base of the skull and is attached to the base of the brain by a short stalk. It weighs about 0.5 g. Galen considered it as a strainer for spinal fluid, and Vesalius later thought it was the source of mucus, lubricating the nasopharynx. Pituitary is from the Latin *pituita,* meaning slime or mucus.

The pituitary body is in reality 2 glands by origin and function:

1. The anterior lobe is ectodermal in origin—derived from an outpouching from the primitive pharynx.

2. The posterior lobe is neural in origin—derived from an outpouching of the base of the brain.

POSTERIOR PITUITARY

Extracts of **posterior pituitary** lobe exhibit the following effects in experimental animals and in man:

1. A pressor effect, owing to arteriolar and capillary vasoconstriction;

2. Direct stimulation of smooth muscle, seen in the intact animal or in preparations of isolated muscles;

3. An antidiuretic action, effected by increasing the tubular and collecting duct resorption of water in the kidney.

The diversity of these effects complicated attempts at therapeutic utilization of unfractionated extracts of the posterior pituitary, and the use of such preparations has been largely superseded by the use of oxytocin (ocytocin) or vasopressin, the 2 hormonal substances that have been isolated from this gland. However, these 2 hormones do not appear to provide a clear-cut separation of the physiologic properties associated with the secretions of the gland. The 2 hormones are closely related octapeptides (Fig. 9–3) with 5 of the amino acid residues in a cyclic structure involving a labile cystine moiety. These similar cyclopeptides are difficult to separate quantitatively, and part of the lack of definitive pharmacologic responses using the hormones isolated from nature has been correctly attributed to impurities. This problem is eliminated when the hormones are prepared synthetically, but their actions, especially those of vasopressin, still show a surprising degree of overlap.

Oxytocin (α-hypophamine) is the uterine-stimulating fraction, and it is relatively free from action on other smooth muscle. It is especially active on the pregnant uterus, which has been sensitized by estrogens. Oxytocin appears to increase the permeability of uterine cell membranes to sodium ion with an effective augmentation of the contracting myofibrils. Some

physiologic involvement by oxytocin in the normal onset of labor is suspected, but further scientific clarification is needed.

Vasopressin (β-hypophamine) is the antidiuretic principle; the pressor effects of this hormone are observed only when large quantities are administered. Vasopressin regulates the threshold for resorption of water by the epithelium of the renal tubules. The hormone is released into the blood when osmoreceptors in the hypothalamic nuclei detect an increased extracellular electrolyte concentration in the serum or a decreased blood volume. The resulting fluid conservation contributes to maintenance of homeostasis.

No clinical conditions have yet been associated with hyperfunction of posterior pituitary. A deficiency state is seen only in the condition of diabetes insipidus, which follows a deficiency of the antidiuretic principle. The increased urine output when drinking is caused physiologically, in part, by a temporary deficiency state because alcohol inhibits the release of vasopressin.

Diabetes insipidus (literally an outpouring of tasteless urine) is characterized by a failure of renal resorption of water—there is a tremendous diuresis and associated

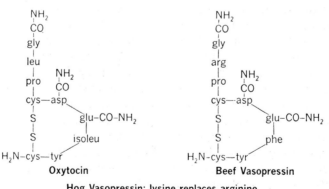

Oxytocin

Beef Vasopressin

Hog Vasopressin: lysine replaces arginine

Fig. 9–3. Structures of oxytocin and vasopressin.

tremendous thirst and water intake. This condition must not be confused with the diabetes mellitus of insulin deficiency.

The biologic half-lives of oxytocin and vasopressin are short, a factor that can be considered an advantage or a disadvantage, depending on therapeutic objectives. Vasopressin is employed in replacement therapy for the management of diabetes insipidus, and one of the concerns in formulation is a need for an increase in the duration of action. Oxytocin is used as a pharmacologic agent for its oxytocic properties, and thus the desired duration of therapy is short.

The relatively small size of these polypeptides provided a focusing point for initial studies on chemical synthesis and structure-activity comparisons that undoubtedly have implications for all physiologically active polypeptides. No prepared analogs, with one possible exception, have been superior in therapeutic properties to the 2 naturally occurring hormones, and most changes in the molecules result in a loss of activity. The one practical development of these studies to date is the commercially feasible synthesis of oxytocin, vasopressin, and related analogs.

The posterior pituitary hormones, oxytocin and vasopressin, are standardized biologically; oxytocin by using chickens or the isolated uterus of nulliparous guinea pigs and vasopressin by using rats. The potency is expressed in arbitrary assay units based on a Posterior Pituitary Reference Standard.

Vasopressin injection is a sterile solution in water for injection of the water-soluble, pressor principle prepared by synthesis or obtained from the posterior lobe of the pituitary. Either 8-L-arginine-vasopressin (argipressin or beef vasopressin) or 8-L-lysine-vasopressin (lypressin or hog vasopressin) meets monographic require-ments, but the slightly more stable lysine-vasopressin is used more commonly.

Vasopressin injection is standardized so that 1 ml possesses a pressor activity equivalent to 20 USP posterior pituitary units. It is used to control neurohypophyseal diabetes insipidus, but is ineffective in the nephrogenic form of the disease. Usual dose, intramuscularly or subcutaneously, is 5 to 10 units, 2 to 4 times a day.

ANALOGOUS PRODUCT. Pitressin®.

The dosage of vasopressin must be adjusted to the needs of the individual patient, but convenient therapy is handicapped to a degree by the relatively rapid inactivation of the hormone in the body. The need to administer 5 to 10 USP units of vasopressin (vasopressin injection), 2 to 4 times daily, is common. Formulation of vasopressin tannate in peanut oil (Pitressin® Tannate) was developed to give a gradual release of the hormone and a longer duration of action; an intramuscular injection of 2.5 to 5 USP units of this preparation may exert the desired action for 48 to 96 hours. Formulations of lypressin (Diapid®) and desmopressin (DDAVP®) are also available for intranasal administration; desmopressin or 1-deamino-8-D-arginine-vasopressin is a synthetic analog that reportedly possesses only a small fraction (1/2000) of the undesirable pressor effect of argipressin and has a long duration of action.

Oxytocin injection is a sterile solution in water for injection of an oxytocic principle prepared by synthesis or obtained from the posterior lobe of the pituitary. Each milliliter possesses an oxytocic activity equivalent to 10 USP posterior pituitary units. Oxytocin is used for induction of labor based on medical indications, but the risk-benefit ratio suggests that its use for elective induction is inappropriate. It can also be used to control postpartum hemorrhage.

The dosage for induction of labor is determined by uterine response; the intravenous infusion is started at a rate of 0.001 to 0.002 units per minute. The dose is increased in similar increments until a contraction pattern that resembles normal labor has been established. The dosage for control of postpartum hemorrhage is 3 to 10 units intramuscularly after delivery of the placenta.

ANALOGOUS PRODUCTS. Pitocin®, Syntocinon®.

An oxytocin nasal spray has been formulated to promote milk ejection in the infrequent occasions when this is a problem in breast feeding.

ANTERIOR PITUITARY

The anterior lobe of the pituitary exerts a profound influence on the growth and development of the body and on its sex characteristics through its stimulating actions on the other endocrine glands. **Anterior pituitary** has been referred to as the "master gland," the "conductor of the endocrine symphony." Primary disturbances in anterior pituitary function may result in widespread endocrine involvement and generalized secondary disturbances. Therapy in such complex situations is far from simple and is associated with unusual potential for undesirable side effects. Effective therapeutic utilization of the hormones of the anterior pituitary is still in an early stage of development.

Hormones with adrenocorticotropic, gonadotropic, and thyrotropic activities are used for therapeutic or diagnostic purposes as is growth hormone (somatropin). Another hormone recognized as originating in the anterior pituitary is prolactin. All of these hormones are glycoproteins or proteins, and they tend to be produced and accumulated in small quantities. Available evidence indicates that, with the exception of adrenocorticotropin, their molecular weights are in the 20,000 to 40,000 range,

considerable interrelationships exist among subunits of the various hormonal substances, and labile disulfide bonds occur in these hormones. These factors contribute to the difficulty in securing concentrated, purified extracts with only a single hormonal activity. Technical barriers to the feasible synthesis of such molecules have further limited the medicinal utilization of the anterior pituitary hormones. They appear to have short biologic half-lives (less than 30 minutes), but preliminary evidence suggests that the length of half-life may vary with the pathologic status.

The gonadotropic hormones present several interesting features. At least 2 gonadotropic hormones are excreted by the anterior pituitary; these hormones elicit distinct responses in females and males, and glycoproteins with similar activities are produced by the chorionic villi of the placenta. The follicle-stimulating hormone (FSH or follitropin) is necessary for maturation of the ovarian follicles in females and for maturation of the seminiferous tubules of the testes in males. Luteinizing hormone (LH or lutropin) or interstitial cell-stimulating hormone is essential for causing ovulation and for the development and maintenance of the corpus luteum in the ovary. In the male, LH is apparently active in the development of the Leydig cells of the testes.

Feedback, hypothalamic, and perhaps other mechanisms stimulate the secretion of the tropic hormones of the anterior pituitary. Hypothalamic releasing factors have received considerable attention recently, and a tripeptide and a decapeptide from the hypothalamus have been shown to cause the release of thyrotropin and gonadotropins, respectively. The latter factor appears to lack specificity and to initiate the release of both FSH and LH. The potential for administration of releasing factors of small molecular size is obvious, but problems with variable response precludes therapeutic application at the current stage of knowledge. The first implication of a releasing factor to achieve therapeutic utility may involve inhibition. Prolactin facilitates development of breast cancer, and the inhibition of prolactin release holds clinical promise. Thyrotropin releasing factor is used for diagnostic purposes.

Adrenocorticotropin, ACTH, or corticotropin is a straight-chain polypeptide containing 39 amino acid residues. A portion of the peptide molecule with 20 amino acid residues has the full biologic activity of this hormone. Corticotropin injection is a sterile preparation of the principle or principles that are derived from the anterior lobe of the pituitary of mammals used for food by man and that exert a tropic influence on the adrenal cortex. Its tropic effects involve primarily glucocorticoids. Corticotropin may be used in collagen diseases, particularly in rheumatoid arthritis and acute rheumatic fever, when the adrenal cortex is functional; it avoids the glucocorticoid-associated problem of atrophy of the adrenal cortex. Usual dose, intramuscularly, is 20 USP units, 4 times a day. It can be administered by intravenous infusion if a rapid response is desired; however, this situation is uncommon because the most frequent objection to the use of corticotropin injection is the short duration of action.

PRESCRIPTION SPECIALTY. Acthar®.

Repository corticotropin injection is corticotropin in a solution of partially hydrolyzed gelatin (Cortigel®, Cortrophin® Gel, Cotropic® Gel, H P Acthar® Gel). This formulation has a prolonged therapeutic effect; its usual intramuscular dose is 40 USP units, once daily. A similar, prolonged duration of action is obtained with a suspension prepared by adsorbing corticotropin on zinc hydroxide (Cortrophin® Zinc).

A pseudomonas polysaccharide (Piromen®) stimulates the pituitary gland to release endogenous ACTH. This endocrine stimulant is used parenterally as an adjuvant in some allergic and dermatologic conditions.

Cosyntropin (Cortrosyn®) is a synthetically prepared peptide subunit of corticotropin and is used as a diagnostic aid in suspected adrenal insufficiency. It contains 24 amino acid residues and presents a lesser risk of allergenic reactions than the natural hormone.

Chorionic gonadotropin (HCG or choriogonadotropin) is a mixture of the gonadotropic principles and is obtained from the urine of pregnant women. This anterior-pituitarylike substance resembles LH in its response and is used as replacement therapy to stimulate descent of the testes in cryptorchidism and to stimulate the development of interstitial cells of the testes in delayed adolescence and hypogonadotropic eunuchoidism. The major indication for withdrawal of therapy or reduction of dosage is sexual precociousness. Other degenerative side effects may be noted in females; hence, chorionic gonadotropin is infrequently used in females although it can be used effectively to maintain the functional integrity of the corpus luteum in some cases of habitual abortion. HCG has been used in weight-loss clinics, but its effectiveness in adjunct therapy for the treatment of obesity has not been demonstrated.

Chorionic gonadotropin is a relatively labile glycoprotein that contains about 12% of galactose. It must be administered parenterally and is formulated in a dry mixture with suitable diluents and buffers to give greater shelf life. Usual dose, intramuscularly, is 500 to 5000 USP units, 3 times a week.

PRESCRIPTION SPECIALTIES. Android-HCG®, Antuitrin S®, A. P. L. Secules®, Chorex®, Follutein®, Glukor®, Gonadex®, Libigen®, Pregnyl®, Stemutrolin®.

Menotropins or urogonadotropin is a purified preparation of gonadotropins obtained from the urine of postmenopausal women. The urine gonadotropin levels are high in such women because atrophic ovaries cannot respond to tropic stimulation, thus precluding feedback suppression. The preparation contains approximately equal amounts of FSH and LH. It is used to enhance fertility in anovulatory women with functional ovaries. The usual dosage regimen involves intramuscular injection of 75 International units each of FSH and LH daily for 9 to 12 days to stimulate follicular growth and maturation. One day after the last menotropins injection, 10,000 units of HCG is administered to simulate a preovulatory LH surge and to induce ovulation.

PRESCRIPTION SPECIALTY. Pergonal®.

Somatropin, somatotropin or growth hormone influences a number of essential growth processes. It stimulates linear growth of bones during development, and its anabolic effects include an increased intracellular transport of amino acids and a net body retention of nitrogen, phosphorus, and potassium. Hypofunction of the growth-stimulating activity in children results in the pituitary dwarf; in adults, such deficiency often produces an increased delicacy of structure, referred to as acromicria.

Growth hormones from various animal sources appear to be more species specific in their activity than do most other hormones. Human pituitary growth hormone contains 190 amino acid residues and 2 disulfide bonds. Although lack of a feasible natural source or a feasible synthetic procedure for this pituitary hormone precluded consideration of therapeutic use for many years, the recent discovery of a human chorionic analog circumvented these logistic barriers.

Somatropin is used to stimulate linear growth in patients with documented pituitary growth hormone deficiency. It is not indicated for use in patients with closed epiphyses. Many interactions, including influences of hormones of the adrenal cortex, gonads, parathyroid, and thyroid, contribute to growth. Therapy with somatropin must be monitored carefully. Use of this hormone is restricted to physicians experienced in the diagnosis and management of patients with pituitary growth hormone deficiency.

The usual dosage regimen of somatropin is 2 International units, intramuscularly, 3 times a week (a minimum of 48 hours between injections) for as long as growth continues. Treatment should be discontinued when the patient has reached a satisfactory adult height, when the epiphyses have fused, or when response to the therapy is no longer satisfactory. Five percent of the patients can be expected to develop neutralizing antibodies and to fail to respond to the hormone.

PRESCRIPTION PRODUCT. Ascellacrin®.

Thyrotropin is the thyrotropic principle of the anterior pituitary. It is obtained from bovine glands and is purified to remove significant amounts of corticotropic, gonadotropic, and other hormones. It can be used in replacement therapy, but it is used primarily as a diagnostic aid in evaluating thyroid function, including distinction between primary and secondary hypothyroidism, or as supportive therapy to facilitate the uptake of ^{131}I in treatment of toxic goiter or thyroid carcinoma. Thyrotropin is available as a lyophilized powder and is administered intramuscularly or subcutaneously, usually in daily doses of 10 International units.

PRESCRIPTION SPECIALTY. Thytropar®.

Protirelin is the synthetic tripeptide, L-pyroglutamyl - L-histidyl-L-prolinamide. Identical to the thyrotropin-releasing factor from the hypothalamus, it is used diagnostically to assist in distinguishing secondary and tertiary hypothyroidism. The usual adult dose is 200 to 500 μg intravenously.

PRESCRIPTION PRODUCT. Thypinone®.

PANCREAS

The bulk of the **pancreas** is an exocrine gland that supplies digestive enzymes to the duodenum. Isolated groups of cells, the islets of Langerhans comprising about 3% of the gland, produce the hormonal substances. **Glucagon** is produced by the α-cells, and **insulin** is formed by the β-cells. Glucagon and insulin are both polypeptide hormones, and they exert counterbalancing actions on carbohydrate metabolism in the body.

Glucagon elicits a hyperglycemic response by increasing adenyl cyclase which, in turn, increases liver phosphorylase activity, a key factor in glycogenolysis. The hypoglycemic action of insulin appears to involve glucokinase, membrane transport, and perhaps other factors associated with normal metabolism of blood glucose. In the normal individual, these hormones function to maintain blood glucose within a physiologically tolerated balance by increasing or decreasing, respectively, the glucose level.

Pathologic conditions related to a deficiency in glucagon formation either do not occur, have an insufficient survival factor to create a medical problem, or are unrecognized. The typical case of a hypofunctioning pancreas gland results in insulin deficiency and the condition known as diabetes mellitus. This condition was described by Auretaeus in the first century A.D. as a siphoning of flesh into urine; it is characterized by a high blood-glucose level (hyperglycemia), excess glucose in the urine (glucosuria), and diuresis, resulting in dehydration and constipation. The primary impairment of glucose metabolism induces a number of secondary metabolic changes. Accumulation in the blood of such metabolites as β-hydroxybutyric acid, ketone bodies, and other breakdown products of fats is common. The untreated diabetic, as a result of such metabolic irregularities, suffers from severe acidosis, depression, coma, and ultimately death.

Treatment of diabetes mellitus with insulin is replacement therapy. Insulin prolongs life in the diabetic and permits a fuller and happier life, but its use does not cure or prevent the pathologic condition. Insulin is especially valuable in preventing the complications of diabetes that are frequently the cause of death: arteriosclerosis with hypertension, nephritis, superficial ulcers and infections, gangrene of the extremities, and gallstones.

Conditions of hyperinsulinism may result from overdosage of insulin, underfeeding, tumors of the pancreas, or certain pituitary or adrenal disturbances. Outstanding symptoms are fatigue, hunger, marked sweating, and convulsions.

In management of diabetes mellitus caused by insulin deficiency, an adequate diet is determined, and the amount and spacing of insulin dosage is established to keep the patient symptom-free and free from glucosuria. The plasma half-life of insulin is approximately 10 minutes; therefore, continuous delivery of the hormone is needed in replacement therapy. This is accomplished by subcutaneous administration of a suspension that is formulated to provide slow release of the insulin. Insulin is a potent drug, and the therapeutic considerations are relatively complex and sophisticated. Dosage must be coordinated with dietary intake, and a regularized eating schedule is necessary to accommodate the programmed delivery of insulin and to avoid drug-induced hypoglycemia. The over-the-counter status of insulin, compared to other drugs, is inconsistent with the inherent complexity and risks of the therapy, but it is indicative of what can be achieved by concerted patient education programs.

One USP unit of insulin can cause the metabolism of approximately 1.5 g of glucose. Occasionally, insulin resistance or tolerance develops, and abnormally large doses of insulin are required to control diabetes. The resistance appears to involve antibody binding to restrict the biologic availability of much of the administered hormone; a high potency insulin (500 units per ml) is available for such cases. The objective of high doses in resistant cases is distinct from such uses in treating schizophrenic states. An insulin overdose in the latter situation is used to induce therapeutically convulsive (hypoglycemic) shock.

Glucagon can be used in the diagnosis of glycogen storage diseases and in the treatment of hypoglycemia associated with improper management of diabetes mellitus or with psychiatrically induced insulin shock. Intravenous administration of glucose can also be used to treat hypoglycemia, but glucagon is more convenient to use with unconscious or uncooperative nonhospitalized patients.

Glucagon is a straight-chained polypeptide containing 29 amino acid residues with a molecular weight of 3485. The amino acid sequence has been determined. The isoelectric point of the hormone is between 7.5 and 8.5. It is soluble in acids and bases, below 3.0 and above 9.5, respectively; these solutions are relatively stable. The alkali stability of glucagon can be used for the selective inactivation of insulin, which is a labile cystine-containing contaminant that is difficult to remove quantitatively in the isolation of this hormone.

Insulin is a polypeptide with a molecular weight of 5734. It contains 48 amino acid residues (including 3 cystine residues) that are arranged in 2 linear chains connected by disulfide linkages. Insulin tends to form dimeric and hexameric forms, a characteristic that resulted in an initial estimate of about 35,000 for the molecular weight of the hormone. This hormone has been studied more extensively than any other polypeptide hormone. One of the interesting observations resulting from these studies is the variation in amino acid residues 8, 9, and 10, depending on the origin of the insulin (Fig. 9–4). The amino acid sequence in these 3 positions has no effect on the normal physiologic properties of the polypeptide. It is always possible that variations in this portion of the molecule could cause an antigenic reaction, and this is the basis for selecting all porcine insulin in cases of suspected insulin hypersensitivity or tolerance. However, most of the early cases of hypersensitivity to insulin preparations can be explained by other foreign proteins that were present in the formulations. The distinctive amino acid residue 30 of the larger peptide chain of human insulin is apparently without physiologic significance because an analog lacking amino acid residues 26 to 30 retains activity.

The disulfide bonds that link the 2 peptide chains are major obstacles to the feasible synthesis of insulin, and the biosynthetic accomplishment of this feat has intrigued scientists. The recent elucidation of proinsulin has clarified significantly the biologic formation of the hormone. Proinsulin is a straight-chain polypeptide containing some 80 amino acid residues and all of the disulfide linkages inherent to insulin. The polypeptide sequences at the amino terminal and carboxylic acid terminal ends of the proinsulin molecule correspond to the 2 chains of insulin, and a proteolytic enzyme in the pancreas apparently cleaves peptide bonds to remove the connecting polypeptide sequence and to form the physiologically active, 2-chained insulin.

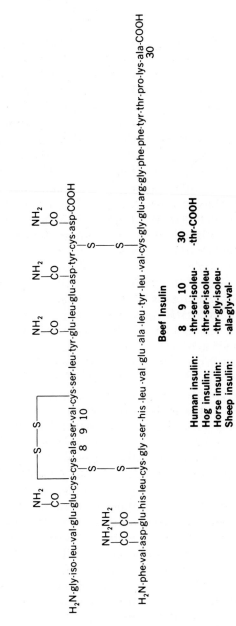

Fig. 9—4. Structures of insulin from several mammals.

Insulin was crystallized in 1926 by the addition of traces of zinc, and crystals of zinc insulin formed the original reference standard of the USP. The isoelectric point of zinc insulin is 5.1 to 5.3. Thus, it is soluble at the alkaline pH of tissue fluids and is rapidly absorbed from subcutaneous injection sites. Insulin is digested by proteolytic enzymes (a common property of polypeptide hormones), and it is ineffective when given orally.

The production of both glucagon and insulin involves isolation of these substances from pancreas glands. The procedures are relatively complex, a situation that is common for the isolation and purification of most peptide molecules. At least 20 major steps are accomplished before a form of insulin suitable for human use is finally developed. Immediately following their removal from slaughtered animals, the raw beef and pork pancreases are frozen to prevent enzymatic destruction of the insulin in the gland. About 8000 pounds of animal pancreases are needed to yield 1 pound of pure zinc insulin crystals.

The first step in actual production involves grinding of the frozen glands. Successive steps include extracting the still-frozen powder with acidic alcohol to obtain the insulin and to suppress enzyme activity, centrifuging the crude extract to separate the liquid from the glandular residue, clarifying the liquid extract containing the insulin and impurities, evaporating in vacuum to remove the alcohol, treating the concentrate to separate the fat, filtering to remove residual fat, adding salt water to precipitate the insulin, redissolving the precipitate, reprecipitating by isoelectric means, buffering to obtain a uniformly soluble product, washing, drying, and pooling the insulin obtained from other lots prepared in the same manner, and finally, determining the potency. Insulin prepared in this manner may be subjected to further purification by ion-exchange chromatography to yield a purified insulin product (NMT 10 parts per million proinsulin contaminant).

A promising development in the commercial production of peptide hormones is the application of recombinant DNA techniques to human insulin production. At the time of this writing (1980), Eli Lilly and Company has earmarked $40 million to build facilities for the production of human insulin by bacteria bearing the genes for human insulin. In initial studies, the genes (DNA), which direct the biosynthesis of the A and B polypeptide chains for human insulin, were made chemically. Each gene was connected to DNA genetically coding for the enzyme β-galactosidase, a step that puts the chemically synthesized insulin gene under the control of a set of genes called the "lac operon." This operon controls β-galactosidase synthesis and secretion. The connected genes were introduced separately into plasmids. The plasmids were then taken up by Escherichia coli, producing one strain that formed the A chain of insulin and another strain that formed the B chain. The addition of lactose to the bacterial cultures switches on the "lac operon" genes. This, in turn, switches on the gene for the production of either the A or the B chain of human insulin because these genes are now linked to the genes for the formation and secretion of β-galactosidase. The β-galactosidase is synthesized with the A and B chain of insulin attached, and these are recovered by chemically cleaving them from the enzyme. Consequently, the A chain of 21 amino acids and the B chain of 30 amino acids are purified separately and the complete insulin molecule is chemically synthesized from the chains by forming 2 disulfide bridges.

This briefly outlined procedure describes the basic methodology that has been employed in preliminary studies. It is anticipated that, in all likelihood, modifications of these techniques will be required before bringing human insulin to the marketplace can be economically and commercially feasible. When this does happen, it is expected that the bacterially produced human insulin will reduce the incidence of allergic reactions exhibited by a small proportion of diabetics to the insulin currently available from animal pancreas glands. In addition, the bacterially produced hormone would relieve the American Diabetes Association's concern regarding a shortage of animal pancreas glands in 10 to 20 years.

Glucagon for injection is a mixture of the hydrochloride with one or more suitable, dry diluents. When the aqueous injection is reconstituted, it has a pH between 2.5 and 3.0 and is usually formulated to contain 1 mg in each ml. Usual parenteral dose is 500 μg to 1 mg, repeated in 20 minutes, if necessary.

Insulin injection, insulin, or insulin hydrochloride is a sterile, acidified, or neutral solution of the active principle of the pancreas that affects the metabolism of glucose. Insulin injection contains 40, 100, or 500 USP insulin units in each ml. It is a prompt-acting preparation with a peak of action at 2 to 4 hours. This is the preparation of choice when glucose tolerance fluctuates rapidly; such situations may include the presence of a severe infection, shock, surgical trauma, or unstable diabetes. Usual dose, for diabetic acidosis, intravenously, is 1 to 2 units per kg of body weight, repeated in 2 hours as necessary; for diabetes, 10 to 20 units, subcutaneously, 3 or 4 times a day according to the needs of the patient.

PROPRIETARY PRODUCT. Regular Iletin®.

Purified pork regular insulin (Regular Iletin II®) is available in 100- and 500-unit formulations for patients who need such products.

Preparations of insulin are marketed in multiple-dose ampuls of varying unitage. Package color of commercial products varies with the unit value. There is increasing emphasis on use of 100-unit insulin formulations to reduce dosage errors. The need for 40-unit insulins is being studied, and the FDA may eventually decertify them.

Protamine zinc insulin suspension or protamine zinc insulin is a sterile suspension, in a phosphate buffer, of insulin modified by the addition of zinc chloride and protamine. The protamine is prepared from the sperm or from the mature testes of fish belonging to the genus Oncorhynchus Suckley, or Salmo Linné (Fam. Salmonidae). Protamine zinc insulin suspension provides 40 or 100 USP insulin units in each ml. It is a prolonged-acting insulin preparation. Usual dose, subcutaneously, is 7 to 20 units once a day.

PROPRIETARY PRODUCT. Protamine, Zinc and Iletin®.

Purified pork protamine zinc insulin (Protamine, Zinc and Iletin II®) is available in a 100-unit formulation.

Protamines are basic proteins; they combine with insulin to form protamine-insulin salts, stabilized by a trace of zinc. This complex has an isoelectric point of approximately 7.3; it is buffered to this point and dispensed in a smooth suspension. When injected subcutaneously, it is insoluble at the pH of tissue fluids and is therefore slowly absorbed to provide a prolonged action. Peak of action occurs at 14 to 20 hours, with some effect manifest over 36 hours.

Globin zinc insulin injection, globin insulin with zinc, or globin zinc insulin is a sterile solution of insulin modified by the addition of zinc chloride and globin. The globin used is obtained from globin hydrochloride prepared from beef blood. Globin zinc insulin injection provides 40 or 100 USP insulin units in each ml. It is an intermediate-acting insulin preparation. Usual dose, subcutaneously, is 10 to 20 units once a day.

Isophane insulin suspension, isophane insulin, or NPH insulin is a sterile suspension, in a phosphate buffer, of insulin made from zinc-insulin crystals modified by the addition of protamine in such a manner that the solid phase of the suspension consists of crystals composed of insulin, protamine, and zinc. It provides 40 or 100 USP insulin units in each ml. It is an intermediate-acting insulin preparation. Usual dose, subcutaneously, is 10 to 20 units, 1 or 2 times a day.

PROPRIETARY PRODUCT. NPH Iletin®.

Purified pork isophane insulin (NPH Iletin II®) is available in a 100-unit formulation.

Both globin zinc insulin and isophane insulin are insoluble at the pH of tissue fluids and are therefore slowed in their absorption rate. Maximum effect occurs at 8 to 12 hours.

Insulin zinc suspension is a type of intermediate-acting insulin preparation. It consists of a mixture of crystalline and amorphous materials (approximately a 7:3 ratio) suspended in an acetate buffer. It provides 40 or 100 USP insulin units in each ml. Usual dose, subcutaneously, is 10 to 20 units, once a day.

PROPRIETARY PRODUCT. Lente Iletin®.

Purified pork zinc insulin (Lente Iletin II®) is available in a 100-unit formulation.

The use of an acetate buffer provides a prolonged duration of action. Achievement of this objective without the addition of foreign proteins, such as globin or protamine, circumvents occasional hypersensitivity problems associated with these additives. The ratio of crystalline and amorphous insulin is selected to give a convenient duration of action of approximately 24 hours.

Extended insulin zinc suspension is a sterile suspension, in an acetate buffer, of insulin modified by the addition of zinc chloride in such a manner that the solid phase of the suspension is crystalline. It provides 40 or 100 USP insulin units in each ml. It is a long-acting insulin preparation; the duration of action is determined by the particle size and persists for over 36 hours. Usual dose, subcutaneously, is 7 to 20 units, once a day.

PROPRIETARY PRODUCT. Ultralente Iletin®.

Prompt insulin zinc suspension is a sterile suspension, in an acetate buffer, of insulin modified by the addition of zinc chloride in such a manner that the solid phase of the suspension is amorphous. It provides 40 or 100 USP insulin units in each ml. It is a rapid-acting insulin preparation; however, its duration of action extends from 12 to 16 hours. Usual dose, subcutaneously, is 10 to 20 units, 1 or 2 times a day.

PROPRIETARY PRODUCT. Semilente Iletin®.

The chief difference between prompt zinc insulin suspension and extended zinc insulin suspension is the size of the particles that make up the solid phase of the suspensions. Prompt zinc insulin suspension has a shorter duration of action. This product is not intended to replace insulin injection in combating diabetic acidosis or in emergencies when immediate action is essential. In such cases, insulin injection should be administered.

PARATHYROID HORMONE AND CALCITONIN

The **parathyroid glands** in man are usually 4 in number, oval, 5 to 6 mm in length, and situated upon or imbedded in the dorsal surface of the thyroid gland. They develop and function independently of thyroid tissue. For a number of years, after their discovery by Sandstrom in 1880, the parathyroids were considered to be remnants of embryonic thyroid tissue.

The parathyroid glands exert a hormonal control over calcium metabolism. Acute deficiency results in tetany when the level of serum calcium falls from normal (10 to 11 mg%) to around 6 to 7 mg%. Fibrillary muscular twitching progresses to the convulsive state, culminating in death by tetanic spasm of the larynx and muscles of respiration.

Parathyroid hyperfunction produces a condition known as Recklinghausen's disease of bone (osteitis fibrosa cystica), characterized by bone pain, marked elevation of serum calcium with fall in serum phosphate, and cystic rarefaction of bones with spontaneous fracture and deformity. The calcium removed from bone is excreted in the urine. A similar picture may result from overdosage with extracts of parathyroid gland. In either case, renal stones and calcification of soft tissues occur.

The **parathyroid hormone (parathyrin)** is a straight-chain polypeptide containing 83 amino acid residues and has a molecular weight of approximately 9500. A portion of the molecule that contains only 35 amino acid residues can elicit the significant physiologic activity of the hormone. The essential 35-amino-acid subunit of human parathyroid hormone differs in 5 or 6 of its amino acid residues from the animal parathyroid hormones that are available through the meat-packing industry. Immunologic recognition of this factor may contribute to the high incidence of tolerance noted in therapy. The hormone has a hypercalcemic action. Its principal effect involves bone resorption and calcium release, but it also promotes absorption of calcium from the gut and renal tubules.

Parathyroid hormone is inactivated in the intestinal tract, but it is used parenterally in medicine for blood-calcium maintenance in cases of parathyroid tetany. Following injection, the blood calcium level rises in about 4 hours, reaching a maximum in about 16 hours and returning to the original level after 24 to 36 hours. Repeated or prolonged administration may establish a complete tolerance with abolition of therapeutic effect. To avoid this, dihydrotachysterol may frequently be substituted; this preparation may be given orally. Adequate intake of calcium, phosphate, and vitamin D_2 (calciferol) must be assured. Some authorities question the justification for using parathyroid hormone for therapeutic purposes, and its future use may be primarily in the diagnostic area.

Parathyroid injection is a sterile solution in water for injection of the water-soluble principle of the parathyroid glands that has the property of increasing the calcium content of the blood. This preparation is biologically assayed and standardized so that 1 ml possesses a potency of not less than 100 USP parathyroid units, each unit representing 1/100 of the amount required to raise the calcium content of 100 ml of the blood serum of normal dogs 1 mg within 16 to 18 hours after administration. Usual dose, parenterally, is 20 to 40 units, 2 times a day.

Calcitonin is produced by the parafollicular or C cells of the thyroid gland, and recent clarification of its function has increased significantly our comprehension of calcium metabolism. This hormone exerts a hypocalcemic effect by suppressing bone resorption. Thus, calcitonin and parathyroid hormone have counterbalancing actions similar to the situations observed with glucagon-insulin and other control mediators of biologic processes.

Calcitonin is a polypeptide containing 32 amino acid residues. The individual amino acid composition of calcitonin from different animals sources varies considerably. The key molecular features for biologic activity appear to include a prolinamide moiety at the carboxyl terminal end of the peptide and a cyclic sub-unit containing 6 amino acid residues, including the ring closing cystine, at the amino terminal end of the molecule. Reduction of the disulfide linkage causes a loss of activity.

Calcitonin can be used to treat Paget's disease (osteitis deformans) and to control hypercalcemia secondary to other osteolytic conditions. The preparation used in therapy is a synthetic salmon calcitonin. Salmon calcitonin elicits 20-fold or more activity on a molar basis than do human or porcine calcitonins; the apparent increased potency may be caused, in part, by a greater affinity for receptor sites and thus a slower rate of degradation and a longer duration of action. Usual maintenance dose for Paget's disease is 50 units subcutaneously per day or every other day. Therapy to control secondary hypercalcemia usually starts with 4 units per kg of body weight every 12 hours, and the dose may be increased, if necessary, up to 8 units per kg every 6 hours. Intramuscular injection and multiple sites are preferred when larger doses are required.

PRESCRIPTION SPECIALTY. Calcimar®.

GASTROINTESTINAL HORMONES

The intestinal mucosa secretes such peptide hormones as cholecystokinin, gastrin, and secretin. These hormones facilitate digestion by stimulating the release by the gastrointestinal tract or the pancreas of various enzymes and other exocrine substances. There is no therapeutic indication for these hormones, but a secretin preparation from porcine duodenal mucosa is used in the diagnosis of pancreatic disorders. Secretin normally increases the bicarbonate content and volume of secretion from the pancreas. It is a linear polypeptide containing 27 amino acid residues; the amino acid sequence has a noticeable similarity to that of glucagon.

Pentagastrin (Peptavlon®), a synthetic pentapeptide with effects similar to those of natural gastrin, is also used for diagnostic purposes. Pentagastrin increases gastrointestinal motility and stimulates the secretion of gastric acid, pepsin, and intrinsic factor; it is used to test gastric secretory function.

READING REFERENCES

Baba, S., Kaneko, T., and Yanaihara, N., eds.: Proinsulin, Insulin, C-Peptide, Amsterdam, Excerpta Medica, 1979.

Butt, W. R.: Hormone Chemistry, 2nd ed., 2 vols., New York, Halsted Press—John Wiley & Sons, Inc., 1975–1976.

Brobeck, J. R., ed.: Best & Taylor's Physiological Basis of Medical Practice, 10th ed., Baltimore, The Williams & Wilkins Co., 1978.

Collu, R., Barbeau, A., Ducharme, J. R., and Rochefort, J.-G., eds.: Central Nervous System Effects of Hypothalamic Hormones and Other Peptides, New York, Raven Press, 1979.

Czech, M. P.: Molecular Basis of Insulin Action, Ann. Rev. Biochem., 46:359, 1977.

Dockray, G. J.: Comparative Biochemistry and Physiology of Gut Hormones, Ann. Rev. Physiol., 41:83, 1979.

Foa, P. P., Bajaj, J. S., and Foa, N. L., eds.: Glucagon: Its Role in Physiology and Clinical Medicine, New York, Springer-Verlag, 1977.

Glass, G. B. J., ed.: Gastrointestinal Hormones, New York, Raven Press, 1980.

Harland, W. A., and Orr, J. S., eds.: Thyroid Hormone Metabolism, New York, Academic Press, Inc., 1975.

Lee, J., and Laycock, J.: Essential Endocrinology, New York, Oxford University Press, 1978.

Li, C. H., ed.: Hormonal Proteins and Peptides, Vols. I–VI, New York, Academic Press, Inc., 1973–1978.

Litwack, G., ed.: Biochemical Actions of Hormones, Vols. I–III, New York, Academic Press, Inc., 1970–1975.

Martin, C. R.: Textbook of Endocrine Physiology, Baltimore, The Williams & Wilkins Co., 1976.

Parsons, J. A., ed.: Peptide Hormones, Baltimore, University Park Press, 1976.

Rabinowitz, D., and Roth, J., eds.: Heterogeneity of Polypeptide Hormones, New York, Academic Press, Inc., 1975.

Saxena, B. B., Beling, C. G., and Gandy, H. M., eds.: Gonadotropins, New York, Wiley-Interscience, 1972.

Tolis, G., Labrie, F., Martin, J. B., and Naftolin, F., eds.: Clinical Neuroendocrinology, New York, Raven Press, 1979.

Williams, R. H., ed.: Textbook of Endocrinology, 5th ed., Philadelphia, W. B. Saunders Co., 1974.

Chapter 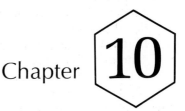 **10**

Enzymes and Other Proteins

ENZYMES

Enzymes are organic catalysts produced by living organisms. They make possible the many complex chemical reactions that make up life processes. Although produced by living organisms, enzymes are lifeless. When isolated, they still exert their characteristic catalytic effect. Although their chemical composition varies, they do exhibit several common properties: (1) enzymes are colloids and are soluble in water and dilute alcohol, but are precipitated by concentrated alcohol; (2) most enzymes act best at temperatures between 35 and 40° C; temperatures above 65° C, especially in the presence of moisture, usually completely destroy them, whereas their activity is negligible at 0° C; (3) certain heavy metals, formaldehyde, and free iodine retard the enzyme's activity. Their activity is markedly affected by the pH of the medium in which they act or by the presence of other substances in this medium. They are usually highly selective in their action.

The enzymes are proteins that range in molecular weight from about 13,000 to as much as 840,000. They are presently classified according to their action by a complex system established by the Commission on Enzymes of the International Union of Biochemistry. Six major classes are recognized, each has 4 to 13 subclasses, and each enzyme is assigned a systematic code number (E.C.) comprised of 4 digits. The major classes in this system are:

1. **Oxidoreductases**—catalyzing oxido-reductions between 2 substances.
2. **Transferases**—catalyzing a transfer of a group, other than hydrogen, between a pair of substrates.
3. **Hydrolases**—catalyzing hydrolysis of ester, ether, peptide, glycosyl, acid-anhydride, C-C, C-halide, or P-N bonds.
4. **Lyases**—catalyzing removal of groups from substrates by mecha-

nisms other than hydrolysis, leaving double bonds.

5. **Isomerases**—catalyzing interconversion of optic, geometric, or positional isomers.

6. **Ligases**—catalyzing linkage of 2 compounds coupled to the breaking of a pyrophosphate bond in ATP or a similar compound.

Because the nomenclature of enzymes was rather well established prior to the promulgation of this system, the well-known trivial names are still ordinarily employed in the pharmaceutic literature. Those encountered with some frequency are:

1. **Esterases,** including lipase, phospholipase, acetylcholinesterase, and others.

2. **Carbohydrases,** including diastase, lactase, maltase, invertase, cellulase, hyaluronidase, glucuronidase, lysozyme, and others.

3. **Nucleases,** including ribonuclease, desoxyribonuclease, nucleophosphatase, and others.

4. **Nuclein deaminases,** including adenase, adenosine deaminase, and others.

5. **Amidases,** including arginase, urease, and others.

6. **Proteolytic enzymes,** including pepsin, trypsin, chymotrypsin, papain, fibrinolysin, streptokinase, urokinase, and others.

Enzymes often occur in combination with inorganic or organic substances that have an important part in the catalytic action. If these are nonprotein organic compounds, they are known as **coenzymes.** If they are inorganic ions, they are referred to as **activators.** Coenzymes are integral components of a large number of enzyme systems. Several vitamins (thiamine chloride, riboflavin, nicotinic acid) are recognized as having a coenzymatic function.

Because enzymes may be recovered from plant and animal cells and because many have been purified, they are utilized as therapeutic agents in addition to their use as controlling factors in certain chemical reactions in industry. Pepsin, pancreatin, and papain are employed therapeutically as digestants; hyaluronidase facilitates the diffusion of injected fluids; streptokinase and streptodornase dissolve clotted blood and purulent accumulations; zymase and rennin are used extensively in the fermentation and cheese industries; and penicillinase inactivates the various penicillins.

Although the terminology is variable, the names used to designate enzymes usually end in -*ase* or -*in.* Some of the more common enzymes are listed in the following classification:

I. THE AMYLOLYTIC ENZYMES OR CARBOHYDRASES

Diastase and amylase are terms applied to 2 well-known amylolytic enzymes. Salivary diastase or **ptyalin** and pancreatic diastase or **amylopsin** are found in the digestive tract of animals; they are sometimes called "animal diastase." **Malt diastase** is formed during the germination of barley grains and converts starch into maltose. It is most active in solutions that are approximately neutral; acidity of pH 4 destroys the enzyme.

Invertase or sucrase is found in yeast and in the intestinal juices. It brings about the hydrolysis of sucrose into glucose and fructose. **Maltase,** which causes the conversion of maltose into glucose, is also found in yeast and the intestinal juices.

Zymase is a fermenting enzyme causing the conversion of monosaccharides (glucose, fructose) into alcohol and carbon dioxide.

Emulsin is an enzyme found in almonds. It causes the hydrolysis of β-glucosides; thus, amygdalin is hydrolyzed into glucose, benzaldehyde, and hydrogen cyanide.

Myrosin is found in white and black mustard; it hydrolyzes sinalbin, sinigrin, and other glycosides.

II. THE ESTERASES

Lipase is a lipolytic enzyme widely distributed in the animal and vegetable kingdoms. It is found in the pancreatic juice of animals and in oily seeds. Lipase causes the hydrolysis of fats into glycerin and fatty acids.

Pectase splits pectin into pectic acid and methyl alcohol.

Steapsin is a lipolytic enzyme capable of digesting dietary fat.

Urease is obtained from soybeans and is used as a laboratory reagent for converting urea to ammonia.

III. THE PROTEOLYTIC ENZYMES

Pepsin is a proteolytic enzyme found in the gastric juice. It is most active at a pH of about 1.8, but in neutral or alkaline media, pepsin is entirely inactive. It converts proteins into proteoses and peptones.

Trypsin is formed when the proenzyme, trypsinogen, is acted on by the enterokinase of the intestinal juices. Trypsin is a proteolytic enzyme that is considerably more active than pepsin, converting proteoses and peptones into polypeptides and amino acids. It acts best in an alkaline medium of about pH 8 and may thus be distinguished from pepsin, which acts only in acid media.

Erepsin is a proteolytic enzyme also found in the intestinal juices. It converts proteoses and peptones into amino acids.

Rennin is a coagulating enzyme present in the mucous membrane of the stomach of mammals. It curdles the soluble casein of milk.

Papain is a mixture of active proteolytic enzymes found in the unripe fruit of the papaya tree. It is a meat tenderizer.

The rationale for oral or parenteral use of proteolytic enzymes in the treatment of traumatically induced inflammation and edema of soft tissues is questionable. Evidence of therapeutic usefulness in such conditions is based solely on the subjective interpretation of results and is, at best, inconclusive.

IV. THE OXIDIZING ENZYMES

Peroxidases are widely distributed in plants. They bring about the oxidation reactions that cause the discoloration of bruised fruits.

Thrombin converts the fibrinogen of the circulating blood into the insoluble fibrin of the blood clot.

Zymase, although splitting monosaccharides, is essentially an oxidizing enzyme because the monosaccharide is split by oxidation.

MALT EXTRACT

Barley is the dried grain of one or more varieties of *Hordeum vulgare* Linné (Fam. Gramineae). Barley is grown throughout the world wherever the climate is favorable.

Malt or malted barley is dried, artificially germinated barley grain. To prepare malt, heaps of barley grain are kept wet with water in a warm room and allowed to germinate until the caulicle protrudes. The grain is then quickly dried. The enzyme diastase in the moist warm grains converts the starch to maltose, thereby stimulating the embryo to growth. The embryo is killed when the grain is dried.

Dry malt resembles barley, but is more crisp, has an agreeable odor, and has a sweet taste. It contains 50 to 70% of the sugar, maltose; 2 to 15% of dextrins; 8% of proteins; diastase; and a peptase enzyme.

Malt is used extensively in the brewing and alcohol industries.

Malt extract is the product obtained by extracting malt, the partially and artificially germinated grain of one or more varieties of *Hordeum vulgare*. The malt is infused with water at 60° C, and the expressed liquid is concentrated at a temperature not exceeding 60° C, preferably under reduced pressure.

Malt extract may be mixed with 10%, by weight, of glycerin. It contains dextrin, maltose, a small amount of glucose, and amylolytic enzymes. It can convert not less than 5 times its weight of starch into water-soluble sugars.

USES AND DOSE. Malt extract is used as an easily digested nutritive and as an aid in digesting starch. Usual dose is 15 g. Many commercial extracts of malt do not contain diastase, which is destroyed by the heat used for their sterilization. Such extracts should not be confused with this product. They are used as bulk-producing laxatives. An example is Maltsupex®.

Diastase is a yellowish white, amorphous powder obtained from an infusion of malt. It can convert 50 times its weight of potato starch into sugars. A related product, Taka-Diastase®, is obtained from the fungus *Aspergillus oryzae* Cohn grown on sterilized wheat bran. It converts 300 times its weight of starch into sugars.

Lactase is an enzyme that hydrolyzes lactose to galactose and glucose. It is obtained commercially from the yeast, *Saccharomyces lactis,* and is used as LactAid® Powder to help patients with lactose intolerance to digest the lactose in milk or milk products.

PEPSIN

Pepsin is a substance containing a proteolytic enzyme obtained from the glandular layer of the fresh stomach of the hog, *Sus scrofa* Linné var. *domesticus* Gray (Fam. Suidae). The generic name *Sus* is from the Greek *Us,* meaning hog; *scrofa* is Latin and means breeding sow; and *domesticus* is Latin and means the household.

Pepsin is prepared by digesting the minced stomach linings with hydrochloric acid. This solution is clarified, partially evaporated, dialyzed, concentrated, and either poured on glass plates to dry, thus forming **scale pepsin,** or carefully evaporated in a vacuum, forming **spongy pepsin.**

Pepsin occurs as lustrous, transparent, or translucent scales, as granular or spongy masses ranging in color from light yellow to light brown, or as fine white or cream-colored amorphous powder. It is free from offensive odor and has a slightly acid or saline taste.

Pepsin digests not less than 3000 and not more than 3500 times its weight of coagulated egg albumin. A pepsin of higher digestive power may be reduced to the standard by admixture with a pepsin of lower power or with lactose. NOTE: Pepsin produced commercially, especially spongy pepsin, often is 4 to 5 times as active as that used medicinally.

Pepsin is administered to assist gastric digestion. It is a proteolytic enzyme and should preferably be given after meals and followed by a dose of hydrochloric acid. Usual dose is 500 mg. It is often combined with pancreatin in product formulations. Pepsin has a long history of use in medicine, but its actual beneficial contribution is poorly documented.

PANCREATIN

Pancreatin is a substance containing enzymes, principally amylase, lipase, and protease. It is obtained from the pancreas of the hog, *Sus scrofa* Linné var. *domesticus* Gray (Fam. Suidae), or of the ox, *Bos taurus* Linné (Fam. Bovidae). The pancreas is a gland that lies directly inside the posterior wall of the abdomen. The fresh glands are minced and extracted by methods similar to those employed in the manufacture of pepsin.

Pancreatin is a cream-colored amorphous powder with a faint, characteristic, but not offensive, odor. Its greatest activity is in neutral or faintly alkaline solution. More than traces of mineral acids or large amounts of alkali hydroxides render pancreatin inert, and an excess of alkali carbonates inhibits its action.

Pancreatin contains, in each mg, not less than 25 USP units of amylase activity, not less than 2 USP units of lipase activity, and not less than 25 USP units of protease activity. Pancreatin of a higher digestive power may be labeled to indicate its strength in whole-number multiples of the 3 minimum activities or may be diluted by appropriate admixture to conform to aforementioned specifications. One USP unit of amylase activity is contained in the amount of pancreatin that digests 1 mg of dry USP Potato Starch Reference Standard, 1 USP unit of lipase activity liberates 1 μEq of acid per minute at a pH of 9 and at 37°C, 1 USP unit of protease activity digests 1 mg of casein, all under specified conditions.

Pancreatin is a digestive aid and is also used in the preparation of predigested foods for invalids. Enteric-coated granules of pancreatin have been used to treat infants with celiac disease and related pancreatic deficiencies. Usual dose is 325 mg to 1 g as tablets, capsules, or granules.

PROPRIETARY PRODUCTS. Elzyme®, Panteric®, Viokase®. Products containing both pepsin and pancreatin in combination with bile salts include Digestozyme®, Donnazyme®, Enzobile®, Entozyme®, Gastroenterase®, Gourmase®, Kanulase®, Mizyme®, Nu'Leven®, Pentazyme®, and Pro-Gestine®. Bilogen®, Co-Bile®, Digestalin®, Digestex®, Digolase®, Enzymet®, Enzypan®, Gasticans®, Milco-Zyme®, Panchola®, Pepsocoll®, Phazyme®, and Zypan® are related products.

PANCRELIPASE

Pancrelipase is essentially a more concentrated form of pancreatin. It contains in each mg not less than 24 USP units of lipase activity, 100 USP units of amylase activity, and 100 USP units of protease activity. Thus the lipase activity is increased 12-fold, but the amylase and protease activity only 4-fold when compared to pancreatin.

Employed as a digestive aid, pancrelipase increases the intestinal absorption of fat, thus aiding in the control of steatorrhea. It is available in the form of capsules, powder packets, and tablets. The usual dose range is 8000 to 24,000 USP units of lipolytic activity prior to each meal or snack, to be determined by the practitioner according to the needs of the patient suffering from pancreatic insufficiency.

PROPRIETARY PRODUCTS. Cotazym®, Ilozyme®, Ku-Zyme HP®, Pancrease®.

RENNIN

Rennin is the partially purified milk-curdling enzyme obtained from the glandular layer of the stomach of the calf, *Bos taurus* Linné (Fam. Bovidae). Rennin may be prepared by macerating the minced glandular layer of the digestive stomach of the calf in 0.5% sodium chloride solution, filtering, acidfying the filtrate with hydrochloric acid, and saturating with sodium chloride. The enzyme is precipitated by the sodium chloride, separated, dried, and powdered.

Rennin occurs as a yellowish white powder, or as yellow grains or scales. It has a characteristic and slightly saline taste and a peculiar, not unpleasant odor. It is usually standardized so that it coagulates approximately 25,000 times its own weight of fresh cow's milk.

Rennin can be used to coagulate milk, thus rendering it more digestible for convalescents. It is also an ingredient in pepsin and rennin elixir (Pepsin Essence). Its principal use, however, is to coagulate milk for the manufacture of cheese.

PAPAIN

Papain is the dried and purified latex of the fruit of *Carica papaya* Linné (Fam. Caricaceae). The papaya tree is indigenous to tropical America and is cultivated in Sri Lanka, Tanzania, Hawaii, and Florida. It attains a height of about 5 or 6 meters. The fruit (Fig. 10–1) grows to a length of about

30 cm and a weight of 5 kg. The epicarp adheres to the orange-colored, fleshy sarcocarp, which surrounds the central cavity. This cavity contains a mass of nearly black seeds.

The full-grown but unripe fruit is subjected to shallow incisions on the 4 sides. The latex flows freely for a few seconds, but soon coagulates. After collection, the coagulated lumps are shredded and dried by the sun or by the use of artificial heat, the latter method yielding the better grade of crude papain. Incisions and collections are made at weekly intervals as long as the fruit exudes the latex. The crude papain is purified by dissolving in water and precipitating with alcohol. Papain has been referred to as "vegetable pepsin" because it contains enzymes somewhat similar to

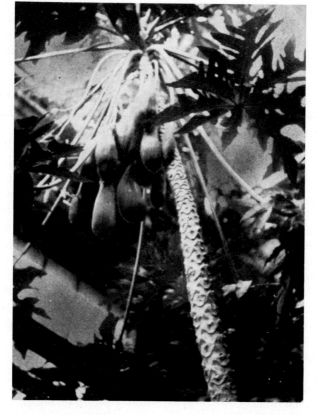

Fig. 10–1. Fruits of *Carica papaya.*

pepsin; however, unlike pepsin, papain acts in acid, neutral, or alkaline media.

Papain contains several enzymes: one or more proteolytic enzymes, among which is peptidase I, capable of converting proteins into dipeptides and polypeptides; a renninlike, coagulating enzyme that acts on the casein of milk; an amylolytic enzyme; a clotting enzyme similar to pectase; and an enzyme that has a feeble activity on fats. It is quite apparent that more than one proteolytic enzyme is present because a single sample of papain yields variable results, depending on the protein used. Although differing in strength in accordance with the method of manufacture, papain can digest about 35 times its own weight of lean meat. For this reason, it is used to tenderize meats. The best grade of papain digests 300 times its own weight of egg albumin.

Papain is used as a digestant for proteins because it has an action much like that of pepsin. It is employed to relieve the symptoms of episiotomy (surgical incision of the vulva for obstetric purposes). In the meat packing industry, papain is used extensively for tenderizing beef.

PROPRIETARY PRODUCTS. Caroid® and Papase®.

BROMELAIN

Bromelain or bromelin is a protein-digesting and milk-clotting enzyme obtained from the juice of the pineapple plant, *Ananas comosus* (Linné) Merr. (Fam. Bromeliaceae). Although this enzyme can appear in the juice of the fruit, it can also occur in the stem of the plant. It differs from papain because it is obtained from both the ripe and unripe fruits.

Bromelain is used as adjunctive therapy to reduce inflammation and edema and to accelerate tissue repair, especially following episiotomy. Its effectiveness in such conditions is apparently owing to depolymerization and permeability modifi-cations that it induces following oral administration. Bromelain is also employed in the production of protein hydrolysates, in tenderizing meats, and in the leather industry.

PRESCRIPTION PRODUCT. Ananase®.

TRYPSIN

Crystallized trypsin is a proteolytic enzyme crystallized from an extract of the pancreas gland of the ox, *Bos taurus* Linné (Fam. Bovidae). When assayed as directed, it contains not less than 2500 USP trypsin units in each mg. It occurs as a white to yellowish white, odorless, crystalline or amorphous powder. The assay involves a spectrophotometric comparison of the solution to be tested to known solutions of measured USP trypsin crystallized reference standard. Similar to other enzymes, crystallized trypsin is stable in the dry state, but rapidly deteriorates in solution form. Thus, it should be stored in tight containers away from excessive heat.

Crystallized trypsin is a proteolytic enzyme. It has been employed orally, topically, or by inhalation or local injection for debridement of necrotic and pyogenic surface lesions. Proof of efficacy of oral and parenteral administration of proteolytic enzymes in such conditions is lacking. The current use of trypsin is primarily topical by aerosol application for wound and ulcer cleansing.

PRESCRIPTION PRODUCT. Granulex®.

CHYMOTRYPSIN

Chymotrypsin is a proteolytic enzyme crystallized from an extract of the pancreas gland of the ox, *Bos taurus* Linné (Fam. Bovidae). It contains not less than 1000 USP chymotrypsin units in each mg. The enzyme occurs as a white to yellowish white, odorless, crystalline or amorphous powder. Chymotrypsin is available as **chymotrypsin for ophthalmic solution.**

This proteolytic enzyme is administered in solution to the posterior chamber of the eye, under the iris, to achieve zonal lysis. One to two ml of a solution containing 75 to 150 units per ml are ordinarily applied. Products, usually in combination with trypsin, are available for oral use.

PRESCRIPTION PRODUCTS. Alpha Chymar®, Avazyme®, Catarase®, Zolyse®.

COMBINATION PRODUCTS. Chymoral®, Orenzyme®.

HYALURONIDASE

Hyaluronidase for injection is a sterile, dry, soluble, enzyme product prepared from mammalian testes and capable of hydrolyzing mucopolysaccharides of the type of hyaluronic acid. Its potency is expressed in USP hyaluronidase units. Hyaluronidase for injection contains not more than 0.25 μg of tyrosine for each USP hyaluronidase unit.

Hyaluronidase is a mucolytic enzyme capable of depolymerizing and catalyzing hyaluronic acid and similar hexosamine-containing polysaccharides. It is also a spreading factor and a diffusing factor. It occurs in human testes, in various bacterial cultures as a metabolic product, in heads of leeches, and in snake venoms. Because of its action on hyaluronic acid, this enzyme promotes diffusion and hastens absorption of subcutaneous infusions.

Hyaluronidase for injection is a spreading agent. Usual dose, hypodermoclysis, is 150 USP units.

PRESCRIPTION PRODUCTS. Alidase®, Wydase®.

STREPTOKINASE AND STREPTODORNASE

Streptokinase and streptodornase are 2 enzymes elaborated by hemolytic streptococci and, in combination, are applied locally or topically wherever clotted blood or fibrinous or purulent accumulations appear following injury to the tissues. Streptokinase breaks down fibrin, whereas streptodornase affects desoxyribonucleic acid and desoxyribonucleoprotein, which are the chief constituents of pus and necrotic tissue.

The enzyme combination is available as an injection for intramuscular use, as a solution or jelly for topical application, and as tablets for buccal and oral administration. The ratio of streptokinase to streptodornase in these preparations is 4:1. For intramuscular injection, 5000 units of streptokinase in combination with 1250 units of streptodornase, twice daily, is recommended. The usual oral dose is 10,000 units of streptokinase in combination with 2500 units of streptodornase, 4 times daily; however, only streptokinase is thought to be active when administered via this route.

PRESCRIPTION SPECIALTY. Varidase®.

Streptokinase is also used for its indirect thrombolytic properties. The enzyme acts on the endogenous fibrinolytic system by converting plasminogen to the proteolytic enzyme plasmin or to fibrinolysin. The latter enzyme then degrades fibrin clots.

Thrombolytic enzymes should be used only by physicians with experience in the management of thrombotic diseases and only in hospitals where clinical and laboratory monitoring can be performed. Streptokinase is indicated for massive pulmonary emboli and for extensive thrombi of the deep veins in adults. There are significant risks of bleeding and other adverse reactions, and diagnoses should be confirmed by objective means before use of the enzyme. It should not be used to treat superficial thrombophlebitis.

Streptokinase is administered by continuous intravenous infusion. The usual dosage regimen is 100,000 units per hour for 24 to 72 hours.

PRESCRIPTION PRODUCT. Streptase®.

UROKINASE

Urokinase is isolated from human urine. This enzyme has thrombolytic activity and is used as an alternate to streptokinase in the treatment of massive pulmonary emboli. Urokinase appears to have a reduced probability of serious allergic reactions, presumably owing to its human origin, but it should be used with appropriate caution. The usual dosage regimen is 4,400 units per kg of body weight per hour for 12 hours by intravenous infusion.

PRESCRIPTION PRODUCT. Abbokinase®.

FIBRINOLYSIN

Fibrinolysin is in the blood serum as a protease and in plasma as the inactive precursor, profibrinolysin (or plasminogen). It is prepared commercially by activating a human blood plasma fraction with streptokinase. In the dried form, fibrinolysin retains its proteolytic activity almost indefinitely; however, in solution form, it rapidly deteriorates. Its enzymatic activity is lost completely when it is exposed to room temperature for 6 to 8 hours. It can attack the protein portions of dead tissues, exudates, and blood clots found in wounds, ulcers, and burns. Fibrinolysin is used primarily in the treatment of blood clots within the cardiovascular system, exclusive of thrombi of the coronary and cerebral arteries. It is administered by intravenous infusion in conditions such as phlebothrombosis, thrombophlebitis, and pulmonary emboli.

PRESCRIPTION PRODUCT. Thrombolysin®.

SUTILAINS

Sutilains is a substance containing proteolytic enzymes derived from the bacterium *Bacillus subtilis*. It contains not less than 2.5 million USP casein units of proteolytic activity per g. This cream-colored powder is applied topically, in ointment form, 2 to 4 times daily, for wound debridement.

PRESCRIPTION PRODUCT. Travase® Ointment contains 82,000 USP casein units of proteolytic activity per g.

COLLAGENASE

Collagenase is an enzyme preparation obtained from fermentative cultures of *Clostridium histolyticum*. It cleaves collagen and is used topically to debride dermal ulcers and severely burned areas. Care should be exercised to avoid heavy metal inactivation of the enzyme; Burow's solution can be used to stop the enzyme action if the risk of bacteremia develops. Available ointments contain 250 units of collagenase activity per g.

PROPRIETARY PRODUCT. Collagenase ABC®, Santyl®.

DESOXYRIBONUCLEASE

Desoxyribonuclease or deoxyribonuclease is a nucleolytic enzyme that is obtained in a highly purified state from pancreatic glands of bovine origin. Like fibrinolysin, it is stable in dry form but rapidly loses its activity in solution form. It can catalyze cleavage of the giant molecules of desoxyribonucleic acid into numerous fragments of smaller size (polynucleotides); thus, it acts against devitalized tissues in purulent states. It is available as a combination product with bovine fibrinolysin.

COMBINATION PRODUCT. Elase®.

L-ASPARAGINASE

L-Asparaginase, an enzyme obtained from cultures of certain strains of *Escherichia coli*, induces hematologic and clinical remissions of short duration in a significant percentage of children with acute leukemia. The antitumor effect may be attributed to degradation by the enzyme of circulating L-asparagine, which results in the death of cells that require exogenous sources of this amino acid for survival. The notable absence of toxicity to normal marrow elements suggests that the effectiveness of the drug is related to a difference in the requirement for L-asparagine between normal cells and some neoplastic cells.

A number of serious adverse reactions are noted with asparaginase, including allergic reactions and fatal anaphylaxis. It is used primarily in combination with other chemotherapeutic agents, such as prednisone and vincristine. Administration is intravenous, usually 1,000 units per kg of body weight daily, or intramuscular, 6,000 units per square meter of body surface at 3-day intervals.

PRESCRIPTION PRODUCT. Elspar®.

OTHER PROTEINS

Proteins are nitrogenous organic substances produced by and associated with living matter. They occur in both plants and animals; those from plants are more easily isolated in crystalline form. Plants usually store proteins in the form of aleurone grains. In animals, proteins occur as living matter, thus making them difficult to obtain in the individual state.

Proteins may be classified into 3 groups: *simple, conjugated,* and *derived.* The simple proteins hydrolyze entirely into amino acids; the conjugated proteins are combinations of a protein and a nonprotein group (the latter is called the prosthetic group); and the derived proteins are degradation products of the proteins. Each of these groups has several subdivisions.

Because they are present in all living matter, proteins are of great importance in biochemistry. They form an important class of food and are equally as essential as carbohydrates and fats. Meat, fish, and eggs are important sources of animal protein foods. Cereal grains, particularly wheat and soybeans, are sources of plant protein foods.

Although proteins are important in metabolism, relatively few isolated proteins are employed as therapeutic agents. Whole glandular products, oil-bearing plant seeds, antitoxins, serums, and globulins contain proteins in combination with other biochemical substances—all these substances possess therapeutic activity, but they are classified in other chapters of the text. Allergens are usually proteinaceous by nature; however, carbohydrates and fats may also produce allergic reactions. Allergens are described in Chapter 14.

Certain proteins are highly poisonous: the plant toxalbumins, **ricin** from castor beans, **robin** from locust bark, and **abrin** from jequirity seeds. Among the poisonous animal proteins are hemolysins from salamanders (*Triturus* sp.) and the various toxins, **neurotoxoids,** from snake venom (see page 417).

The following drugs are comprised of proteins, modified proteins, and amino acids; their therapeutic applications are extremely varied. They are grouped together according to homogeneity of origin rather than similarity of function.

GELATIN

Gelatin is a product obtained by the partial hydrolysis of collagen derived from the skin, white connective tissue, and bones of animals. Commercially, gelatin is prepared from the suitable by-products of slaughtered cattle, sheep, and hogs. Bones are first decalcified by treatment with hydrochloric acid. The materials are extracted with boiling water and steam under pressure until the collagen is hydrolyzed. The solution is then filtered by electroosmosis, concentrated under reduced pressure, allowed to gel, and rapidly dried on netting in currents of warm air.

Gelatin occurs in sheets, flakes, shreds, or as a coarse or fine powder. It is faintly yellow or amber and has a slight, characteristic odor and taste. When dry, gelatin is stable in the air, but when moist or in solution, it is subject to bacterial decomposition. Gelatin is insoluble in cold water but swells and softens when immersed in cold water, gradually absorbing from 5 to 10 times its weight of water. It is soluble in hot water and insoluble in most immiscible solutions and in volatile and fixed oils.

Commercially, gelatin is available as 2 types: A and B. Type A exhibits an isoelectric point between pH 7 and 9 and is incompatible with anionic compounds such as acacia, tragacanth, and agar. Type B, on the other hand, should be used when such mixtures are desired because it exhibits an isoelectric point between pH 4.7 and 5.

If gelatin is intended for use in the manufacture of capsules to contain medication or for the coating of tablets, it may be colored with a certified color, may contain various additives, and may have any suitable gel strength.

Gelatin contains amino acids: alanine, arginine, aspartic acid, cystine, cysteine, glutamic acid, glycine, histidine, hydroxyproline, isoleucine, leucine, lysine, methionine, phenylalanine, proline, serine, threonine, tyrosine, and valine. Because only traces of other important amino acids are present and tryptophan is absent, gelatin is an incomplete nutritional protein. The gelatinizing constituent is known as chondrin and the adhesive substance is known as glutin.

Gelatin is a pharmaceutic aid (encapsulating agent, suspending agent, tablet binder, and coating agent). Combined with glycerin, it forms glycerinated gelatin; as such, it is employed as a vehicle and also for the manufacture of suppositories. Zinc oxide is added to form zinc gelatin, which is used as a topical protectant. In addition, gelatin is a nutrient and is extensively used for the preparation of commercial food products and for bacteriologic culture media.

ABSORBABLE GELATIN SPONGE

Absorbable gelatin sponge is a sterile, absorbable, water-insoluble, gelatin-base sponge. It consists of a light, nearly white, porous, pliable, nonantigenic matrix prepared from purified, specially treated gelatin and is sterilized by heat. Even when handled roughly, this product shows little tendency to disintegrate. It absorbs about 50 times its weight of water and about 45 times its weight of blood.

Control of capillary oozing and of bleeding from veins is effected through the use of absorbable gelatin sponge applied in the dry form or saturated with sterile, isotonic sodium chloride solution or sterile thrombin solution. The sponge is applied to the bleeding area and held for 10 to 15 seconds, after which it is left in place.

Absorbable gelatin sponge is a local hemostatic. It is applied topically in operative wounds.

COMMERCIAL PRODUCT. Gelfoam®. This is supplied as individual sponges, dental packs, prostatectomy cones, and powder intended for a variety of uses (Fig. 10–2).

ABSORBABLE GELATIN FILM

Absorbable gelatin film is a specially prepared gelatin product used in neurosurgery and in thoracic and ocular surgery. It consists of a thin, pliable, nonantigenic, absorbable film of purified gelatin. In the dry state, it resembles cellophane in appearance and stiffness and occurs in pieces about 25 × 50 mm or 100 × 125 mm in size and about 0.075 mm in thickness. When moistened by immersion in salt solution, it is easily cut into the

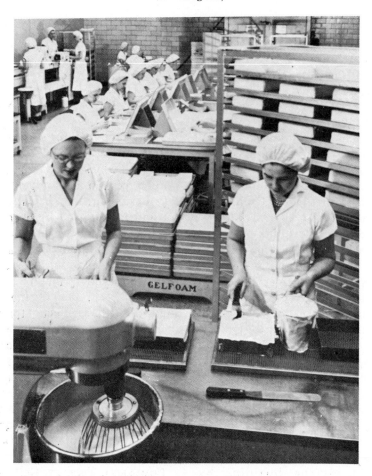

Fig. 10–2. Complete operation of the manufacture of Gelfoam: preparing the gelatin (foreground), filling molds, baking, cutting the finished product into desired shapes, packaging, and sterilizing. (Photo, courtesy of The Upjohn Company.)

shape needed to fit into the contours of the incision.

COMMERCIAL PRODUCT. Gelfilm®.

MICROFIBRILLAR COLLAGEN

Microfibrillar collagen is a fibrous, water-insoluble material prepared from purified bovine corium collagen. It is an absorbable, topical hemostatic agent that is used in surgical procedures when control of bleeding by ligature or other conventional means is ineffective or impractical.

It is applied dry and directly onto the bleeding surface; the microfibrillar collagen attracts platelets that adhere to the fibrils and trigger the formation of thrombi.

PROPRIETARY PRODUCT. Avitene®.

ABSORBABLE SURGICAL SUTURE

Absorbable surgical suture is a sterile strand prepared from collagen derived from healthy mammals or from a synthetic polymer. It can be absorbed by living mammalian tissue but may be treated to modify its resistance to absorption. It may be impregnated with a suitable antimicrobial agent and may be colored by a color additive approved by the federal Food and Drug Administration.

The USP lists specifications for labeling, length, diameter, tensile strength, and other requirements. This product is also known as **catgut suture, surgical catgut,** and **surgical gut.**

NONABSORBABLE SURGICAL SUTURE

Nonabsorbable surgical suture is a strand of material that is suitably resistant to the action of living mammalian tissue. It may be composed of either natural or synthetic fibers; in some cases, metal wire is employed. The label must contain detailed information about the product.

PENICILLAMINE

Penicillamine is D-3-mercaptovaline or β,β-dimethylcystine. It is a degradation product of penicillin-type antibiotics. This substance is a metal-chelating agent employed in Wilson's disease (hepatolenticular degeneration) to promote urinary excretion of excess copper. It is also useful in treating lead poisoning, and for reasons unknown, it is sometimes useful in cases of severe active rheumatoid arthritis that are refractory to conventional therapy. The usual dose in Wilson's disease is 250 mg, 4 times a day; a single daily dose of up to 1.5 g is used in rheumatoid arthritis.

PRESCRIPTION PRODUCT. Cuprimine®.

HEPARIN SODIUM

Heparin sodium or heparin is a mixture of active principles and has the ability to prolong the clotting time of blood. It is usually obtained from the lungs, intestinal mucosa, or other suitable tissues of domestic mammals used for food by man. It inhibits the formation of fibrin clots.

The chief use of heparin is for patients in whom slower blood coagulation is desired. Usual dose, intravenously, is 5000 to 10,000 USP units, 4 to 6 times a day; infusion, 20,000 to 40,000 units per liter at a rate of 15 to 30 units per minute. The drug may also be injected subcutaneously, 8000 to 10,000 units, 3 times daily.

PRESCRIPTION SPECIALTIES. Heprinar®, Liquaemin® Sodium, Lipo-Hepin®, and Panheprin®.

PROTAMINE SULFATE

Protamine sulfate is a purified mixture of simple protein principles obtained from the sperm or testes of suitable species of fish, usually those belonging to the genera *Oncorhynchus* Suckley, *Salmo* Linné, or *Trutta* Jordan et Evermann (Fam. Salmonidae). It has the property of neutralizing heparin. Each mg of protamine sulfate neutralizes not less than 80 USP units of heparin activity derived from lung tissue and not less than 100 USP units of heparin activity derived from intestinal mucosa.

Protamine sulfate is a fine, white or off-white, amorphous or crystalline powder that is sparingly soluble in water. It is an antidote to heparin and is administered intravenously. The usual dose, intravenously, is 1 mg for each 90 or 115 USP units of heparin activity, derived from beef lung tissue or porcine intestinal mucosa, respectively, in 1 to 3 minutes, up to a maximum of 50 mg in any 10-minute period, repeated as necessary.

Protamine sulfate for injection is a sterile mixture of protamine sulfate with one or more suitable dry diluents. **Protamine sulfate injection** is a sterile isotonic solution of protamine sulfate.

PROTEIN HYDROLYSATE INJECTION

Protein hydrolysate injection is a sterile solution of amino acids and short-chain peptides that represents the approximate nutritive equivalent of the casein, lactalbumin, plasma, fibrin, or other suitable protein from which it is derived by acid, enzymatic, or other method of hydrolysis. This preparation must have not less than 50% of the total nitrogen present in the form of α-amino nitrogen; for this reason, it may be modified by partial removal and restoration of the amino acids or by addition of one or more amino acids.

This drug is intended for use when the patient is unable to ingest or digest food to supply the nitrogen necessary to replace that amount lost through tissue metabolism.

Protein hydrolysate injection is a parenteral nutrient. Usual dose, intravenously, is 2 to 3 liters of a 5% solution daily.

PRESCRIPTION PRODUCTS. Amigen®, Aminosol®, Travamin®.

LEVODOPA

Levodopa or 3-hydroxy-L-tyrosine is an amino acid that occurs in the seeds of *Vicia faba* Linné (Fam. Leguminosae), commonly referred to as the horse bean, the velvet bean, or the broad bean. Isolation of the compound from protein hydrolysate is somewhat difficult owing to its tendency to become oxidized; therefore, synthetic methods of production are employed. An efficient microbial conversion of L-tyrosine to levodopa has been reported.

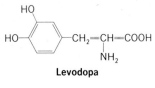

Levodopa

Large oral doses of levodopa have been effective in relieving parkinsonism; improvement in patients receiving up to 8 g daily ranges from modest to dramatic. Most symptoms are relieved to some degree, but akinesia and rigidity respond more readily than tremor. The major adverse effects noted include transitory nausea and vomiting, orthostatic faintness, and transient depression of granulocytes.

Symptoms of parkinsonism appear to be related to the depletion of striatal dopamine. Exogenously administered dopamine is either destroyed or does not cross the blood-brain barrier, but levodopa, the biosynthetic precursor of dopamine, does cross the blood-brain barrier. The action of levodopa presumably involves the decarboxylation in the neural ganglia of the amino acid to give the amine.

The usual dose, initially, is 250 mg, 2 to 4 times a day, gradually increasing the total daily dose in increments of 100 to 750 mg every 3 to 7 days as tolerated. The usual dose range is 500 mg to 8 g daily. Administration takes place in the form of capsules or tablets.

PRESCRIPTION PRODUCTS. Bendopa®, Dopar®, Larodopa®.

READING REFERENCES

Bohak, Z., and Sharon, N., eds.: *Biotechnical Applications of Proteins and Enzymes*, New York, Academic Press, Inc., 1977.

Boyer, P. D., ed.: *The Enzymes*, 3rd ed., Vols. I–XIII, New York, Academic Press, Inc., 1970–1976.

Colowick, S. P., and Kaplan, N. O., eds.: *Methods in Enzymology*, Vols. I–LXVIII, New York, Academic Press, Inc., 1955–1979.

Dixon, M., and Webb, E. C.: *Enzymes*, 3rd ed., London, Longman Group Ltd., 1979.

Ferdinand, W.: *The Enzyme Molecule*, New York, John Wiley & Sons, Inc., 1976.

Magnusson, S., Ottesen, M., Foltmann, B., Danø, K., and Neurath, H., eds.: *Regulatory Proteolytic Enzymes and Their Inhibitors*, New York, Pergamon Press, 1978.

Neurath, H., and Hill, R. L., eds.: *Proteins*, 3rd ed., Vols. I–IV, New York, Academic Press, Inc., 1975–1979.

Nord, F. F., and Meister, E., eds.: *Advances in Enzymology*, Vols. I–L, New York, John Wiley & Sons, Inc., 1941–1979.

Ory, R. L., and St. Angelo, A. L., eds.: *Enzymes in Food and Beverage Processing*, Washington, D.C., American Chemical Society, 1977.

Ruyssen, R., and Lauwers, A., eds.: *Pharmaceutical Enzymes*, Gent, E. Story-Scientia, 1978.

Schulz, G. E., and Schirmer, R. H.: *Principles of Protein Structure*, New York, Springer-Verlag, 1979.

Scrimgeour, K. G.: *Chemistry and Control of Enzyme Reactions*, New York, Academic Press, Inc., 1977.

Wolf, M., and Ransberger, K.: *Enzyme Therapy*, New York, Vantage Press, 1972.

Chapter **11**

Vitamins and Vitamin-containing Drugs

Vitamins are organic compounds necessary to the normal growth and the maintenance of life in animals, including man. They do not furnish energy and are not utilized as building units for the structure of the organism, but they are essential for the regulation of metabolic processes. In their capacity as metabolic regulators, vitamins act in a number of different ways. Some (A, C, E, K, niacin) function as redox agents, others (B_1, B_2, B_6, B_{12}, D) as coenzymes or enzyme activators, and others (biotin, folic acid) as nuclear agents. Some vitamins combine 2 or more of these activities with other metabolic roles. When the natural supply of vitamins is lacking, a number of deficiency diseases occur. Thus, vitamins are therapeutic agents of value in the prophylaxis and treatment of these diseases.

The definition of vitamins has been criticized. The substances that are called "vitamins" exert no vitamin activity as such, but become active only after chemical transformation into other compounds. Thiamine, riboflavin, and niacin are constituents of enzyme systems that each have a different catalytic activity.

Vitamins are derived from a variety of sources, both plant and animal. They are usually isolated, concentrated, and purified for use as drugs; many of them are now synthesized. Varying widely in chemical constitution, vitamins have little in common except that they are called "vitamins." Some are relatively simple (niacin), others are quite complex (folic acid), and still others are related to the sterols (calciferol). Their applications in therapeutics also differ, e.g., in xerophthalmia, beriberi, scurvy, rickets, and other diseases; in promoting blood clotting; in stimulating growth; in preventing anemia; in diminishing capillary fragility; and in numerous other conditions.

FISH LIVER OILS

Cod liver oil is the partially destearinated fixed oil obtained from the fresh livers of *Gadus morrhua* Linné and other species of the Family Gadidae. The generic name *Gadus* is from the Greek *gados*, meaning codfish, and *morrhua* is the Latin name of the codfish. Codfish inhabit the northern Atlantic Ocean, coming to its shores to spawn in the late winter and spring.

The principal fishing grounds are located from New England north to Nova Scotia and Newfoundland and along the coast of Norway. Fishing is done by trap nets, hand-lines, and set-lines. In the early days, the fish were cleaned on shipboard; the edible portion was salted, and the separated livers were thrown into barrels where, through a process of "rotting," the tissue disintegrated and the oil rose to the top. Today, for the production of medicinal oil, the fish are brought to the fish houses a few hours after they are caught, the livers are removed with care, and the gallbladders are completely separated. The livers are steamed in closed kettles, and the oil rises to the top and is collected. The air above the oil is replaced by carbon dioxide to prevent oxidation. The oil is strained, decanted into tin-lined containers, and chilled to a temperature below −5° C. During this chilling process, the stearin separates out as a solid, and the lighter oil is decanted and filtered. Finally, the oil is adjusted to a definite vitamin content by admixture, if necessary, of different lots of the oil with higher or lower vitamin values. The liver-marc is often resteamed and pressed for a further yield of oil that is used for technical purposes.

Cod liver oil was exported from Norway as early as the Middle Ages. Its use, however, was technical only. It was introduced into medicine during the middle of the eighteenth century.

Cod liver oil is a thin, oily liquid that has a peculiar, slightly fishy, but not rancid, odor and a fishy taste. It is slightly soluble in alcohol but freely soluble in ether, chloroform, carbon disulfide, and ethyl acetate.

The medicinal constituents of cod liver oil are vitamin A (the growth-promoting, antixerophthalmic vitamin) and vitamin D (the antirachitic vitamin). The oil consists of glyceryl esters of unsaturated (about 85%) and saturated (about 15%) fatty acids. (A sterile solution of the sodium salts of the fatty acids, sodium morrhuate injection, is employed as a sclerosing agent, see page 98.) The unsaturated acids include oleic, linoleic, gadoleic, and palmitoleic. The saturated acids include myristic, palmitic, and traces of stearic. Bile salts and the alkaloids, morrhuine and aselline, should be absent. The presence of the former indicates contamination of the livers with gallbladders, and the presence of the latter indicates decomposition.

STANDARDS AND TESTS. Cod liver oil contains in each gram not less than 255 μg (850 USP units) of vitamin A and not less than 2.125 μg (85 USP units) of vitamin D.

The vitamin A content of cod liver oil was formerly determined by the amount necessary to cure induced vitamin A starvation in young albino rats, but at the present time, a spectrophotometric assay following chromatographic methods is employed. The vitamin D potency is determined by the degree of restoration on the proximal end of the tibia or on the distal end of the radius or ulna of albino rats under the influence of controlled vitamin D starvation. This test is known as the "Line Test."

Cod liver oil may be flavored by the addition of not more than 1% of a suitable flavoring substance or a mixture of such substances.

Cod liver oil should be preserved in tight containers, preferably in a cool place. It may be bottled or packaged in containers from which air has been expelled by the production of a vacuum or by an inert gas.

USES AND DOSE. Cod liver oil is employed for its content of antixerophthalmic and antirachitic vitamins. It is used principally for the cure and prevention of rickets; the vitamin D helps to utilize calcium in the formation of bones and teeth. Because of its vitamin A content, cod liver oil is valuable as a "flesh builder" in wasting diseases and as a "growth promoter" in children. Usual dose is 5 ml containing 1170 μg (3900 USP units) of vitamin A and 9.7 μg (386 USP units) of vitamin D. NOTE: Cod liver oil containing more than the minimum requirements for both vitamin A and vitamin D may be administered in proportionately smaller doses.

Halibut liver oil or oleum hippoglossi is the fixed oil obtained from the fresh or suitably preserved livers of halibut species of the genus *Hippoglossus* Linné (Fam. Pleuronectidae). The name halibut is from *hali,* meaning holy, and *butte,* meaning flounder, and refers to a flounder eaten on holy days. The term *hippoglossus* is from the Greek *hippos* meaning horse, and *glossus,* meaning tongue, and refers to the flat shape of the fish. The halibut inhabits the oceans of the northern hemispheres where commercial fishing is carried on by handlines or set-lines. The livers are processed in much the same way as codfish livers.

The principal constituents of halibut liver oil are vitamins A and D. Olein, palmitin, and cholesterol make up the body of the oil.

STANDARDS AND TESTS. Halibut liver oil contains in each gram not less than 18 mg (60,000 USP units) of vitamin A and not less than 15 μg (600 USP units) of vitamin D.

USES AND DOSE. Halibut liver oil is used therapeutically because of its anti-xerophthalmic vitamin content. Although its use parallels that for cod liver oil, its high vitamin potency permits administration of much smaller doses. It is often prescribed as halibut liver oil capsules. Usual dose is 0.1 ml (1.5 mg or 5000 USP units of vitamin A) daily.

VITAMIN A

Vitamin A, the anti-infective, anti-xerophthalmic vitamin, and its naturally occurring isomer, **neovitamin A** (5-*cis*-vitamin A) are both found in cod liver oil and in other fish liver oils. They have a molecular weight of 286.44 and bear the formula $C_{20}H_{30}O$. Vitamin A occurs as yellow prisms with a melting point of 62 to 64° C and an absorption maximum of 324 to 325 nm; neovitamin A consists of pale yellow needles with a melting point of 58 to 60° C and an absorption maximum of 328 nm. In addition, **hepaxanthin** (vitamin A epoxide) may be obtained from cod liver oil or by formation from vitamin A; it is a viscous yellow oil and has a molecular weight of 302.44, the formula $C_{20}H_{30}O_2$, and an absorption maximum of 272 nm.

Vitamin A and neovitamin A are found in the unsaponifiable fraction of fish oils; are resistant to heat in the absence of air, acids, and alkalies; are destroyed by oxidation at all temperatures; and are unstable to light. They may occur as free alcohols or as esters (acetate, palmitate), which are more stable to oxidation.

Vitamin A has the following structural formula:

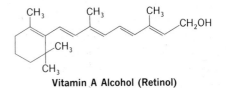

Vitamin A Alcohol (Retinol)

A group of substances of plant origin, known as **natural carotenes, provitamin A substances,** or **carotenoids** and including α-, β-, and γ-carotene and cryptoxanthin, are converted in the liver of animals to vitamin A. A few years ago, the carotene content of certain lichens was shown to be a good source of provitamin A materials. Such carotenes and carotenoids consist of dark red crystals that are insoluble in water, acids, and alkalies, but sensitive to oxidation.

Beta-carotene has been proved effective in reducing photosensitivity in individuals with erythropoietic protoporphyria. It does not act as a sunscreen in normal individuals and should not be used for that effect. However, β-carotene does provide a novel and safe approach to the treatment of a specific type of photosensitivity. When ingested over a period of several weeks, the drug produces carotenemia, a yellowing of the skin often first observed in the palms of the hands or on the soles of the feet. The mode of action has not been established, but is no doubt related to the coloration of the skin. During the course of therapy, elevated blood-carotene levels are observed, but vitamin A levels do not rise above normal.

tective effect is not total, but varies with each individual.

Prescription Product. Solatene®.

Biosynthesis of Vitamin A. Vitamin A, per se, is neither accumulated in plants nor synthesized by them. However, its carotenoid precursors are apparently biosynthesized only by plants. Consequently, the vitamin results when a carotenoid of plant origin is ingested and subsequently metabolized by an animal.

The carotenoid precursors are C_{40} isoprenoid compounds (tetraterpenes) and, like other terpene derivatives, are formed via the acetate-mevalonic acid pathway. For convenience, most of the studies on carotenoid biosynthesis have been carried out with microorganisms, but studies utilizing tissues of higher plants have yielded similar results.

Feeding of mevalonic acid-2-^{14}C to cultures of *Phycomyces blakesleeanus* resulted in the production of β-carotene labeled in the anticipated positions.

Although the exact sequence of intermediates remains to be determined, experiments indicate that a molecule of farnesyl pyrophosphate condenses with a molecule of isopentenyl pyrophosphate to form the C_{20} compound, geranylgeranyl pyrophos-

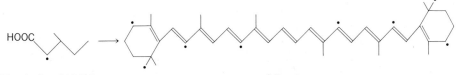

Mevalonic acid-2-^{14}C   *β*-Carotene

The usual adult dose of β-carotene is 50 to 500 mg per day, adjusted according to the severity of the symptoms and to the response of the patient. Increased exposure to sunlight should not occur until the patient first appears carotenemic, 2 to 6 weeks after initiation of therapy. The pro-

phate. This compound then undergoes nonreductive dimerization (head-to-tail) to yield the C_{40} compound, phytoene, which apparently functions as a common precursor for the various carotenoids. Oxygenated carotenoids (xanthophylls) arise from the hydrocarbon types.

In spite of extensive investigations of the conversion of β-carotene and its isomers to vitamin A, the mechanism of this reaction has not been established. It occurs in the intestinal wall and involves central fission of the molecules followed by terminal oxidation.

The following biologic functions of vitamin A may be listed:

1. It is specific in the prevention and cure of xerophthalmia and nyctalopia.

2. It prevents hyperkeratosis of the skin, which may occur in severe cases of vitamin A deficiency.

3. It is useful in overcoming retardation of growth and development when this condition is caused by vitamin A deficiency (Fig. 11–1).

4. It is of value for increasing resistance of the body to infection only when body reserves have been exhausted and vitamin A has been inadequately ingested.

Excessive doses of vitamin A produce toxic symptoms. These range from headache, drowsiness, nausea, loss of hair, and diarrhea in adults, to dermatitis, weight loss, and skeletal pain in infants. Individual differences in sensitivity exist, but prolonged daily dose administration exceeding 25,000 USP units should be closely supervised. Recovery is rapid, usually occurring within 72 hours after withdrawal of excess intake, and permanent effects are rare. Because of this potential toxicity of vitamin A, the FDA currently restricts oral preparations containing more than 10,000 units per dose (or recommended daily intake) to prescription use.

DAILY REQUIREMENTS. Adults, 5000 units; pregnant and lactating mothers, 6000 to 8000 units; children, 2000 to 3500 units.

Fish liver oils, egg yolk, cream, cheese, butter, and milk are sources of vitamin A; green leafy vegetables, apricots, carrots, and sweet potatoes are sources of carotene; yellow corn and egg yolk are sources of cryptoxanthin.

Vitamin A or oleovitamin A is a substance that contains a suitable form of retinol ($C_{20}H_{30}O$; vitamin A alcohol) and possesses vitamin A activity equivalent to not less than 95% of that declared on the label. It may consist of retinol or esters of retinol formed from edible fatty acids, principally acetic and palmitic acids. It may be diluted with edible oils, or it may be incorporated

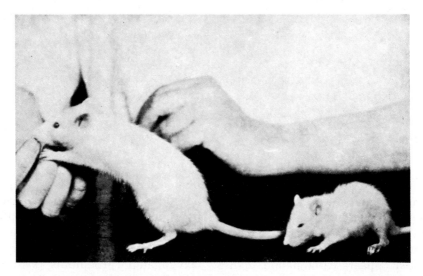

Fig. 11–1. Two rats of equal weight were placed on a vitamin A starvation diet: one was fed cod liver oil, the other received none. (Photo, courtesy of Parke, Davis & Co.)

in solid edible carriers or excipients. Vitamin A may contain suitable antimicrobial agents, dispersants, and anti-oxidants. It is a yellow to red oily liquid that may solidify when refrigerated. It may be nearly odorless or may have a fishy odor, but it has no rancid odor or taste. It is unstable to air and light.

Vitamin A is assayed spectrophotometrically, although 1 USP vitamin A unit represents the specific biologic activity of 0.3 μg of the all-*trans* isomer of retinol. Classed as an antixerophthalmic vitamin, its usual prophylactic dose is 1.5 mg (5000 USP vitamin A units) once a day; therapeutic, 3 to 15 mg (10,000 to 50,000 units) once a day.

PROPRIETARY PRODUCTS. Alphalin® and Aquasol A®.

VITAMIN D

The antirachitic vitamin occurs in a number of forms. Four crystalline D vitamers have been isolated, and at least 10 provitamins D are known. For humans, most of the vitamin D activity is supplied from animal sources or from sunshine.

Biosynthesis of Vitamin D. Vitamins of this class derive from $\Delta^{5,7}$-sterols, especially ergosterol and 7-dehydrocholesterol, by complex photochemical reactions. Biosynthesis of the sterol precursors takes place via the acetate-mevalonic acid pathway previously outlined in Chapter 7, Steroids.

Vitamin D$_2$ is formed by exposing ergosterol to ultraviolet irradiation or other energy. It is:

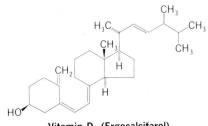
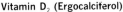

Vitamin D$_2$ (Ergocalciferol)

Vitamin D$_3$ is the natural vitamin D found in fish oils and formed in the skin of man and animals following exposure to sunlight. It may be formed by the irradiation of 7-dehydrocholesterol and has the following formula:

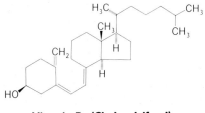
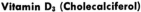

Vitamin D$_3$ (Cholecalciferol)

Vitamins D$_2$ and D$_3$ are known as vitamers. They are white crystalline substances, soluble in fats and organic solvents, and stable to heat and aeration. They exhibit characteristic absorption spectra with a maximum of 265 nm. Vitamin D$_2$ melts at 115 to 118° C and vitamin D$_3$ at 84 to 88° C.

Vitamin D$_4$ is 22, 23-dihydrovitamin D$_2$; its biologic activity does not appear to be significant.

The ultraviolet irradiation of ergosterol, a sterol of vegetable origin found principally in yeast and ergot, produces a series of chemical reactions yielding the following products: ergosterol → lumisterol → tachysterol → ergocalciferol → toxisterol → supresterols 1 and 2.

In the production of ergocalciferol (vitamin D$_2$), it is important that the conditions of irradiation permit the production of ergocalciferol to the exclusion of the toxic "overirradiation" products, such as toxisterol. In the past, certain irradiated ergosterol products were contaminated with toxisterol because proper consideration was not given to the degree of irradiation.

Drugs and foods are assayed for vitamin D by the rat curative "Line Test" and also by chromatographic-spectrophotometric assay. A color reaction with antimony trichloride and ultraviolet absorption are used for certain high-potency products, but in general, these are not applicable to food products.

Vitamin D aids in the utilization of calcium and phosphorus. It is essential to the development and maintenance of strong teeth and bones. Rickets in children and osteomalacia in adults are remedied and prevented by an adequate vitamin D intake. Vitamin D requirements are increased during pregnancy and lactation. One USP unit is equivalent to 0.025 μg of crystalline vitamin D_3 (cholecalciferol).

Of all the vitamins, vitamin D has the most serious toxic potential when administered in excessive doses. Adult doses of 100,000 USP units or more per day may lead to elevated serum levels of calcium and phosphorus and to attendant complications including metastatic calcification, renal failure, hypertension, and gastrointestinal symptoms. All forms of vitamin D are potentially dangerous. For this reason, the FDA has restricted to prescription use all oral preparations containing vitamin D in excess of 400 units per dose or recommended daily intake.

DAILY REQUIREMENTS. Infants, children, and pregnant or lactating women, 10 μg (400 units). Other adults have little need for vitamin D in the diet.

SOURCES. Cod liver oil and other fish oils; butter, cream, and liver; milk and cereals fortified with vitamin D; the activating action of sunlight or ultraviolet light on the skin.

Ergocalciferol, calciferol, or vitamin D_2 is 9,10-secoergosta-5,7,10(19),22,tetraen-3β-ol. It may be formed by exposing ergosterol to ultraviolet irradiation or other energy. It occurs as white, odorless crystals affected by air and light. It is insoluble in water but soluble in alcohol, chloroform, ether, and fatty oils. Ergocalciferol is an antirachitic vitamin. Usual daily dose is, in rickets: prophylactic, 10 μg (400 USP units), therapeutic, 300 μg to 1.25 mg (12,000 to 50,000 units); in hypocalcemic tetany, 1.25 to 10 mg (50,000 to 400,000 units).

PRESCRIPTION PRODUCTS. Drisdol®, Deltalin®, and Geltabs®.

Cholecalciferol, activated 7-dehydrocholesterol, or vitamin D_3 is 9,10-secocholesta-5,7,10(19)-trien-3β-ol. It may be formed by the irradiation of 7-dehydrocholesterol and resembles ergocalciferol in appearance and physical properties. It is an antirachitic vitamin. Usual dose is the same as for ergocalciferol. This vitamin is the only member of the D-group that occurs naturally in higher animals.

Oleovitamin A and D is a solution of vitamin A and vitamin D in fish liver oil or in an edible vegetable oil.

The label of the container of oleovitamin A and D should indicate the content of vitamin A in mg per g or in USP units of vitamin A per g. The label should further state whether the product contains ergocalciferol, cholecalciferol, or vitamin D from a natural source. The vitamin D content should be stated either in μg per g or in USP units of vitamin D per g. Usual dose is determined by the physician according to the needs of the patient.

Dihydrotachysterol or 9,10-secoergosta-5,7,22-trien-3β-ol, a steroid closely related to ergocalciferol, is prepared by the reduction of tachysterol. It occurs as colorless or white crystals, or as a white crystalline powder. Although it possesses only weak antirachitic activity, it is employed as a calcium-regulating steroid and is useful in the treatment of hypoparathyroidism, sprue, severe infantile diarrhea, and tetany. Usual dose range is: initial, 800 μg to 2.4 mg daily; maintenance, 200 μg to 1 mg daily.

PRESCRIPTION PRODUCT. Hytakerol®.

DRIED YEAST

Yeasts are unicellular organisms and are usually regarded as greatly reduced sac fungi. They feed on sugars, splitting them to form alcohols and carbon dioxide. Hence, yeasts are important in the alcohol industry and also in the making of bread, where the liberated carbon dioxide tends to swell the dough, making it porous and "light." Yeast is also used medicinally as a source of vitamin B.

Brewer's yeast is a viscid, semifluid, frothy mass containing the living cells of *Saccharomyces cerevisiae* Hansen (Fam. Saccharomycetaceae), or of other species of *Saccharomyces* associated with bacteria and molds. Pure strains of yeast may be grown in suitable culture media containing sucrose and certain salts or proteins.

When yeast is grown at a temperature of 15 to 20° C, the cells are larger, tend to "bud" and form chains of cells, and rise to the top of the fermenting mass. This growth is known as "top" yeast. If the temperature is kept near or below 10° C, the yeast cells are smaller, do not bud, and apparently reproduce from spores. The cells tend to remain in the lower portion of the fermenting mass and constitute "bottom" yeast.

Compressed yeast is brewer's yeast or purer strains of yeast, partially dried by expression of water and admixed with a starchy or absorbent base. These yeast "cakes" wrapped in air-proof foil maintain the life of the yeast cells for a relatively long period of time.

Dried yeast consists of the dried cells of any suitable strain of *Saccharomyces cerevisiae* or *Candida utilis* (Henneberg) Lodder and Kreger-Van Rij (Fam. Cryptococcaceae), commonly called torula yeast. Dried yeast may be obtained by growing suitable strains of the above species in media, other than those required for beer production, under appropriate environmental conditions. Such yeasts, properly designated as to species, are commonly known as "primary dried yeasts."

Dried yeast may also be obtained as a by-product of brewing beer. The yeasts are washed to free them of beer residues; sometimes the washing procedure may include the use of one or more alkaline solutions to remove the insoluble acidic bitter resins left on the yeast cells by the hops. Such washed and dried yeasts are commonly known as "brewer's dried yeasts" or, if the acidic bitter resins are removed, "debittered dried yeasts."

Dried yeast occurs as yellowish white to weak yellowish orange flakes, granules, or powder with an odor and taste characteristic of the type. Because the cells are dead, dried yeast is inactive in fermenting power.

Yeast contains a number of enzymes, including zymase, diastase, and invertase; nucleoproteins; glycogen; and the vitamins of the B complex.

Dried yeast contains not less than 45% of protein and, in each gram, the equivalent of not less than 120 μg of thiamine hydrochloride, 40 μg of riboflavin, and 300 μg of niacin. The live bacteria count does not exceed 7500 per g, and the mold count does not exceed 50 per g.

USE AND DOSE. Dried yeast is a natural source of protein and B-complex vitamins. It is used almost exclusively for its vitamin B-complex content. Usual dose is 10 g, 4 times a day.

VITAMIN B COMPLEX

Vitamin B complex includes a number of dietary essentials that are found in significant quantities in liver and yeast. Originally, these natural extracts were thought to contain only one vitamin, but as research progressed, several components were eventually isolated. In an early classification, the "B complex" was subdivided into vitamins B_1 and B_2; the former was thermolabile and the latter thermostable. The structures of at least 12 and possibly more substances recognized as members of this group are known. The vitamin status of some of them, although included in the group, is not clearly established. The members of the group have little in common from a chemical standpoint.

THIAMINE

Thiamine hydrochloride or vitamin B$_1$ occurs as small, white crystals or as a crystalline powder. It decomposes at 248° C and, in dry form, is relatively stable to heat and light. In aqueous solution, the pH is about 3.1, and such solutions may be sterilized by heating for 20 minutes at 120° C or for 1 hour at 100° C without appreciable loss of potency. In foods, however, there is some destruction of the vitamin during cooking.

Thiamine hydrochloride is assayed fluorometrically. It occurs in nature in the free form or as thiamine pyrophosphate (cocarboxylase) or as the cocarboxylase protein complex.

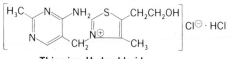

Thiamine Hydrochloride

Studies with the enzyme systems in bakers' yeast have elucidated the final steps in the biosynthesis of thiamine. These involve reactions between a pyrimidine pyrophosphate and a thiazole monophosphate to form first thiamine monophosphate and then thiamine. However, the origin of the pyrimidine and thiazole moieties remains obscure. The pyrimidine structure may derive from the same precursors as other pyrimidines, e.g., purine bases, q.v., but experimental evidence is lacking.

Vitamin B$_1$ has a fundamental function in intermediate carbohydrate metabolism in all living cells and is therefore essential for the normal functioning of all body organs and tissues. In the body, thiamine is converted to the pyrophosphate, cocarboxylase, which functions as a coenzyme in the decarboxylation of pyruvic acid to form acetyl-CoA and carbon dioxide. The vitamin is not stored in the body to any appreciable extent; the excess is largely eliminated or destroyed. Marked deficiency symptoms that respond to thiamine therapy are emotional hypersensitivity, loss of appetite, susceptibility to fatigue, muscular weakness, and beriberi. Symptoms of mild or subacute thiamine deficiency are less clearly defined.

DAILY REQUIREMENT. Adults, 1 to 1.4 mg; children, 0.6 to 1.1 mg. Exact requirements vary according to body weight, caloric intake, intestinal synthesis, and fat content of the diet. Needs are increased during pregnancy and lactation.

Thiamine occurs in enriched cereals, whole grain cereals, milk, legumes, and meats. Special sources include yeast, liver concentrates, and synthetic thiamine.

Thiamine hydrochloride, aneurine hydrochloride, thiamin chloride, vitamin B$_1$, or vitamin B$_1$ hydrochloride is a water-soluble vitamin (enzyme cofactor). It is a member of the vitamin B complex. Usual dose is, orally or intramuscularly, prophylactic, 5 to 10 mg daily; therapeutic, 10 to 20 (35) mg, 3 times a day.

PROPRIETARY PRODUCT. Betalin S® and Bewon, Elixir®.

Thiamine mononitrate, thiamine nitrate, or vitamin B$_1$ mononitrate is similar to thiamine hydrochloride in therapeutic use and dose.

RIBOFLAVIN

Riboflavin, vitamin B$_2$, vitamin G, or lactoflavin was first identified in milk and, because of its yellow color, was known as "lactochrome" and later as "lactoflavin." It occurs naturally in the free form or in various chemical complexes with protein, phosphoric acid, adenine, or nucleic acid.

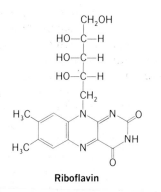

Riboflavin

Riboflavin is slightly soluble in water and in alcohol; it is insoluble in lipoidal solvents. It crystallizes from absolute alcohol as yellow, needle-shaped crystals that melt with decomposition at 280° C. Although it is stable to dry heat and to oxidation, it is sensitive to light. It is stable in acid solution, but unstable in alkaline solution. In solution, riboflavin possesses an intense greenish yellow fluorescence. When exposed to light in acid solution, the vitamin is changed to lumichrome. When irradiated in alkaline solution, a degradative split occurs yielding a new pigment, lumiflavin. Neither lumichrome nor lumiflavin possesses physiologic activity. The vitamin is assayed fluorometrically.

Many of the details of riboflavin biosynthesis are still unknown, although it has been shown to originate from a purine precursor. Available evidence indicates that guanine, or a metabolic equivalent, is converted via intermediates not yet established with certainty to 6,7-dimethyl-8-ribityllumazine (DMRL). This compound yields a C_4 fragment or possibly 2 C_2 fragments, which, in turn, recombines with another molecule of DMRL to form riboflavin.

Riboflavin, following its ingestion, combines with phosphoric acid and protein to form an enzyme called "Warbug's Yellow Enzyme" or "the yellow oxidation enzyme." Apparently riboflavin cannot be synthesized by animal cells and therefore must be supplied in the diet. Riboflavin functions, as the yellow enzyme, in tissue oxidation. Deficiency symptoms are characterized by cheilosis, glossitis, and peeling of the skin. Ocular disturbances are characterized by itching, burning, and a sensation of roughness of the eyes accompanied by mild photophobia.

DAILY REQUIREMENT. Adult, 1.5 to 1.7 mg; children, 0.6 to 1.2 mg. These requirements are related to caloric intake and protein levels. They are increased during pregnancy and lactation.

Milk, egg yolk, liver, meats, green leafy vegetables, and bread contain riboflavin.

Riboflavin or vitamin B₂ is a water-soluble vitamin (enzyme cofactor). Usual dose is, daily, orally or parenterally, prophylactic, 2 mg; therapeutic, 5 to 10 mg.

NIACIN AND NIACINAMIDE

Niacin or nicotinic acid and niacinamide or nicotinamide. The names niacin and niacinamide are utilized in the pharmaceutic literature because they do not have the phonetic similarity to nicotine as do the chemical names.

They have the following structural formulas:

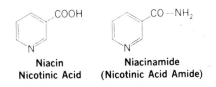

Niacin
Nicotinic Acid

Niacinamide
(Nicotinic Acid Amide)

These compounds have been known since 1867, and their presence in animal tissues was recognized in 1912. No dietary importance was attached to them, however, until 1937 when it was reported that liver, a source rich in niacin, cured "black tongue" in dogs, which had long been considered to have a counterpart in the human disease known as pellagra.

Niacin occurs as colorless, odorless needles or as a crystalline powder; it melts between 234 and 237° C. It is soluble in water and alcohol, but is insoluble in lipoidal solvents. It is quite stable in dry form and in solution. The amide, also a colorless, crystalline powder, is slightly hygroscopic and has a slightly bitter taste; it melts between 128 and 131° C and is more soluble in water and alcohol than in the acid. It is quite stable in dry form and in solution. Prolonged exposure to light should be avoided.

Biosynthesis of Nicotinic Acid. This vitamin originates via one pathway in certain higher plants and bacteria and via an entirely different pathway in animals and certain fungi. The first route involves a reaction between aspartic acid and glyceraldehyde-3-phosphate, as has been noted in the discussion of nicotinic acid as a nicotine precursor in *Nicotiana* species (see page 199). Animals and fungi employ an alternate route that utilizes tryptophan as a precursor and leads to nicotinic acid

by a number of seemingly devious but well-documented reactions (Fig. 11–2).

In nature, the vitamin is found as the free acid or as its amide, chemically bound in a number of enzyme systems. Niacinamide is the functional group in coenzymes I and II, nicotinamide adenine dinucleotide and nicotinamide adenine dinucleotide phosphate, respectively. These compounds have an important function in tissue respiration, in carbohydrate metabolism, and in fermentations by transporting hydrogen.

The potency of niacin is expressed on a weight basis. The compound, particularly in admixture, may be assayed microbiologically, but a chemical colorimetric method using cyanogen bromide and various amines is now ordinarily employed. Although most of the symptoms of pellagra are owing to a deficiency of niacin, it is now believed that the various manifestations of the disease are not all caused by the deficiency of a single vitamin. The appropriate administration of niacin leads to a disappearance of the alimentary, dermal, and other lesions characteristic of the disease, but the vitamin does not influence the polyneuritis or

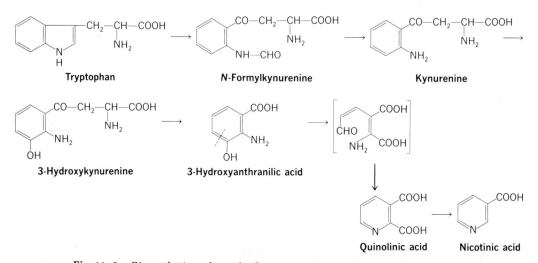

Fig. 11–2. Biosynthetic pathway leading to nicotinic acid in animals and fungi.

cheilosis so frequently observed in pellagrous patients. These patients require the administration of thiamine and riboflavin.

DAILY REQUIREMENTS. Adults, 13 to 18 mg; children, 8 to 15 mg.

Niacin occurs in meats, liver, eggs, milk, cereals, and nuts. In addition, 4 cups of strong coffee provide an adequate daily intake.

Niacin, nicotinic acid, or 3-pyridine-carboxylic acid is a water-soluble vitamin (enzyme cofactor). It is an effective but transient peripheral vasodilator. Usual dose is, requirement, orally, 20 mg daily; therapeutic, orally and parenterally, 50 mg, 3 to 10 times a day.

Niacinamide, nicotinamide, or nicotinic acid amide does not possess the vasodilator activity of niacin, but is otherwise similar. Usual dose is, prophylactic, orally and parenterally, 10 to 20 mg, once a day; therapeutic, orally, 50 mg, 3 to 10 times a day, parenterally, 25 to 50 mg, 2 to 10 times a day.

PANTOTHENIC ACID

Pantothenic acid is the designation for the factor in the vitamin B complex that is necessary for the proper growth of animals. It is also known as the "chick antidermatitis factor."

It is dextrorotatory and is usually marketed as the calcium salt, **calcium D(+)-pantothenate;** however, the racemic form is also available.

The acid itself is a viscous oily liquid, soluble in water and some organic solvents, but insoluble in benzene and chroroform. Pantothenic acid is unstable toward acids, alkalies, and prolonged heating when in aqueous solution. The calcium salt is relatively thermostable, but is unstable towards alkalies, acids, ferric salts, and calcium precipitants. The salt is a white, crystalline powder.

Biosynthesis of Pantothenic Acid. Examination of the structure of this vitamin reveals that it is a compound molecule composed of the amino acid, β-alanine, and a substituted butyric acid designated pantoic acid. Experimental evidence reveals that pantothenic acid derives from β-alanine and α-ketoisovaleric acid.

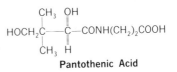

$$HOCH_2C \overset{\overset{\displaystyle CH_3}{|}}{\underset{\underset{\displaystyle CH_3}{|}}{\;}} \overset{\overset{\displaystyle OH}{|}}{\underset{\underset{\displaystyle H}{|}}{C}} CONH(CH_2)_2COOH$$

Pantothenic Acid

The potency of this vitamin is usually expressed in milligrams of the acid. It is assayed by a microbiologic method employing *Lactobacillus plantarum.*

Although pantothenic acid is found in most living tissue, its definite role is unknown, and no definite pantothenic acid deficiency has been demonstrated in human beings.

DAILY REQUIREMENT. Unknown, but estimated to be 10 to 15 mg for adults. No data are available for children.

Liver, kidney, yeast, milk, cereals, legumes, and nuts contain pantothenic acid.

Calcium pantothenate or calcium D(+)-pantothenate is the calcium salt of the dextrorotatory isomer of pantothenic acid. It is a water-soluble vitamin (enzyme cofactor). Usual dose is 10 mg, once a day.

Racemic calcium pantothenate or calcium (±)-pantothenate is a mixture of the calcium salts of the dextrorotatory and levorotatory isomers of pantothenic acid. Its physiologic activity is approximately one-half that of calcium pantothenate. Usual dose is 20 mg (equivalent to approximately 10 mg of dextrorotatory calcium pantothenate).

PROPRIETARY PRODUCT. Pantholin®.

PYRIDOXINE

Pyridoxine or vitamin B$_6$ consists of a group in which pyridoxine is one of three members. The 3 forms known at the present time are as follows:

human beings, a diagnosis based on clinical symptoms is impossible. Pyridoxine deficiency may accompany other deficiencies of the B complex, however. The failure of patients suffering from B-complex deficiency to recover com-

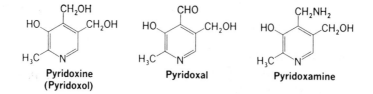

Pyridoxine
(Pyridoxol)   Pyridoxal   Pyridoxamine

The 3 forms are about equally active for rats but not for microorganisms. Pyridoxine hydrochloride melts at 204 to 208° C, is soluble in water, alcohol, and acetone, and is slightly soluble in other organic solvents. It is stable toward heat, concentrated acid, and alkali, but is destroyed by light. Potencies of pyridoxine are expressed in milligrams or micrograms. Biologic methods of assay are either microbiologic, spectrophotometric, or titrimetric. Microbiologic procedures use *Lactobacillus helveticus*, *Streptococcus faecalis*, and *Saccharomyces carlsbergensis*.

Investigations of the biosynthesis of pyridoxine have been hindered by the failure of investigators to find biologic systems that produce pyridoxine in workable quantities. Consequently, it is impossible to make a definite statement regarding its production in living organisms.

Pyridoxine appears to be related to the metabolism of fats and amino acids. Its exact biologic function is, however, not fully understood. Rats deprived of pyridoxine develop a symmetric dermatitis (acrodynia) and fail to grow. Dogs and other animals develop microcytic anemia and exhibit a degeneration of striated and cardiac muscles.

Because no definite vitamin B$_6$ deficiency syndrome has been recognized in

pletely when riboflavin and nicotinic acid were administered has been noted. Such patients continued to complain of extreme nervousness, irritability, insomnia, abdominal pain, and difficulty in walking. Parenteral administration of pyridoxine hydrochloride in such patients has supposedly produced dramatic relief.

DAILY REQUIREMENT. Unknown, but recommended daily allowances are, adults, 2 mg; children, 0.5 to 1.2 mg. Meats, seafoods, cereals, legumes, and yeast contain pyridoxine.

Pyridoxine hydrochloride is a vitamin B-complex component. It functions as a water-soluble vitamin (enzyme cofactor). Usual dose is, orally and parenterally, prophylactic, 2 mg, once a day; therapeutic, 10 to 150 mg, 1 to 3 times a day.

PROPRIETARY PRODUCT. Hexa-Betalin®.

INOSITOL

Inositol, a member of the vitamin B complex, has the following formula:

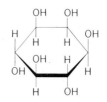

Of the 8 possible isomers, only one (meso-inositol) is optically inactive. This optically inactive isomer is the only isomer that is active as a growth factor. It occurs in the free form and in various complexes, such as phytin and liposterol. Inositol is soluble in water and insoluble in petroleum ether and in absolute alcohol. It is stable toward heat, strong acids, and alkalies. The anhydrous form melts at 225 to 226° C. Amounts of inositol are expressed in milligrams rather than in units. Microbiologic methods employing *Saccharomyces cerevisiae* or *Neurospora sitophila* have been used.

The structural similarities of glucose and inositol indicate that the former compound is a possible biosynthetic precursor of the vitamin. Experiments have shown that glucose can function in this way, but indirectly because different carbon atoms of the sugar are incorporated in different degrees. The suggestion that inositol is formed via condensation of a C_2 fragment with a C_4 fragment requires verification.

The nutritional status of inositol is controversial. Under certain conditions it appears to prevent alopecia, to have lipotropic activity, and to influence gastric motility. Conflicting observations indicate that inositol is not a dietary essential or that the substance may be involved in intestinal flora activity. Because no specific deficiency syndromes in man have been attributed to inositol, its exact role in human metabolism is unknown.

Daily Requirement. Unknown. Inositol occurs in cereals, citrus fruits, certain meats, milk, and yeast.

Inositol, *i*-inositol, or *meso*-inositol is 1,2,3,5/4,6-cyclohexanehexol. It is isolated from liver and is widely distributed in nature; however, most of the commercial supply is synthetic. It is a vitamin B-complex component and is also a lipotropic. Usual dose is 2 g.

PARA-AMINOBENZOIC ACID

Para-aminobenzoic acid has long been known as a synthetic organic chemical compound and has the following formula:

It has also been recognized as a component of the B complex, but only for those animals that do not use preformed folic acid with its p-aminobenzoyl moiety. Because human beings do utilize folic acid, p-aminobenzoic acid is not a vitamin for them, and its use as a nutritional supplement is not justified. The substance occurs in the free state or in the acetylated or conjugated form. It is soluble in boiling water and alcohol and stable toward acids and alkalies. The colorless crystals melt at 187 to 188° C. It is destroyed by ferric salts and oxidizing agents. Potency is expressed in terms of milligrams of p-aminobenzoic acid. Both chemical and microbiologic methods have been used in the assay of this compound; however, the chemical method is officially recognized.

Para-aminobenzoic acid is probably derived biosynthetically from shikimic acid, but direct evidence of the incorporation of the carbon atoms of the suspected precursor into the vitamin is lacking. The nitrogen atom of the vitamin arises from the amide nitrogen of glutamine.

Removal of p-aminobenzoic acid from the diet causes achromotrichia in rats and failure of growth in chicks. It is active in neutralizing the bacteriostatic effect of some sulfa drugs. It is employed topically as a sunscreen in the form of a 0.5 to 5% solution.

DAILY REQUIREMENT. None for human beings. Meats and vegetables contain p-aminobenzoic acid.

Aminobenzoic acid, para-aminobenzoic acid, or PABA is usually produced synthetically although it is present in natural products. It is considered a member of the vitamin B complex for certain animals. In humans, it is administered with salicylates in the treatment of rheumatic fever to prolong the effect of the salicylates. Usual dose is, orally, in combination with salicylates, 600 mg, 4 to 6 times a day.

BIOTIN

Biotin or vitamin H is the yeast growth or the anti-egg-white injury factor.

Free biotin is somewhat water- and alcohol-soluble, but is relatively insoluble in ether, chloroform, and petroleum ether. The substance is heat stable and does not decompose when heated with acids or alkalies. The pure vitamin melts at 231 to 232° C, whereas its methyl ester melts at 166 to 167° C. Biotin is active in both animals and microorganisms, and the methyl ester is active for animals but not for all microorganisms. Amounts of biotin are expressed in milligrams, and microbiologic methods of assay employ *Lactobacillus plantarum* or *Saccharomyces cerevisiae.*

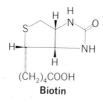
Biotin

Recent studies have confirmed that pimelic acid is a precursor of biotin. Details of the biosynthetic pathway are unknown. Desthiobiotin may be an immediate precursor of biotin, but experimental data are equivocal on this point.

Biotin deficiency symptoms have not as yet been definitely established because the compound is produced by intestinal flora and excreted in the feces in amounts 2 to 5 times greater than the dietary intake. The vitamin, however, is claimed to be necessary for the maintenance of health. It is thought to be present in minute amounts in every living cell. Some of the symptoms that reflect a deficiency of biotin are said to be seborrheic dermatitis, pallor of the skin, mental depression, and muscular pains. Avidin, a raw-egg-white protein, induces biotin deficiency by forming a nonabsorbable avidin-biotin complex.

The biotin content of cancerous tumors is higher than that of normal tissues.

DAILY REQUIREMENT. Unknown but estimated to be 150 to 300 μg. Egg yolk, liver, kidney, yeast, grains, and milk contain biotin.

CHOLINE

Choline, as a component of lecithin and as a phospholipid, has been known for many years. It has the following formula:

$$\left| (CH_3)_3 \overset{\oplus}{-}N-CH_2-CH_2-OH \right| OH^{\ominus}$$

Some authorities have recognized it as a member of the B complex, but this classification is questioned by others. Choline is marketed as the chloride, bitartrate, and dihydrogen citrate. Choline and choline salts are freely soluble in water and alcohol, but are insoluble in ether, benzene, and petroleum ether. They are stable to heat in acid solution, but are unstable in alkaline solution. They are extremely hygroscopic. Potencies are expressed in milligrams of choline. Colorimetric and microbiologic procedures have been used as methods of assays.

BIOSYNTHESIS OF CHOLINE. Choline originates from serine by decarboxylation and

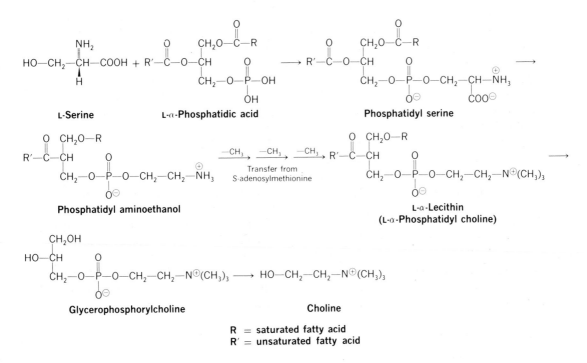

Fig. 11–3. Biosynthesis of choline.

stepwise N-methylation of the resulting aminoethanol. However, these reactions do not take place with the compounds per se, but with their phosphatidyl derivatives, thereby resulting in the formation of lecithin, which yields choline on hydrolysis (Fig. 11–3).

Choline is the basic constituent of lecithin. It affects the fat transport and, indirectly, the carbohydrate metabolism. Deficiency of choline leads to hemorrhagic kidney degeneration. It is one of the pancreatic factors that prevents development of fatty livers in depancreatized animals. Choline is useful in the treatment of cirrhosis of human liver.

DAILY REQUIREMENT. Unknown. Choline occurs in egg yolk, heart, liver, sweetbreads, milk, fish, root vegetables, fruits, and grains.

Choline dihydrogen citrate is (2-hydroxyethyl)trimethylammonium dihydrogen citrate. Although it is sometimes considered to be a member of the vitamin B complex, it is used as a lipotropic. Usual dose is 2 g.

PROPRIETARY PRODUCT. Cholinate®.

CYANOCOBALAMIN

Cyanocobalamin or vitamin B_{12} is a crystalline compound isolated originally from liver extract; it represents the active principle of liver that is effective in the treatment of pernicious anemia. It occurs as dark red crystals or as a crystalline or amorphous powder; when anhydrous, it is hygroscopic and may absorb about 12% of water if exposed to the air. It is a metabolic product of *Streptomyces griseus*.

A rapid spectrophotometric assay for vitamin B_{12} has now largely replaced earlier microbiologic procedures involving

Lactobacillus leichmannii or other organisms.

Experiments have shown that the porphyrin-like corrin ring of cyanocobalamin originates from succinyl-CoA and glycine. These compounds react to form α-amino-β-ketoadipic acid, δ-aminolevulinic acid, porphobilinogen, and, ultimately, the porphyrin moiety of B_{12}. Methyl groups on the porphyrin ring derive from methionine, and the aminopropanol portion of B_{12} derives from threonine.

Cyanocobalamin may occur as several vitamers (B_{12a}, B_{12b}, B_{12c}, B_{12d}), which are designated as cobalamins. The word "cobalamin" is from the term "cobalt-vitamin." (The cobalt is responsible for the red color).

dose is, intramuscularly or subcutaneously, maintenance, 100 μg, once a month or every other month; therapeutic, 100 μg, once or twice a week. The recommended allowances of cyanocobalamin are: adults, 5 to 6 μg per day; children, 2 to 5 μg per day. Cyanocobalamin injection is available commercially.

PRESCRIPTION SPECIALTIES. Betalin 12 Crystalline®, Rubramin PC®, Redisol®, and many others.

Cyanocobalamin Co 57 capsules and solution and cyanocobalamin Co 60 capsules and solution are products containing radioactive cobalt in their molecular structures. The specific activity of these preparations is not less than 0.5 μCi per μg of cyanocobalamin. When calculating dos-

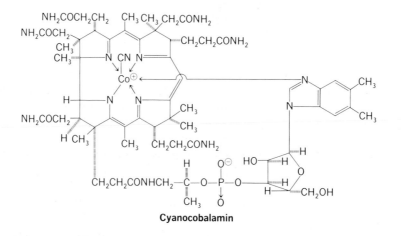

Cyanocobalamin

USES AND DOSE. Cyanocobalamin is a water-soluble hematopoietic vitamin. It functions as a coenzyme in the synthesis of nucleic acids, proteins, and lipids and specifically helps to maintain epithelial cells and the myelin sheath of nerves. A significant role is also played in leukopoiesis and, with folic acid, in erythropoiesis. Cyanocobalamin serves as a standard for comparison of the activity of other antianemic products (see page 323). Usual

age, a correction should be made for radioactive decay because the radioactive half-life of ^{57}Co is 270 days and that of ^{60}Co is 5.27 years. NOTE: The expiration date for the capsules and solutions of both radioactive substances is not later than 6 months after date of standardization.

The administration of radioactive cyanocobalamin to patients suffering from pernicious anemia causes practically all of the compound to bind to plasma proteins, rather than to be excreted to a large degree in the urine, as occurs in normal individuals. Thus, these preparations serve a useful function in the detection of pernicious anemia.

USE AND DOSE. Cyanocobalamin Co 57 and Cyanocobalamin Co 60 preparations are classed as diagnostic aids in determining pernicious anemia. Usual dose of cyanocobalamin Co 57 is the equivalent of 0.5 μCi; of cyanocobalamin Co 60, 0.5 to 2 μg, containing not more than 1 μCi.

PRESCRIPTION PRODUCTS. Rubratope-57® and Rubratope-60®.

Vitamin B$_{12}$ with intrinsic factor concentrate is vitamin B$_{12}$ that is made more readily absorbable from the gastrointestinal tract of patients with pernicious anemia by combination with suitable preparations of the stomach or intestine of domestic animals used for food by man.

PRESCRIPTION PRODUCTS. Trinsicon®, Pronemia®, Perrihemin®, and Ferritrinsic® are a few of the many products containing vitamin B$_{12}$ and intrinsic factor concentrate in combination with other vitamins.

Hydroxocobalamin or vitamin B$_{12a}$ is an analog of cyanocobalamin in which the cyano radical has been replaced by a hydroxyl group. Although it occurs naturally as a fermentation product, hydroxocobalamin is also produced commercially by semisynthesis from cyanocobalamin.

USES AND DOSE. Hydroxocobalamin is said to produce slightly higher and more prolonged blood levels on intramuscular injection than does cyanocobalamin, but the clinical significance of this is slight. Usual dose is, intramuscularly, maintenance, 50 μg every 2 weeks or 100 μg monthly; therapeutic, 50 μg, 2 or 3 times weekly.

PRESCRIPTION SPECIALTY. Neo-Betalin 12®.

FOLIC ACID

Folic acid, folacin, or pteroylglutamic acid is a natural vitamin conjugate found in plant and animal tissues. Because it was originally isolated from leafy vegetables, the name "folic" acid was applied. This vitamin is one of the B-complex group and is related to several growth factors, such as B$_c$, *Lactobacillus casei* factor, and vitamin M. Whereas folic acid is composed of one molecule of glutamic acid, the others contain several molecules.

BIOSYNTHESIS OF FOLIC ACID. The pteridine ring of folic acid is apparently biosynthesized either from purine or a purine equivalent via an intermediate that is either 2-amino-4-hydroxypteridine-6-carboxaldehyde or a closely related compound. The p-aminobenzoic acid moiety derives from shikimic acid. A molecule of glutamic aid completes the structure of the vitamin (Fig. 11–4).

It occurs as a yellow or yellowish orange, odorless, crystalline powder and is slightly soluble in water. Deficiency of this vitamin causes retardation of growth and macrocytic anemia in the chick and the rat. It is present in liver extract.

USES AND DOSE. Folic acid is a B-complex vitamin that has hematopoietic properties. It functions as a coenzyme in such different vital metabolic reactions as purine and pyrimidine synthesis, histidine and tryptophan metabolism, erythropoiesis, leukopoiesis, and cell and organ growth and maintenance. Usual dose is, orally or parenterally, maintenance, 100 to 250 μg, once a day; therapeutic, 250 μg to 1 mg, once a day. The estimated recommended allowance, adults or children, is 0.4 mg per day. In the human being, this amount is normally provided by intestinal synthesis, but in conditions such as illness or pregnancy, additional amounts are required.

The FDA ruled that all products containing more than 0.4 mg of folic acid must be considered prescription items and must not be sold over the counter. This restriction was imposed because large doses of folic acid can induce an incomplete and

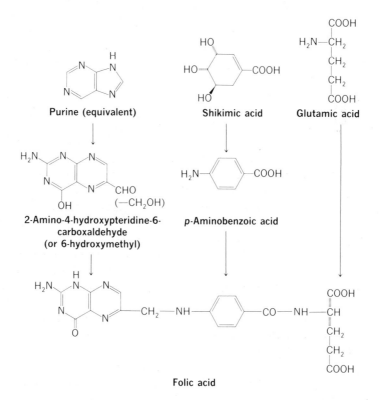

Fig. 11–4. Biosynthesis of folic acid.

temporary hematopoietic response in pernicious anemia, possibly causing the physician to overlook the basic disorder. Moreover, folic acid alone does not affect the progressive neurologic lesions associated with the disease, which may become serious and irreversible. These lesions can be treated effectively with a combination of folic acid and cyanocobalamin.

PRESCRIPTION SPECIALTIES Folvite® is a folic acid product; in combination, folic acid is present in many "antistress" formulas and in "multivitamin" preparations.

VITAMIN C

Ascorbic acid or vitamin C is found naturally in several forms: as the reduced form

(ascorbic acid), as the oxidized form (dehydroascorbic acid), and as ascorbinogen (the protein complex). Ascorbic acid is called the antiscorbutic factor.

The formula for the reduced form is as follows:

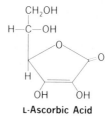

L-Ascorbic Acid

whereas the oxidized form has the following structure:

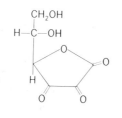

L-Dehydroascorbic Acid

Ascorbic acid is an optically active compound, but only the levo-form is biologically active. It is an odorless, white, crystalline substance that slowly darkens when exposed to light. It melts at 190 to 192°C and is soluble in water, alcohol, and propylene glycol, but is insoluble in ether and benzene. Dry ascorbic acid is fairly stable, but aqueous solutions are rapidly decomposed when exposed to air. Ascorbic acid is a relatively strong reducing agent; it is reversibly oxidized to dehydroascorbic acid. The latter can be further oxidized to 2,3,diketo-L-gulonic acid, which is inactive. Alkalies accelerate both oxidations, but acids retard them. Because ascorbic acid is the least stable of all vitamins, special consideration must be given to this factor when planning diets.

The potency is expressed in milligrams of ascorbic acid. Although bioassay methods based on the curative or preventive effect of ascorbic acid continue to be used, the official assay involves titration with standard dichlorophenol-indophenol solution.

As was long suspected on the basis of structural similarities, ascorbic acid is derived from hexoses. Both D-glucose and D-galactose function as precursors of the vitamin in both plants and animals (except primates and guinea pigs). In each case, the pathway involves uronic acid and lactone intermediates.

Vitamin C is essential for the proper formation and maintenance of intercellular material in tissues, especially of bones and teeth. It prevents and cures scurvy and is claimed by some authorities to be valuable in increasing resistance to infection. It has definitely been established as clinically important in the healing of wounds. Ascorbic acid is an important factor in preventing oxidation and rancidity in foodstuffs.

The assertion of Linus Pauling that the daily ingestion of large doses (1 to 4 g) of ascorbic acid is useful in preventing and treating the common cold has resulted in much partisanship and little satisfactory evidence. Recent research has revealed that (1) large amounts of ascorbic acid can be stored in leukocytes and platelets, (2) determination of plasma levels alone is insufficient for establishing tissue utilization, (3) ascorbic acid is involved in histamine detoxification and protects against some consequences of stress, and (4) large doses stimulate the microsomal enzyme system, which facilitates the destruction of various organic compounds including ascorbic acid itself. However, it must be concluded that, at present, the utility of megadoses of ascorbic acid in treating and preventing the common cold is only by inference.

DAILY REQUIREMENT. Adults, 55 to 60 mg; children, 40 mg; additional amounts are required in such cases as pregnancy, lactation, infection, stress, allergies, and old age.

Fresh fruits, potatoes, green leafy vegetables, and seafoods contain vitamin C.

Ascorbic acid or vitamin C is prepared synthetically, but it is a common vitamin in citrus fruits, tomatoes, and other fruits. It is an antiscorbutic vitamin and is available as ascorbic acid tablets and as ascorbic acid injection. Usual dose is, orally or parenterally, maintenance, 60 mg, once a day; therapeutic, 100 to 250 mg, 1 or 2 times a day.

PROPRIETARY PRODUCTS. Ascorbicap®, Cecon®, Cevalin®, and Ce-Vi-Sol®.

VITAMIN E

Vitamin E designates various forms of alpha tocopherol. It includes (+)- or (±)-alpha tocopherol, their acetate or acid succinate esters, and preparations of these compounds (except the acid succinate ester) in suitable vehicles. It must be labeled to indicate the chemical form or forms present, their weight in milligrams, and equivalents in terms of International units of vitamin E. In nature, α-tocopherol is accompanied by several structurally related vitamers, including β- γ-, and δ-tocopherol. These possess similar, but lesser (0.1 to 0.01) vitamin E potencies.

The structural formulas are as follows:

One International unit of vitamin E is equivalent to 1 mg of pure (±)-α-tocopherol acetate. Gas chromatographic assay methods are now generally employed.

No definitive experiments have been reported on the biosynthesis of vitamin E. However, from an inspection of the structures of the tocopherols and comparison to analogous structures, one may conclude that this type of vitamin derives via the acetate-mevalonic acid pathway.

Vitamin E is essential for the normal course of pregnancy in rats and also for normal growth and the prevention of paralysis in rats. In human nutrition, it apparently helps to insure cellular mem-

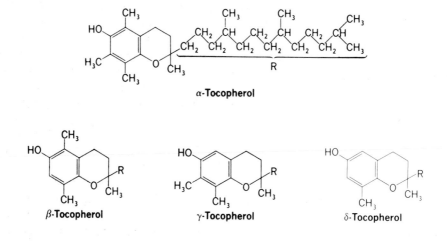

α-Tocopherol

β-Tocopherol   γ-Tocopherol   δ-Tocopherol

All 4 compounds are odorless oils that are insoluble in water, but soluble in alcohol, ether, and other fat solvents. They are stable to heat in the absence of oxygen, stable to strong acids and visible light, but unstable to ultraviolet light, alkalies, and oxidation. The tocopherols are antioxidants (the *delta* compound is significantly more effective than any of the others), but they are destroyed by rancid fats. The esters of the tocopherols are more stable than the free alcohols. Tocopherols are used to stabilize vitamin A preparations.

brane integrity, probably by mechanisms that include the conversion of free radicals, the destructive products of oxidative deterioration of unsaturated fatty acids, to less harmful, nonreactive forms. It has not been proven to be therapeutically effective in restoring sexual potency, preventing abortion, reversing or preventing the onset of senility, or treating cardiovascular disease, and the promotion of vitamin E for these and similar conditions must be considered as fraudulent. In fact, the megadoses of several thousand International units that have been recommended for such purposes by faddists have recently been shown to produce deleterious effects in small animals.

DOSAGE. The usual prophylactic dose of vitamin E ranges from 5 to 30 International units. The therapeutic dose is determined by the physician according to the needs of the patient. Recommended allowances are, adults, 25 to 30 IU per day; children, 10 to 15 IU per day.

Vitamin E occurs in wheat germ oil, cottonseed oil, green leafy vegetables, egg yolk, and meat.

PROPRIETARY PRODUCTS. Because of the different forms of vitamin E that are available commercially, as well as the recent "faddism" connected with this vitamin, proprietary products are especially numerous. A few selected examples are Aquasol E®, Ecofrol®, Eprolin®, and E-Ferol Succinate®.

VITAMIN K

Vitamin K, the coagulation vitamin, occurs naturally in 2 forms: vitamin K_1 and vitamin K_2. Many synthetic compounds of related chemical constitution also have vitamin K activity.

Although experimental proof is lacking, examination of the structures of the 2 forms of vitamin K leads to the conclusion that biosynthesis takes place via the acetate-mevalonic acid pathway.

Vitamin K is said to be necessary for the formation of prothrombin in the liver. Because prothrombin is an essential constituent for the normal clotting of the blood, vitamin K has an indirect function in that process. A deficiency of prothrombin (hypoprothrombinemia) results in a prolongation of the clotting time.

Deficiency of vitamin K is seldom owing to dietary origin. Because vitamin K is formed by microorganisms in the intestines, it seems reasonable to conclude that normal humans are largely independent of a dietary supply. Inadequate absorption does occur in cases of obstruction, jaundice, diarrhea, and during the excessive use of laxatives.

The special use of vitamin K lies in its prevention of hemorrhagic disease of the newborn.

Definite daily requirements have not as yet been determined because they are normally met by the quantities of vitamin K synthesized by intestinal bacteria. The therapeutic dose for the cure or prophylaxis of prothrombinopenia is 5 to 25 mg daily. The effect is tested after about 8 hours, and the dosage is increased if no perceptible rise of the prothrombin level has occurred. Toxic effects have been noted in animals following the administration of large doses.

Vitamin K occurs in green leafy materials, such as spinach and kale, and in tomatoes and vegetable oils.

Phytonadione, 2-methyl-3-phytyl-1,4-naphthoquinone, phylloquinone, or vitamin K_1 may be obtained from alfalfa, spinach, and other green vegetables. It occurs as a clear, yellow, viscous, odorless or nearly odorless liquid; it is stable in air but decomposes when exposed to sunlight. The formula follows:

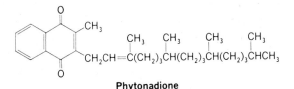

Phytonadione

USE AND DOSE. Phytonadione is a pro-thrombogenic vitamin. Usual dose is, orally, 10 mg; intramuscularly, 5 mg. Doses of up to 50 mg may be administered in cases of toxicity owing to bishydroxy-coumarin and related drugs.

PRESCRIPTION PRODUCTS. Mephyton® and Konakion®.

Vitamin K₂ is a yellow, crystalline solid obtained from putrefied fish meal. It has the following structure:

PRESCRIPTION PRODUCT. Hescor-K® contains menadione in combination with hesperidin and ascorbic acid.

Menadione sodium bisulfite or 2-methyl-1,4-naphthoquinone sodium bisulfite is a prothrombogenic vitamin and is employed in large doses as an antidote to coumarin anticoagulants. Usual dose is, intravenously and subcutaneously, 2 mg daily; up to 100 mg to counteract coumarin anticoagulation.

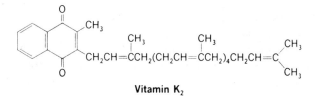

Vitamin K₂

Menadione, menaphthene, menaphthone, or 2-methyl-1,4-naphthoquinone is a synthetic substitute for vitamin K. It occurs as a bright yellow, crystalline powder. It is nearly odorless but is affected by sunlight. The structural formula is:

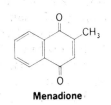

Menadione

USE AND DOSE. Menadione is a prothrombogenic vitamin. Usual dose is, orally and intramuscularly, 2 mg daily. CAUTION: Menadione powder is irritating to the respiratory tract and to the skin; a solution in alcohol has vesicant properties.

PRESCRIPTION PRODUCT. Hykinone Solution®.

Menadiol sodium diphosphate is a water-soluble vitamin K analog; chemically, it is 2-methyl-1,4-naphthalenediol bis (dihydrogen phosphate) tetrasodium salt. It is a prothrombogenic vitamin and is used in the prevention and treatment of hypoprothrombinemia. Usual dose is, parenterally, 5 mg, once a day.

PRESCRIPTION PRODUCTS. Kappadione® and Synkayvite®.

MULTIVITAMIN THERAPY

Diets deficient in one vitamin are likely to be deficient in several, and conditions that hinder the absorption of one vitamin may likewise interfere with the absorption of others. Inadequate vitamin intake can result not only from a poor diet but also from alcoholism, increased needs during pregnancy and lactation, prolonged broad-spectrum antibiotic therapy, and the course of parenteral nutrition. Poor absorption of ingested vitamins occurs frequently in elderly persons, chronically ill persons, and others who suffer from infections, reduced bile flow, intestinal disease, diarrhea, and the like. For these reasons, the supplementation of diets with multivitamin preparations does have a rational basis in certain circumstances.

Decavitamin capsules and decavitamin tablets serve as model multivitamin preparations, providing 10 vitamins for which recommended allowances have been established and one vitamin for which there is no such recommendation. Each capsule or tablet contains the labeled amounts of vitamins A, B_1, B_2, B_6, B_{12}, C, D, E, calcium pantothenate, folic acid, and niacinamide. Usual dose is 1 capsule or tablet daily.

PROPRIETARY PRODUCTS. (Some of these may differ slightly from the composition of Decavitamin.) Multicebrin®, Unicaps®, Theragran®, Theracebrin®.

Hexavitamin capsules and hexavitamin tablets each contain the following specified amounts of 6 vitamins: vitamin A, 1.5 mg; B_1, 2 mg; B_2, 3 mg; C, 75 mg; D, 10 mg; niacinamide, 20 mg. Usual dose is determined by the practitioner according to the needs of the patient.

PROPRIETARY PRODUCT. Hepicebrin®.

LIVER AND STOMACH

These organs serve an endocrine function in collaborating to produce one or more principles essential to adequate functioning of the erythropoietic bone marrow. They also serve other less clearly defined functions. The essential substance is referred to as the "antianemia principle" (AAP) or the "erythrocyte-maturing factor" (EMF).

Deficiency in the supply or utilization of the principle(s) leads to complex disturbances centering around a severe anemia and characterized by one or more of the following:

1. Pernicious anemia (addisonian anemia). This condition was first described by Combe in 1822 and later by Addison in 1849.

2. Gastrointestinal disturbances: smoothing and inflammation of the tongue, digestive disturbances, and diarrhea associated with lack of gastric hydrochloric acid.

3. Nervous disturbances involving particularly the spinal cord and the peripheral nerves.

4. Bone marrow changes, with a cessation of erythrocyte maturation at the stage of abnormal megaloblasts.

In untreated cases, the disease progresses by repeated episodes of these changes to a fatal termination. Adequate replacement therapy is available in oral or parenteral preparations containing the essential principle prepared from the stomachs or livers (or both) of domesticated food animals.

Under conditions of normal function, the elaboration of this essential principle may be outlined as follows:

1. An adequate diet contains a substance designated as the "extrinsic factor," now designated as vitamin B_{12} (cyanocobalamin) and its precursors.

2. Gastric and duodenal glands secrete a substance known as the "intrinsic factor," which is necessary for the absorption of vitamin B_{12} from the intestinal tract.

3. The antianemic principle, vitamin B_{12}, is stored in the liver and other tissues, pending release to the bone marrow and other organs.

Pernicious anemia may result from defects at any point between the dietary intake and the utilization of the hormone in the bone marrow. The most common defects lie in an inadequate production of intrinsic factor and in an inadequate absorption of the interaction product from the small intestine.

Minot and Murphy in 1926 showed that the daily oral ingestion of 200 to 400 g of whole liver resulted in remission of pernicious anemia and the maintenance of a normal erythrocyte and marrow picture. This whole liver must be ingested raw or, at most, lightly cooked because the active principle is destroyed by more thorough cooking. Preparations in use at present are the results of improvements in the extraction of the intrinsic factor from the livers and stomachs of food animals.

The active material in liver extracts possesses the properties of a peptide with a molecular weight greater than 5000. It is water-soluble, stable at $100°$ C at pH 5, and is readily absorbed from the intestine or from intramuscular injection sites.

Oral liver extracts are relatively expensive, often unpleasant to the point of nauseating, and slow and relatively uncertain in their action. In severe cases, particularly if complicated by nausea, vomiting, diarrhea, or established nervous system changes, oral therapy is frequently inadequate.

Liver injection is a preparation containing a partially purified extract of liver. It contains the soluble, relatively thermostable fraction of mammalian livers that increases the number of red corpuscles in the blood of persons affected with pernicious anemia. It is classified as a hematopoietic substance and contains, among other compounds, vitamin B_{12}, folic acid, and folinic acid. Its potency is expressed on the basis of vitamin B_{12} activity. Available preparations possess activity equivalent to 1 or 2 μg of cyanocobalamin in each ml. Usual dose is, intramuscularly, a minimum of 1 μg daily, preferably administered as 7 to 15 μg weekly.

PRESCRIPTION SPECIALTY. Pernaemon®.

Stomach concentrate is prepared from the mucosal glands of porcine stomach walls. It contains the intrinsic factor that increases the number of red corpuscles in the blood of people affected by pernicious anemia. The intrinsic factor-containing stomach concentrate is combined with liver extract (Extralin®); with liver extract and vitamins B_1, B_2, and B_{12} (Extalin B®); and with vitamin B_{12} and folic acid (Extralin F®) for oral administration.

Two general points must be considered in the therapeutic use of these antianemia preparations of liver and stomach:

1. Their use is replacement therapy— not curative. Relapses may be expected after cessation of therapy.

2. Pernicious anemia is caused by a specific deficiency, relieved by the specific antianemia factor. The popular addition of vitamins, iron, and other factors to therapy is justified only on the basis of an established need for them—they are of no specific value in pernicious anemia.

READING REFERENCES

Arnstein, H. R. V., and Wrighton, R. J., eds.: The Cobalamins, Baltimore, The Williams & Wilkins Co., 1971.

Baker, H., and Frank, O.: Clinical Vitaminology, New York, Interscience Publishers, 1968.

Bernfeld, P., ed.: Biogenesis of Natural Compounds, 2nd ed., New York, Pergamon Press, Inc., 1967.

Blakley, R. L.: The Biochemistry of Folic Acid and Related Pteridines, Amsterdam, North-Holland Publishing Co., 1969.

Goodhart, R. S., and Shils, M. E.: Modern Nutrition in Health and Disease, 5th ed., Philadelphia, Lea & Febiger, 1973.

György, P., and Person, W. N.: The Vitamins, 2nd ed., Vols. VI–VII, New York, Academic Press, Inc., 1967.

Hashmi, M.: Assay of Vitamins in Pharmaceutical Preparations, London, John Wiley & Sons Ltd., 1973.

Kutsky, R. J.: Handbook of Vitamins and Hormones, New York, Van Nostrand Reinhold Co., 1973.

Levy, J. V., and Bach-y-Rita, P.: *Vitamins: Their Use and Abuse*, New York, Liveright, 1976.

Lewin, S.: *Vitamin C: Its Molecular Biology and Medical Potential*, New York, Academic Press, Inc., 1976.

Marks, J.: *A Guide to the Vitamins*, Baltimore, University Park Press, 1975.

Morton, R. A., ed.: *Fat-Soluble Vitamins*, Oxford, Pergamon Press Ltd., 1970.

Noyes, R.: *Vitamin B$_{12}$ Manufacture*, Park Ridge, New Jersey, Noyes Development Corp., 1969.

Rubel, T.: *Vitamin E Manufacture*, Park Ridge, New Jersey, Noyes Development Corp., 1969.

Sebrell, W. H., Jr., and Harris, R. S., eds.: *The Vitamins*, 2nd ed., Vols. I–III, V, New York, Academic Press, Inc., 1967–1972.

Chapter 12

Antibiotics

Antibiotics probably represent the greatest single contribution of drug therapy in the past half-century, a period characterized by unprecedented advancements in health care. This group of drugs provides effective control of many human microbial pathogens that previously caused prolonged incapacitation or death without appreciable regard for age, economic status, or physical fitness.

The word "antibiotic" is derived from the term antibiosis, which literally means "against life" (*anti*—against, *bios*—life). A measure of the significant and spectacular contribution of antibiotics to therapy is indicated by the common inclusion of the word in the layman's vocabulary. Most people have an accurate, or at least a functional, general concept of the word, but workers intimately involved in the antibiotic field find considerable difficulty in drafting a precise definition. The varied scientific concepts of this word reflect the viewpoints of scientific specialists, a rapidly expanding field of knowledge about all aspects of antibiotics and their applications, and such factors as a recognition of the lack of definitive separation for conditions previously considered etiologically distinct (e.g., certain neoplastic conditions and viral infections).

The most widely accepted concept defines an antibiotic as a chemical substance produced by a microorganism that has the capacity, in low concentration, to inhibit selectively or even to destroy bacteria and other microorganisms through an antimetabolic mechanism. Essentially all definitions limit antibiotics to biologic constituents that exert their action in low concentrations. This definition excludes microbial metabolites, such as ethanol, that are active against protoplasmic functions at higher concentrations. The definition of the term may be expanded by including higher plants as a source and tumors as a site of action. The concept of antibiotics as used by health-care professionals, exclusive of some individuals practicing in experimental clinics and hospitals, is limited for practical purposes to commercially available substances. Fortunately, this reduces confusion resulting from special research objectives or "antibiotics" that are too toxic for feasible therapy. A logical case can be made for including the antiplasmodial activity of quinine under an antibiotic designation, but the arbitrary exclusion of quinine from most antibiotic concepts has caused little confusion for the practitioner. The selective action of some naturally occurring compounds on the abnormal metabolism and cells of neoplasms may create greater problems in the future. Practitioners must maintain a flexible approach toward the scope of antibiotics to accommodate the applications of scientific advances.

DEVELOPMENTAL HISTORY

The history and development of antibiotics as therapeutic agents are similar to the patterns noted for other types of drugs. Relatively ineffective attempts to use materials that are now recognized as having antibiotic associations can be detected in folk medicine and in prepenicillin scientific literature. Development in the antibiotic field since 1940 is characterized by a practical blending of empiric observation and increasingly sophisticated manipulations of biologic and chemical factors. This familiar pattern is frequently overlooked because an aura of twentieth-century miracle drugs has surrounded the antibiotics.

Reports, some dating back 2500 years, indicate that various ancient and primitive peoples applied moldy bread, soybean curds, and other materials to boils and wounds liable to infection; this can be considered a folk-medicine type of antibiotic therapy. Pasteur demonstrated bacterial antagonism shortly after he established the bacterial etiology of infectious disease. During the 1880s, attempts were made to utilize antagonism to achieve an ecologic control of the human microbial flora by introducing selected nonpathogenic organisms. Pyocyanase, a crude mixture of metabolites extracted from *Pseudomonas aeruginosa*, became available around the

turn of the century and could be considered the first commercial antibiotic. Pyocyanase, at best, was a poor antibiotic by modern standards, but its failure to achieve wide acceptance as a therapeutic agent can be related, in part, to variable composition of the crude mixture and the resultant lack of reproducible or predictable therapeutic responses.

Establishment of the therapeutic feasibility of penicillin antagonism in the early 1940s stimulated the intensive efforts that have culminated in the high level of current antibiotic development. Numerous approaches to the production and use of antibiotics have been used concurrently in the past, and practical considerations of biologic, chemical, and economic factors will undoubtedly dictate a similar situation in the predictable future.

The progressive trend in the logistic aspects of antibiotic development can be illustrated by the following sequence of objectives: (1) Screen diverse sources of microorganisms for detection of useful antagonism. (2) Select improved microbial mutants, determine optimal environmental and nutritional conditions, and develop suitable procedures for recovering antibiotics from cultures. (3) Direct or induce the formation of specific, desired metabolites. (4) Modify the fermentative metabolites by biologic or chemical manipulations to yield more useful antibiotic substances. (5) Develop procedures for total synthesis of antibiotics for possible economic advantage.

Initially, antibiotic therapy was commonly employed in a wide range of microbial infections with only limited logic or design. However, with the accumulation of experience and the availability of a greater variety of antibiotics, the trend has moved toward a more precise diagnosis of the pathogenic organism, including a consideration of sensitivity variations with certain pathogens, and a more conservative use of these valuable therapeutic agents.

Production of commercial quantities of the various antibiotics involves many different approaches and procedures to accommodate the individual biologic idiosyncrasies of the producing organisms and the chemical characteristics of the individual antibiotics. A detailed consideration of antibiotic production is obviously a subject for specialized study. Fortunately, the health-science practitioner only needs a general knowledge of the production procedures and of the significance of key manipulations. This background provides a basis for understanding the scientific limits and economic components of these therapeutic agents and for comprehending readily the types of research developments that will lead to future advances and change.

SCREENING FOR ANTIBIOTICS

In searching for new antibiotics, relatively simple and rapid methods have been developed for screening microorganisms for antibiotic-producing ability. Soil samples are commonly employed in the screen because they are a rich source of antibiotic-producing organisms (Fig. 12–1). Most of these organisms are members of a group of branching, procaryotic microorganisms that occupy a position in their morphologic characteristics between fungi and bacteria. They are placed in the taxonomic order Actinomycetales and are given the common name actinomycetes. A compilation of the microbial sources of antibiotics discovered in the United States and Japan between 1953 and 1970 reveals that approximately 85% are produced by actinomycetes, 11% by fungi, and 4% by bacteria. These facts do not detract from the significance of antibiotics from other organisms and sources, but they do suggest a greater probability for the discovery of new useful antibiotics from soil microorganisms. The antibiotics currently used in therapy are produced by surprisingly few groups of distantly related organisms. The important genera and their consensus taxonomic relations are as follows:

Phylum Schizomycophyta
   Class Schizomycetes
      Order Eubacteriales (bacteria)

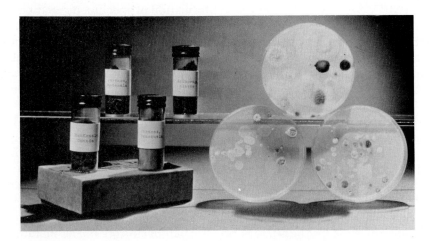

Fig. 12–1. Soil samples from various parts of the world and agar plates showing colonies of soil flora. (Photo, courtesy of Eli Lilly & Co.)

Family Bacillaceae
    Genus *Bacillus*
Order Actinomycetales (actino-
    mycetes)
    Family Streptomycetaceae
        Genus *Micromonospora*
        Genus *Streptomyces*
Phylum Eumycophyta (fungi)
  Class Ascomycetes
    Order Aspergillales
      Family Aspergillaceae
        Genus *Penicillium*
  Form-Class Deuteromycetes (Fungi
    Imperfecti)
    Form-Order Moniliales
      Form-Family Moniliaceae
        Form-Genus *Cephalosporium*

A general method for screening first involves treating the soil sample with chemicals that inhibit the growth of interfering bacteria and fungi but do not affect actinomycetes. Cycloheximide is an antifungal antibiotic often employed for this purpose, and a 1:140 dilution of phenol is used as an antibacterial agent. Varying dilutions of the treated soil sample are streaked on agar plates containing medium that supports the growth of actinomycetes. After incubation for 3 to 7 days at 25 to 30° C, the plates are examined for characteristic colonies of actinomycetes. These colonies are then selectively transferred onto fresh medium. Giant colonies of the selected organisms are grown, and plugs are cut from the colonies that include not only the organism, but also the underlying agar. If the organism produces an antibiotic, it should diffuse into the agar medium. The plugs are placed on an agar plate that has been seeded with a test organism that gives an indication of the potential usefulness of the antibiotic. For example, activity against gram-positive bacteria can be determined with *Staphylococcus aureus* or *Bacillus subtilis*, activity against gram-negative bac-

teria with *Escherichia coli* or *Salmonella typhi*, and antifungal activity with *Neurospora crassa*. The test plates are incubated under conditions appropriate for maximal growth of the test organism, and if after incubation there is a clear zone around the plug of the actinomycete, it can be assumed that an antibiotic in the plug inhibited the growth of the test organism (Fig. 12–2).

The next step in the screening procedure is to determine whether the chemical substance that produced the inhibition is a new antibiotic or a known compound. A rapid method that has been developed for this determination is termed bioautography. This assay employs paper chromatography or thin-layer chromatography and a biologic assay. An extract containing

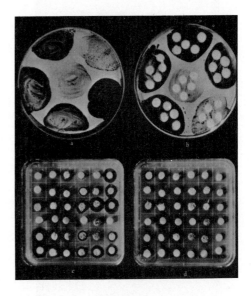

Fig. 12–2. A method for the detection of antibiotic-producing organisms: *a*, giant colonies growing on an agar plate; *b*, giant colonies with plugs removed; *c*, plugs from giant colonies showing zones of inhibition (clear zone around plug) on test plate seeded with *Staphylococcus aureus*, indicating antibiotic activity against gram-positive bacteria; *d*, plugs on test plate seeded with *Escherichia coli* showing fewer zones of inhibition, indicating little antibiotic activity against gram-negative bacilli. (Photo, courtesy of Eli Lilly & Co.)

the newly discovered antibiotic is chromatographed along with reference, known antibiotics using several different solvent systems. Because each antibiotic would possess a characteristic mobility on the chromatogram in a given solvent system, a comparison of the mobilities of the unknown antibiotic with those of known antibiotics in several solvent systems would indicate whether the newly discovered antibiotic was a known compound. The detection of the antibiotics on the developed chromatogram using chemical detection methods is difficult because the antibiotics are widely diverse chemi-

cally; consequently, a biologic method is used to detect the antibiotics. By placing the developed chromatogram on an agar medium that has been seeded with an appropriate test organism, the antibiotics diffuse from the paper into the agar, and after incubation, clear zones on the agar owing to inhibition of growth of the test organism indicate the position of the antibiotics on the chromatogram (Fig. 12–3).

After it is established that a microorganism has been isolated that produces a new antibiotic, quantitative assays must be employed to monitor the antibiotic titer through the various processes of production and isolation. The 2 most commonly employed assays, the turbidimetric (tube dilution) assay and the plate (agar diffusion) assay, require the use of a test organism as in bioautography. In the turbidimetric assay, the test organism is grown in test tubes that contain different concentrations of the antibiotic. There is a direct relationship of the concentration of antibiotic to the growth of the test organism, and by measuring the growth of the organism, which is indicated by the turbidity of the contents of the test tube, the antibiotic titer can be determined. Clear tubes indicate a higher antibiotic concentration than do turbid tubes, and the lowest concentration of antibiotic that completely prevents the appearance of turbidity is known as the **minimum inhibitory concentration** (MIC) (Fig. 12–4).

In the plate assay, filter paper discs are impregnated with solutions of antibiotic of varying concentration, allowed to dry, placed on agar medium seeded with an appropriate test organism, and incubated. As the concentration of the antibiotic increases, the diffusion of the antibiotic through the agar medium increases; therefore, the size of the clear zone of growth inhibition around the filter paper disc is related to the concentration of antibiotic (Fig. 12–5).

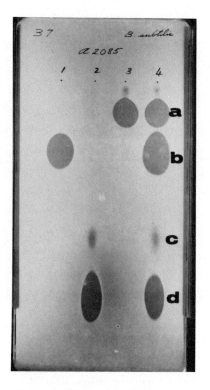

Fig. 12–3. A bioautograph with *Bacillus subtilis* as the test organism. The zones of inhibition indicate the following antibiotics were separated on the paper chromatogram: *a*, cephalexin; *b*, cephaloridine; *c*, desacetylcephalothin; *d*, cephalothin. (Photo, courtesy of Eli Lilly & Co.)

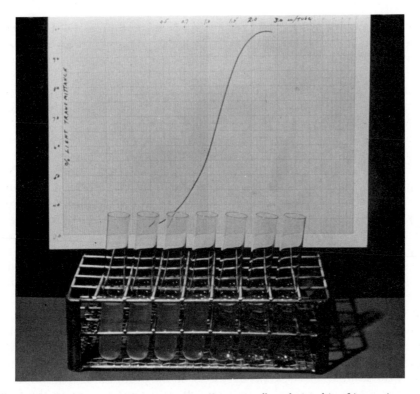

Fig. 12–4. Turbidimetric assay tubes with curve illustrating the relationship of increasing percent light transmittance on the y axis and increasing concentration of antibiotic on the x axis. (Photo, courtesy of Eli Lilly & Co.)

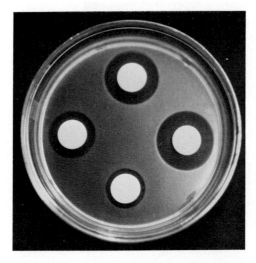

Fig. 12–5. A microbiologic assay plate showing zones of inhibition of varying size owing to different concentrations of antibiotic on the filter paper discs. The disc on the right contains the greatest concentration of antibiotic. (Photo, courtesy of Eli Lilly & Co.)

COMMERCIAL PRODUCTION

When a new antibiotic has been discovered, investigations into the chemical, physical, and biologic properties of the antibiotic are required before the decision to produce the antibiotic commercially can be made. Two important requirements for production are: (1) the organism must produce the antibiotic in submerged culture as opposed to surface culture and (2) the organism must excrete the antibiotic into the culture medium. However, some antibiotics, such as those of the polyene group, are retained in the cells of the organism and require special extraction procedures for recovery. These requirements are important considerations in production costs which, in turn, determine whether the antibiotic can compete with other antibiotics for a portion of the market. Other considerations are chemical stability, the minimum inhibitory concentration against strains of pathogenic organisms, toxic manifestations in mammals, and activity in vivo.

The commercial production of antibiotics is an excellent example of the benefits that can be achieved from a multidisciplinary approach to solving a technologic problem. One must be impressed when one thinks, on the one hand, of an obscure microorganism growing in soil and, on the other hand, the product of that microorganism—a pure crystalline chemical substance used to save a human life. The transition from one to the other has required the most diligent application of the sciences of microbiology, chemistry, and engineering.

Commercial fermentative production of an antibiotic almost always involves growth of the producing organism in aerated tanks holding thousands of gallons of nutrient medium. Spores or occasionally vegetative growth from a stock culture of the organism are used to start the fermentation process. It is important to maintain stock cultures (e.g., by lyophilization) that require transfer as infrequently as possible because repeated transfer may select for those cells of the organism that are poor producers of antibiotic (Fig. 12–6). The several hundred gallons of vegetative growth that are necessary for inoculating the large fermentation tanks are obtained by successively transferring the organism to increasingly larger volumes of nutrient (Fig. 12–7). The use of a large standard inoculum reduces the incubation time required for production of the antibiotic, lessens the chance for costly contamination by foreign microorganisms, and provides the best possible opportunity for control of subtle environmental and nutritional factors that influence the antibiotic yield.

In the production of antibiotics there are often distinct phases in the fermentative process. These phases can be divided into

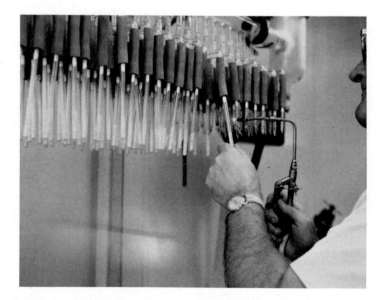

Fig. 12–6. In stock culture maintenance, the lyophilized cultures of antibiotic-producing organisms are preserved in small, sealed, glass tubes. The freeze-dried pellets in the small glass tubes will be used to start antibiotic production. (Photo, courtesy of Eli Lilly & Co.)

Stock Culture
↓
Liquid Medium Cultures
(in one-liter flasks)
| Several flasks
↓
Bazooka (a special device
used to transfer aseptically
into fermentation tanks)
↓
Inoculum Tank (also called
Seed Tank or Bump Tank)
↓
Production Tank (usually 10×
the volume of Inoculum Tank—
some tanks are as large 100,000
gallons and six stories high)

Fig. 12–7. The scale-up procedure in the commercial production of antibiotics.

the growth phase of the organism, which is also termed the trophophase, and the antibiotic production phase, also termed the idiophase. Figure 12–8 illustrates these phases in the course of a typical penicillin fermentation carried out in a culture medium containing glucose and lactose as the sources of carbon nutrition, corn steep

liquor for nitrogen sources, and phosphate buffer. During the growth phase, the culture becomes thick owing to the formation of aggregates of fungal cells called mycelium. Growth is indicated in the figure by the curve showing an increase in mycelial nitrogen and lasts from the beginning of the culture period to approximately 1 day later (0 to 24 hours). During the growth phase, glucose rather than lactose is preferentially utilized because it can be used directly as a source of carbon. In the growth process, ammonia is liberated by deamination of amino acids of the corn steep liquor. This liberation raises the pH of the medium to 7, the optimum pH for penicillin stability, and buffers in the medium maintain the pH close to neutrality.

Penicillin production increases rapidly between 24 to 80 hours. At the start of the antibiotic production phase, glucose has been used up, and the fungus then uses lactose for a carbon source. Little additional growth occurs because the lactose

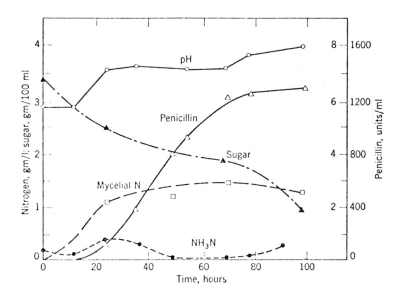

Fig. 12–8. Chemical changes, mycelial growth, and penicillin production in a typical penicillin fermentation. (Reprinted with permission from Brown and Petersen, 1950. Industrial and Engineering Chemistry, 42:1769–1774. Copyright by the American Chemical Society.)

cannot be utilized until it is hydrolyzed to glucose and galactose. The decreased availability of a carbon source is thought to be the triggering mechanism for penicillin production.

INCREASING COMMERCIAL YIELD

Considerable effort is devoted to determining the optimal environmental and nutritional conditions for antibiotic production. Optimal conditions for antibiotic formation are frequently quite different from those for maximum vegetative growth. Factors that are often observed to have qualitative or quantitative importance for antibiotic production include sources of nutritional carbon and nitrogen, ratio of carbon/nitrogen nutrients, mineral composition of medium, incubation temperature, initial pH and control of pH during the fermentation period, rate and method of aeration, and addition and timing of addition of special growth- and antibiotic-promoting substances. Selection of optimal fermentation conditions is usually based on empiric observations, but careful attention to such factors is often critical. For example, some strains of *Bacillus subtilis* produce optimal yields of bacitracin when the C/N ratio is about 15; at lower ratios the yield is less, and when the ratio is reduced to approximately 6, licheniformin, a related but commercially undesired antibiotic, is produced.

The practical benefit of adding special chemicals to the fermentation cultures has probably achieved only a small fraction of its ultimate potential, but some examples will show the practical utility of this general approach. It was observed at a fairly early stage in the development of penicillin production that the addition of phenylacetamide or related compounds to the culture medium had a minor beneficial effect on the yield of penicillin substances and had a major influence on the composi-

tion of the penicillin mixture. The presence of phenylacetic acid derivatives in the nutrient mixture favored the formation of penicillin G; this reduced the problems of using a mixture of unknown or variable composition and the cost of separating the individual antibiotic substances. Use of various acyl moieties to direct the fermentative formation of other penicillins (e.g., penicillin V) achieved limited commercial success, but semisynthetic techniques have superseded this approach to the production of specialized penicillins.

The use of mercaptothiazole in cultures of *Streptomyces aureofaciens* emphasizes that additives can be beneficial without being incorporated into the antibiotic molecule. Strains of this actinomycete usually produce both chlortetracycline and tetracycline; the proportions depend to some degree on the availability of chloride ion in the culture medium. Tetracycline has the greater therapeutic utility, but the resolution of mixtures of these 2 tetracyclines is costly. Because the organism tends to be a chloride scavenger and because chloride ion is one of the most difficult ions to exclude quantitatively from water and nutrients, control of the presence of this ion in the nutrient medium to favor the production of tetracycline is not commercially feasible. However, the addition to the fermentation mixture of mercaptothiazole or any other compound that presumably inhibits chlorination favors tetracycline production.

Some additives may increase antibiotic production through an enzyme induction effect. For example, the addition of methionine to a cephalosporin C fermentation during the trophophase stimulates the production of the antibiotic. Because methionine does not serve as a biosynthetic precursor to the antibiotic, as compared to the role of phenylacetic acid in penicillin G biosynthesis, it is assumed that methionine stimulates the production of the cephalosporin C biosynthetic enzymes.

Conversely, it has been demonstrated that in penicillin fermentation, lysine in the culture medium inhibits antibiotic production. Penicillin and lysine are end products of a branched biosynthetic pathway in which α-aminoadipic acid is a common precursor. Lysine production is regulated either by inhibition or repression of the enzymes required for the production of α-aminoadipic acid, which ultimately results in a decrease in penicillin formation.

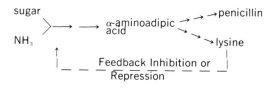

Another important approach to increasing the yield of antibiotic is mutation and strain selection. Mutation induced by exposing the parent strain to ultraviolet light, x rays, or various mutagenic chemicals, such as nitrogen mustards and analogs of purines and pyrimidines, is the major approach for selecting improved strains, but a search of natural sources for new wild-type or different species that produce the antibiotic in higher yield than the original producing organism is also employed. In the case of induced mutations, lethal levels of the mutagen are adjusted so that approximately 90 to 99% of the cells of the organism are killed. Mutants that produce a higher yield of antibiotic are selected from the surviving cells. Penicillin production offers a good illustration of the potential success of these approaches. Penicillin antagonism was observed originally with a culture of *Penicillium notatum* Westling, which produced in surface culture 4 mg of penicillin per liter of culture medium. No

mutants of *P. notatum* were found in the early selection process which would give a satisfactory yield of pencillin in submerged fermentation; however, in 1944, through natural selection, a strain of *P. chrysogenum* Thom was discovered which yielded penicillin in the amount of 40 mg per liter. Subsequently, by utilizing procedures of mutation and strain selection, the yield has been increased to 21,000 mg per liter.

RECOVERY AND ISOLATION

Most of the commercially important antibiotics are excreted readily into the nutrient medium where they accumulate. In cases such as certain of the peptide antibiotics where the antibiotic is retained endocellularly until the cells reach an advanced physiologic age, the fermentation period is terminated when most of the cell membranes have undergone lysis or have lost their selective retention property. Thus, isolation of antibiotic substances is basically recovery from the culture broth. The fundamental approaches that are usually considered are selective precipitation, selective adsorption, or selective extraction with an immiscible solvent. The chemical characteristics of various antibiotics and their accompanying metabolites govern the manipulations that will be effective in any given situation. Ideally, the initial isolation procedure should be as efficient and selective as possible to give the best yield and to facilitate subsequent purification, but economic considerations commonly dictate a compromise procedure.

Precipitation is theoretically one of the best ways to recover a substance from a large volume of an aqueous mixture, but this approach has not proved commercially satisfactory for any of the therapeutically important antibiotics. The most nearly feasible application of this approach probably involves polymyxin. Polymyxin forms an insoluble helianthate complex when helianthine (methyl orange) is added to the culture broth, but this antibiotic can be recovered more economically by using an adsorption procedure. Lack of selectivity and recoverability from the precipitated complex is the most commonly cited technical disadvantage to the practical utility of this general method.

Liquid-liquid extraction using some water-immiscible organic solvent is the approach utilized for most antibiotics. This procedure lacks a high degree of selectivity with most solvents that are sufficiently inexpensive to be employed on a commercial scale. It is also relatively inefficient because antibiotic substances tend to be fairly polar molecules. However, the economic advantage of easy adaptation to a chemical engineering flow process more than offsets these limitations in most cases unless the antibiotic molecule is so polar that the partition coefficient favors the aqueous phase.

Highly polar antibiotics, such as neomycin and other aminoglycoside antibiotics, are usually recovered from the culture broth by adsorption on some suitable adsorbent. Many adsorbents remove antibiotics of this type from culture broths with varying degrees of selectivity. The major limitation to selecting adsorbents is the need to recover the antibiotics by reversing the adsorption without using extreme conditions that would be destructive. Use of charcoal of controlled activity grades and elution of the antibiotic with dilute acid is a typical example of this isolation approach.

Once the crude antibiotic has been recovered from the nutrient broth, it is subjected to chromatography, recrystallization, or other standard manipulations to effect an appropriate degree of purification. It should be noted that attainment of chemical purity is usually considered im-

practical and unnecessary for therapeutic purposes. Extraneous metabolites, such as foreign proteins that cause undesirable side effects, are routinely excluded during purification, but separation of closely related antibiotic molecules is often unfeasible. Most fermentatively produced antibiotics used in therapy are actually mixtures of closely related compounds with one of the metabolites comprising the majority of the mixture. This practical approach permits reproducible therapeutic responses because a given antibiotic molecule always accounts for most of the mixture; it also provides the most economic materials for drug formulations because the inefficiency and expense of total separation of similar chemical molecules, the relative concentrations of which are unequal, can be avoided. The presence of up to 6% chlortetracycline in commercial tetracycline represents a practical application of such purification considerations. Accepted standards of purity for antibiotics and antibiotic preparations are established by the Food and Drug Administration. Qualitative and quantitative evaluations of antibiotic preparations for adherence to established standards utilize both biologically and chemically based tests. Colorimetric and spectrophotometric approaches and definitive measurements have largely replaced microbiologic assay and arbitrary units for quantitative purposes. However, biologic tests are still employed to detect the presence of pyrogens in parenteral antibiotic formulations. The objectives and approaches of most tests for evaluation of antibiotic preparations are not significantly different from those used to insure the standards of other drugs.

The one unusual aspect of evaluating antibiotics is associated with the need to guarantee sterility in parenteral preparations. Masking of the presence of microbial contaminants through bacteriostatic action of the antibiotic must be precluded. Three basic approaches can be used to eliminate the antibiotic masking of microbial contaminants. Preparations containing antibiotics that are inactivated readily by biologic or chemical means may be subjected to the appropriate treatment before testing for sterility. Penicillinase inactivation of penicillin G and hydroxylamine hydrochloride inactivation of streptomycin illustrate this approach. Parenteral solutions of all antibiotics, especially those containing the more stable antibiotics, can be evaluated by diluting the preparation such that the antibiotic level is below the minimum threshold concentration for activity or by initially removing any microorganisms with a sterile millipore filter in a manipulation that separates the organisms from the antibiotic.

MANIPULATIVE FORMULATIONS

Effective use of many drug substances can be enhanced through various manipulations in pharmaceutic formulations. Antibiotics are no exception. Three approaches for the protection of labile antibiotic molecules, the use of insoluble derivatives to eliminate objectionable tastes and thus gain patient acceptance for certain oral formulations, and the use of either soluble or insoluble salts to facilitate the desired delivery of the therapeutic agent illustrate the practical utilization of manipulative formulations for various antibiotics.

Buffers in oral penicillin G preparations reduce the destructive effect of gastric acidity, and enteric coatings of some oral erythromycin formulations protect the macrolactone ring of this antibiotic until it passes through the acidic environment of the stomach and into the small intestine where it is absorbed. Erythromycin estolate (the dodecyl sulfate salt of the pro-

pionyl ester) and triacetyloleandomycin are much more insoluble than the parent macrolide antibiotics. This property makes a dual contribution to oral suspensions of these antibiotic substances. The insolubility helps to avoid the extremely bitter taste of these drugs and to protect them until they reach the lower intestine.

The glucoheptonate and lactobionate salts of erythromycin are used to increase the solubility of the antibiotic sufficiently to permit intravenous administration. The relatively insoluble benzathine and procaine salts of some penicillins are used intramuscularly for repository effects. When benzathine penicillin G is used in oral suspensions, this insolubility characteristic contributes a stability factor.

THERAPY AND UNDERLYING BIOLOGIC FACTORS

Various antibiotics are widely employed for the effective control of most serious infections, but prophylactic administration of antibiotics to individuals is rarely justified. Effective antibiotic therapy involves the correct diagnosis of the pathogen and the proper selection of an antibiotic. Diagnostic bacteriologic examination is usually a minimum basis for rational therapy. Exceptions include diseases such as scarlet fever, typhoid fever, or other conditions characterized by clinical symptoms that are indicative of a specific microbial etiology. Interim antibiotic therapy is usually initiated on a calculated judgment basis in acute cases of meningitis, pneumonia, urinary tract infections, and similar conditions with multiple possible causes pending bacteriologic diagnosis; the therapeutic approach is modified as necessary upon confirmation of the causative organism.

In order for the physician to exercise clinical judgment properly, he must have a knowledge of the bacteriologic statistics of

Table 12–1. A Summary of Common Pathogens That Cause Infections That Can Be Treated with Antibiotics

Pathogenic Organism	Disease Produced
Gram-positive cocci	
Staphylococcus aureus	cellulitis, impetigo, septicemia, endocarditis, meningitis, osteomyelitis, pneumonia, food poisoning, furunculosis
Streptococcus pyogenes β-hemolytic group A	scarlet fever, rheumatic fever, erysipelas, pharnygitis, impetigo
Streptococcus faecalis	subacute bacterial endocarditis, urinary tract infection
Streptococcus pneumoniae	pneumonia, meningitis, otitis
Gram-positive bacilli	
Bacillus anthracis	anthrax
Clostridium tetani	tetanus
Clostridium perfringens	gas gangrene
Clostridium botulinum	food poisoning (botulism)
Corynebacterium diphtheriae	diphtheria
Gram-negative cocci	
Neisseria meningitidis	meningitis
Neisseria gonorrhoeae	gonorrhea
Gram-negative bacilli	
Bacteroides fragilis	abscesses of abdomen, lung, brain
Bordetella pertussis	whooping cough
Brucella abortus, B. melitensis, and B. suis	brucellosis
Enterobacter aerogenes	pneumonia, wound infections, urinary tract infection
Escherichia coli	urinary tract infection, septicemia, respiratory infections, peritonitis
Haemophilus influenzae	respiratory infections, meningitis, otitis
Klebsiella pneumoniae	pneumonia, urinary tract infection, septicemia
Legionella pneumophila	Legionnaire's disease
Proteus vulgaris	urinary tract infection, septicemia
Pseudomonas aeruginosa	urinary tract infection, pneumonia, burn-wound infection, septicemia
Salmonella typhi	typhoid fever
Salmonella species	food poisoning (salmonellosis)
Shigella dysenteriae	bacillary dysentery
Vibrio cholerae	asiatic dysentery
Yersinia pestis	bubonic plague
Acid-fast bacilli	
Mycobacterium leprae	leprosy
Mycobacterium tuberculosis	tuberculosis
Spirochetes	
Treponema pallidum	syphilis
Fungi	
Blastomyces dermatitidis	North American blastomycosis
Candida albicans	candidiasis (moniliasis)
Coccidioides immitis	coccidioidomycosis (San Joaquin fever)
Cryptococcus neoformans	cryptococcosis
Histoplasma capsulatum	histoplasmosis

Table 12–1.   A Summary of Common Pathogens That Cause Infections That Can Be
Treated with Antibiotics (continued)

Pathogenic Organism	Disease Produced
Epidermophyton, Microsporum, and Trichophyton (various species)	dermatomycoses (ringworm, athlete's foot)
Miscellaneous, Rickettsiae, Large Viruses	
Mycoplasma pneumoniae	respiratory infections
Rickettsia typhi	endemic typhus
Rickettsia prowazekii	epidemic typhus
Rickettsia rickettsii	Rocky Mountain spotted fever
Chlamydia trachomatis	trachoma
Chlamydia psittaci	psittacosis (parrot fever)

infection, i.e., he must know what organisms most often produce a certain type of infection in particular areas of the body and in patients at a particular age. For example, in cases of bacterial meningitis in adults, the most common causative organisms are Neisseria meningitidis and Streptococcus pneumoniae. In children under 10 years of age, Haemophilus influenzae is also a common causative agent; however, in infants less than 1 month of age, coliform bacteria such as species of Escherichia, Klebsiella, and Enterobacter are added to the list of common causative agents (Table 12–1).

It should be emphasized, however, that rational antibiotic therapy depends first on isolating and identifying the pathogenic organism from the focus of infection and then on determining the sensitivity of that strain or organism against properly selected antibiotics known to be potentially active against the organism. Antibiotics with antibacterial activity are often classified into 2 broad categories on the basis of inhibiting predominantly gram-negative or gram-positive bacteria. Knowledge that a given antibiotic or group of antibiotics is characterized by a gram-negative or a gram-positive spectrum has

some therapeutic utility, especially for selecting an antibiotic for initiating therapy in the absence of definitive bacteriologic data and for considering alternate antibiotic approaches. When the pathogen is known or strongly suspected, selection of an effective antibiotic can frequently be based on the knowledge that the spectrum of an antibiotic includes a specific microorganism. However, judicious selection of an effective antibiotic for control of Escherichia coli and many pathogenic species of Klebsiella, Proteus, Pseudomonas, and Staphylococcus necessitates individual determination of susceptibility because various strains of these pathogens have different antibiotic sensitivities.

Many pathogens are susceptible to more than one commercially available antibiotic. The choice of antibiotic for any given therapeutic situation must be based on composite considerations of a number of factors and is rarely unequivocal. Properties frequently cited for a clinically ideal antibiotic include a complete freedom from acute and chronic toxicities; an optimal activity near pH 7 that is not influenced by serum, other body fluids, or pus; sufficient solubility in aqueous fluids to facilitate good distribution to all body tissues; chemical stability; efficient absorption following oral administration; no tendency to induce the development of resistant strains of pathogens; and a low expense factor. No known antibiotic possesses all of these ideal characteristics. The naturally occurring penicillins probably most nearly approach many of these properties for therapeutic situations where their spectrum is adequate because these penicillins tend to have a rapid onset of systemic activity when orally administered, cause a low incidence of toxicity, and are inexpensive. However, serious penicillin hypersensitivities contraindicate the use of these antibiotics in some individuals, and the development of resistance by some pathogens is a definite therapeutic concern. Cost is never a major or exclusive criterion for selection of a first-choice antibiotic for therapeutic purposes, but if all other factors are equal, the least expensive therapeutic approach (not necessarily the least expensive unit formulation) serves the best interests of the patient.

Properties of the antibiotic per se are not the only considerations in selecting the best therapeutic agent. Such factors as age and secondary debilitating conditions may influence the use or choice of antibiotics in specific situations. The following examples illustrate generally the situations that may be encountered. Gradual development of normal renal function during the neonatal period necessitates adjustment in the dosage and administration interval when employing antibiotics that are eliminated by the kidneys. An antibiotic that is excreted in the urine also must be used cautiously for systemic purposes in adult patients with renal complications, and chloramphenicol is usually considered an antibiotic of last resort when an infection is accompanied by hematopoietic abnormalities. When serious gastrointestinal complications would contribute to erratic absorption upon oral administration, the parenteral features of an antibiotic become dominant.

Data are being accumulated on the modes and mechanisms of action of various antibiotics, on the bases for toxicities in antibiotic therapy, and on the details of resistance. The available information is sufficient to rationalize scientifically many developments that may be observed during therapy. A consideration of these factors will undoubtedly provide a basis for more effective and precise antibiotic therapy in the future when more complete knowledge becomes available.

MODES AND MECHANISMS OF ACTION

A number of different classification schemes could be used to categorize the selective toxicity of antibiotics for susceptible microorganisms. The recognition of 4 general modes of action, namely, inhibition of microbial cell-wall formation, biosynthesis of some essential protein, disruption of deoxyribonucleic acid metabolism, and alteration of normal function of the cellular membrane, is satisfactory pending the accumulation of more data. It is frequently difficult to distinguish primary from referred responses in preliminary attempts to determine the mode of antibiotic action. When more detailed information becomes available, current concepts on the mode of action of a few antibiotics (Table 12–2) may be altered, and the relative therapeutic importance of alternate modes of action will be clarified for antibiotics that give experimental indications for more than one general basis for their antagonistic effects.

The mechanism of action of an antibiotic, as contrasted to the general mode of action, is frequently an individualistic feature, and distinctive mechanisms of action are often observed for 2 antibiotics with the

Table 12–2. General Mode of Antibiotic
Action

Inhibition of cell wall formation	Inhibition of protein biosynthesis
Bacitracin	Chloramphenicol
Cephalosporins	Clindamycin
Cycloserine	Erythromycin
Penicillins	Gentamicin
Vancomycin	Kanamycin
	Lincomycin
	Neomycin
Disruption of deoxyribonucleic acid metabolism	Oleandomycin
	Paromomycin
	Spectinomycin
	Streptomycin
Actinomycin D	Tetracyclines
Doxorubicin	
Mithramycin	
Mitomycin C	
Novobiocin	
Rifampin	Alteration in cellular membrane function
Bleomycin	
	Amphotericin B
	Candicidin
	Gramicidin
	Nystatin
	Polymyxin

same mode of action. Precise knowledge of the mechanism of action offers a tremendous potential for sophisticated developments in antibiotic therapy. Sufficient information is available on the mechanism of action of certain antibiotics that interfere with cell-wall formation and protein biosynthesis to show representative patterns of biologic involvement.

Inhibition of cell-wall formation involves the disruption of mucopeptide synthesis. Gram-positive bacteria are particularly susceptible to antibiotics that inhibit mucopeptide formation because they possess a cell wall that contains a relatively thick mucopeptide layer to provide structural support of the cytoplasm. The mucopeptide layer is known variously as

murein, glycopeptide, or peptidoglycan, and because of the nature of its chemical structure, it is tough and fibrous. Support is required because gram-positive bacteria concentrate low-molecular-weight metabolites such as amino acids and nucleotides, which impart a high internal osmotic pressure. On the other hand, gram-negative bacteria have a relatively low internal osmotic pressure with a thin layer of mucopeptide.

The synthesis of mucopeptide occurs in distinct steps. The first step is a series of reactions inside the cell that result in the production of the basic building units (uridine diphospho-N-acetyl-muramyl-pentapeptide). Cycloserine inhibits the formation of the pentapeptide portion of the building block. In the next step, the building units are carried to the outside of the cell membrane. During this process, the units are linked covalently to the preexisting cell wall. Vancomycin and bacitracin inhibit this step of the biosynthesis. The final stage of the biosynthesis is the cross-linking of linear molecules to form the highly cross-linked, 3-dimensional mucopeptide. The last reaction in mucopeptide formation is catalyzed by a transpeptidase that splits the terminal D-alanine residues of the pentapeptide of the building unit and forms a peptide bond between the terminal glycine of a pentaglycine bridge and the penultimate D-alanine of a mucopeptide strand (Fig. 12–9). Therefore, each polypeptide side chain of each repeating building unit becomes covalently linked to the side chains of neighboring mucopeptide strands. The penicillins and the cephalosporins are competitive inhibitors of this transpeptidation. Although the precise mechanism is not known, it appears that the penicillin or cephalosporin molecule occupies the D-alanyl-D-alanine substrate site of the transpeptidase and irreversibly inactivates the enzyme.

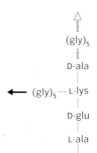

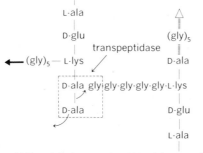

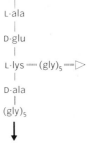

Fig. 12–9. Partial structure of bacterial cell wall mucopeptide showing polysaccharides composed of polymeric chains of alternating units of N-acetylglucosamine and N-acetylmuramic acid. The peptide chains crosslink the polysaccharide chains to make a rigid 3-dimensional structure. The last step in mucopeptide formation is catalyzed by a transpeptidase that splits off the terminal D-alanine and forms a peptide bond between the penultimate D-alanine and the glycine of a pentaglycine bridge.

In recent years, evidence has shown that, in addition to the disruption of cell-wall formation by the inhibition of mucopeptide synthesis, penicillin can cause rapid lysis of the bacterial cell by inducing the action of bacterial autolysins (mucopeptide hydrolases). The penicillin molecule apparently binds to the autolysins to displace or in some other way release a lipoteichoic acid that normally inhibits the bacterial autolysin.

Formation of an essential protein may be blocked at any of the basic stages of protein biosynthesis. The antibiotic could adversely influence the replication and synthesis of DNA, the transcription of the genetic code and the specific sequential synthesis of DNA, the transcription of the genetic code and the specific sequential synthesis of mRNA, or the synthesis and assembly of the ribosomes. All of these biologic processes are fundamental for the eventual synthesis of a protein, but many constituents that act at these levels tend to be relatively toxic. Most of the therapeutically useful (more selectively toxic) antibiotics that act on protein biosynthesis

influence in some manner the normal assembly of the amino acids into proteins at the surface of the mRNA-ribosome complex.

The ribosomes found in bacteria have a sedimentation coefficient of 70S, and they are composed of 2 particles of different size, the 50S and the 30S ribosomal subunits. Each subunit is composed of

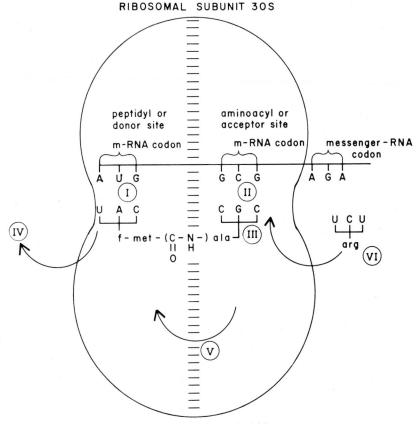

Fig. 12–10. Sequence of events of protein synthesis on the 70S ribosome:

   I. Formation of initiation complex. Involves the binding of the first aminoacyl-tRNA to the ribosome. In bacteria, the first amino acid bound is formylmethionine (f-met).
  II. Binding of the next aminoacyl-tRNA to aminoacyl site.
 III. Formation of peptide bond catalyzed by a ribosome-bound peptidyl transferase.
  IV. Release of formylmethionine-specific tRNA.
   V. The peptidyl-tRNA (f-met-ala-tRNA) moves to the peptidyl site. This is called the translocation step, and the mRNA shifts to the next codon.
  VI. The aminoacyl site is free and available for the next addition of aminoacyl-tRNA which, in this case, is arginine-tRNA.

ribosomal RNA and a number of different proteins. Antibiotic action to inhibit protein biosynthesis can be focused on the events that take place on the ribosomes. These are initiation, binding of aminoacyl-tRNA, peptide bond formation, translocation, and termination (Fig. 12–10).

Streptomycin and, most likely, the other aminoglycoside antibiotics (neomycin, kanamycin, and gentamicin) bind to the 30S subunit and effectively inhibit initiation. All of these antibiotics induce some misreading of the mRNA. The tetracyclines interfere with the binding of aminoacyl-tRNA to the acceptor site of the 30S subunit. Chloramphenicol binds to the 50S subunit where it disrupts the function of peptidyl transferase. Erythromycin also binds to the 50S subunit. It does not inhibit peptide bond formation, but it does block translocation.

The antitumor antibiotics and others disrupt DNA metabolism. Actinomycin D and mithramycin bind through hydrogen bonding to guanine residues of the DNA double helix. Mitomycin C covalently cross-links between the complementary strands of the DNA double helix. These complexes of the drug with the DNA template block the transcription of RNA by DNA-dependent RNA polymerase which, in turn, is responsible for the antitumor effect.

Other antibiotics affect the permeability of the cell membrane in a way that causes leakage of cytoplasmic solutes. The 2 most important groups of these drugs are the polyene antibiotics, amphotericin B, nystatin, and candicidin, and the peptide antibiotics, gramicidin and the polymyxins. The polyene antibiotics are antifungal agents that affect the membranes of eucaryotic cells but have no activity on bacteria. This difference in sensitivity of different organisms to these antibiotics is determined by the presence of sterols in the cell membrane of eucaryotic cells. The polyenes bind to the membrane and the extent of binding is proportional to the amount of sterol present. The peptide antibiotics also bind to the cell membrane and disturb membrane function; however, because these antibiotics are active against bacteria, sterols are not required for binding.

BASES OF TOXICITY

One limitation to the therapeutic use of an antibiotic substance is mammalian toxicity. The manifestation of such adverse reactions varies greatly with different antibiotic molecules. Basically, these side effects are an extension to mammalian biologic processes of the mechanisms of antibiotic action, hypersensitivity, or a pharmacologic action that is independent of the antibiotic activity of the molecule. An antibiotic that acts by inhibiting protein synthesis in susceptible microorganisms is potentially toxic to mammalian systems involving the same or related essential proteins. Theoretically, the safest antibiotic inhibits an essential process, such as cell-wall formation, that is unique to the microorganism. Actual situations usually follow the theoretic considerations, as illustrated by the relative safety of the penicillins and the relative toxicity of chloramphenicol. However, some degree of deviation from the ideal is probably universal because antibiotic molecules normally lack absolute specificity or the ability to influence only one biochemical reaction. In the case of penicillins, hypersensitization with serious consequences precludes the use of these antibiotics in some individuals. Many antibiotic molecules are characterized by reactive functional groups, and hypersensitivity may be a problem with molecules containing functional oxygen groups that can react with proteins to yield a potentially antigenic hapteneprotein molecule. Toxicity caused by some independent pharmacologic property of the antibiotic is usually difficult to predict; this type of complication must be evaluated individually for each antibiotic.

In addition to any adverse pharmacologic action of an antibiotic per se, indirect toxicities can be observed with these therapeutic agents. The most common type of indirect antibiotic-induced toxicity is associated with an alteration in the ecologic balance of the intestinal flora. This problem is greatest with the broad-spectrum antibiotics because a major portion of the intestinal flora may be suppressed. Candida albicans is an example of the slow-growing, unsusceptible microorganism that may become a dominant component of the intestinal flora following the administration of antibiotics. The body frequently has no prior adaptation or tolerance to the level of foreign metabolites resulting from the unusual proliferation of such organisms; the toxicity is usually manifest as gastrointestinal disturbances rather than as acute toxicities.

MODES OF RESISTANCE

Antibiotic resistance is a major therapeutic concern. One practical way to circumvent this problem, at least for short-term purposes, is to develop and use new antibiotics, but experts are concerned justifiably about the practicality of long-term developmental aspects of this approach. Resistance to antibiotics may result through spontaneous or induced genetic mutation. However, many of the practical problems have developed via the process of selection or, in other words, favoring through the use of antibiotics the small frequency of organisms of antibiotic-resistant genotype that exists naturally in the antibiotic-sensitive, wild population. Spontaneous mutation is believed to make only a minor contribution to the total problem of antibiotic resistance. Bacterial cells can acquire genetic material from other bacterial cells through the processes of transformation, transduction, and conjugation. Transformation, which is a process by which DNA from a lysed bacterial cell is inserted directly into a recipient cell, makes no substantial contribution to the clinical problem of drug resistance. Transduction, or the phage-induced transfer of resistant determinant sections of bacterial DNA, is believed to be an important factor in the emergence of drug-resistant strains of Staphylococcus. Conjugation is a widely recognized mechanism for transmitting resistance among gram-negative bacilli of clinical concern. Conjugation of compatible cells (which may represent different species or even genera) provides a means for direct transfer of R-factor genes residing on bacterial episomes, and great danger lies in the fact that bacterial episomes may contain genetic information for multiple resistance.

Multiple mechanisms of resistance to many antibiotics appear to exist, and the lack of precise information in many cases makes general categorization difficult. However, some modes of resistance that can be noted include:

1. Enzymatic inactivation of the antibiotic;
2. Altered permeability of the pathogen to the antibiotic;
3. Development of altered, less sensitive enzymes or of alternate metabolic pathways in the pathogen.

The β-lactamase inactivation of penicillins and cephalosporins is by far the best documented mechanism leading to antibiotic resistance. The significance of penicillinase was recognized at an early date in antibiotic therapy, and the semisynthetic penicillins are a direct result of efforts to avoid the specificity of this enzyme. A penicillin amidase also occurs in some microorganisms; this amidase yields the inactive 6-aminopenicillanic acid, but this type of penicillin inactivation does not appear to contribute significantly as a means of pathogenic resistance in any actual therapeutic problem.

Gram-negative bacteria bearing any of several R-factors for multiple resistance can enzymatically inactivate aminoglycoside antibiotics by forming either phosphoryl, adenyl, or acetyl derivatives of these antibiotics.

Altered permeability is a frequently mentioned mode of resistance. Actual substantiation of this type of involvement is limited. Tetracycline resistance in *Escherichia coli* appears to be related to a decrease in the ability of the bacterial cells to take up the antibiotic. Another possible example is chloramphenicol. One biochemical basis of resistance to this antibiotic is an acquired selective impermeability of cellular membranes of some organisms; however, it is also known that certain strains of *E. coli* that are resistant to chloramphenicol enzymatically inactivate the antibiotic by acetylation.

Resistance caused by the development of altered enzymes or metabolic pathways is poorly documented in the current scientific literature. This general mode of resistance is recognized, e.g., certain resistant strains of *Bacillus subtilis* that fail to bind erythromycin at the 50S subunits on the ribosomes, but the overall therapeutic significance of this type of resistance is relatively unknown.

ANTIBIOTICS DERIVED FROM AMINO ACID METABOLISM

The commercially available and therapeutically useful antibiotics can be classified on the basis of the biosynthetic origin of the antibiotic molecules. These useful microbial metabolites are products of amino acid, acetate, and carbohydrate metabolism. Only one of the basic groups of metabolites is involved in the formation of most medicinally important antibiotics, but in the case of some, such as the macrolides, precursors from diverse metabolic origins are combined to yield the antibiotic molecule.

Antibiotics derived from amino acids include the penicillins, the cephalosporins, chloramphenicol, cycloserine, dactinomycin, and the polypeptide antibiotics (e.g., bacitracin, polymyxin). Considerations of chronology, sophisticated state of current development, and significance suggest the penicillins for initial monographic coverage.

PENICILLINS

Penicillin antagonism attracted the attention of Sir Alexander Fleming in 1928. Fleming was studying staphylococci at St. Mary's College in London when he noticed a zone of inhibition surrounding a *Penicillium* contaminant in one of his cultures. The *Penicillium* was initially identified as *P. rubrum*, but was later determined to be *P. notatum*. Interest in this antagonism remained largely academic until after 1940. In 1938, Florey and Chain at Oxford University first isolated a crude penicillin mixture from the mold, and during the early 1940s, the therapeutic potential of penicillin was demonstrated.

Conditions in England during the first half of World War II were such that efforts to determine suitable procedures for producing commercial quantities of the antibiotic were conducted primarily in the United States. Significant early discoveries included the influence of nutrient composition on penicillin production and the discovery of a strain of *P. chrysogenum* which would produce the antibiotic in submerged fermentation. The presence of phenylpropanoid or phenylacetyl derivatives in the nutrient medium favored the formation of benzylpenicillin (penicillin G). Other penicillins could be formed by adding the appropriate precursor moieties to the fermentation cultures; penicillin V is an example of a therapeutically useful penicillin that was prepared initially by this type of manipulated biologic process (Fig. 12–11).

Discovery in the late 1950s of a strain of *P. chrysogenum* that accumulated high yields of 6-aminopenicillanic acid provided an alternate approach to preparing unusual penicillins, such as penicillin V, and provided an opportunity for even greater modification in the antibiotic molecules. 6-Aminopenicillanic acid has

no significant antibiotic activity per se, but this biologically prepared substance can be chemically acylated to give a wide variety of active molecules. Ampicillin, amoxicillin, carbenicillin, cloxacillin, cyclacillin, dicloxacillin, hetacillin, methicillin, nafcillin, oxacillin, and ticarcillin are therapeutically utilized semisynthetic penicillins that have been selected for various advantages offered by their chemical, physical, or spectral properties. Structures of the commercially available penicillins are shown in Figure 12–12.

BIOSYNTHESIS OF PENICILLINS. The amino acids cysteine and valine are incorporated

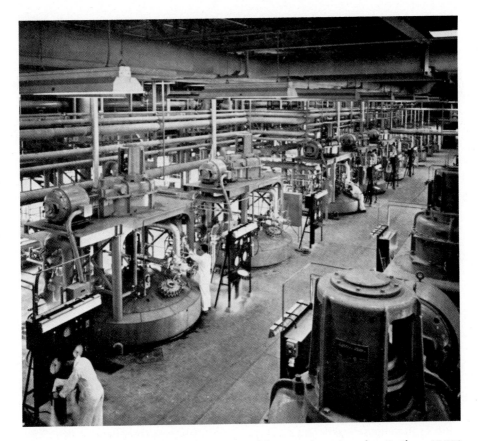

Fig. 12–11. Antibiotic fermentation area. Final fermentation takes place in these 18,000-gallon tanks. The tanks are 30 feet high but are buried to within a few feet of their tops. A maze of pipes carries water, steam, and air into the area. Storage tanks of 30,000-gallon capacity are located nearby. (Photo, courtesy of Eli Lilly & Co.)

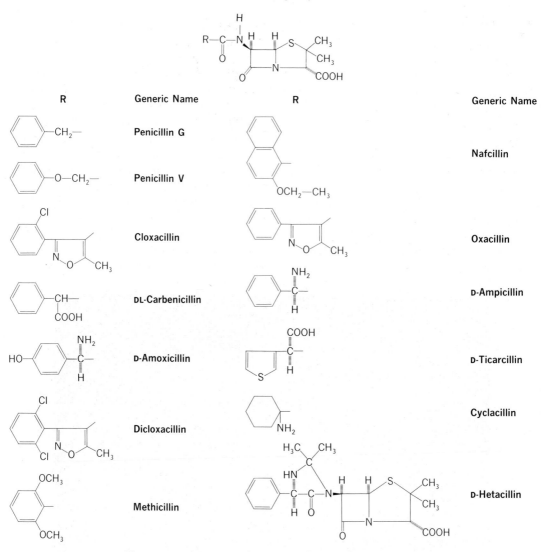

Fig. 12–12. Structures of commercially available penicillins.

into the 6-aminopenicillanic acid portion of penicillin molecules, and the acyl group of penicillin G is derived from phenylacetic acid. Many of the details of the biosynthetic pathway require further clarification. It is generally believed that terminal steps in the pathway involve introduction of the characteristic acyl group, and the action of an acyl transferase on isopenicillin N is suspected (Fig. 12–13). The tripeptide, δ-(α-aminoadipyl)-cys-

teinylvaline, is the presumed precursor of isopenicillin N, and dehydrogenation involving the mercapto function and one of the methyl groups of the valine residue of some metabolite of this tripeptide appears to yield the nucleus of cephalosporin C.

PROPERTIES OF THE PENICILLINS. The chemical structure of the penicillin nucleus is unusual and is characterized by a 4-membered β-lactam ring fused to a

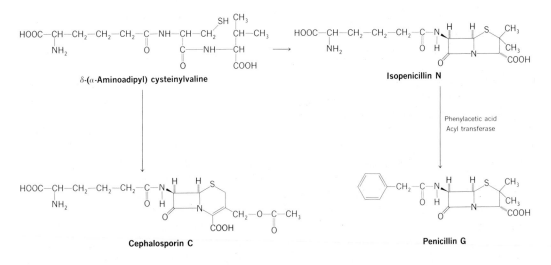

Fig. 12–13. Biosynthesis of penicillin G and cephalosporin C.

thiazolidine ring. This ring system contains 3 asymmetric carbon atoms in a fixed spatial arrangement, and any disruption of this arrangement by rupturing either the β-lactam ring or the thiazolidine ring results in a complete loss of antimicrobial activity. Unfortunately, the 4-membered β-lactam ring has considerable biologic and chemical lability, which has created a number of problems in the therapeutic utilization of these antibiotics. Biologically, microorganisms resistant to the action of penicillin G produce a β-lactamase (penicillinase) which hydrolyzes the β-lactam ring to form inactive penicilloic acid (Fig. 12–14). Chemically, penicillin G is rapidly inactivated when the pH is more acid than 5 or more alkaline than 8. In acidic conditions, penicillin G is converted to penillic acid and to penicilloic

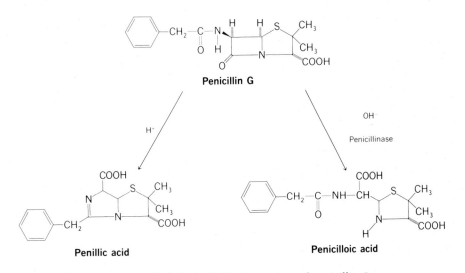

Fig. 12–14. Hydrolysis of β-lactam system of penicillin G.

acid in alkali (Fig. 12–14). Ideally, aqueous solutions of penicillin G salts should be buffered at pH 6.8 for maximum stability. Penicillins are also inactivated by metal ions, such as zinc and copper, and by oxidizing agents. The need for penicillin antibiotics with inherent stability in gastric fluids and with resistance to penicillinase prompted the search for and development of other penicillins. Ampicillin and penicillin V are characterized by a significant degree of acid stability, and cloxacillin, dicloxacillin, nafcillin, and oxacillin are both acid-stable and penicillinase-resistant. In the case of the penicillins with increased stability in gastric acid, the introduction of an electron-attracting group into the side chain in close proximity to the amide linkage inhibits the participation of the side-chain amide carbonyl in the electron displacement caused by the acid proton. Penicillins resistant to the action of penicillinase possess side chains with acyl groups that protect the β-lactam ring through steric hindrance.

Definite proof of the structure of penicillin was not established until 1949. The need for quantitation of penicillin antibiotics prior to complete elucidation of their chemistry and prior to feasible approaches for resolving or avoiding mixtures of penicillins resulted in the use of microbiologic assay. Microbiologic assay still has some utility in evaluating certain antibiotics, and biologic units are used to express quantitation for penicillin G and penicillin V. Sodium penicillin G is currently accepted as the reference standard; 1 unit is the antibiotic activity of 0.6 μg of sodium penicillin G reference standard. Microbial assays must be conducted under carefully controlled conditions, and alternate procedures frequently offer some advantages at the present time for quantitation of chemical availability. However, therapeutic efficacy is best determined biologically. *Staphylococcus aureus* ATCC* No. 29737 is used as the control test organism for all commercially available penicillins and cephalosporins, except ampicillin, carbenicillin, and ticarcillin. These penicillins have an extended spectrum of antimicrobial activity. *Micrococcus luteus* ATCC No. 9341 is used as a test organism for ampicillin. Carbenicillin is assayed with *Pseudomonas aeruginosa* ATCC No. 25619 and ticarcillin with *Pseudomonas aeruginosa* ATCC No. 29336.

USE OF PENICILLINS. Penicillin G is considered the agent of first choice against many pathogenic gram-positive bacteria. These include *Bacillus anthracis, Clostridium tetani, Clostridium perfringens, Staphylococcus aureus,* β-hemolytic group A *Streptococcus, Streptococcus pneumoniae,* and *Streptococcus faecalis*. In addition, penicillin is the drug of choice in treating syphilis (*Treponema pallidum*) and infections caused by the gram-negative cocci, *Neisseria gonorrhoeae* and *Neisseria meningitidis*.

Intramuscular or intravenous injection is the usual method of administration for penicillin G. The water-soluble sodium or potassium salts are available for this purpose as are the repository forms, which are water-insoluble salts of high-molecular-weight amines such as procaine and benzathine.

Penicillin G is destroyed by gastric acid, and therefore absorption after oral administration is irregular and variable; consequently, the penicillin of choice for oral administration is penicillin V, which is less susceptible than penicillin G to degradation by gastric acid and produces blood levels 2 to 5 times higher than does penicillin G. The patient should also be cautioned to take the antibiotic on an empty stomach

*American Type Culture Collection, 12301 Parklawn Drive, Rockville, Md. 20852.

(1 hour before or 2 hours after eating) because food inhibits its absorption.

In vitro sensitivity tests have shown that strains of group A *Streptococcus* have a sensitivity to penicillin G as low as 0.006 μg per ml; and the MIC range for other bacteria causing infections in which penicillin G is recommended is 0.01 to 2.0 μg per ml. The rapid intravenous administration of sodium or potassium penicillin G results in an immediate high blood level; however, after 1 hour, only 10% of the original dose remains in the blood owing to both distribution and elimination of the drug. Therefore, to maintain therapeutic blood levels in life-threatening infections, the antibiotic is administered by continuous infusion, preferably with a constant-infusion pump rather than by the constant-drip method.

After intramuscular injection of sodium or potassium penicillin G, a peak blood level is obtained within 30 minutes. Then the serum level falls rapidly with a usual half-life of only 30 minutes. It is important to remember that the height of the blood-level peak and the length of time during which penicillin may be demonstrated in the blood depend on the dose and also can vary from person to person.

In order to maintain therapeutic blood levels of penicillin G, 2 approaches are utilized. One approach interferes with the excretion of the antibiotic in the tubules of the kidney. When probenecid is used with penicillin, penicillin serum concentrations are approximately doubled. The supposed mechanism involves the hydrolysis of probenecid in the body to yield benzoic acid, which is conjugated in the liver with glycine to provide β-aminohippuric acid, which, in turn, competes with penicillin for renal excretion.

A more widely used approach for maintaining therapeutic blood levels delays absorption by employing repository penicillins. After intramuscular injection of an aqueous suspension of procaine penicillin G, a peak blood level is obtained in about 2 hours, and if an adult dose of at least 600,000 units is used, detectable levels are maintained in most patients for at least 24 hours. Benzathine penicillin G is less water soluble than the procaine salt, and, following intramuscular injection of 600,000 units in an aqueous suspension, serum concentrations of 0.018 to 0.06 μg per ml persist for up to 2 weeks.

Resistance to penicillin G occurs fairly frequently among strains of *Staphylococcus aureus*. For this reason, if it is not known whether the infecting organism is a penicillinase producer, a penicillinase-resistant semisynthetic penicillin is normally the antibiotic of first choice until a culture-sensitivity test can be performed. Among the penicillinase-resistant semisynthetic penicillins exists essentially equivalent antimicrobial activity against pathogenic gram-positive cocci with MICs of 0.05 to 1.0 μg per ml; however, in general they are less effective than penicillin G against these organisms.

Ampicillin, amoxicillin, carbenicillin, cyclacillin, and ticarcillin are extended spectrum penicillins and have activity against certain pathogenic gram-negative bacilli against which penicillin G has little activity at normal therapeutic doses. For this reason, ampicillin and amoxicillin are useful in the treatment of *Escherichia*, *Haemophilus*, *Salmonella* and *Shigella* infections as well as of those infections caused by gram-negative cocci and gram-positive organisms. Carbenicillin and ticarcillin are important in treating *Enterobacter*, *Escherichia*, *Proteus*, and *Pseudomonas aeruginosa* infections. The most recently marketed extended-spectrum penicillin, cyclacillin, has been approved for use against gram-positive cocci, *Haemophilus*, and urinary tract infections caused by *Escherichia coli* and *Proteus mirabilis*.

A possible explanation for the extension of the antimicrobial spectrum of some of the penicillins such as ampicillin is that these antibiotics penetrate to the site of action more readily than does penicillin G. The mucopeptide layer of the cell wall of gram-negative organisms lies behind layers of polysaccharide, protein, and lipid, which serve as a penetration barrier to penicillin G but not to the extended-spectrum penicillins. In the wild type *Escherichia coli* with an intact penetration barrier, the MIC for penicillin G is 200 μg per ml as opposed to 2 μg per ml for ampicillin; however, if the penetration barrier is removed through mutation, penicillin G exhibits an MIC of 5 μg per ml and ampicillin an MIC of 0.5 μg per ml against the mutant strain.

The penicillins act by inhibiting mucopeptide formation in bacterial cell walls (see page 341). Presumably, the lack of comparable metabolism in zoologic systems contributes to the relatively low incidence of serious side effects with these antibiotics. The most frequent adverse reactions are allergic responses, and the occasional incidence of anaphylactic shock can be fatal in the absence of emergency treatment. Epinephrine is usually administered for symptomatic control in penicillin shock.

In the early years of penicillin therapy, many of the cases of hypersensitivity were attributed correctly to foreign proteins, and the frequency of such reactions was reduced by improved purification procedures. However, impurities are not responsible for all penicillin reactions. Penicillin acts as a hapten and combines with body proteins to form an antigen which, in this case, is an allergen. Cross-sensitivity occurs among all compounds with the penicillin nucleus; however, there is experimental and clinical evidence that some semisynthetic penicillins are less allergenic. Sensitization is usually owing to a previous treatment with penicillin, but some people get an allergic reaction when first treated owing to a hidden contact such as consumption of milk containing penicillin as a result of veterinary treatment. A history of hypersensitivity to penicillin is an indication to use alternate antibiotics for control of penicillin-susceptible pathogens.

Penicillin G potassium or potassium benzyl penicillin is normally formulated with suitable buffer systems. Solid formulations have an expiration date that is not later than 5 years from the time the lot was released by the manufacturer. Sterile aqueous solutions may be stored in a refrigerator for 3 or 7 days (the latter if an approved sodium citrate buffer is used) without significant loss of potency, and the appropriate storage period must be stated on the label.

Penicillin G potassium may be administered orally, intramuscularly, or intravenously. One mg of pure penicillin G potassium is equivalent to 1595 units. The usual dose is 200,000 to 500,000 units, 3 or 4 times daily orally and 500,000 to 1 million units intravenously, 6 to 8 times a day. Daily doses of 10 million units or more are given by intravenous infusion, and up to 100 million units daily may be administered by this method. The dose range varies widely, depending on the pathogen being treated, the extent of the infection, and other clinical conditions.

PRESCRIPTION PRODUCTS. Numerous preparations of penicillin G potassium are available, including Sugracillin®, Pentids®, and Pfizerpen®.

Penicillin G sodium or sodium benzyl penicillin is normally formulated with suitable buffer systems. Solid preparations have an expiration date that is not later than 5 years from the time the lot was released by the manufacturer, and sterile aqueous solutions may be stored in a refrigerator for 3 days without significant loss of potency. Pure penicillin G sodium is used as the reference standard for microbial assays of the penicillins, and 1 mg is equivalent to 1667 units. Penicillin G sodium is used orally, intramuscularly, or intravenously in the same manner as the potassium salt. A wide range in dosage will be encountered; the usual dose is considered to be 400,000 units, 4 times a day, orally or intramuscularly, and 10 million units daily, intravenously.

Penicillin G procaine is the slightly soluble procaine salt of penicillin G. One mg of pure penicillin G procaine is equivalent to 1009 units.

This antibiotic is used intramuscularly and has the advantage of prolonged action owing to slow absorption. It is formulated in an aqueous suspension. The usual intramuscular dose is 300,000 to 600,000 units, 1 or 2 times a day.

PRESCRIPTION PRODUCTS. Crysticillin A. S.®, Duracillin A. S.®, Wycillin®, Pfizerpen-A.S.®.

Penicillin G benzathine or N,N'-dibenzylethylenediamine dipenicillin G is a slightly soluble salt of penicillin that is used intramuscularly for its unusually prolonged duration of action and orally for its resistance to gastric inactivation. One mg of pure penicillin G benzathine is equivalent to 1211 units, and commercial material must have a potency of not less than 1050 units per mg. The usual dose, intramuscularly, is 1.2 million to 2.4 million units as a single dose or 600,000 to 1.2 million units, 2 times a month to 3 times a week. The oral dose is 400,000 to 600,000 units, 4 to 6 times a day.

PRESCRIPTION PRODUCTS. Bicillin®, Permapen®.

Penicillin V or phenoxymethyl penicillin and penicillin V potassium or phenoxymethyl penicillin potassium are relatively acid-stable. The potassium salt is soluble in water, and this appears to favor better absorption following oral administration. However, both forms of this penicillin gave good blood levels, the average ranging from 2 to 5 times higher than the levels obtainable with comparable oral doses of penicillin G. One mg of pure phenoxymethyl penicillin is equivalent to 1695 units, and 1 mg of the pure potassium salt equals 1530 units. Quantities are usually expressed on a weight basis for preparations of these penicillins, and the usual oral dose is 125 to 500 mg (200,000 to 800,000 units), 3 or 4 times a day.

PRESCRIPTION PRODUCTS. Free acid: V-cillin®; potassium salt: Ledercillin VK®, Pen-Vee K®, V-Cillin K®, Veetids®, Pfizerpen VK®.

Cloxacillin, dicloxacillin, methicillin, nafcillin, and oxacillin are semisynthetic penicillins that are not inactivated by penicillinase. They are recommended primarily for treatment of staphylococcal infections resistant to other penicillins. Methicillin is acid-labile and must be administered parenterally. The other 4 penicillins are stable in gastric acidity. Nafcillin and oxacillin are available in formulations for oral and parenteral administration; cloxacillin and dicloxacillin are only used orally. All of these penicillins are employed as sodium salts.

Cloxacillin, dicloxacillin, nafcillin, and oxacillin are characterized by a high degree of binding to serum protein, but approximately only 20% of methicillin in blood is bound to serum proteins. Dicloxacillin is absorbed more readily than the other penicillinase-resistant penicillins that are administered orally. However, food interferes sufficiently with the absorption of all of these penicillins, including dicloxacillin, to prompt the recommendation that they be administered before meals in order to obtain satisfactory blood levels. A 500-mg oral dose of oxacillin results in a peak blood level of 2.6 μg per ml in 1 hour. When compared to oxacillin at the same dose, cloxacillin provides a 2-fold greater blood level, and dicloxacillin effects a 4 times greater blood level. The usual doses are 1 g, intramuscularly or intravenously, 4 to 6 times a day for methicillin; 250 mg to 1 g, orally, 4 to 6 times a day and 500 mg to 1 g, intramuscularly or intravenously, 4 to 6 times a day for nafcillin; 500 mg to 1 g, orally, 4 to 6 times a day and 250 mg to 1 g, intravenously or intramuscularly, 4 to 6 times a day for oxacillin; 250 to 500 mg, orally, 4 times a day for cloxacillin; and 125 to 250 mg, orally, 4 times a day for dicloxacillin.

PRESCRIPTION PRODUCTS. Cloxacillin: Tegopen®; dicloxacillin: Dynapen®, Pathocil®, Veracillin®; methicillin: Staphcillin®, Azapen®; nafcillin: Unipen®; oxacillin: Prostaphlin®, Bactocill®.

Ampicillin or aminobenzyl penicillin is an acid-stable, readily absorbed semi-synthetic penicillin. It is inactivated by penicillinase, but has an unusual spectrum of activity for a penicillin. It is active against most of the bacteria sensitive to penicillin G, but also has greater activity against certain gram-negative bacilli than does penicillin G. The L-isomer of ampicillin is only about as active as penicillin G against gram-negative bacteria. The D-isomer shows increased activity; therefore, the D-isomer is used in therapy. Ampicillin has special clinical value for treatment of infections caused by *Haemophilus influenzae, Salmonella* species, and *Shigella* species. This antibiotic controls effectively nonpenicillinase-forming strains of *Proteus mirabilis* and *Escherichia coli,* but the high frequency of penicillinase formation by these pathogens limits the clinical effectiveness of ampicillin with respect to these species. The in vitro MICs for ampicillin range from 0.25 μg per ml for strains of *Haemophilus influenzae* to 5 μg per ml for sensitive strains of *Escherichia coli*. A 250-mg oral dose of ampicillin results in a peak blood level of 1.8 μg per ml reached in 2 hours; therefore, it is important to use high doses to treat *E. coli* infections. The sodium salt of ampicillin is used in parenteral formulations, and oral dosage forms normally utilize the free acid. The usual dose is 250 to 500 mg, orally, 4 times a day and 500 mg, intramuscularly or intravenously, 4 times a day.

PRESCRIPTION PRODUCTS. Amcill®, Omnipen®, Penbritin®, Pensyn®, Polycillin®, Principen®, Totacillin®.

Hetacillin is prepared by a reaction of ampicillin with acetone. It undergoes hydrolysis in solution both in vivo and in vitro with the formation of ampicillin; consequently, hetacillin has antibacterial activity identical to that of ampicillin. A 225-mg oral dose of hetacillin provides a 1.7 to 2.1 μg per ml peak blood level of ampicillin. The usual dose is 225 to 450 mg, orally, 4 times a day.

PRESCRIPTION PRODUCT. Versapen®.

Amoxicillin is the p-hydroxy derivative of ampicillin. It is stable in the presence of gastric acid and better absorbed from the gastrointestinal tract in the presence of food than is ampicillin. Amoxicillin has antibacterial activity similar to that of ampicillin. A 250-mg oral dose gives a peak blood level of 4.3 μg per ml. The usual dose is 250 to 500 mg, orally, 3 times a day.

PRESCRIPTION PRODUCTS. Amoxil®, Larotid®, Polymox®.

Carbenicillin disodium is a carboxybenzyl penicillin with increased antibacterial activity against gram-negative bacilli. The D- and L-isomers display only slight differences in biologic activity and undergo rapid interconversion when in solution; therefore, the racemic mixture is used. Carbenicillin is the drug of choice in the treatment of *Pseudomonas aeruginosa* infections and is an alternate antibiotic in *Escherichia coli, Enterobacter,* and *Proteus* infections. The antibiotic can be administered in sufficient dosage (up to 40 g daily) to obtain serum concentrations exceeding 50 to 60 μg per ml. Such concentrations inhibit most *Pseudomonas aeruginosa* strains. The usual dose, intramuscularly or intravenously, is the equivalent of 1 to 2 g of carbenicillin, 4 times a day and, by intravenous infusion, up to 40 g a day. Carbenicillin indanyl sodium is also available for oral administration. The usual dose is 382 to 764 mg, 4 times a day.

Prescription Products. Carbenicillin Disodium: Geopen®, Pyopen®; Carbenicillin Indanyl Sodium: Geocillin®.

Ticarcillin disodium is the thienyl analog of carbenicillin and has the same antimicrobial spectrum and indications as does carbenicillin. Evidence suggests that it is somewhat more active than carbenicillin, particularly against *Pseudomonas aeruginosa*. The usual dose for uncomplicated urinary tract infections is 1 g every 6 hours, either intramuscularly or intravenously. For urinary tract infections with complications, the intravenous dose is 150 to 200 mg per kg per day in divided doses every 4 or 8 hours. For systemic infections, the adult intravenous dose is 200 to 300 mg per kg of body weight daily in divided doses every 3, 4, or 6 hours.

Prescription Product. Ticar®.

Cyclacillin is the most recently approved penicillin for therapeutic use. It is acid-stable and rapidly and well absorbed from the gastrointestinal tract. The peak concentration after a 500-mg dose is 4 times higher than that of ampicillin and about 1½ times the peak concentration of oral amoxicillin. Whereas cyclacillin has an antimicrobial spectrum similar to that of ampicillin, it has less activity in vitro than ampicillin against many organisms. It has been approved for treatment of respiratory tract infections, otitis media, skin infections caused by gram-positive cocci and

Haemophilus influenzae, and urinary tract infections caused by *Escherichia coli* and *Proteus mirabilis*. The usual dose range is 250 to 500 mg, 4 times daily.

Prescription Product. Cyclapen®.

CEPHALOSPORINS AND CEPHAMYCINS

In 1945, Brotzu isolated a microorganism from sea water collected near a sewage outlet off the coast of Sardinia and noted its antagonism to both gram-positive and gram-negative bacteria. The organism was identified as *Cephalosporium acremonium*. Abraham and his coworkers at Oxford reported the isolation of 3 substances with antibiotic activity from cultures of this organism during 1955 and 1956. These metabolites were a steroid (cephalosporin P) that has achieved no therapeutic significance, penicillin N and cephalosporin C. Cephalosporin C is biosynthetically related to the penicillins (see page 347) and resembles these antibiotics in many of its biologic and chemical properties. The major difference is a 7-aminocephalosporanic acid nucleus which has a fused dihydrothiazine *beta*-lactam ring system rather than the fused thiazolidine *beta*-lactam system of 6-aminopenicillanic acid. The degree of antibacterial activity of cephalosporin C is only moderate and it is not used therapeutically. However, it is produced by fermentation in large quantities to serve as a starting material for the chemical production of the semisynthetic cephalosporin antibiotics (Fig. 12–15).

The cephamycins are *beta*-lactam antibiotics that are closely related chemically to the cephalosporins. They are produced by actinomycetes rather than fungi and are 7-α-methoxycephalosporins. Cephamycin C, which is produced by *Streptomyces lactamdurans*, serves as a starting material for

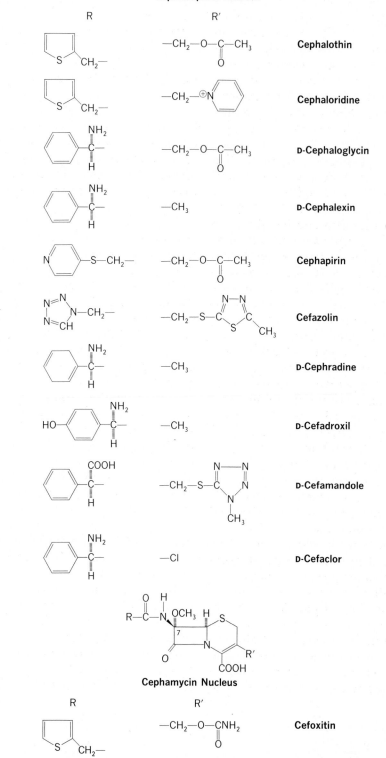

Fig. 12–15. Structures of commercially available cephalosporin and cephamycin antibiotics.

the chemical synthesis of cefoxitin, the only cephamycin antibiotic currently available for therapeutic use.

Cephalothin, cephaloridine, cefazolin, cephapirin, cephradine, cephaloglycin, cephalexin, cefadroxil, cefamandole, and **cefaclor** have antibacterial activity similar to that of ampicillin. They are effective against gram-positive bacteria including penicillinase-producing *Staphylococcus* (Table 12–3). The cephalosporin antibiotics are resistant to penicillinase, but they are inactivated by another β-lactamase, cephalosporinase. Certain gram-negative organisms, including *Neisseria, Haemophilus, Salmonella, Shigella, Escherichia coli, Proteus mirabilis* and some strains of *Klebsiella pneumoniae,* are sensitive to the cephalosporins. Species of *Enterobacter* and *Pseudomonas* as well as most indole-producing species of *Proteus* are resistant. The susceptibility of *Haemophilus in-* *fluenzae* is quite variable and, generally, cephalosporins are less active against this organism than are the extended-spectrum penicillins such as ampicillin. The cephalosporins penetrate most tissues well except that, unlike the penicillins, they are unpredictable in the manner in which they cross the blood-brain barrier; consequently, the cephalosporins should never be considered an adequate substitute for the penicillins in treating meningitis. For most of the parenterally used cephalosporins (cephalothin, cephaloridine, cefazolin, cephapirin), the in vitro MIC values may vary slightly with a particular antibiotic; however, they are essentially equivalent. The MIC values for these antibiotics range from 0.007 μg per ml for strains of *Streptococcus* to 16 μg per ml for strains of *Haemophilus influenzae.* Cefamandole is purported to be more resistant than most other cephalosporins to the

Table 12–3. Therapeutically Important Cephalosporin and Cephamycin Antibiotics

Generic Name	Prescription Products	Usual Dose	Peak Blood Levels
Parenteral:			
(intravenous or intramuscular)			
Cephalothin sodium	Keflin®	500 mg to 1 g, 4 to 6 times daily	9 μg/ml[a]
Cephaloridine	Loridine®	500 mg every 8 hours	19 μg/ml[a]
Cefazolin sodium	Kefzol®, Ancef®	500 mg to 1 g, 3 to 4 times daily	32 μg/ml[a]
Cephapirin sodium	Cefadyl®	500 mg to 1 g, 4 to 6 times daily	10 μg/ml[a]
Cephradine	Velosef®	500 mg to 1 g, 4 times daily	5 μg/ml[a]
Cefamandole naftate	Mandol®	500 mg to 1 g, 3 to 6 times daily	14 μg/ml[a]
Cefoxitin	Mefoxin®	1 to 2 g, 3 to 6 times daily	11 μg/ml[a]
Oral:			
Cephaloglycin dihydrate	Kafocin®	250 mg every 6 hours	——
Cephalexin monohydrate	Keflex®	250 mg, 4 times daily	9 μg/ml[b]
Cephradine	Velosef®, Anspor®	250 to 500 mg, 4 times daily	9 μg/ml[b]
Cefadroxil monohydrate	Duricef®	500 mg to 1 g, 2 times daily	9 μg/ml[b]
Cefaclor	Ceclor®	250 mg, 3 times daily	6 μg/ml[b]

[a] 30 minutes after a 500-mg intramuscular dose.
[b] 1 hour after a 250-mg oral dose.

cephalosporinases produced by gram-negative bacilli of the Enterobacteriaceae and by *Haemophilus influenzae*. In this regard, it has shown activity against many ampicillin-resistant strains of *Haemophilus influenzae*. The cephalosporins used orally, namely, cephaloglycin, cephalexin, cefadroxil, cefaclor, and cephradine, which is also used parenterally, are less effective than the parenteral cephalosporins against *Escherichia coli*, *Proteus mirabilis*, and species of *Klebsiella*. Cephalexin, cefadroxil, and cephradine can be used to treat infections caused by gram-positive bacteria, and because of the high concentration of these antibiotics excreted in the urine, e.g., 1000 μg per ml following a 250-mg oral dose of cephalexin, they are used to treat urinary tract infections caused by *Escherichia coli*, *Proteus mirabilis*, and *Klebsiella* species. For the same reason, cephaloglycin's main use is the treatment of urinary tract infections. Because of a prolonged excretion, cefadroxil has the advantage of providing a more sustained serum and urine concentration than is obtained with other oral cephalosporins. Clinical studies indicate that cefadroxil, 1 g twice daily, is as effective as cephalexin, 500 mg 4 times daily. Cefaclor is more active in vitro against *Haemophilus influenzae* than are other available oral cephalosporins.

The cephalosporins inhibit cell-wall formation, and this general mode of action explains their relatively low toxicity. Hypersensitivity is a frequent side effect of the cephalosporins, and some cross-sensitivity in patients allergic to penicillin necessitates care in administering cephalosporins to individuals allergic to penicillin. Cephaloridine in doses above 4 g daily can damage the renal tubules; therefore, patients with impaired renal function should be given an alternate antibiotic. Cephalothin can cause thrombophlebitis when administered intrave-nously in doses larger than 6 g daily for periods longer than 3 days; also, intramuscular injection of this antibiotic may be painful. Cefamandole produces less severe pain on intramuscular injection, but because some pain may be produced, the use of the intramuscular route of administration may be restricted. Cefazolin is the first cephalosporin marketed that seems to be devoid of these undesirable side effects and is fast becoming the parenteral cephalosporin of choice.

Cefoxitin has resistance to many of the β-lactamases that can hydrolyze the commonly used cephalosporins. This resistance is owing to the steric hindrance around the 7-position of the cephamycin nucleus because of the 7 α-methoxy group. This drug is available only for parenteral use because it is not absorbed from the gastrointestinal tract. Intramuscular injection of cefoxitin is less painful than cephalothin. The antimicrobial spectrum of cefoxitin is similar to that of cefamandole.

CHLORAMPHENICOL

Chloramphenicol was originally obtained from a culture of *Streptomyces venezuelae* Burkholder that was isolated in 1947 from a soil sample collected near Caracas, Venezuela. Because the organism had not been described previously, Burkholder applied the name *venezuelae* to the species. This antibiotic attracted considerable attention because it was the first truly broad-spectrum antibiotic discovered. Its spectrum of action includes gram-negative and gram-positive bacteria, a number of rickettsial pathogens, and a few viruses.

Chemically, chloramphenicol proved to be fairly simple. Its most unusual feature was the presence of a nitro group on a normal biologic metabolite. The molecular skeleton of the antibiotic suggested a biosynthetic origin via phenylpropanoid metabolism. Experimental studies with radioactive precursors have confirmed a shikimic acid-phenylpropanoid pathway for the biosynthesis of chloramphenicol, but the pathway apparently branches from normal phenylpropanoid metabolism prior to the formation of phenylalanine or tyrosine. p-Aminophenylpyruvic acid has been suggested as an early metabolite in the biosynthetic pathway, and subsequent steps involving transamination, hydroxylation, acylation, reduction of the carboxyl group, and terminal oxidation of the amino group are suspected (Fig. 12–16).

The relative simplicity of the chloramphenicol molecule led to the early development of feasible synthetic procedures for commercial production of the antibiotic. This antibiotic is unique with respect to the successful development of totally synthetic means for commercial production. Four isomers exist; the active one is D(−)-threo-2,2-dichloro-N-[β-hydroxy-α-(hydroxymethyl)-p-nitrophenethyl]acetamide.

Chloramphenicol acts by inhibiting protein synthesis at the ribosome level. It binds preferentially to the 50S subunit of microbial 70S ribosomes and disrupts peptidyl transferase, the enzyme that catalyzes peptide bond formation. Other types of involvement can be detected experimentally, but their significance for therapeutic application of the antibiotic is unknown. The relative lack of affinity for mammalian 80S ribosomes presumably explains the low incidence of adverse reactions with chloramphenicol. However, occasional development of aplastic anemia (estimated to be 1:25,000 or less) and related blood dyscrasias, which may be irreversible and fatal, introduces a serious limitation on the therapeutic utility of this antibiotic. When chloramphenicol is employed, the blood picture should be monitored daily or on alternate days for evidence of changes in the reticulocytes or other abnormalities. Biochemical details of the toxicities have not been clarified fully, but microbial reduction by the gut flora of the nitro func-

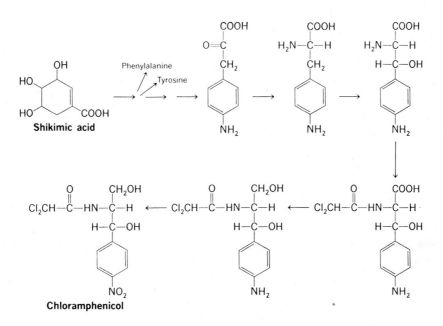

Fig. 12–16. Biosynthesis of chloramphenicol.

tion in a low percentage of the ingested chloramphenicol may be a contributing factor.

Other antibiotics now provide alternate means of controlling many pathogens formerly controlled only by chloramphenicol, which should be used only in serious infections caused by susceptible organisms when other less dangerous antibiotics are ineffective or contraindicated. Chloramphenicol may still be the drug of choice for acute typhoid fever, other severe *Salmonella* infections, and certain *Bacteroides* strains. Penicillin hypersensitivity and renal insufficiency present considerations that could favor the use of chloramphenicol over ampicillin and tetracycline, respectively. Microbial resistance to chloramphenicol is characterized in many cases by acetylation of the antibiotic. The greatest resistance problem occurs with *Pseudomonas*, but episomal R-factor transfer causes some resistance in other gram-negative bacteria.

Chloramphenicol is stable, but esters of the antibiotic are employed in certain pharmaceutic formulations for solubility purposes. These esters are hydrolyzed in the body to release the physiologically active molecule. The insoluble palmitate ester is used in some oral formulations to avoid the bitter taste of the antibiotic, and the monosodium succinate ester is used for greater water solubility in preparations for intravenous use. The usual dose is the equivalent of 50 mg of chloramphenicol per kg of body weight daily in 4 divided oral doses or intravenously in 2 or 3 divided doses. The antibiotic is absorbed readily on oral administration; the usual dose gives blood levels of approximately 10 μg per ml in 2 to 4 hours. The MIC range for most clinically sensitive bacteria is 0.2 to 2.0 μg per ml, but higher doses of the antibiotic are required occasionally for pathogens with an MIC in the 15 to 50 μg per ml range. Chloramphenicol is 60% pro-

tein bound in the blood, diffuses readily into other body tissues and fluids, and has a normal biologic half-life between 2 and 5 hours. Hepatic conjugation with glucuronic acid inactivates approximately 90% of the antibiotic prior to tubular excretion. The balance of the antibiotic is eliminated in free form by glomerular filtration; rapid renal clearance yields urine concentrations of active chloramphenicol that are adequate for therapeutic purposes, but this antibiotic is rarely indicated for urinary tract infections.

PRESCRIPTION PRODUCTS. Chloromycetin®, Mychel®.

LINCOMYCIN AND CLINDAMYCIN

Lincomycin is produced by *Streptomyces lincolnensis*. It has an amide function in the molecule and may be derived by a combination of amino acid and carbohydrate metabolites. **Clindamycin** (7-chloro-7-deoxylincomycin) is synthetically derived from lincomycin. These antibiotics have primarily gram-positive spectra, including pneumococci, staphylococci, and streptococci, with the exception of *Streptococcus faecalis*; the anaerobic spectra (both gram-negative and gram-positive) are also recognized as distinctive and significant. Clindamycin appears slightly more effective quantitatively than lincomycin; the MICs for most bacteria susceptible to clindamycin are in the 0.01 to 3.1 μg per ml range compared with a range of 0.02 to 6.2 μg per ml for lincomycin.

These antibiotics inhibit protein synthesis by a mechanism related closely to that of chloramphenicol and erythromycin. They all bind to the same site on the 50S subunit of 70S ribosomes. Erythromycin has a greater affinity for the site and thus effectively antagonizes the action of clindamycin or lincomycin. The absence of aerobic gram-negative spectra for clindamycin and lincomycin may relate to their inability to penetrate the cell walls of these bacteria. Microbial resistance to clindamycin and lincomycin slowly develops, but resistant strains are commonly resistant to multiple antibiotics, especially to erythromycin.

These antibiotics yield effective serum levels readily and exhibit no appreciable protein binding or accumulation, but their significant biologic properties show some variation. Clindamycin is more rapidly and completely absorbed and is more readily eliminated from the body. The usual 500-mg dose of lincomycin gives a peak serum level of 1.8 to 5.3 μg per ml in 4 hours and has a normal half-life in the 4 to 6 hour range. Food does reduce the serum levels that are achieved with lincomycin, and administration on an empty stomach is recommended to avoid this problem; an extended half-life necessitates dosage adjustment in cases of renal disease or hepatic complication. Food does not influence the absorption of clindamycin, and the slight extension of antibiotic half-life with hepatic or renal dysfunction tends to be insignificant clinically. The usual 300-mg dose of clindamycin gives a peak serum level of 2.6 to 3.6 μg per ml in 1 to 2 hours, and the normal half-life is between 2 and 4 hours.

Both clindamycin and lincomycin can cause severe colitis and pseudomembranous colitis, which may end fatally. It is recommended that their use be reserved for serious infections caused by susceptible anaerobic bacteria or by pneumococci, staphylococci, or streptococci in patients with mitigating considerations, such as penicillin hypersensitivity. Distribution of these antibiotics in bone also favors their use in staphylococcal osteomyelitis.

Lincomycin is available in formulations of the HCl salt, and the usual adult dose is the equivalent of 500 mg of the antibiotic orally, 3 or 4 times a day, 600 mg intramus-

cularly, 1 or 2 times a day, and 600 mg by intravenous infusion (over a period of not less than 1 hour) every 8 to 12 hours.

Prescription Product. Lincocin®.

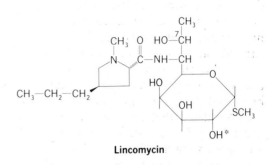

Lincomycin

*Esterified (palmitate or phosphate) in some formulations of clindamycin.

Clindamycin is available in formulations of the HCl salt (capsules) and of the HCl salt of the palmitate ester (suspension) for oral administration and of the phosphate ester for parenteral use. The palmitate and phosphate esters are inactive per se, but they are readily hydrolyzed to clindamycin in the body; gradual hydrolysis of the phosphate ester following intramuscular administration gives a flattened, delayed peak serum concentration and half-life of approximately 5 hours. The usual adult dose is the equivalent of 150 to 450 mg of the antibiotic, orally, 4 times a day and 300 mg, intramuscularly or intravenously, 2 to 4 times daily. The usual pediatric dose is the equivalent of 8 to 25 mg per kg per day divided into 3 or 4 equal doses.

Prescription Product. Cleocin®.

CYCLOSERINE

Cycloserine or D-4-amino-3-isoxazolidinone is probably the simplest metabolite with useful antibiotic activity. It can be produced by cultures of *Streptomyces orchidaceus* or by synthesis. Cycloserine has a fairly broad spectrum of activity, but its therapeutic utility is associated with its inhibitory effect on *Mycobacterium tuberculosis*. This antibiotic inhibits alanine racemase. The inhibitory action precludes the incorporation of D-alanine into the pentapeptide side chain of the murein component of bacterial cell walls, and this presumably accounts for its antibiotic activity. Cycloserine sometimes causes an increase in the protein content of the cerebrospinal fluid, and this explains in part the CNS effects that may occur when doses exceed 1 g daily. Manifestations of these side effects are usually mental confusion, drowsiness, and coma; rare cases of psychosis or convulsions are known.

Cycloserine is considered an antibiotic of second choice and is most frequently employed in combination with isoniazid in treating tubercular patients who fail to respond to streptomycin. Cycloserine is readily absorbed following oral administration and is excreted rather rapidly via the kidneys without metabolic alteration. The usual dose is 250 mg twice a day; the blood level should be monitored, and the dosage adjusted to keep the serum level below 30 μg per ml.

PRESCRIPTION PRODUCT. Seromycin®.

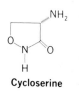

Cycloserine

DACTINOMYCIN

Dactinomycin or actinomycin D is obtained from selected strains of *Streptomyces antibioticus*. The molecule contains a phenoxazone chromophore that is linked to 2 cyclic polypeptides. The N-methyl amino acids, sarcosine and N-methylvaline, are present in the cyclo-

peptide portions of the antibiotic; this type of amino acid metabolite is uncommon in the plant kingdom. Biosynthetic studies indicate that the phenoxazone portion of the molecule arises from 2 molecules of tryptophan, presumably via the well-established pathway involving 3-hydroxyanthranilic acid.

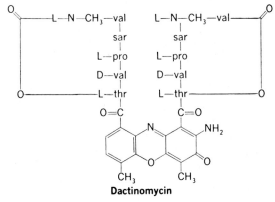

Dactinomycin

Dactinomycin is an antineoplastic agent and is used for hospital treatment of Wilms's tumor and several other types of carcinoma and sarcoma. Nausea is common with intravenous administration of dactinomycin, and the best tolerance is obtained in isolated metastases when a perfusion technique can be employed. The drug is available as a lyophilized powder with mannitol. The usual adult dosage regimen is 10 to 15 μg per kg of body weight daily for 5 days by intravenous infusion; therapy is repeated at 4- to 6-week intervals and may involve concurrent administration of other antineoplastic agents.

PRESCRIPTION PRODUCT. Cosmegen®.

VIDARABINE

Vidarabine is a purine nucleoside obtained from cultures of a strain of *Streptomyces antibioticus*. It has antiviral activity against *Herpes simplex* virus types 1 and 2. It is indicated for treatment of encephalitis caused by the *Herpes simplex* virus; if treatment is initiated early, the mortality rate can be reduced from 70% to the 28% range. It acts by inhibiting viral DNA synthesis. Vidarabine is teratogenic to laboratory animals, and a safe dose for the human embryo or fetus has not been established.

Vidarabine is administered by slow intravenous infusion. It is rapidly deaminated in the body to arabinosylhypoxanthine, a metabolite that has significantly less antiviral activity than does vidarabine. Excretion is renal, primarily as the deaminated metabolite; arabinosylhypoxanthine has a half-life of 3.3 hours.

The usual dosage regimen is 15 mg per kg of body weight per day by intravenous infusion over 12 to 24 hours for 10 days.

PRESCRIPTION PRODUCT. Vira-A®.

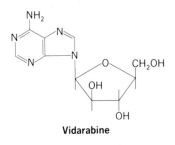

Vidarabine

POLYPEPTIDE ANTIBIOTICS

A fairly large number of **polypeptides** of bacterial origin, which contain both D- and L-amino acids, have antibiotic activity. However, only a few of these metabolites have therapeutic utility. These antibiotics are not absorbed from the intestinal tract, and nephrotoxicity is a potential problem if they are used systemically. Most of the useful peptide antibiotics have a predominantly gram-positive spectrum; exceptions include the strongly basic polymyxins, which are active primarily against gram-negative organisms, and the antineoplastic bleomycin. These peptides have a surfactant property, and the polymyxins exert their effect by interacting with the lipid-rich anionic bacterial cell membrane. However, inhibition of mucopeptide synthesis in cell-wall formation by bacitracin appears to be more significant than membrane disruption for the action of this antibiotic, and inhibition of DNA synthesis is probably the most significant involvement of bleomycin.

The polypeptide antibiotics tend to occur as mixtures of closely related compounds. Components of these mixtures often differ in only 1 or 2 amino acid residues; resolution of such mixtures is not feasible for therapeutic purposes. The use of selected strains of producing organisms controls the composition of commercial mixtures to a degree, and use of microbial assay for quantitation provides a reliable indication of therapeutic response against susceptible organisms.

Polymyxin B is a mixture of antibiotics produced by *Bacillus polymyxa* (Prazmowski) Migula. The mixture contains minimal amounts of the more toxic polymyxins A, C, and D, but the polymyxin B component is actually a mixture of polymyxins B_1 and B_2. Polymyxins B_1 and B_2 contain 10 amino acid residues in common and differ only in a 6-methyloctanoic acid residue in polymyxin B_1 and an isooctanoic acid residue in polymyxin B_2. Both molecules have a cyclopeptidic structure and contain 6 residues of α,γ-diaminobutyric acid. This latter feature gives a strongly basic character to the polymyxin antibiotics.

Polymyxin B is normally employed as the sulfate salt, which must have a potency of not less than 6000 units per mg. *Bordetella bronchiseptica* ATCC No. 4617 is used as the test organism for microbial assay of polymyxin B and the related colistin.

Polymyxin B is not absorbed when administered orally and was formerly employed for control of infections of the intestinal tract caused by *Shigella, Pseudomonas aeruginosa, and Escherichia coli.* It is used topically in ointments (usually 5,000 or 10,000 units per g) and ophthalmic solutions (10,000 units per ml) and parenterally as an alternate antibiotic. Nephro- and neurotoxicities occur fairly frequently when polymyxin B sulfate is used systemically, but it has some limited utility in serious infections of *Pseudomonas aeruginosa* and certain coliform bacilli that do not respond to other antibiotics, such as carbenicillin or gentamicin. Polymyxin is excreted renally and is useful in controlling resistant infections of the urinary tract.

Biopharmaceutic considerations for the polymyxins are complex, and the available data lack significant utility in evaluating therapeutic situations. The antibiotic binds to bacterial and mammalian cell membranes and persists in various body tissues long after it has disappeared from the serum. The in vitro MIC for most sensitive bacteria is in the lower end of the 0.02 to 4.0 μg per ml range.

The usual adult dose is, by intravenous infusion, 7500 to 12,500 units per kg of body weight in 300 to 500 ml of 5% dextrose injection, 2 times a day; it can also be administered intramuscularly or intrathecally. The dose should be reduced in persons with renal impairment; the high incidence of toxic manifestations in obese patients also suggests need for deviation from a dosage regimen based exclusively on weight.

PRESCRIPTION PRODUCT. Aerosporin®.

Colistin is obtained from cultures of *Bacillus polymyxa* var. *colistinus* and contains primarily colistin A (polymyxin E) with a small amount of colistin B. This antibiotic has essentially the same spectrum and therapeutic utility as polymyxin B. The sulfate salt is used orally and topically, and the sodium salt of a methane sulfonate derivative (colistimethate) is used parenterally.

The colistimethate is inactive, but active compounds are released in the body. Colistimethate is considered the polymyxin formulation of choice for intramuscular administration. It is less painful, gives higher serum levels (6 to 25 μg per ml), is poorly bound to cell membranes, and has a shorter half-life (6 to 12 hours). It is claimed to have less systemic toxicity; however, it is not free from nephro- and neurotoxicities, and special caution is necessary in cases of existing renal dysfunction.

The usual dose of colistin is, orally, 5 to 15 mg per kg of body weight daily in 3 divided doses and, intramuscularly or intravenously, 1.25 mg per kg, 2 to 4 times a day.

PRESCRIPTION PRODUCTS. Sulfate salt: Coly-Mycin S®; colistimethate: Coly-Mycin M®.

Bacitracin is produced by an organism of the licheniformis group of *Bacillus subtilis* Cohn & Prazmowski and is a mixture of at least 5 polypeptides. The major component of the mixture is bacitracin A, which is a dodecylpeptide with 5 of the amino acid residues arranged in a cyclic structure. Bacitracin must have a potency of not less than 40 units per mg, unless it is intended for parenteral use; in the latter case, the potency must be not less than 50 units per mg. Bacitracin is assayed microbiologically using *Micrococcus flavus* ATCC No. 10240 or *Sarcina subflava* ATCC No. 7468.

This antibiotic is active against a wide range of gram-positive bacteria. Bacitracin or zinc bacitracin is a component in many ointment formulations for the control of topical infections; ointments usually contain 500 units per g. Parenteral formulations of bacitracin are available, but systemic use is rarely justified owing to problems of nephrotoxicity and to the increasing availability of less toxic alternate antibiotics. Indications for systemic use are restricted to infants with staphylococcal pneumonia and empyema caused by susceptible organisms; it should be used only where adequate laboratory facilities are available and when constant supervision of the patient is possible. It is administered intramuscularly, 2 or 3 times a day, using a dosage regimen based on age and body weight.

Tyrothricin is a mixture of polypeptide antibiotics produced by *Bacillus brevis* Dubos. The peptides of tyrothricin can be grouped into 2 major categories called **gramicidin** and **tyrocidin.** At least 3 polypeptides representing each group are present in commercial tyrothricin. The tyrocidins are basic, usually occur in tyrothricin mixtures as the HCl salts, and constitute the majority of the mixtures.

The neutral gramicidins are most active against gram-positive cocci and usually account for 20 to 25% of tyrothricin mixtures. Gramicidin is soluble in an acetone-ether mixture, and this solvent can be used to dissolve selectively the gramicidin fraction. Gramicidin is a component in a number of formulations for control of topical infections and has replaced tyrothricin for such purposes.

Capreomycin is a mixture of peptides produced by *Streptomyces capreolus.* Capreomycin I is the major component (80 to 90%); capreomycin II accounts for most of the balance of the mixture. Frequent nephrotoxicity is observed with therapeutic use of this antibiotic. Ototoxicity with irreversible auditory impairment and changes in hepatic function are also encountered.

The antibiotic is used as an alternate

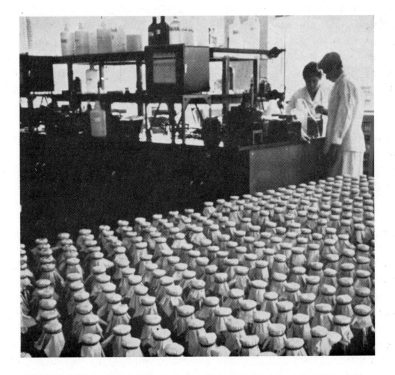

Fig. 12–17. Each sealed flask contains a culture of a microorganism. Culture Laboratory, Pfizer Medical Research Laboratories, Groton, Connecticut (Photo, courtesy of Charles Pfizer & Company, Inc.)

antitubercular agent in susceptible strains of *Mycobacterium tuberculosis* when other primary agents, such as streptomycin, are ineffective. It is administered intramuscularly as the sulfate salt, and the usual dose is the equivalent of 1 g of the antibiotic daily for 2 to 4 months, then 1 g, 2 or 3 times a week.

PRESCRIPTION PRODUCT. Capastat®.

Vancomycin is produced by *Streptomyces orientalis*. The chemical identity of this antibiotic has not been fully clarified, but it is a glucopeptide. The molecular weight is estimated to be 785, and polymeric forms probably explain earlier estimates of 1560 and 3200. The antibiotic contains organically bound chlorine and yields glucose and several amino acids on hydrolysis. It is assayed microbiologically using *Bacillus subtilis* ATCC No. 6633.

Vancomycin has a gram-positive spectrum, and the HCl salt is used primarily as an alternate antibiotic for treating septicemia or endocarditis caused by straphylococci that are resistant to other antibiotics. The antibiotic is not absorbed orally, but oral administration is used occasionally for the treatment of staphylococcal enterocolitis. Vancomycin acts on bacterial cell walls by inhibiting murein biosynthesis at some step after formation of the nucleotide pentapeptide.

Intramuscular administration is painful and frequently associated with local necrosis; thus, systemic therapy with vancomycin employs intravenous infusion over a period of 20 to 30 minutes. The usual parenteral dose is 500 mg, 4 times a day. This dosage regimen maintains a serum level of 10 μg per ml or more for 1 to 2 hours from the time of injection; most sensitive bacteria have MICs in the 0.2 to 5.0 μg per ml range. The antibiotic has a half-life of approximately 6 hours and is excreted renally. Ototoxicity is the most frequently encountered side effect; the risk is increased with the high doses, prolonged therapy, or renal insufficiency.

PRESCRIPTION PRODUCT. Vancocin®.

Bleomycin is a mixture of antineoplastic glycopeptides produced by *Streptomyces verticillus*. The mixture can be separated into A and B fractions, and more than a dozen individual components have been reported. Bleomycin A_2 is the major constituent, comprising between 60 and 70% of the mixture. Bleomycin B_2 (25 to 32%) is the second major constituent, and material intended for medicinal use must contain not more than 1% of bleomycin B_4. Bleomycin is standardized biologically, and the potency is expressed in units; bleomycin sulfate contains not less than 1.5 units and not more than 2 units of bleomycin per mg.

Bleomycin appears most useful for its palliative effect in some squamous cell carcinomas, but it is useful in lymphomas, testicular carcinomas, and some soft tissue sarcomas. Its low myelosuppressive action may offer clinical advantages. However, pulmonary toxicity frequently necessitates discontinuation of therapy. Bleomycin is preferentially concentrated in tumors, and a bleomycin-technetium 99m complex has diagnostic potential as a tumor-scanning agent.

Bleomycin is administered parenterally as the sulfate salt. The usual dosage regimen is 0.25 to 0.5 units per kg of body weight once or twice weekly.

PRESCRIPTION PRODUCT. Blenoxane®.

ANTIBIOTICS DERIVED FROM ACETATE METABOLISM

Acetate metabolism normally involves head-to-tail condensation of 2 carbon units or the formation of some type of isoprenoid compound. Both types of metabolism are basic to most protoplasmic systems, as evidenced by the ubiquitous distribution of fatty acids and certain steroids. However, biosynthetically minor deviations at key stages of normal acetate metabolism can result in uncommon metabolites, some of which have antibiotic activity. The therapeutically useful antibiotics derived from acetate metabolism include the tetracyclines, 2 macrolides, a few polyenes, and griseofulvin. These antibiotics are derived from polyketides, and their formation deviates from the fatty acid pathway by a disruption or lack of the normal reduction-dehydration-reduction sequence as the chain elongates. Subsequent metabolic steps yield the characteristic constituents.

TETRACYCLINES

The **tetracyclines** are a group of actinomycete antibiotics that have a broad spectrum and considerable therapeutic utility (Fig. 12–18). Chlortetracycline was discovered by Duggar in 1948 from *Streptomyces aureofaciens*. *S. rimosus* yielded oxytetracycline in 1950, and tetracycline was found in the antibiotic mixture from *S. aureofaciens* in 1953. The latter observation resulted in patent problems, cross-licensing agreements, a number of legal challenges, and a major governmental in-

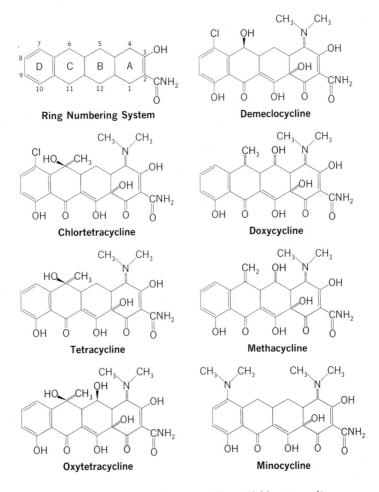

Fig. 12–18. Structures of commercially available tetracyclines.

vestigation. Other minor tetracyclines occur in fermentation mixtures, but only 7-chloro-6-demethyltetracycline (demeclocycline) is currently used in therapy.

Developments in the selection of mutant strains and in manipulations to control chlorination and methylation have proven useful in the fermentative production of various tetracyclines. The presence of aminopterin or other methylation inhibitors in the nutrient mixture favors the formation of 6-demethyltetracyclines, and compounds such as mercaptothiazole aid tetracycline production by inhibiting chlorination. Initially, tetracycline was prepared in commercial quantities by catalytic dehalogenation (hydrogenolysis) of chlortetracycline, but fermentation procedures are currently more advantageous. Doxycycline, methacycline, and minocycline, however, are semisynthetic antibiotics that are prepared by chemical modification of oxytetracycline or tetracycline.

BIOSYNTHESIS OF TETRACYCLINES. Studies with radioactive compounds have confirmed that tetracycline antibiotics originate through acetate-malonate metabolism. Mutant strains of tetracycline-producing organisms have been selected for genetic blocks in the biosynthetic pathway and have been used to clarify a number of the sequential steps.

It is believed that a malonamyl-CoA residue serves as a primer and that 8 malonate units undergo stepwise condensations with the addition of C_2 units and decarboxylation to yield a linear C_{19} polyketide (Fig. 12–19). Carbonyl-methylene condensations yield the tetracyclic pretetramide nucleus. Methylation of the C-6 position of the pretetramide is an early step in the biosynthesis of most tetracyclines, but this step is omitted in the formation of the naturally occurring demethyltetracyclines. Hydroxylation of the C-4 position and dearomatization to yield a 4-keto intermediate appears to precede 7-chlorination. Halogenation must precede introduction of the 4-amino group, which is methylated stepwise. Terminal reactions in the biosynthetic sequence are hydroxylation at C-6 and reduction of a double bond in ring B. The 5-hydroxy group in oxytetracycline is probably introduced before the reduction of ring B; it is interesting to note that the presence of a 7-halogen substituent apparently inhibits 5-hydroxylation.

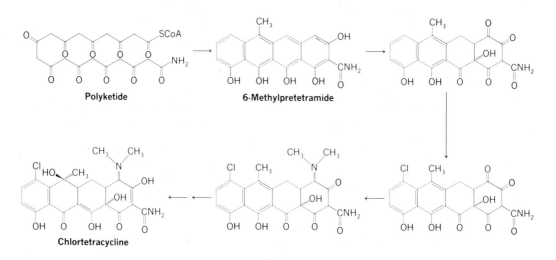

Fig. 12–19. Biosynthesis of chlortetracycline.

PROPERTIES AND USES OF THE TETRACYCLINES. All tetracyclines are reasonably stable and are absorbed adequately upon oral administration. These amphoteric substances are most stable in acid and least stable in alkali. The tetracycline antibiotics are usually employed as the HCl salts. Chlortetracycline is the least stable of these antibiotics, but it is sufficiently stable for satisfactory oral usage.

Calcium ions in dairy products tend to cause erratic and unsatisfactory absorption of the tetracyclines. Best absorption is obtained when caution is used in scheduling the administration of these antibiotics to avoid interference from heavy metal ions in foods or in such preparations as aluminum hydroxide-containing antacids. Phosphate combinations may be used in tetracycline formulations to reduce the impact of heavy metal ions on absorption. Demeclocycline, doxycycline, and methacycline are absorbed more readily than the other tetracycline antibiotics, their absorption is influenced to a lesser degree by food and milk, their slower renal clearance favors prolonged maintenance of blood levels, and they appear to be the tetracyclines of choice when absorption is a problem. The biologic properties of minocycline resemble those of demeclocycline, doxycycline, and methacycline, but it is considered a specialty tetracycline at this time. The indication for parenteral use of tetracycline antibiotics is uncommon.

The tetracyclines have a broad spectrum of activity that includes gram-negative and gram-positive bacteria, rickettsia, some of the larger viruses, and some intestinal amebae. Tetracyclines are often considered the antibiotics of choice for treatment of brucellosis, cholera, relapsing fever, and infections caused by *Chlamydia, Mycoplasma, Yersinia (Pasteurella)*, and rickettsia. The tetracyclines are effective, alternate-choice antibiotics for treating a large number of other infections. The action spectra for the various tetracyclines are qualitatively comparable, but lower median MICs may favor the use of doxycycline or minocycline in some cases. Normal serum levels on oral regimens are 2 to 4 μg per ml.

The usual serum half-lives of the various tetracyclines are 5 to 6 hours for chlortetracycline, 8 to 9 hours for tetracycline, 9 to 10 hours for oxytetracycline, 12 to 14 hours for demeclocycline and methacycline, and 17 to 19 hours for doxycycline and minocycline. These antibiotics are eliminated by biliary excretion, glomerular filtration, and metabolism. There is extensive enterohepatic recycling of the tetracycline antibiotics, even after parenteral administration. Urinary excretion usually accounts for 20 to 50% of the tetracyclines; the rate of renal clearance is slowest for doxycycline and minocycline. Metabolic degradation of these antibiotics is relatively insignificant, except for chlortetracycline and doxycycline; doxycycline does not accumulate in patients with renal impairment and is the indicated tetracycline in such cases.

Resistance to the tetracyclines developed slowly, but it has become a serious clinical consideration, especially with pneumococci, staphylococci, streptococci, and such gram-negative pathogens as *Escherichia coli* and *Shigella* species. It has been suggested that penicillins, unless specifically contraindicated, should be selected in preference to the tetracyclines for treating susceptible coccal infections. Tetracycline resistance is characterized by an increasing median MIC for strains of various pathogens; the mechanism appears to involve decreased cell permeability to the antibiotics.

Tetracyclines exert their action by inhibiting protein synthesis. The antibiotics interfere with the binding of aminoacyl-tRNA to acceptor sites on the 30S subunit of microbial 70S ribosomes. Tetracyclines can also attack mammalian 80S ribosomes, but preferential penetration and concentration of these antibiotics in bacterial cells presumably explain the infrequent occurrence of major side effects.

The most frequently encountered adverse effect of tetracycline therapy is alteration of the intestinal flora; this is usually manifest by an overgrowth of *Candida albicans*. Hypersensitivities may occur; the most serious is a photosensitivity that occurs most often with demeclocycline. The staining of teeth by deposition of tetracyclines in the calcium complex is a basis for selecting alternate antibiotics when treating children during the second dentition period. Hepatotoxicity can also occur, especially in pregnant women, and is usually associated with high blood levels resulting from parenteral administration or renal deficiency. The ability of some tetracyclines to complex with calcium ion can depress plasma prothrombin activity, and patients who are also on anticoagulant drugs may require dosage adjustment.

Chlortetracycline or 7-chlorotetracycline was the first tetracycline antibiotic available for therapeutic purposes. Satisfactory results can be obtained with this antibiotic, and it is still available in formulations for topical use, including ophthalmic purposes. Therapeutic use of other tetracycline antibiotics has replaced its oral and intravenous uses in human medicine, but chlortetracycline is still employed in veterinary medicine.

PRESCRIPTION PRODUCT. Aureomycin®.

Tetracycline is the least expensive and most commonly utilized tetracycline antibiotic. It is available in a large number of formulations of the tetracycline base, HCl salt, and phosphate complex. Usual dosage schedules are based on the equivalence to tetracycline HCl and are: 250 to 500 mg, orally, 4 times a day; 250 mg, intramuscularly, once a day or 100 mg, 3 times a day by this route; and 250 to 500 mg, intrave-

nously, 2 times a day. Preparations for topical use are also available.

Low oral doses of tetracycline (250 mg per day) have been used successfully to treat chronic severe cases of acne. The scientific basis for this therapeutic use is unclear. It may be a combination of antibiotic activity reducing slightly the skin population of *Staphylococcus epidermidis* and *Corynebacterium acnes* and of the potential inhibiting effect of tetracycline on bacterial lipase from the latter species. It is believed that acne lesions are related to the irritation caused by free fatty acids in the sebum. Risks of *Candida* superinfection or other toxic responses are minimal with the low dosage regimen, but the prospects for encouraging the selection of resistant strains should preclude the use of tetracycline in trivial cases of acne.

PRESCRIPTION PRODUCTS. Achromycin®, Amtet®, Bio-Tetra®, Bristacycline®, Centet®, Cyclopar®, Deltamycin®, Desamycin®, Duratet®, G-Mycin®, Maytrex®, M-Tetra®, Nor-Tet®, Paltet®, Panmycin®, Partrex®, Piracaps®, Retet®, Robitet®, Sumycin®, Tet®, Teline®, Tetra-Bid®, Tetra-C®, Tetra-Co®, Tetracap®, Tetrachel®, Tetracyn®, Tetralan®, Tetram®, Tri-Tet®; phosphate complex: Tetrex®.

Oxytetracycline or 5-hydroxytetracycline is available in various formulations for oral, parenteral, and topical purposes. The insoluble calcium salt is used in oral suspensions, and the HCl salt is usually employed in other oral dosage forms. The usual dosage schedule is the same as that for tetracycline.

PRESCRIPTION PRODUCTS. Oxlopar®, Terramycin®, Tetramine®, Uri-Tet®.

Demeclocycline or 7-chloro-6-demethyltetracycline has greater acid stability than the tetracyclines with a 6-methyl substituent. The better absorption and slower excretion by the body of this tetracycline antibiotic provide blood levels that offer some special therapeutic advantages. Demeclocycline is used orally and is available in various formulations of the free base and the HCl salt. The usual dose is 600 mg daily in 2 or 4 divided doses.

PRESCRIPTION PRODUCT. Declomycin®.

Doxycycline or 6-deoxy-5-hydroxy-tetracycline is prepared from oxytetracycline by chemical dehydration and reduction. It is readily absorbed following oral administration, slow excretion gives prolonged blood levels, and no significant accumulation is noted with renal impairment. A suspension of doxycycline base is used orally, and formulations of the water-soluble doxycycline hyclate are available for oral and intravenous administration. The usual oral dosage regimen is the equivalent of 100 mg of the antibiotic 2 times a day for 1 day, then 50 to 100 mg 2 times a day. The usual intravenous schedule is 200 mg on the first day, administered in 1 or 2 infusions, then 100 or 200 mg daily, depending on the severity of infection.

PRESCRIPTION PRODUCTS. Doxychel®, Vibramycin®.

Methacycline is prepared from oxytetracycline by chemical dehydration; it has a methylene function in the 6-position. The utility of methacycline is associated with good oral absorption and a prolonged serum half-life. It is used orally as the HCl salt, and the usual dose is 600 mg daily in 2 or 4 divided doses.

PRESCRIPTION PRODUCT. Rondomycin®.

Minocycline is prepared by reductive methylation of 7-nitro-6-demethyl-6-deoxytetracycline. It is readily absorbed from the intestinal tract, has a slow renal clearance to give prolonged blood levels, and is characterized by lower MICs than other tetracycline antibiotics for some pathogens. Minocycline is especially useful for treating *Neisseria gonorrhoeae*, carrier states of *N. meningitidis,* and tetracycline-resistant strains of staphylococci

when penicillin is contraindicated. It is used as the HCl salt, and the usual oral or intravenous regimen involves a loading dose equivalent to 200 mg of the antibiotic, then 100 mg, 2 times a day.

PRESCRIPTION PRODUCTS. Minocin®, Vectrin®.

ANTINEOPLASTIC ANTHRACYCLINE DERIVATIVES

The attention of medical investigators has been attracted to acetate-derived polycyclic metabolites of actinomycetes other than the tetracycline antibiotics. Doxorubicin and mithramycin are 2 such metabolites; they both occur as glycosides and have been judged to have utility in treating some neoplastic conditions.

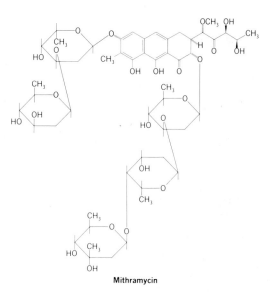

Mithramycin

Mithramycin is produced by *Streptomyces agrillaceus* and *S. plicatus.* Mithramycin inhibits DNA replication by forming a stable cross-link between the 2 strands of double-stranded DNA. It is indicated primarily for treatment of disseminated testicular carcinoma when surgery and radiation are contraindicated. Severe toxic reactions restrict administration of mithramycin to selected hospitalized patients, and the therapeutic response tends to be inconsistent. The usual antineoplastic dosage regimen is, by intravenous infusion, 25 to 30 μg per kg of body weight in 1 liter of 5% dextrose injection over a period of 4 to 6 hours once a day for 8 to 10 days or until hematologic or biochemical toxicities require discontinuation. Mithramycin can also be considered for symptomatic control in patients with hypercalcemia and hypercalciuria secondary to a variety of advanced neoplasms.

The antibiotic is unstable, and the lyophilized preparations should be stored at a temperature between 2 and 8° C. Once reconstituted, any unused solution must be discarded.

PRESCRIPTION PRODUCT. Mithracin®.

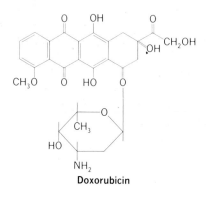
Doxorubicin

Doxorubicin is produced by *Streptomyces peucetius* var. *caesius*. It causes remission in a wide range of solid tumors, but unfortunately, the remission is short lived in many cases. It appears to show special promise for breast cancer and for solid lung tumors in children. Doxorubicin inhibits DNA-dependent RNA synthesis and exhibits a high incidence of bone marrow depression and other side effects, such as severe local tissue necrosis and serious irreversible myocardial damage. Complications associated with altered

blood coagulation, leg-vein thromboses, and pulmonary infarcts are claimed to present fewer problems with doxorubicin than with daunomycin, a related experimental drug produced by the same actinomycete species.

Doxorubicin is administered intravenously as the HCl salt. It is excreted in the bile, and enterohepatic recycling gives an extended blood level. Slow renal elimination gives a red coloration to the urine for 1 or 2 days after administration of the drug. The recommended adult dose is 60 to 75 mg per square meter of body surface at 21-day intervals.

PRESCRIPTION PRODUCT. Adriamycin®.

MITOMYCIN

Mitomycin C is one of the antineoplastic substances produced by *Streptomyces caespitosus*. It is not significantly more effective than other anticancer agents, and it causes more serious adverse reactions than most. It is considered useful in the treatment of disseminated adenocarcinoma of the stomach or pancreas and is an alternate drug in advanced metastatic conditions of various types that have become resistant to other chemotherapeutic agents. The response rate has been low, as anticipated in such high-risk situations, and remission is usually of short duration.

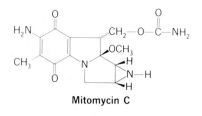
Mitomycin C

Mitomycin C is inactive per se; the active form is produced metabolically in situ and apparently acts as an alkylating agent to suppress DNA synthesis. Local tissue necrosis may occur, but severe bone marrow depression is the most serious side effect. The usual dosage regimen is, intravenously, 20 mg per square meter of body surface either as a single dose or as divided doses over 10 days.

PRESCRIPTION PRODUCT. Mutamycin®.

MACROLIDE ANTIBIOTICS

Macrolide antibiotics are characterized by a macrolactone ring that is glycosidically linked to one or more sugars. Biosynthetic studies have established that the macrolactone ring is formed by a condensation of acetate and/or propionate units, apparently via malonyl-CoA and 2-methylmalonyl-CoA. Methyl substituents on the lactone ring appear to be residual from incorporation of propionate units rather than from terminal biologic methylation. The sugar components of these antibiotics are usually deoxysugars, at least one sugar residue is routinely an aminosugar, and both N-methyl and O-methyl groups of methionine origin are common. Experimental data suggest that these uncommon sugars are derived from glucose. Thus, the macrolides must be considered as products of both acetate and carbohydrate metabolism. It is suspected that glycosidation is a terminal reaction in the pathway.

Erythromycin and oleandomycin (Fig. 12–20) are the only macrolide antibacterial agents currently used in therapy. They are produced by actinomycete fermentation, and the large number of asymmetric centers in these antibiotics (19 in erythromycin A) suggests that the potential for chemical modification to develop analogs with improved antibiotic activity is limited and that total chemical synthesis will undoubtedly never become feasible. The macrolactone ring is unstable in gastric acidity, a factor that must be considered when devising pharmaceutic formulations. Enteric coating can be used to deliver the antibiotic to the intestinal tract where it is readily absorbed. The use of insoluble esters, which are hydrolyzed in the intestine and elsewhere in the body, also protect the macrolide antibiotics. This approach offers the additional advantage of masking the bitter taste of these antibiotics in oral suspensions. Erythromycin is absorbed readily from the rectum and may be administered by this route.

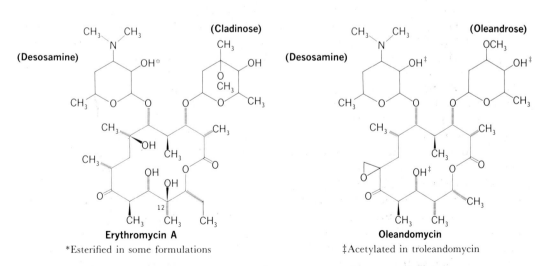

Erythromycin A
*Esterified in some formulations

Oleandomycin
‡Acetylated in troleandomycin

Fig. 12–20. Structures of erythromycin and oleandomycin.

Erythromycin and oleandomycin have predominantly gram-positive spectra that resemble the spectra of the penicillins and lincomycin. Erythromycin is slightly more active than oleandomycin, but these antibiotics both have utility, primarily in treating pneumococcal and hemolytic streptococcal infections when penicillins are contraindicated or ineffective. Erythromycin appears to be the antibiotic of choice when treating infections of *Legionnella pneumophila*.

Staphylococci frequently become resistant to the macrolides, and this introduces a practical limitation on their therapeutic applications to many strains of these pathogens. Several mechanisms of bacterial resistance to macrolides appear to exist. A lack of effective antibiotic penetration of cell membrane explains the relative insensitivity of most gram-negative bacteria to these antibiotics, and similar permeability considerations seem to characterize some resistant strains of normally susceptible species. Destruction of the antibiotics is not a known factor in resistance, but evidence in some cases suggests antibiotic-induced change in the ribosomal structure and an R-factor transfer.

The macrolides exert their action by inhibiting the synthesis of essential proteins. Most of the experimental information has been obtained with erythromycin. It binds to the 50S subunit of microbial 70S ribosomes; it does not inhibit peptide bond formation, but it does block the translocation of the peptidyl-tRNA from the acceptor site to the donor site.

Adverse reactions, except for hepatotoxicity, are uncommon with the macrolide antibiotics. The hepatotoxicity is associated with use of formulations of erythromycin estolate and triacetyloleandomycin for longer than 10 days. It appears to be a function of these macrolide derivatives rather than of the antibiotics per se, may result from a combined chemical-hypersensitivity mechanism, and is reversible upon cessation of therapy. Recognition of the risk of hepatotoxicity with erythromycin estolate and of the lack of special therapeutic advantages of this derivative prompted the FDA to remove adult dosage forms of this ester from the market. Because the risk of hepatotoxicity appears to be less in young children, pediatric dosage forms of erythromycin estolate were not included in the recall process.

Erythromycin was isolated in 1952 from cultures of *Streptomyces erythreus*. The commercial product is primarily erythromycin A, but it also contains small amounts of 2 related antibiotics that have been designated erythromycins B and C. Erythromycin B lacks the 12-hydroxyl group that is present in erythromycin A, and erythromycin C has a hydroxyl group rather than a methoxy group in the sugar corresponding to cladinose.

Erythromycin on oral administration is absorbed primarily in the lower intestinal tract, and absorption is most efficient for lipid-soluble nonionized forms. Food somewhat retards absorption, and plasma levels vary depending on the form of the drug and on whether it is administered to a fasting patient. The highest levels are obtained with fasting patients and the estolate form of the antibiotic, but most therapeutic needs are met satisfactorily by any of the available formulations and without excluding rigorously the impact of food. There are analytic problems in evaluating effective in vivo levels of erythromycin formulations, and considerable uncontrolled data can be noted in the literature. When the ester form is employed, a relatively large portion (65 to 80% for erythromycin estolate) of the drug is still unhydrolyzed at the time of peak serum level and thus is inactive.

Normal peak serum levels that have been reported for the usual oral dosage regimens of erythromycin are between 0.3 and

5.0 μg per ml. The antibiotic is distributed with unusual efficiency into most body fluids and tissues, except the cerebrospinal fluid. Pertinent MICs for erythromycin range from 0.01 to 3.1 μg per ml, with most susceptible gram-positive cocci falling in the lower end of the range; pathogens such as *Haemophilus influenzae* and *Neisseria* species have higher MICs and have more strains that are not susceptible to concentrations ordinarily achieved in therapy.

The normal serum half-life of erythromycin is approximately 1.5 hours, and this is not prolonged greatly in anuria. Some erythromycin is excreted by the kidney (2.5 to 10%), there is extensive enterohepatic recycling, and most of the antibiotic is metabolized prior to elimination. The key involvement of hepatic metabolism may prompt the need for dosage reduction in cases of severe liver disease.

Erythromycin is used orally in various formulations of the free base, the stearate salt, and the ethylsuccinate ester. The lauryl sulfate salt of the propionate ester (estolate) is used in pediatric dosage forms. The soluble glucoheptonate (gluceptate) and lactobionate salts are used for intravenous administration. Ointments (0.5 and 1.0%) are also available for topical purposes. The usual dose, as the equivalent of erythromycin, is 250 mg, orally, 4 times a day for the free base and stearate preparations; 400 mg, orally, 4 times a day for the ethylsuccinate; and 250 mg, intravenously, 4 times a day, for the gluceptate and lactobionate.

PRESCRIPTION PRODUCTS. Delta-E®, E-Mycin®, Ilotycin®, Robimycin®, RP-Mycin®; estolate: Ilosone®; gluceptate: Ilotycin®; ethylsuccinate: E.E.S.®, Pediamycin®; lactobionate: Erythrocin®; stearate: Bristamycin®, Erypar®, Erythrocin®, Ethril®, Pfizer-E®, Romycin®, Wintrocin®.

Oleandomycin was isolated in 1954 from a strain of *Streptomyces antibioticus*.

The insoluble triacetyl ester of oleandomycin (troleandomycin) is available in formulations for oral administration. The usual dose is 250 to 500 mg, orally, 4 times a day. The biologic and chemical properties and the therapeutic considerations for troleandomycin are essentially the same as those for comparable erythromycin formulations. Troleandomycin is an alternate for erythromycin, but it offers no advantage over erythromycin.

PRESCRIPTION PRODUCT. Tao®.

POLYENES

The designation **polyene,** for practical considerations in medicine and pharmacy, refers to a group of amphoteric actinomycete metabolites that are characterized by a series of conjugated double bonds. These metabolites are unsaturated macrolides with macrolactone rings that are considerably larger than those of erythromycin and oleandomycin. They are usually categorized on the basis of the number of conjugated double bonds in the molecules. Nystatin and natamycin, tetraenes, and amphotericin B and candicidin, heptaenes, are the polyenes used in therapy. The polyenes have no antibacterial activity, and their therapeutic utility is related to their antifungal action. The biologic activity of these antibiotics is determined with various strains of *Saccharomyces cerevisiae*.

The polyenes are fairly unstable, poorly absorbed from the intestinal tract, and reasonably toxic when administered systemically. They are insoluble, and this property sufficiently protects these antibiotics from inactivation to permit local action in the intestinal tract following oral administration. Limited solubility precludes intramuscular administration of amphotericin B, the only polyene currently recommended for systemic use; therefore, this antibiotic is given by slow intravenous infusion of a formulation that contains sodium deoxycholate to form a colloidal suspension of the polyene.

The polyenes act by destroying the integrity of the cellular membrane of susceptible organisms, and this action may be related to the binding of the polyenes to steroids in the membranes and the formation of aqueous pores. Such a mechanism of action would explain the absence of antibacterial activity because bacterial membranes lack a steroid component. This type of interference with biologic processes may also account for at least one of the adverse reactions observed with systemic use of the polyenes; hemolytic anemia may result directly or indirectly from alteration in the formation or function of cholesterol-containing erythrocyte membranes. The most frequently observed toxicity with systemic use of amphotericin B is nephrotoxicity. Nephrotoxicity with this antibiotic is almost routine, is usually reversible upon cessation of therapy, and must be balanced against the need for control of systemic mycoses in justifying initiation and continuation of therapy in individual cases.

Candida albicans is susceptible to the polyenes, and control of *Candida* overgrowth induced by broad-spectrum antibiotic therapy is a major use of these antifungal agents. Use of polyenes to control *Candida* infections of such origin is justified, but routine incorporation of a polyene in formulations of tetracyclines for prophylactic purposes has been challenged. The challenge is based, in part, on a concern for consequences of any increase in resistance to the polyenes and on a recognition that no alternate antifungal agents are currently available for treatment of systemic candidiasis.

Amphotericin B is produced by *Streptomyces nodosus,* and the commercial product must contain not less than 750 μg of amphotericin B per mg. The less active amphotericin A, a tetraene that is also present in the polyene fraction from cultures of this actinomycete, forms a soluble complex with calcium chloride; this manipulation is used in the commercial preparation of amphotericin B.

Amphotericin B can be used for topical purposes, but its special therapeutic utility is intravenous administration for treatment of potentially life-threatening, disseminated mycotic infections, such as blastomycosis, systemic candidiasis, coccidioidomycosis, cryptococcosis, histoplasmosis, and moniliasis. The MICs of susceptible fungi range from 0.03 to 1.0 μg per ml. This antibiotic is slowly eliminated from the body; the plasma half-life is about 24 hours, and the elimination half-life of this strongly protein-bound drug is estimated to be 15 days. Effective blood levels can be maintained with daily administration of a relatively small dose. The usual initial dose is 250 μg per kg of body weight

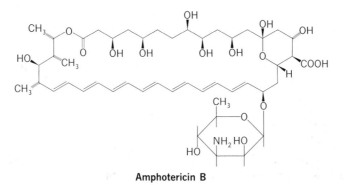

Amphotericin B

daily, and most regimens call for an increase in the dose every 2 to 4 days for 4 to 8 weeks. Under no circumstances should a total daily dosage exceed 1.5 mg per kg. The antibiotic is administered by slow intravenous infusion over a period of 6 hours.

Experimental studies suggest that the action of amphotericin B on cell membranes may have potential use in an interesting type of synergistic combination

must contain not less than 4400 units of activity per mg. It is available in formulations for treatment of cutaneous, intestinal, and vaginal infections of *Candida*. MICs range from 1.5 to 6.5 μg per ml. The usual dose is 500,000 to 1 million units, orally, 3 times a day or 100,000 units, intravaginally, 1 or 2 times a day.

PRESCRIPTION PRODUCTS. Candex®, Korostatin®, Mycostatin®, Nilstat®, O–V Statin®.

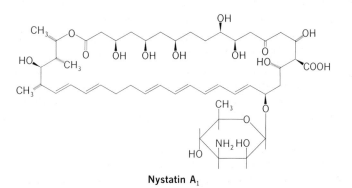

Nystatin A$_1$

therapy. The absence of an antifungal spectrum for a number of antibiotics that interfere with protein or RNA synthesis appears to relate to the lack of antibiotic penetration into the fungal cell. A low concentration of amphotericin B in combinations with other selected antibiotics, such as rifampin and tetracycline, seems to facilitate membrane passage of the normally excluded antibiotics; this synergistic action may open new improved therapeutic approaches for treatment of fungal infections.

PRESCRIPTION PRODUCT. Fungizone®.

Candicidin is a mixture of heptaenes produced by a strain of *Streptomyces griseus*. It is available in ointment and suppository formulations for control of vaginal candidiasis. Usually, a 3-mg dose is inserted twice daily for 14 days.

PRESCRIPTION PRODUCT. Vanobid®.

Nystatin is a tetraene produced by *Streptomyces noursei*. The commercial material

Natamycin is a tetraene produced by *Streptomyces natalensis*. It is available as a 5% ophthalmic suspension and is used to treat fungal blepharitis, conjunctivitis, and keratitis caused by susceptible organisms, including species of *Aspergillus, Candida, Cephalosporium, Fusarium,* and *Penicillium*. It is the drug of choice for keratitis caused by *Fusarium solani*, an infection occurring in hot, humid climates that frequently leads to blindness.

One drop of the suspension is instilled in the conjunctival sac at intervals of 1 or 2 hours; the frequency of application can be reduced to 1 drop, 6 to 8 times daily after 3 or 4 days, but therapy normally should be continued for 14 to 21 days.

GRISEOFULVIN

Griseofulvin was isolated from cultures of *Penicillium griseofulvum* in 1939, and it was utilized initially in plant pathology for its antifungal activity. Its value in therapeutic control of dermatophytes was not recognized until 1958.

Griseofulvin is also produced by a number of other *Penicillium* species, including *P. janczewski, P. nigrum,* and *P. patulum.* It arises biosynthetically from head-to-tail condensation of 7 acetate units. A polyketide is generally considered the basic precursor (Fig. 12–21), and griseophenone C has been identified as an early intermediate in the pathway. Subsequent methylation and chlorination are believed to precede the oxidative coupling of the benzophenone to the spiran, dehydrogriseofulvin. Presumably, the last step is reduction to yield griseofulvin.

Griseofulvin is stable and only slightly soluble in water. The insolubility of the drug leads to considerable variation in absorption upon oral administration. A microcrystalline form (predominantly particles approximately 4 μm in diameter) of griseofulvin is used, and absorption can be facilitated further by administration with a high lipid meal. It is usually employed systemically for control of some dermatophytes belonging to the genera *Epidermophyton, Microsporium,* and *Trichophyton.* Griseofulvin is incorporated preferentially into keratin; this factor explains the unusual oral administration of an antibiotic for dermatomycoses and griseofulvin's lack of therapeutic efficacy in deep mycoses. Sensitive fungi exhibit an unusually narrow range of MICs (0.22 to 0.44 μg per ml). The biologic potency of griseofulvin is measured with *Microsporium gypseum* ATCC No. 14683.

Further studies are necessary to establish conclusively the means by which griseofulvin exerts its antifungal action. Some type of inhibition of fungal mitosis has been implicated.

Griseofulvin is administered orally, and the usual dose is 250 mg, 2 times a day. A 3- to 4-week treatment period is adequate for many conditions, but continued therapy for 6 to 12 months is necessary in some cases (e.g., infections of the fingernails or toenails). Griseofulvin is generally free of serious side effects; the most frequently encountered adverse reactions involve hypersensitivity, including occasional photosensitive reactions.

PRESCRIPTION PRODUCTS. Fulvicin®, Grifulvin®, Grisactin®, grisOwen®, Gris-PEG®.

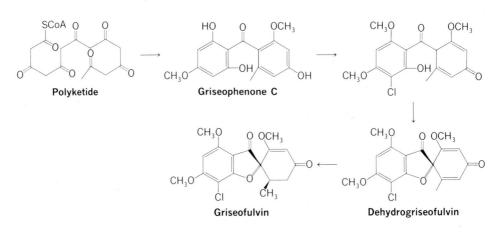

Fig. 12–21. Biosynthesis of griseofulvin.

RIFAMPIN

Rifampin is a semisynthetic antibiotic that is derived from rifamycin B, a metabolite of *Streptomyces mediterranei*. Rifampin has a distinctive macrocyclic lactam structure. The antibiotic inhibits DNA-dependent RNA-polymerase activity in susceptible cells. It has a good gram-positive and a moderate gram-negative spectrum, but its clinical significance is based primarily on the sensitivity of *Mycobacterium tuberculosis* to the antibiotic. It is recommended for treatment of pulmonary tuberculosis; it should be used in combination with at least one other antitubercular agent to avoid selective development of resistant strains of the tubercle bacillus. Rifampin is also useful in the treatment of asymptomatic carriers of *Neisseria meningitidis* when the risk of meningococcal meningitis is high.

deacetylated in the liver to give an antimicrobially active metabolite, and most of the antibiotic is in the deacetyl form when it is ultimately eliminated in the feces. Enterohepatic recycling of rifampin is extensive, but the deacetyl form is not reabsorbed after biliary excretion.

Rifampin is relatively free of toxicity. The most serious adverse reactions involve liver dysfunction, and the increased risk of toxicity in persons with liver damage, such as chronic alcoholics, may preclude the use of this antibiotic. Unfortunately, there is a high incidence of tuberculosis among alcoholics.

Rifampin is administered orally, and the usual dose is 600 mg, once a day. It should be taken 1 hour before or 2 hours after meals to avoid food interference with absorption. Patients should be advised that the antibiotic may color stools, urine, saliva, sweat, or tears a red-orange.

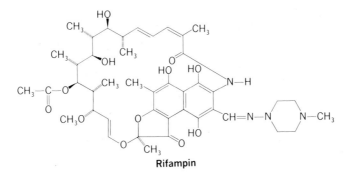

Rifampin

Rifampin, in contrast to the naturally occurring rifamycins, is absorbed adequately on oral administration. Peak serum levels with usual dosage regimens are 4 to 32 μg per ml in 2 to 4 hours; the MICs of sensitive strains of M. tuberculosis have been reported to range between 0.006 and 0.5 μg per ml. The biologic half-life of rifampin is approximately 3 hours. Urinary excretion may account for elimination of up to 20% of the drug, but biliary excretion is the major pathway. Rifampin is gradually

PRESCRIPTION PRODUCTS. Rifadin®, Rimactane®.

NOVOBIOCIN

Novobiocin is produced by *Streptomyces niveus* and *S. spheroides*. The structure of novobiocin suggests an unusual biosynthetic origin for this antibiotic; it appears to involve moieties derived from amino acid, acetate, and carbohydrate metabolic pathways.

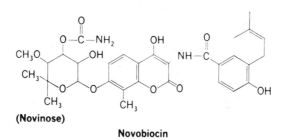

(Novinose)

Novobiocin

The activity spectrum for novobiocin is predominantly gram-positive. Staphylococci tend to be unusually sensitive to this antibiotic (MIC range of 0.1 to 2.0 μg per ml, but resistance develops rapidly), and it has been used an an alternate means for controlling penicillin-resistant staphylococci. However, novobiocin has a high incidence of adverse reactions (hypersensitivity, hepatic dysfunction, and blood dyscrasias), and it is recommended only for use in serious infections when other less toxic drugs are ineffective or contraindicated. The penicillinase-resistant penicillins and other available antibiotics have obviated much of the former need for novobiocin; a number of authorities feel that its use can no longer be justified.

It is absorbed rapidly following oral administration. Peak serum levels of 10 to 20 μg per ml are achieved in 2 to 4 hours, and the normal plasma half-life is between 2 to 4 hours. Renal elimination is insignificant (approximately 3%); excretion is primarily biliary, and there is some recycling. The hepatic toxicity of novobiocin may be explained, in part, by its interference with glucuronyl transferase and the consequent disruption in normal biliary excretion of various glucuronide conjugates. Strong protein binding of novobiocin and displacement of other substances from binding sites also create a high risk for drug-drug interactions.

Novobiocin is available as the sodium salt for oral administration. The usual dose is 250 mg every 6 hours.

Prescription Product. Albamycin®.

ANTIBIOTICS DERIVED FROM CARBOHYDRATE METABOLISM

Carbohydrates provide the basic metabolic substrate for the formation of essentially all microbial products, but this category of antibiotic substances is restricted to compounds that are derived directly from carbohydrate precursors and retain a recognizable carbohydrate character. The therapeutically useful antibiotics derived from **carbohydrate metabolism** include amikacin, gentamicin, kanamycin, neomycin, paromomycin, spectinomycin, streptomycin, and tobramycin.

The chemical and biologic properties of these antibiotics are similar. Common chemical properties include water solubility, a strongly basic character, and stability. The antibiotic molecules, except spectinomycin, routinely have 2 to 3 uncommon sugars linked glycosidically to an amino-substituted cyclohexanyl aglycone. The designation, aminoglycoside antibiotics, is used as a generic term for these compounds. Normally, antibiotic mixtures of closely related molecules are obtained by fermentation, and resolution of the individual components is infeasible and unnecessary for therapeutic purposes. Amikacin is different because it is a semisynthetic material produced from kanamycin A. Spectinomycin is technically an aminocyclitol derivative rather than an aminoglycoside, but a number of its key properties are similar to those of the aminoglycoside antibiotics.

The aminoglycoside antibiotics have a wide spectrum of activity, including many gram-negative and gram-positive bacteria. These antibiotics are not absorbed following oral administration, and their systemic use is limited by nephro- and ototoxicities. The consequences of ototoxicity may be unusually serious. These antibiotics tend to damage both the auditory and vestibular branches of the eighth cranial nerve. Vestibular involvement is observed more frequently, especially with gentamicin and streptomycin. Symptoms include nausea, vertigo, and even vomiting, but recovery is usually complete when therapy is discontinued. Damage of the auditory branch results in irreversible loss of hearing; auditory toxicity appears to be more common with kanamycin and neomycin.

The aminoglycoside antibiotics act on the 30S subunit of 70S ribosomal systems to induce specific misreading of the genetic codon and to inhibit the formation of essential bacterial proteins. The misreading of coded information yields proteins that lack the distinctive physiologic function of normal microbial proteins, but blockage of protein synthesis is believed to be the more therapeutically important mechanism of action. The detailed mechanism(s) for clinically significant inhibition of protein synthesis by the various aminoglycoside antibiotics has (have) not been clarified; this may be distinctive for different antibiotics and/or pathogens.

Emergence of resistant strains, especially of gram-negative bacilli, staphylococci, and mycobacteria, is becoming an increasing problem with the aminoglycoside antibiotics and has contributed, in part, to a decreasing therapeutic utility, especially for kanamycin, neomycin, and streptomycin. Known mechanisms of resistance include chromosomal involvement (alteration of the reactive site on the 30S ribosomal subunit), plastid transfer of extrachromosomal R-factors, and exclusion of the antibiotic from the bacterial cell. The greatest clinical problems are associated with resistance caused by R-factor transfer; enzymatic inactivation of one or more of the aminoglycosides is accomplished by acetylation, adenylation, or phosphorylation. Cross-resistance among the various aminoglycoside antibiotics is often complete, but no or only partial cross-resistance is observed with some bacteria, depending on the nature of the metabolic inactivation that is involved. For example, if streptomycin is inactivated by phosphorylation of the 3-hydroxyl function of 2-deoxy-N-methylglucosamine, cross-resistance can be expected with kanamycin and paromomycin; if the same position is adenylated, cross-resistance occurs with spectinomycin.

The need for therapeutic control of gram-negative organisms and mycobacteria contributes to the therapeutic importance of the aminoglycoside antibiotics. However, the high incidence of resistance and the considerable variation that has been noted in some biologic properties of the antibiotics require efforts greater than normal with the administration of these drugs to insure effective utilization. Strain sensitivity should be determined routinely, and blood levels should be monitored periodically. A serum plasma level between 4 and 16 μg per ml is usually desired for most aminoglycoside antibiotics and most pathogens, and dosage regimens should be adjusted individually as needed. There is considerable variation in the absorption of these antibiotics on intramuscular administration, and renal conditions have an unusually profound influence on their excretion, which is predominantly by glomerular filtration. Renal impairment can increase the biologic half-life from 2 or 3 hours to several days; in such cases, drastic adjustments in the dosage regimen must be made to avoid prolonged high serum levels and the associated increased risks of toxic reactions.

STREPTOMYCIN

Recognition of the therapeutic potential of penicillin stimulated an intensive search for other antibiotic substances. A special objective of these efforts was the discovery of antibiotics antagonistic to gram-negative bacteria. **Streptomycin** was isolated from a strain of *Streptomyces griseus* by Waksman and coworkers in 1944 after they had noted the in vitro inhibitory effect of metabolites of this species on gram-negative bacteria.

ponents are derived from D-glucose. No definitive information is available on the linking of the 3 components, but it is probably a terminal phase of the biosynthetic sequence. Detailed knowledge on the formation of individual moieties of aminoglycoside antibiotics is limited, but a general indication of the metabolic relationships of glucose to the various moieties can be gained from the biosynthetic origins of the streptomycin components (Fig. 12–22).

The nephro- and ototoxicities common to the aminoglycoside antibiotics are encountered with the systemic use of streptomycin. The high incidence of hypersensitivity to streptomycin, even on topical contact, is less serious. Hypersensitivity is not a major adverse response to aminoglycoside antibiotics as a group, and it is probably related in this instance to hap-

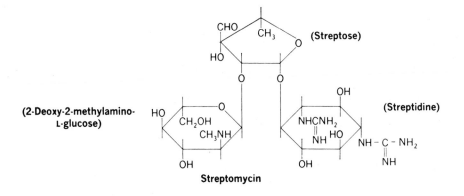

Streptomycin

Because streptomycin was the first aminoglycoside antibiotic to be discovered, studies on its origin and properties provide the basis for much of the current knowledge about this group of antibiotics. Components of streptomycin include streptidine and the disaccharide, streptobiosamine, which contains the sugar residues, 2-deoxy-2-methylamino-L-glucose and streptose. Biosynthetic studies have shown that all 3 of these com-

tene formation involving the formyl group of the streptose unit in streptomycin.

The potential toxicity associated with systemic use of streptomycin is such that the antibiotic is considered for therapeutic use only when satisfactory alternatives are unavailable. *Mycobacterium tuberculosis* is refractory to most antibiotic therapy, and tuberculosis is the major condition requiring systemic administration for which streptomycin is the first-choice antibiotic.

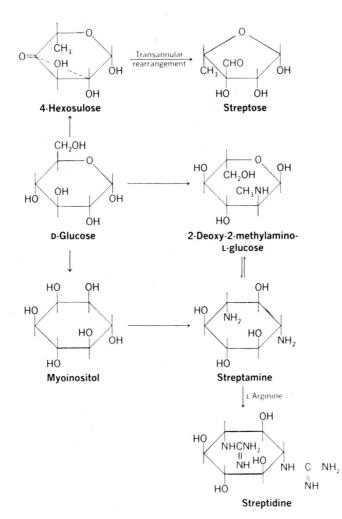

Fig. 12–22. Biosynthesis of components of streptomycin.

In treatment of tuberculosis, streptomycin is normally combined with ethambutol and isoniazid to achieve the best results. Justification is lacking for earlier claims that dihydrostreptomycin, which can be prepared fermentatively with S. humidus or chemically from streptomycin by catalytic reduction of the formyl substituent on the streptose unit, could be used with streptomycin to reduce toxicity. The incidence of serious auditory impairment is now recognized to be greater with dihydrostreptomycin than with streptomycin.

Streptomycin has some value in controlling *Yersinia pestis* (plague) and *Francisella tularensis* (tularemia); in such cases, it is usually combined with a sulfonamide. Combined streptomycin-penicillin and streptomycin-tetracycline therapeutic approaches are sometimes indicated in bacterial endocarditis and brucellosis, respectively.

The antimicrobial activity of streptomycin and other aminoglycoside antibiotics is significantly greater in slightly alkaline conditions than in acidic environments, a factor that can be exploited beneficially in urinary tract infections. The MIC of streptomycin for *M. tuberculosis* is approximately 0.5 μg per ml; many sensitive gram-negative bacteria have MICs in the 2 to 4 μg per ml range. A 1-g intramuscular dose usually gives peak serum levels of 25 to 50 μg per ml in 1 to 2 hours; the normal half-life is 2.5 to 3 hours. Peak serum levels are not as reliable an indicator of potential ototoxicity with streptomycin as are the 24-hour levels following daily injections; toxicity risks increase with 24-hour levels exceeding 3 μg per ml. Because serum levels are prolonged in patients with kidney impairment, peak serum levels should not exceed 20 to 25 μg per ml in such cases.

Streptomycin is available in formulations of its sulfate salt. The biologic efficacy of streptomycin and preparations of this antibiotic can be measured with *Bacillus subtilis* ATCC No. 6633 or *Klebsiella* *pneumoniae* ATCC No. 10031. The usual intramuscular dose is the equivalent of 1 g of streptomycin, once a day.

NEOMYCIN AND PAROMOMYCIN

Neomycin and paromomycin are mixtures of chemically related aminoglycoside antibiotics that were isolated, respectively, from *Streptomyces fradiae* in 1949 and *S. rimosus* var. *paromomycinus* in 1959. The antibiotic molecules contain a 2-deoxystreptamine unit and 3 sugar residues (Fig. 12–23). Neomycin is a mixture of at least 3 antibiotic compounds. Neomycin B is the main component of the mixture. Neomycin C differs from neomycin B only in the stereochemistry of the aminomethyl group in the aminosugar that is linked to the ribose residue. Neomycin A or neamine has only a single sugar residue (neosamine C) linked to the deoxystreptamine aglycone.

Paromomycin consists of at least 2 different antibiotics. These compounds have been designated paromomycins I and II,

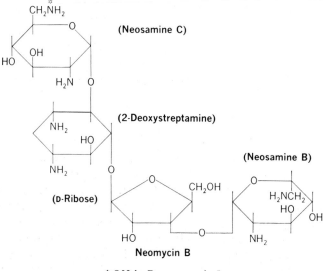

Fig. 21–23. Structures of neomycin B and paromomycin I.

and they are analogs of neomycins B and C, respectively. Paromomycin I is the major component in the mixture, and the paromomycins differ from the neomycins by the replacement of one amino group with a hydroxyl function.

These antibiotics are stable, not absorbed following oral administration, and have the activity spectrum that is generally characteristic of the aminoglycoside antibiotics. Neomycin or other aminoglycoside antibiotics can be taken orally to control intestinal infections by susceptible organisms or for pre- or postoperative reduction of the intestinal flora. Such practices favor emergence of resistant strains. Anaerobic bacteria, the major component of the bowel flora, are not sensitive to these antibiotics. Many authorities recommend restriction of oral administration to serious conditions and high risk situations.

The MICs for such intestinal pathogens as *Escherichia coli* and *Shigella* species are approximately 8 μg per ml. Paromomycin also has therapeutic utility in treating intestinal amebiasis. *Klebsiella pneumoniae* ATCC No. 10031 or *Staphylococcus epidermidis* ATCC No. 12228 can be used as a microbial test organism for evaluating neomycin and paromomycin.

Neomycin is available in formulations of the sulfate salt for oral and topical use. Neomycin is frequently a component (0.35%) in formulations for control of topical infections; these formulations are usually combinations of neomycin and such agents as bacitracin or polymyxin B, which discourage the emergence of resistant strains. This antibiotic is used orally for preoperative reduction of the intestinal flora and for control of intestinal infections. The usual dosage for intestinal infections is the equivalent of 8.75 mg of neomycin per kg of body weight, every 6 hours, for 2 to 3 days. Preoperative use normally involves oral administration of 700 mg of neomycin every hour for 4 doses,

then 700 mg every 4 hours for the balance of 24 hours.

PRESCRIPTION PRODUCTS. Mycifradin®, Neobiotic®.

Paromomycin is available in formulations of the sulfate salt for oral administration. This antibiotic should be taken with meals. The usual dosage regimen is the equivalent of 25 to 35 mg of paromomycin per kg of body weight daily, taken in 3 divided doses for 5 to 10 days.

PRESCRIPTION PRODUCTS. Humatin®.

KANAMYCIN

Kanamycin was isolated from *Streptomyces kanamyceticus* in 1957 and is a mixture of at least 3 aminoglycoside antibiotics. These antibiotics contain 2 aminosugars that are linked individually to a 2-deoxystreptamine aglycone. Kanamycin A is the major component of the mixture (Fig. 12–24).

Kanamycin has an activity spectrum that is comparable to the other aminoglycoside antibiotics. It is used orally for control of infections and for preoperative treatment. The coliform bacteria are sensitive to kanamycin, and *Proteus* species are usually more susceptible to it than to the older aminoglycoside antibiotics. MICs for sensitive gram-negative bacilli usually fall in the 4 to 8 μg per ml range. Kanamycin can be used parenterally for treatment of serious gram-negative infections when susceptible strains are involved. Emerging resistance has become a problem, and gentamicin and tobramycin have replaced kanamycin for systemic treatment of most gram-negative pathogens.

Kanamycin is available in formulations of the sulfate salt for intramuscular, intravenous, and oral use. *Staphylococcus aureus* ATCC No. 6538-P is used for microbiologic assay of this antibiotic. The usual dose for control of intestinal infections is the equivalent of 1 g of kanamycin,

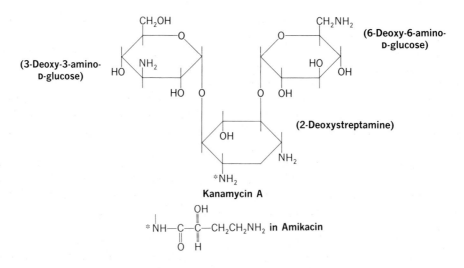

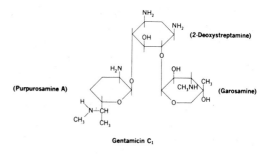

Fig. 12–24. Structures of kanamycin A and amikacin.

3 or 4 times a day. The usual dosage schedule for preoperative treatment is 1 g every hour for 4 doses, then 1 g every 6 hours for 36 to 72 hours. The usual parenteral dosage regimen is up to 15 mg per kg of body weight daily, intramuscularly or by intravenous infusion, in 2, 3, or 4 divided doses. Intramuscular administration gives peak serum levels of approximately 20 μg per ml in 1 to 2 hours; the normal half-life is between 2 and 4 hours.

PRESCRIPTION PRODUCTS. Kantrex®, Klebcil®.

GENTAMICIN

Gentamicin is produced by *Micromonospora purpurea*, an actinomycete. The antibiotic mixture used in medicine consists primarily of gentamicin C_1, C_{1A}, and C_2. Gentamicin C_1 is the major component (approximately 60%). These antibiotic substances contain 2 aminosugar residues and a 2-deoxystreptamine unit. Gentamicin is inhibitory to pathogenic species of such enterobacteria as *Enterobacter*, *Escherichia*, and *Klebsiella* and to *Proteus* and *Serratia* species in lower concentra-

tions (usual MIC, 1 to 2 μg per ml) than other aminoglycoside antibiotics exclusive of tobramycin. It also has a clinically significant activity against *Pseudomonas aeruginosa* (MIC 2 to 8 μg per ml); combined carbenicillin-gentamicin therapy may have special utility in controlling systemic *Pseudomonas* infections. Gentamicin is available in formulations (0.1 and 0.3%) for topical use, but its principal use is parenteral for treatment of serious gram-negative infections caused by sensitive organisms.

Resistance to gentamicin occurs, but cross-resistance with other aminoglycoside antibiotics is often absent in clinical situations; the lack of cross-resistance is presumably related to R-factor-induced inactivation involving specific chemical sites that are not found in the gentamicin molecule (e.g., inactivation by adenylation or esterification of 3-hydroxyl function of a glucosamine moiety).

Gentamicin is rapidly absorbed on intramuscular administration and is readily distributed into various body tissues. Peak serum levels are often achieved in less than 1 hour, and the normal serum half-life is approximately 2 hours. It has been observed that dosage regimens based arbitrarily on mg per kg of body weight result in widely varying plasma levels that may be ineffectively low or dangerously high; for this reason, monitoring of plasma levels and individualization of dosage regimens are highly recommended with this antibiotic. The risk of ototoxicity increases greatly with prolonged serum levels greater than 10 to 12 μg per ml, and trough levels above 2 μg per ml should be avoided.

Gentamicin is available as the sulfate salt, and the usual adult dose is the equivalent of 1 mg of gentamicin per kg of body weight, intramuscularly or intravenously, 3 times a day.

PRESCRIPTION PRODUCT. Garamycin®.

TOBRAMYCIN

Tobramycin or nebramycin factor 6 is the single-component antibiotic that is separated from the nebramycin complex produced by *Streptomyces tenebrarius*. This antibiotic substance contains 2 aminosugar residues and a 2-deoxystreptamine unit; it is structurally related to kanamycin B, differing only in the absence of the 3-hydroxyl function in the kanosamine residue.

Tobramycin was approved in mid-1975 for general medical use. It has biologic properties and clinical indications that are similar to those for gentamicin. Tobramycin may give slightly lower tissue levels than gentamicin, and *Proteus vulgaris* and *Pseudomonas* species are more sensitive in vitro to tobramycin; however, these differences appear to lack significance in clinical situations.

Tobramycin is available as the sulfate salt, and the usual adult dose is the equivalent of 1 mg of tobramycin per kg of body weight, intramuscularly or intravenously, 3 times a day.

PRESCRIPTION PRODUCT. Nebcin®.

AMIKACIN

Amikacin is a semisynthetic aminoglycoside antibiotic derived from kanamycin A by acylation of the 1-amino group of the deoxystreptamine moiety to add an L-(−)-4-amino-2-hydroxybutyryl substituent (Fig. 12–24). The terminal amino group in this substituent is apparently essential for activity; amikacin is active

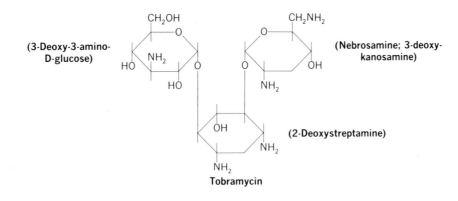

Tobramycin

against many strains of pathogens that inactivate gentamicin, tobramycin, and
other aminoglycoside antibiotics by enzymatic N-acetylation. Pathogens resistant
to amikacin are invariably resistant to
other known aminoglycoside antibiotics, a
consideration that has prompted some authorities to recommend its conservative or
restricted use.

Amikacin is readily absorbed following
intramuscular administration, and its
normal serum half-life is approximately 2
hours. Risks of ototoxicity suggest that the
peak serum level should not exceed 35 μg
per ml and that trough levels should not
exceed 5 μg per ml. A serum level of 8 μg
per ml is adequate to exceed the MICs of
90% of the strains of *Escherichia coli*, *Enterobacter*, *Klebsiella*, and *Proteus*. Levels
of 25 μg per ml are required to reach 90% of
the MICs for strains of *Pseudomonas*, *Serratia*, and *Staphylococcus aureus*.

Amikacin is available as the sulfate salt.
The usual dosage regimen for patients
with normal renal function is 15 mg per kg
of body weight daily, intramuscularly or
by intravenous infusion, in 2 or 3 divided
doses.

PRESCRIPTION PRODUCT. Amikin®.

SPECTINOMYCIN

Spectinomycin is produced by *Streptomyces spectabilis* and *S. flavopersicus*.
The antibiotic molecule is a glycoside, but
it is not technically an aminoglycoside. An
aminocyclitol aglycone is glycosidically

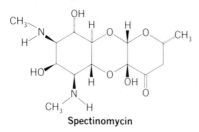

Spectinomycin

linked to a neutral deoxysugar. The dry
antibiotic powder is stable for long periods
of time.

A number of the biologic properties of
spectinomycin resemble those of the
aminoglycoside antibiotics. It is not absorbed on oral administration, is excreted
after injection in an active form by
glomerular filtration, and acts by inhibiting protein synthesis through a mechanism involving the 30S subunit of the 70S
ribosomal system. Spectinomycin has a
broad antibacterial spectrum, but its only
clinical indication is treatment of
gonorrhea. Susceptible strains of *Neisseria
gonorrhoeae* (MIC range of 7.5 to 20 μg per
ml) are frequently controlled by a single
parenteral dose of this antibiotic, a feature
that is unusually advantageous for treatment of a venereal disease. This obviates
many of the problems related to social
stigma and mobile patient populations.
Resistance to spectinomycin is known,
and concern about facilitating the
emergence of more resistance prompts
some authorities to favor restricting the
use of spectinomycin to cases in which
penicillin is ineffective or contraindicated.
Cross-resistance between penicillin and
spectinomycin is unknown.

Spectinomycin is available as the pen-
tahydrate of the dihydrochloride salt. The
usual dose is 2 to 4 g intramuscularly; the
higher dose is routinely recommended for
female patients. Peak serum concentrations of 100 to 160 μg per ml occur in
approximately 1 hour, 8-hour serum levels
are 15 to 30 μg per ml, and total elimination of the antibiotic normally occurs
within 48 hours. The most frequently observed adverse response is pain at the site
of injection; dividing the dose between 2
sites, especially with larger doses of the
antibiotic, has reduced this problem. Neph-
ro- and ototoxicities have not been reported; this may be an inherent property of

spectinomycin or it may reflect the short duration of the normal therapeutic regimen.

Prescription Product. Trobicin®.

READING REFERENCES

Carter, S. K., and Crooke, S. T., eds.: *Mitomycin C, Current Status and New Developments,* New York, Academic Press, Inc., 1979.

Carter, S. K., Crooke, S. T., and Umezawa, H.: *Bleomycin, Current Status and New Developments,* New York, Academic Press, Inc., 1978.

Flynn, E. H., ed.: *Cephalosporins and Penicillins,* New York, Academic Press, Inc., 1974.

Franklin, T. J., and Snow, G. A.: *Biochemistry of Antimicrobial Action,* 2nd ed., New York, Academic Press, Inc., 1975.

Garrod, L. P., Lambert, H. P., and O'Grady, F.: *Antibiotic and Chemotherapy,* 4th ed., Edinburgh, Churchill Livingstone, 1973.

Ghuysen, J. M.: *The Bacterial DD-Carboxypeptidase-Transpeptidase Enzyme System: A New Insight into the Mode of Action of Penicillin,* Tokyo, University of Tokyo Press, 1977.

Glasby, J. S.: *Encyclopaedia of Antibiotics,* 2nd ed., New York, John Wiley & Sons, Inc., 1979.

Gottlieb, D., Shaw, P. D., Corcoran, J. W., and Hahn, F. E., eds.: *Antibiotics,* Vols. I–III, V–1 and V–2, Berlin, Springer-Verlag, 1967–1979.

Kagan, B. M., ed.: *Antimicrobial Therapy,* 3rd ed., Philadelphia, W. B. Saunders Co., 1980.

Kucers, A., and Bennett, N. McK.: *The Use of Antibiotics,* 3rd ed., Philadelphia, J. B. Lippincott Co., 1979.

Medoff, G., and Kobayashi, G. S.: Amphotericin B: Old Drug, New Therapy, JAMA, *232*(6):619, 1975.

Mitscher, L. A.: *The Chemistry of the Tetracycline Antibiotics,* New York, Marcel Dekker, Inc., 1978.

Mitsuhashi, S., and Hashimoto, H., eds.: *Microbial Drug Resistance,* Baltimore, University Park Press, 1976.

Perlman, D., ed.: *Structure-Activity Relationships among the Semisynthetic Antibiotics,* New York, Academic Press, Inc., 1977.

Pratt, W. B.: *Chemotherapy of Infection,* New York, Oxford University Press, 1977.

Smith, H.: *Antibiotics in Clinical Practice,* 3rd ed., Baltimore, University Park Press, 1977.

Storm, D. R., Rosenthal, K. S., and Swanson, P. E.: Polymyxin and Related Peptide Antibiotics, Ann. Rev. Biochem., 46:723, 1977.

Tereshin, I. M.: *Polyene Antibiotics: Present and Future,* Tokyo, University of Tokyo Press, 1976.

Tomasz, A.: From Penicillin-Binding Proteins to the Lysis and Death of Bacteria: A 1979 View, Rev. Infect. Dis., 1(3):434, 1979.

Waksman, S. A.: The Actinomycetes, Vols. I–III, Baltimore, The Williams & Wilkins Co., 1959–1962.

Waksman, S. A.: *The Actinomycetes: A Summary of Current Knowledge,* New York, The Ronald Press Co., 1967.

Weinstein, M. J., and Wagman, G. H., eds.: *Antibiotics—Isolation, Separation and Purification,* Amsterdam, Elsevier Scientific Publishing Co., 1978.

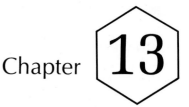

Chapter **13**

Biologics

The inclusive term **"biologic"** may encompass any product derived from a living plant or animal source. However, strictly interpreted, biologics are substances defined by the Bureau of Biologics of the Federal Food and Drug Administration under the Public Health Service Act of 1944, as amended. The law refers to "any virus, therapeutic serum, toxin, antitoxin or analogous product," and it has been interpreted to include a lengthy list of such products as vaccines of bacterial, rickettsial, and viral origin, immune serums for the prevention or treatment of disease, various miscellaneous and diagnostic products, human blood, and products derived from human blood. Such substances as insulin, liver extract, and antibiotic products are not classified as biologics. Much of this reasoning depends on legal definitions and considerations.

The broad term "biologics" thus includes the immunizing biologics that are derivatives of animals (serums, antitoxins, globulins) or of microscopic plant organisms (vaccines, toxins, toxoids, tuberculins), that either directly or indirectly confer a state of protection against pathogenic microorganisms. Because these products do not affect the microorganisms directly, they cannot be considered chemotherapeutic agents; nor can they be classified with the antibiotics.

Biologics can be classified into 2 general categories, antigens and antibodies. An antigen is the material that provokes the immune response, and it can be defined under 3 categories: biologic, chemical, and physical.

Biologically, an antigen is a substance that, when introduced into the tissue of man or other vertebrates, causes the formation of antibodies. These antibodies then react specifically with the antigen that stimulated their production. Therefore, an antigen possesses 2 biologic properties: (1) immunogenicity, the capacity to induce antibody formation, and (2) specificity, governed by small chemical sites on the antigen molecule called the antigenic determinants. The antibody combines with one or more of these sites. Another important biologic concept of the antigen is that it must be considered foreign by the antibody-forming host.

Chemically, antigens are usually protein; however, some high-molecular-weight polysaccharides are antigenic.

Physically, antigens must possess a high molecular weight. A weight of more than 10,000 is required. The high molecular weight is associated with the biologic property of immunogenicity—the capacity to induce antibody formation.

Examples of antigens that are directly concerned in infectious disease are exotoxins, proteins and polysaccharides on the cell surface and capsules of bacteria, and the protein coat of virus particles. Microorganisms contain not one, but many antigens which, in turn, may contain many antigenic determinants.

Compounds with a molecular weight lower than 10,000 can be partial antigens. They are called haptens. Because of their low molecular weight, they cannot induce the formation of antibodies by themselves.

They lack the property of immunogenicity. However, they can attach to host proteins to form a complete antigen which will induce the formation of antibodies specific for the particular hapten. Drugs, or their breakdown products, may act as haptens, and this action is the basis of many drug allergies, e.g., penicillin allergy (see page 432).

Antibodies are found predominately in the serum fraction of the blood, although they also exist in other body fluids and in association with other tissues like lymph nodes and mucous membranes. When serum proteins are separated by electrophoresis, the 4 predominant fractions obtained are serum albumin and alpha, beta, and gamma globulins. The antibodies occur predominately in the gamma

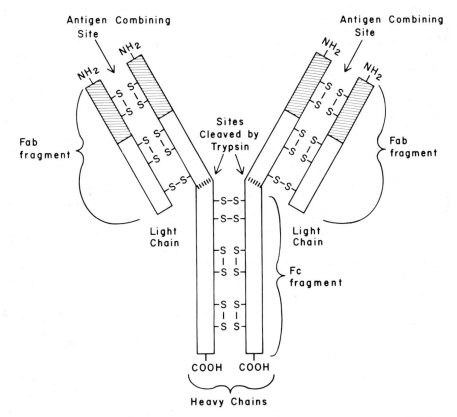

Fig. 13–1. A schematic representation of the structure of immunoglobulin G (IgG); ▨ designates amino acid variable region; ▭ designates amino acid constant region.

globulin fraction and are called immuno-globulins. On the basis of their physical, chemical, and immunologic properties, the immunoglobulins can be separated into 5 subclasses: IgA, IgD, IgE, IgG, and IgM. IgG is the most abundant of the serum immunoglobulins, and the major part (up to 80%) of the serum antibody found after bacterial and viral infections belongs to this class of antibodies. Immunoglobulin G has a molecular weight of approximately 150,000 and contains about 1400 amino acids. These acids are not linked in 1 continuous chain, but are arranged in 4 polypeptide chains—2 heavy and 2 light. Each pair has identical structures. The chains are connected by disulfide bonds, which help impart a tertiary structure to the molecule (Fig. 13–1). With trypsin, the peptides can be cleaved into 2 antigen-binding fragments (Fab) and a third fragment, which cannot combine with antigen and crystallizes in neutral salt solutions (Fc). The 2 antigen-binding fragments are identical and arise from the amino-terminal ends of the 4 peptide chains. Each fragment contains the amino-terminal portion of one light chain and one heavy chain, and studies have shown that the amino acid composition of these portions of the peptide chains is variable from one antibody to another. The amino acid composition of the portion of the peptide chains representing the carboxy-terminal ends that make up the Fc fragment is relatively constant among different antibodies. The variability in the Fab region of the molecule may reflect the unique structure of each specific antibody against a specific antigen.

Because of the 2 combining sites on the IgG molecule, these antibodies are particularly well adapted to form macromolecular lattices with antigens and are usually good precipitating antibodies. The Fc fragments of human IgG contain various sites that are important in specialized functions of the immunoglobulin. One site facilitates placental transmission, one site fixes the antibody to cells in the skin and other tissue when injected into a different animal species, and one site fixes the complement. Complement is a complex of serum proteins and is required for the completion of certain antigen-antibody reactions, including the lysis of bacterial cells or erythrocytes by antibody.

When the newborn infant begins its own antibody production, the first immunoglobulin to appear is IgM. Molecules of IgM are pentamers of the basic 4-chain immunoglobulin unit such as that found in IgG. The 4-chain units are linked by disulfide bonds like a 5-pointed star. The antigen-binding sites point outward. Because of the increased number of possible binding sites on a single antibody molecule, IgM can react with closely spaced antigenic determinants on the surface of cells, thereby making this antibody efficient in agglutinating or clumping erythrocytes and bacteria. For example, the ABO blood group antibodies are of the IgM type.

IgA, IgD, and IgE are found in relatively low concentrations in the blood serum. IgA is the predominate immunoglobulin in external secretions, such as saliva and secretions of the respiratory and gastrointestinal tracts. These antibodies probably form a specific defense mechanism in these areas of the body. IgE antibodies have an affinity for the surfaces of cells, which may be mediated by a cell attachment site on the Fc fragments in the molecule. Antigen reacting with cell-bound IgE molecules leads to cell damage, subsequent histamine release, and the symptoms of immediate hypersensitivity, such as asthma, hay fever, anaphylaxis, and skin eruptions (see Chapter 14). Immunoglobulin D is in the lowest concentration in the serum. IgD's specific role may be as an antigen receptor on antibody-producing cells that are designed for triggering the production of antibody.

Immunity is classified into 2 major types: **natural (innate) immunity** and **acquired immunity.** The term natural or innate means the defense mechanisms that are present in the body because of race, species specificity, and a multitude of other factors not easily defined, but does not include any mechanisms especially developed during the lifetime of the individual. Thus, natural immunity is endowed at birth and is retained because of an individual's constitution.

On the other hand, acquired immunity is quite specific and generally is subdivided into 2 classes: **active immunity** and **passive immunity,** each of which is further subdivided as follows:

Acquired immunity
1. Activity immunity
   a. Naturally acquired active immunity
   b. Artificially acquired active immunity
2. Passive immunity
   a. Naturally acquired passive immunity
   b. Artificially acquired passive immunity

Active immunity means the specific immunity developed by an individual in response to the introduction of antigenic substances into the body. In this type of immunity, the antigenic substances may be received by the body in a natural manner (naturally acquired active immunity) or they may be received by the body through the administration of a vaccine or toxoid (artificially acquired active immunity). In the first instance, recovery from an infection, such as measles or scarlet fever, produces an immunity that is acquired naturally, is developed rather slowly, and is usually long-lasting. In the second case, the immunity may be produced as the re-

sponse to a series of injections (of typhoid or pertussis vaccine, for example), thus stimulating the body cells to make their own antibodies and producing an immunity that is acquired artificially, is developed gradually, and is usually longlasting.

Depending on the nature of the antigen and the site of injection, antibody can be detected in the serum several days after the first injection of antigen. The antibody titer rises gradually to a low peak after the first and immediately subsequent injections and then falls slowly over a period of months (Fig. 13–2). A second injection of antigen, administered while antibodies from the first stimulus are still present, results in a rapid rise to a much higher peak than with the first injection. The second injection cannot be too close in time to the first injection. If so, there is no additional effect on antibody production. The antibodies disappear much more slowly after the second stimulus than after the first. The rapid rise of antibody titer following a second administration of the antigen (the booster shot) presumably indicates that the antibody-producing cells have been primed by the first contact with antigen and, therefore, respond more effectively and more quickly when they encounter the antigen a second time. This phenomenon is termed the recall or anam-

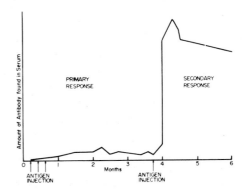

Fig. 13–2. An illustration of the recall or anamnestic phenomenon in antibody production.

nestic phenomenon and has great practical significance in immunization against infectious disease.

The origin of serum antibodies is now believed to be certain lymphocytes called B cells (so named because they were first described as originating from the bursa of Fabricius of chickens) which arise from the bone marrow or a bursa-equivalent organ in man. This is known as the humoral system of immunity because the B cells circulate in the body fluids, primarily in blood. The B-cell system handles most of the infectious organisms that are bacteria. Companion to the B-cell system is another lymphocyte population, the T cells. These cells originate in the bone marrow but depend on the thymus gland for their differentiation. The T cells are the agents of cellular immunity, more stationary than the B cells, and seldom found circulating in the blood. Cellular immunity resists infections by fungi, acid-fast bacilli such as *Mycobacterium tuberculosis*, and viruses. T cells are also responsible for delayed hypersensitivity, e.g., tuberculin reactions and poison ivy dermatitis, and serve as the sentinels of immune surveillance against cancer and the mediators of graft rejection.

The B and T cells act in cooperation with one another; however, the exact mechanism of this cooperation is still to be determined.

Passive immunity is the type developed by the introduction of preformed antibodies (not antigens) into the body. In this type, the body cells are not stimulated to produce their own antibodies. Because the immunity acquired by the individual is not self-developed, but is passed from one individual (or animal) to another, the term passive immunity is applied. The immunity developed in a newly born infant through transmission of the antibodies from the blood of the mother is an example of naturally acquired passive immunity; it is produced quickly but is not long-lasting. The injection of immunizing biologics containing preformed antibodies in forms such as diphtheria antitoxin or gamma globulin, produces artificially acquired passive immunity which, again, is produced quickly but is not long-lasting.

Obviously, certain biologics are intended for **prophylactic or preventive therapy,** whereas others are serviceable as **therapeutic or curative measures.** Vaccines and toxoids in their preventive capacities do not offer immediate protection to the patient; antitoxins, serums, and globulins give instant protection to the patient.

The importance of vaccination cannot be stressed too highly; its value has been proved beyond question. Smallpox has been eliminated from the United States because of the compulsory state laws requiring vaccination of children of preschool age. Typhoid fever and epidemic typhus fever were nonexistent among the armed personnel during the recent wars, an outstanding medical accomplishment related primarily to rigid vaccination schedules maintained by military and naval medical staffs. Conceivably, any disease could be eradicated anywhere in the world if such proper preventive measures as sanitation, vaccination, and education were instituted. At the present time, many childhood diseases can be effectively prevented by utilizing the recommended immunization schedule illustrated in Table 13–1.

Antibiotics are currently available for controlling many infectious diseases, but antitoxins and related passive immunologic agents are still useful in treating infections caused by viruses and other pathogens that fail to respond to antibiotics. Also, the unique utility of antibody-containing biologics for prophylactic purposes must be emphasized. It is infeasible and undesirable to use antibiotics for prophylaxis. These reasons suggest that biologics must be accorded a special place

Table 13–1. Recommended Immunization Schedule

Immunizing Agent	Preferred Age for Initial Dose	Dosage for Primary Immunization	Booster
Adsorbed Diphtheria and Tetanus Toxoids and Pertussis Vaccine[1] (DTP)	2 to 3 months	0.5 ml, intramuscularly, repeated twice at 4 to 6 week intervals.	0.5 ml 1 year after primary and 4 to 5 years later. Td every 10 years thereafter.
Adsorbed Tetanus and Diphtheria Toxoids for Adult Use (Td)	7 years and over	0.5 ml, intramuscularly, repeated once after 4 to 6 weeks.	0.5 ml 1 year after primary and every 10 years thereafter.
Live Oral Poliovirus Vaccine, Trivalent	2 to 3 months	Two doses given at not less than 8-week intervals (in the volume indicated in the labeling), and a third, reinforcing dose 8 to 12 months later.	One dose at entry into school.
Live Attenuated Measles Virus Vaccine[2]	15 months of age or older	0.5 ml subcutaneously	None recommended.
Live Rubella Virus Vaccine[2]	Between age 15 months and puberty	0.5 ml subcutaneously	None recommended.
Live Mumps Virus Vaccine[2]	15 months of age or older	0.5 ml subcutaneously	None recommended.

[1] For primary immunization or boosters over age 6, use Td.
[2] May be given in bivalent or trivalent vaccine.

among medicinally useful materials obtained from natural sources.

All biologics are "dated," i.e., carry an expiration date on the label of the package, because they do not retain their potency for an indefinite period. Specific regulations govern the determination of the expiration date for given biologic formulations. For example, diphtheria antitoxin can have a 5-year expiration date provided the preparation has a 20% excess of potency. Dried formulations of smallpox vaccine have an expiration limit of 18 months from the date of issue, but the expiration date of liquid smallpox vaccine is not more than 3 months from date of issue. Whether the potency of the biologic is still existent near the end of the expiration time depends on the methods of storage.

The nature of biologic products requires that they be refrigerated during storage.

They represent either living or dead microorganisms or their metabolic products as well as the active components of the blood of animals. To insure their activity as immunogenic materials, they should be stored at a temperature ranging from 2 to 8°C. In certain instances, lower temperatures are indicated. Liquid smallpox vaccine and yellow fever vaccine should be stored at a temperature no higher than 5°C and preferably lower than 0°C; live poliomyelitis vaccine should be preserved at a temperature below −10°C. Because biologics are usually stored in mechanically operated refrigerators, they may occasionally become frozen. Provided the container is not broken, such freezing does not affect the potency of the product unless the label states otherwise.

All immunizing biologics must comply with the identity, safety, sterility, and potency tests and other requirements for the individual product in accordance with the Food and Drug Regulations—Code of Federal Regulations, as administered by the Bureau of Biologics of the FDA. Each lot of the product must be released individually before its distribution. The labeling must correspond to certain specifications. It must bear the name of the product, the lot number, and expiration date; the manufacturer's name, license number, and address; and a statement regarding storage and refrigeration. Biologics are to be dispensed in the unopened container in which they were placed by the manufacturer.

In addition to the commercially available biologics, the Center for Disease Control (CDC), U.S. Public Health Service can supply various rare immunologic agents in emergency situations. These products are available through Immunobiologics, Bureau of Laboratories, CDC, Atlanta, Georgia, 30333.

VACCINES

Vaccines may contain living, attenuated, or killed viruses, killed rickettsiae, or attenuated or killed bacteria, and they are used as inoculations to stimulate the production of antibodies.

Primary active immunity from vaccination develops more slowly than the incubation period of most infections and must be induced prior to exposure to the infectious agent; therefore, the general action of vaccines should be considered prophylactic. One exception is the rabies vaccination. Because the rabies virus has a median incubation period of 35 days in man, there is usually sufficient time for protective antibodies to develop when the vaccine is administered postexposure.

Nonliving vaccines provide protection for only a limited time, and repeated vaccination is required to maintain protection against typhoid fever, cholera, plague, and typhus. Active immunization with living agents is generally preferable to immunization with killed vaccines because of a superior and more long-lived immune response. For example, a single vaccination of measles, rubella, or mumps vaccine is sufficient to produce a long-lasting if not permanent immunity. Multiple immunizations are recommended for polio because interference among the 3 simultaneously administered virus types present in the trivalent vaccine could prevent completely successful primary immunization.

The benefits of active immunization far outweigh the dangers associated with the use of vaccines; however, precautionary measures should be followed to insure optimum effectiveness with a minimum of adverse reactions. Use of vaccines is contraindicated under conditions in which the immune response may be depressed, such as during therapy involving corticosteroids, antineoplastic agents, immunosuppressive agents, or radiation; in patients with immunoglobulin deficiency (agammaglobulinemia and dysgammaglobulinemia); and in patients with latent or active infections.

Active immunization may cause fever, malaise, and soreness at injection sites. Some reactions are relatively specific for a particular vaccine, such as arthralgia and arthritis following rubella vaccine or convulsions following pertussis vaccine. During the 1976 "swine flu" immunization program in the United States, there was an 8-fold increase in postimmunization Guillain-Barré syndrome (acute febrile polyneuritis) in comparison to unvaccinated controls. This complication arises within 8 weeks of immunization and has resulted in a 5% mortality rate among patients who developed the syndrome.

Allergic reactions may result either from the organism constituting the vaccine or from a protein incorporated into the vaccine during manufacture, e.g., egg protein from chick embryo tissue cultures. Consequently, a careful history of the patient should be taken before vaccination to detect possible hypersensitivity to the protein to be injected.

VIRAL VACCINES

Viral vaccines for prophylaxis against mumps, rubella, rubeola, smallpox, and yellow fever contain living viruses. Inactivated or killed viruses are used in influenza and rabies vaccines. Preparations containing live attenuated or killed viruses are available for immunization against poliomyelitis.

The cultivation of viruses poses a problem because they are completely dependent on living cells for their sustenance. No method of growing viruses in artificial culture media is known. Viruses for smallpox vaccine and for rabies vaccine have been obtained for years from vesicular tissues of vaccinated calves and brain tissues of infected rabbits, respectively, but this approach has limited utility for many viruses. The use of living chick or duck embryos for viral culture offers advantages in some cases, but the development of techniques for tissue culture of mammalian cells provided the major basic advancement necessary for significant expansion in the practical use of many viral vaccines. A number of viruses currently employed in viral vaccines are grown on tissue cultures prepared from chick embryo, monkey kidney, or human diploid cells. Primary tissue cultures have created some problems, especially because of the need for large numbers of monkeys and because of the continuous need for extensive tests, with resulting expense and delays, to insure the absence of undesirable simian viruses in each monkey kidney donor. It appears that advancements will be forthcoming and will permit indefinite

propagation of suitable cell lines. The use of tissue cultures of human cells has now become a reality (see page 399).

SMALLPOX VACCINE

Smallpox vaccine is the living virus of vaccinia (cowpox) that has been grown in the skin of a vaccinated bovine calf. It is available in dried and in liquid form; the latter consists of a smooth, aqueous suspension of infected tissue that contains 40 to 60% of glycerin or of sorbitol, and may contain not more than 0.5% of phenol as a preservative.

The pioneering work of Dr. Edward Jenner in England in 1796 established that when a mild case of cowpox (vaccinia) is developed by a person, the same person is immune to smallpox. Using this information, he inoculated a young boy with pus from a milkmaid infected with cowpox. Two months later, the boy was inoculated with pus from a patient infected with smallpox, but no disease developed. Immunity had been established.

The calf is prepared by washing and shaving its belly, then scarifying the epidermis so that serum oozes through the cuts. The "seed virus" is inoculated into the scarifications merely by hand rubbing (the workers are protected by rubber surgical gloves). The calf is maintained in an aseptic stall and given food and water during the growth of the virus. The vesicles that develop are removed at the time of maximum potency (Fig. 13–3), thoroughly triturated, and either made into a smooth suspension with an aqueous solution of glycerin or sorbitol or reduced to a dried pellet.

The animal must be in good health prior to inoculation. After the virus is harvested, the animal is killed and a necropsy is performed. If the organs show no effects of disease from other causes, the virus is deemed satisfactory for manufacture.

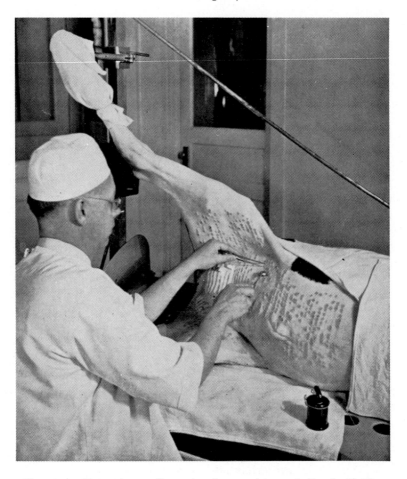

Fig. 13–3. Harvesting smallpox virus from vesicles on belly of calf. (Photo, courtesy of Eli Lilly & Company.)

Smallpox vaccine should be dispensed in the containers in which it was placed by the manufacturer. Liquid vaccine should be kept below 0° C during storage and in shipment because it loses potency rapidly at higher temperatures. Dried vaccine should be kept at a temperature between 2 and 8° C.

USE AND DOSE. Smallpox vaccine is a specific immunizing agent and is used as a prophylactic before the infection occurs. It creates active immunity that usually lasts for about 7 years. Usual dose is, percutaneous, contents of 1 capillary tube, by the multiple-puncture method. In the United States, routine immunization against smallpox is no longer recommended by the Public Health Service because adverse reactions to primary vaccinations can cause death (less than 1 per 100,000 vaccinations). Also, the disease has now undergone complete worldwide eradication.

PRESCRIPTION PRODUCT. Dryvax®.

RABIES VACCINES

Rabies vaccine is a sterile preparation of killed, fixed virus of rabies in dried form.

The virus is obtained from duck embryos that have been infected with fixed rabies virus.

In addition to his other famous accomplishments, Louis Pasteur is also associated with rabies. Pasteur was able to "fix" the virus of rabies by passing it from an infected dog to the brain of a rabbit and then from one rabbit to another until a uniformity was established that resulted in attenuated virulence for man. In the first immunization against rabies in 1885, Pasteur used such a fixed virus to achieve active immunity.

The Pasteur treatment is not a curative treatment, but it actually accomplishes the same result because immunization of a patient bitten by a rabid animal proceeds more quickly than the incubation period of the disease. Because the treatment consists of a series of daily injections for 14 days, the development of antibodies probably inhibits the growth of the virus.

Rabies vaccine of duck embryo origin contains little or no myelin, the "paralytic" factor that causes rabies treatment paralysis. On the other hand, brain tissue, formerly used in the preparation of the vaccine, contains a significant amount of myelin. Of prime importance in immunization against rabies is the early development of antibodies; with duck embryo vaccine, antibodies can be demonstrated in patients by the tenth day of treatment. However, patients treated with duck embryo vaccine may develop allergic reactions if they are hypersensitive to egg protein. Duck vaccine is sometimes called "avianized" vaccine.

Rabies vaccine is usually available in packages containing 7 individual doses and should be stored at a temperature between 2 and 8° C. The dried vaccine may have an 18-month expiration date.

Use. The vaccine is an active immunizing agent and is recommended primarily for the prevention of rabies in persons bitten by an animal supposed or known to be rabid. However, the vaccine of duck embryo origin may be used occasionally for pre-exposure immunization for veterinarians or other high-risk individuals. Postexposure immunization should be started as quickly as possible after the wound has been inflicted; the usual administration schedule is a subcutaneous injection once a day for 14 days. Rabies immune globulin should be administered at the time of the first dose of vaccine for additional protection, particularly in the case of a bite from a wild animal.

Diploid rabies vaccine is a new vaccine prepared from virus grown in cultures of human diploid embryo lung tissue. Because it contains much less foreign protein than does the duck embryo vaccine, more antigen can be given in each dose and with less chance of side effects. Studies of the new vaccine, which requires only 4 to 6 doses postexposure, show that it is more effective than the duck embryo vaccine.

YELLOW FEVER VACCINE

Yellow fever vaccine is an attenuated strain of living yellow fever virus, selected for high antigenic activity and safety. It is prepared by culturing the virus in the living embryo of the domestic fowl (Gallus domesticus) (Fig. 13–4). The virus-infected, chick-embryo pulp is suspended in water and, after appropriate aseptic processing, is distributed in suitable quantities into ampuls and dried from the frozen state. Afterward, the ampuls are filled with dry nitrogen and flame-sealed. The expiration date of this vaccine is not longer than 1 year from the date of issue, and it must be stored at a temperature preferably below 0° C but never above 5° C. Yellow fever vaccine should be hydrated immediately before use. It does not contain human serum.

Yellow fever or "yellow jack" was con-

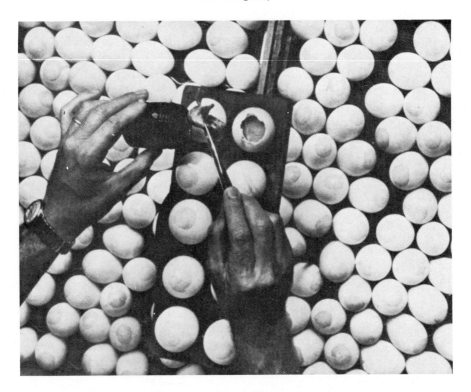

Fig. 13–4.   Preparation of vaccine from virus-infected chick embryo. (Photo, courtesy of Eli Lilly & Company.)

sidered an endemic disease in certain tropical regions, including the Caribbean Islands and Central America. Work on the Panama Canal was abandoned by the French because of the terrific death toll caused by yellow fever. Through the heroism of Walter Reed, Carlos Finlay, and numerous volunteers among the American troops stationed in Cuba during the Spanish-American war, the *Aëdes* mosquito was finally proved to be the vector of the disease. Further investigation was necessary to determine that the cause of yellow fever was a noncultivatable, filter-passing virus.

USE AND DOSE. Yellow fever vaccine is an active immunizing agent that is used to develop active immunity against the disease. Usual dose, subcutaneously, is 0.5 ml. The use of yellow fever vaccine in the United States is limited largely to persons planning to travel through parts of the world where yellow fever is endemic.

INFLUENZA VIRUS VACCINE

Influenza virus vaccine is a sterile, aqueous suspension of suitably inactivated influenza virus types A and B, either individually or combined, or virus subunits prepared from the extra-embryonic fluid of influenza virus-infected chick embryo. The strains of influenza virus used in the preparation of this vaccine are those designated for the particular season by the Bureau of Biologics of the Federal FDA. It contains a suitable preservative and may contain an adsorbent, such as aluminum phosphate or protamine. During the commercial preparation of the vaccine, the virus growths are collected, concentrated, refined by ultracentrifugation, and inactivated by ultraviolet irradiation.

Each lot of influenza virus vaccine must be tested to determine its potency; its power to stimulate the formation of specific virus-neutralizing antibodies in mice is correlated with the potency. Each ml is labeled according to the number of CCA units it contains; the unit refers to the chicken red-cell agglutination titer. This vaccine must be stored at a temperature between 2 and 8°C, and the expiration date is not longer than 18 months from the date of issue.

USE AND DOSE. Influenza virus vaccine is an active immunizing agent. Its usual dose is, intramuscularly or subcutaneously, 2 injections of 0.5 ml, as specified in the labeling, 6 to 8 weeks apart. Annual vaccination is recommended for individuals in high-risk categories, e.g., those with chronic, debilitating disease; those who are immunocompromised; and those over 65 years of age.

Influenza viruses have a high degree of strain specificity and of genetic instability. These factors require a continual reevaluation of the components of influenza virus vaccine and result in periodic infections of epidemic proportions even among immunized persons. Most available vaccines are bivalent and contain types A and B virus strains.

PRESCRIPTION PRODUCTS. Fluax®, Fluogen®.

POLIOMYELITIS VACCINES

Poliovirus vaccine inactivated is a sterile suspension of inactivated poliomyelitis virus of types 1, 2, and 3. The virus

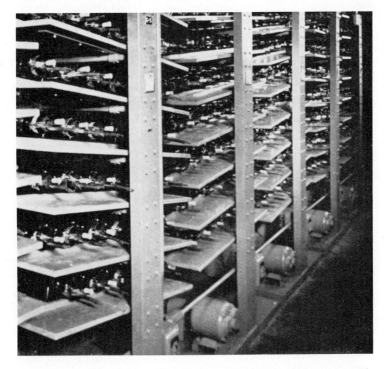

Fig. 13–5. Polio vaccine. The virus-inoculated tissue cultures are gently rocked for 6 days at 35° C (approximately body temperature) in a special incubator room. (Tile and Till, courtesy of Eli Lilly & Company.)

strains are grown separately in primary cultures of Rhesus monkey kidney tissues bathed by a complex nutrient fluid containing more than 60 ingredients (Fig. 13–5). After incubation, the virus is harvested by decanting the nutrient fluid that is clarified by filtration; then, formaldehyde in a concentration of 1:4000 is added. The formaldehyde-treated virus is maintained at 36°C at pH 7 until all viruses are killed (Fig. 13–6). A series of elaborate tests is performed to ascertain that all viruses are inactivated. Following these quality control tests, the formaldehyde is neutralized and a preservative is added

(Fig. 13–7). The 3 types of virus are then pooled, and the resultant mixture is the trivalent vaccine (Fig. 13–8).

In addition to the 3 types of poliomyelitis virus that have been cultured and identified, other paralysis-producing strains undoubtedly exist. In general, however, poliomyelitis epidemics of major proportions have been caused by type 1 (Brunhilde). Type 3 (Leon) has proved to be the etiologic agent in less frequent epidemics, and type 2 (Lansing) has been concerned only in sporadic cases. Immunization with one type of virus does not offer protection against the other types;

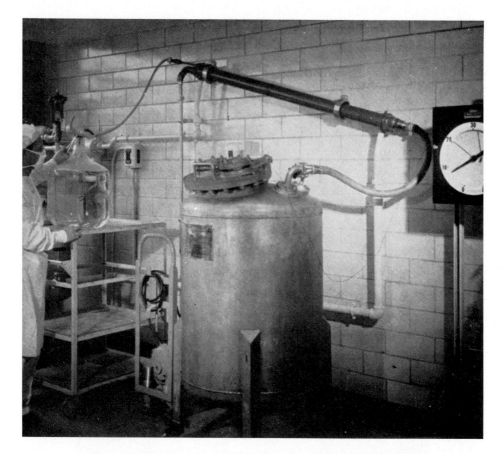

Fig. 13–6. Salk polio vaccine. After the virus has been filtered and proven free of unwanted bacteria and viruses, formaldehyde from bottle at left is added for inactivation as the virus suspension is heated from refrigerator temperatures to 36°C. Thermometer reading of 7.5°C indicates that passage through heat exchanger has just begun. (Tile and Till, courtesy of Eli Lilly & Co.)

thus, the current vaccine is a trivalent preparation. Improved strains of the various viral types are the object of continuous selection studies; the type 1 Mahoney strain, type 2 MEF-1 strain, and type 3 Saukett strain are now used in preparing poliomyelitis vaccines.

Landsteiner and Popper, in 1908, first transmitted and isolated poliomyelitis virus experimentally in monkeys. It was subsequently ascertained that monkeys that had survived one attack of poliomyelitis were resistant to further attacks; furthermore, blood serum from such monkeys neutralized the virus in vitro. Still later, this observation resulted in the successful attempt to induce passive immunity through the use of serum obtained from immune donors.

During 1948, Dr. John F. Enders and his associates at Harvard University originated a method of cultivating polio virus in vitro on animal tissues other than nervous tissue. Then, in 1953, Dr. Jonas Salk

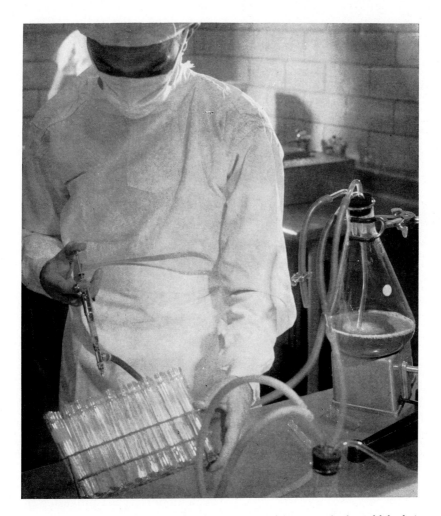

Fig. 13–7. Salk polio vaccine. After inactivation of the virus, the formaldehyde is neutralized. Special tissue culture technique is used to prove that the virus is entirely inactivated. (Tile and Till, courtesy of Eli Lilly & Company.)

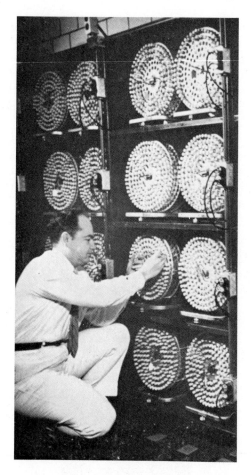

Fig. 13–8. Polio vaccine. All 3 types of vaccine are mixed together to make the final product. This mixture is again tested to be sure no active viruses are present. (Courtesy of Eli Lilly & Company.)

received 1 or more injections of the vaccine; 210,000 received placebo injections consisting of a nutrient medium similar to but not used for actual growth of the virus organisms; and the remaining 1.18 million were observed as controls. Vaccination consisted of an initial intramuscular injection of 1 ml of vaccine followed by a second 1-ml injection 1 week later and a third 1-ml injection about 4 weeks after the second. (NOTE: *The time intervals for active immunization have changed.*) The mass inoculations covered a total of 217 selected areas in 44 states of the United States and 48 areas of Canada and Finland.

The results of this carefully controlled study encouraged the National Foundation for Infantile Paralysis to purchase sufficient vaccine to inoculate approximately 9 million school children during 1955. The success of the mass polio vaccinations in both 1954 and 1955 received international prominence, not only for the enthusiastic response from the children's parents and for the cooperative spirit of the biologic manufacturers, but also for the ingenuity and tireless efforts of Dr. Jonas Salk. (Poliovirus vaccine inactivated is more commonly referred to as Salk polio vaccine.)

USE AND DOSE. Poliovirus vaccine inactivated is an active immunizing agent that has definite value in creating active immunity to the disease. Usual dose, intramuscularly or subcutaneously, is 3 injections of 1 ml, 4 or more weeks apart, and a fourth, reinforcing dose of 1 ml, 6 to 12 months later.

Poliovirus vaccine live oral is a preparation of one or a combination of the 3 types of live, attenuated polioviruses. The virus strains are grown separately in primary cultures of monkey kidney tissue. It has been manufactured and tested in a manner suited only for oral administration and is free from any known microbial agent other than the attenuated poliovirus or polio-

and his coworkers at the University of Pittsburgh perfected the roller-tissue method of polio virus culture, as well as the final detoxified form of polio vaccine. The Nobel Prize was awarded to Dr. Enders for his achievement in virus cultivation; international acclaim was bestowed on Dr. Salk for his development of the vaccine and its success in the extensive inoculation tests.

Field trials using polio vaccine were conducted during 1954 on a total of 1.83 million school children of which 440,000 viruses intended to be present. This vaccine is commonly called **trivalent oral polio vaccine (TOPV)** and contains one or all of types 1, 2, or 3 Sabin poliovirus strains.

Three scientists working independently developed procedures for the manufacture of this vaccine: Dr. Albert Sabin of the University of Cincinnati, Dr. Harold Cox of Lederle Laboratories, and Dr. Hilary Koprowski of the Wistar Institute of Philadelphia. The results of large-scale trials extending over a period of several years indicated that oral polio vaccine has longer-lasting immunity, greater ease of administration, and presumably lower costs of production than the Salk polio vaccine. The tests involved more than 13 million people in countries outside of the United States. Extensive domestic trials were performed in the Dade County, Florida; Minneapolis; Cincinnati; and Rochester, New York areas. In the Dade County field trials, the vaccine was incorporated into a cherry-flavored oral preparation that was designed to immunize against all 3 strains of poliomyelitis.

Safety tests conducted by the U.S. Department of Public Health resulted in the announcement of August, 1960 that the Sabin formula was the most "suitable for use in the United States." Licensed manufacture of this trivalent vaccine began early in 1963; quantity production was reached later that year.

The manufacture of poliovirus vaccine live oral is similar to that of poliovirus vaccine inactivated (Salk) because the virus strains are grown separately in monkey tissue cultures. However, the viruses are not killed by treatment with formaldehyde as is done with Salk vaccine; instead, the viruses are attenuated. Therefore, the Sabin oral vaccine should never be administered parenterally.

Live poliovirus vaccines offer protection against strains of poliomyelitis virus that cause paralysis. The attenuated live virus, when present in the intestinal tract, multiplies and produces a localized resistance to reinfection by the same type of virus, thus stimulating the production of type-specific serum antibodies. The development of such localized resistance to the growth of the virus affords a protection that is independent of specific, circulating antibodies. Salk vaccine provides protection against paralytic poliomyelitis through the stimulation of serum antibodies specific for types 1, 2, and 3 poliovirus, but does not cause inhibition of viral growth in the intestine that characterizes Sabin vaccine.

Poliovirus vaccine live oral is generally frozen. When stored at a temperature of $-10°$ C, the expiration date is not later than 1 year after date of manufacture or date of issue.

USE AND DOSE. Poliovirus vaccine live oral is an active immunizing agent. When administered orally, it effectively develops immunity to the poliovirus, Sabin strains types 1, 2, and 3. The usual administration schedule involves an initial administration of 2 doses at not less than 8-week intervals. A third, reinforcing dose is administered 8 to 12 months later. The volume of vaccine indicated on the label as representing one dose is generally placed on a cube of sugar, which is eaten by the individual to be immunized. The immunization schedule should be carried out in the winter and spring to avoid the summer peak of other intestinal enteroviruses that may interfere with the desired immunologic response.

PRESCRIPTION PRODUCT. Orimune®.

MEASLES VACCINES

Vaccines containing live attenuated rubeola (measles) and rubella (German measles) viruses are available for active immunization. Viruses for production of these vaccines are grown on cultures of either avian embryo tissue or human diploid cell tissue. The vaccines are available in a lyophilized form. They should be stored at a temperature between 2 and 8° C and have a 1-year expiration date.

Measles virus vaccine live or rubeola vaccine is prepared from attenuated viruses derived from the original Edmonston B strain. The Enders strain is a modified Edmonston strain, and it is claimed to have a high degree of antigenicity with a low incidence of adverse reactions; coadministration of immune globulin may not be necessary with vaccines employing this strain. The rubeola virus is grown on cultures of chicken embryo tissue.

Rubeola vaccine is recommended for active immunization of children 15 months of age or older. Use in infants under 15 months of age is not recommended. Good immunity is obtained with a single subcutaneous injection of 0.5 ml of the reconstituted vaccine.

PRESCRIPTION PRODUCTS. Attenuvax®, M-Vac®.

Rubella virus vaccine live is prepared from the Wistar Institute RA 27/3 strain grown on human diploid cell tissue. Rubella vaccine is recommended for active immunization against German measles for children aged 1 to puberty and for certain other individuals. This vaccine should not be administered to pregnant or immediate postpartum women, and special caution must be exercised if it is given to sexually active females. Precautions must be taken to eliminate the possibility of pregnancy in women of child-bearing age for at least 3 months following immunization. Immunity is obtained with a single 0.5-ml subcutaneous injection of the reconstituted vaccine. Use in infants under 1 year of age is not recommended.

PRESCRIPTION PRODUCT. Meruvax II®.

MUMPS VACCINE

Mumps virus vaccine live is prepared with the B-level Jeryl Lynn strain of the virus, which is grown in cell cultures of chicken embryo tissue. It provides active immunity for at least 10 years after immunization and is particularly valuable to susceptible individuals approaching puberty and to adults. It is not recommended for infants less than 1 year old because they may retain maternal mumps antibodies that may interfere with the immune response. The vaccine is available in a lyophilized form; immunization involves a single subcutaneous injection.

PRESCRIPTION PRODUCT. Mumpsvax®.

COMBINATION VIRUS VACCINES

Combination live virus vaccines containing either measles virus and rubella virus, rubella virus and mumps virus, or measles virus, rubella virus, and mumps virus are available. These combination vaccines are administered subcutaneously in a dose of 0.5 ml of the reconstituted vaccine to children 15 months of age or older. Use in infants under 15 months of age is not recommended.

PRESCRIPTION PRODUCTS. Live measles and rubella virus vaccine: M-R-VAX II®; live rubella and mumps virus vaccine: Biavax II®; live measles, mumps, and rubella virus vaccine: M-M-R II®.

RICKETTSIAL VACCINES

Rickettsiae are cultured in chick embryos or in monkey kidney tissue cultures in a manner similar to that for viruses. They cannot be grown in artificial culture media and must be subjected to the same precautions as viruses. At the present time, epidemic typhus fever vaccine is the only rickettsial vaccine produced commercially in the United States. Murine typhus, tsutsugamushi fever, and other rickettsial diseases as well as epidemic typhus, are of considerable importance in other parts of the world. Vaccines are available in these problem areas for all of these rickettsial diseases.

TYPHUS VACCINE

Typhus vaccine is a sterile suspension of the killed rickettsial organisms of a strain or strains of epidemic typhus rickettsiae (Rickettsia prowazekii) selected for antigenic efficiency. The rickettsial organisms are obtained by culturing in the yolk-sac membrane of the developing embryo of the domestic fowl (Gallus domesticus). Typhus vaccine consists of refined material derived from an aqueous suspension of infected yolk-sac membrane, and the rickettsiae are killed by a suitable chemical agent. This vaccine is also known as **epidemic typhus vaccine.**

Typhus vaccine must be stored at a temperature between 2 and 8° C. The expiration date is not later than 18 months after the date of issue.

USE AND DOSE. An active immunizing agent for epidemic typhus fever, the vaccine is administered as a prophylactic measure particularly to travelers to the highland and mountainous areas of Asia. The usual administration involves 2 subcutaneous injections of 0.5 ml, as specified in the labeling, 4 or more weeks apart, followed by 0.5 ml every 6 to 12 months for as long as protection is desired.

BACTERIAL VACCINES

Bacterial vaccines consist of suspensions of attenuated or, more commonly, killed pathogenic bacteria in isotonic sodium chloride solution or other suitable diluents. The strains of bacteria employed in preparation of the vaccines must be selected for high antigenicity, and a measure of the potency of a vaccine may be expressed as the number of organisms per unit volume or as biologic reference units. Suspensions of young, living organisms grown in standard culture media are killed chemically, by application of moist heat at a temperature slightly above the thermal deathpoint, or by exposure to ultraviolet light.

The smooth or "S" strains of bacteria are uniformly more antigenic than the rough or "R" strains. Occasionally, stock cultures lose their antigenic qualities, and care must be exercised in a biologic manufacturer's laboratory to insure the use of suitable strains.

Good immunologic responses are obtained with the following bacterial vaccines: cholera, pertussis, plague, and typhoid. The effectiveness of BCG vaccine, meningitis vaccines, and pneumococcal vaccine is still being evaluated.

TYPHOID VACCINE

Typhoid vaccine is a sterile suspension containing killed typhoid bacilli (Salmonella typhi) of a strain selected for high antigenic efficiency. It contains approximately 1 billion typhoid organisms in each ml and not more than 35 μg of total nitrogen.

Typhoid vaccine has been called enteric vaccine because it prevents the effect of the disease on the intestinal tract. Because typhoid fever organisms occur in sewage, any flood that inundates the water supply of a city is a potential cause of an epidemic of the disease. Public health authorities have prevented serious outbreaks of disease through the encouragement of typhoid vaccination procedures.

USE AND DOSE. Typhoid vaccine is an active immunizing agent for producing immunization against typhoid fever. The usual immunization schedule involves two 0.5-ml subcutaneous injections, at least 4 weeks apart, followed by 0.5 ml every 3 years thereafter. Booster injections are recommended when danger of typhoid fever occurs.

CHOLERA VACCINE

Cholera vaccine is a sterile suspension of killed cholera vibrios (*Vibrio cholerae*) in isotonic sodium chloride solution or other suitable diluent. It is prepared from equal portions of suspensions of cholera vibrios of the Inaba and Ogawa strains. The Inaba strain possesses an antigenic value not less than that of N.I.H. Inaba strain 35-A-3, and the Ogawa strain possesses an antigenic value not less than that of N.I.H. Ogawa strain 41. At the time of manufacture, cholera vaccine contains approximately 8 billion cholera organisms in each ml. This vaccine should be stored at a temperature between 2 and 8° C, and the expiration date is not longer than 18 months from the date of issue.

Statistically, the results reported on cholera vaccination in various parts of the world are sufficiently satisfactory to warrant its continued use in reducing morbidity and mortality from cholera.

USE AND DOSE. Cholera vaccine is an active immunizing agent in the development of immunity to the disease. Usual adult dose, subcutaneously or intramuscularly, is 0.5 ml, and then 1 ml, 4 weeks later; 0.5 ml dose repeated every 6 months, if necessary.

PLAGUE VACCINE

Plague vaccine is a sterile suspension, in an isotonic sodium chloride solution or other suitable diluent, of killed plague bacilli (*Yersinia pestis*) of a strain selected for high antigenic efficiency. It contains approximately 2 billion plague bacilli in each ml.

The bacteria causing bubonic and pneumonic plague in man are named *Yersinia* in honor of the Swiss bacteriologist Yersin, who was the first to isolate and identify the disease-causing organism. Rats serve as an animal reservoir for the organisms, but the disease is transmitted to humans through the bite of fleas that infest the rats. With rat control and large scale vaccination, plague could be eliminated. In the United States, plague bacilli have been found in wild animals and their fleas in 15 western states.

USE AND DOSE. Plague vaccine is an active immunizing agent and is used to produce immunity to the disease. Its use is generally restricted to travelers to southeastern Asia and to persons who have frequent contact with wild rodents in plague enzootic areas, such as the southwestern United States. The usual immunization schedule involves two 0.5-ml intramuscular injections, at least 4 weeks apart, then 0.2 ml, 4 to 12 weeks later.

PERTUSSIS VACCINE

Pertussis vaccine is a sterile bacterial fraction or suspension of killed pertussis bacilli (*Bordetella pertussis*) of a strain or strains selected for high antigenic efficiency. It has a potency of 12 protective units per individual immunizing dose, based on U.S. Standard Pertussis Vaccine. This vaccine should be stored at a temperature between 2 and 8° C and must be protected against freezing. The expiration date is not later than 18 months from the date of issue.

Bordetella pertussis is the organism that causes the disease known as whooping cough or pertussis. The cough is probably caused by a toxin in the bacterial body that also appears in filtrates of bacterial cultures. The organisms attach themselves to the cilia of epithelial cells in the trachea, and the irritation produced provokes the cough spasm.

USE AND DOSE. Pertussis vaccine is an active immunizing agent used to create immunity. Usual dose, subcutaneously, is 3 injections usually of 0.5 ml or 1 ml, as specified in the labeling, at least 3 to 4 weeks apart.

Adsorbed pertussis vaccine consists of pertussis vaccine that has been precipitated or adsorbed by the addition of aluminum hydroxide or aluminum phosphate and resuspended. It corresponds to all of the requirements for pertussis vaccine, but it contains not more than 850 μg of aluminum in the volume stated in the labeling to constitute 1 injection.

USE AND DOSE. Same as for pertussis vaccine, except that the administration is by the intramuscular route.

Pertussis vaccine may be combined with diphtheria and tetanus toxoids to give a multiple immunizing agent (Tri-Immunol®, Triogen®, Triple Antigen®). Simultaneous immunization with these preparations is recommended primarily for infants and children under 6 years of age.

TUBERCULOSIS VACCINES

Studies of the effectiveness of vaccines to produce immunity to tuberculosis are constantly in progress. The vaccine known as BCG (prepared from Bacillus Calmette-Guérin) is a freeze-dried preparation of the culture of an attenuated strain of bovine tuberculosis originally isolated by 2 bacteriologists, Calmette and Guérin. This vaccine has provided bacteriologists and immunologists with a subject of controversy for years. The chief point of difference concerned the relative safety of the vaccine, but refinements in the processing and improvements in the testing have now assured a safe, nontoxic product for human use.

BCG VACCINE

BCG vaccine is a dried, living culture of the bacillus Calmette-Guérin strain of *Mycobacterium tuberculosis* var. *bovis*. The culture is grown in a suitable medium from a seed strain of known history that has been maintained to preserve its capacity for conferring immunity.

The expiration date of BCG vaccine is up to 1 year if it is stored at 5° C. This vaccine should be used within 2 hours after reconstitution. BCG vaccine has been accepted by European physicians for a number of years, and endorsement by American investigators was forthcoming during the 1950s. Immunologic protection against tuberculosis is only relative and is not permanent or predictable. The vaccine is recommended primarily for use for people whose exposure to tuberculosis is unusually high or when other means of control are inadequate. It should be used only with individuals who give a negative tuberculin skin test.

USE AND DOSE. BCG vaccine is an active immunizing agent against tuberculosis. It is administered intradermally as the reconstituted vaccine in doses of 0.1 ml.

OTHER BACTERIAL VACCINES

Meningococcal polysaccharide vaccines contain the specific bacterial capsular polysaccharides for *Neisseria meningitidis* serogroup A and serogroup C. Monovalent vaccines for each serogroup are available. A bivalent vaccine with both serogroups included is also available. The presence in human serum of antibodies to meningococcal polysaccharide antigens is strongly correlated with immunity to meningococcal meningitis. The use of meningococcal polysaccharide vaccine, group A, is indicated for children over 3 months of age and for adult populations at risk in epidemic or highly endemic areas. The group C vaccine and the bivalent vaccine are used for children over 2 years of age and for military recruits and adult populations at risk in epidemic areas.

The immunizing dose is a single subcutaneous injection of 0.5 ml containing 50 μg of meningococcal polysaccharide.

PRESCRIPTION PRODUCTS. Group A, Menomune-A®; Group C, Meningovax-C® and Menomune-C®; Groups A and C, Menomune-A/C®.

Pneumococcal vaccine, polyvalent affords protection against the 14 most prevalent capsular types of pneumococci, which account for at least 80% of pneumococcal disease. It is prepared by isolating and purifying the polysaccharide antigens from strains of Streptococcus pneumoniae that contain these serotypes. Its use is indicated for persons 2 years of age or older in whom there is an increased risk of morbidity and mortality from pneumococcal pneumonia. These special groups include persons with chronic physical conditions, persons in chronic care facilities, and persons convalescing from severe disease.

It is administered as a single 0.5-ml dose that is given either subcutaneously or intramuscularly.

PRESCRIPTION PRODUCTS. Pneumovax®, Pnu-Imune®.

DIAGNOSTIC ANTIGENS

A number of antigen-containing preparations are employed as diagnostic aids to determine whether an individual has developed hypersensitivity to certain types of organisms. Hypersensitivity is usually the result of a previous infection caused by the specific etiologic agent. Small quantities of the diagnostic preparations are usually injected intradermally, and the developing reaction is usually read at 48

hours, although observations at 24 hours and at 72 hours are often helpful. The usual type of positive response is a localized, well-defined wheal accompanied by erythema.

Antigen-containing diagnostic preparations that are commonly available include the tuberculins, histoplasmin, coccidioidin, and mumps skin test antigen. Other preparations that are occasionally used for diagnostic purposes are formulated and employed on the same basic principles.

TUBERCULINS

Tuberculins are preparations obtained in a number of ways from the human and bovine strains of the tubercle bacillus. The active substance of the tuberculin, which is apparently an albuminous derivative insoluble in alcohol, is elaborated by the organisms during their multiplication. In both human and veterinary practice, tuberculin may be applied as a diagnostic agent to determine whether the person or animal is or has been infected with Mycobacterium. The tuberculin may be applied by intracutaneous injection, by rubbing into the scarified skin, by dropping into the eye, or by other methods. In each case, a marked redness or inflammation indicates a positive reaction. A positive test does not necessarily indicate the presence of an active infection, but indicates that further evaluation should be done.

OLD TUBERCULIN

Old tuberculin, concentrated tuberculin, crude tuberculin, or tuberculin-Koch is a sterile solution of the concentrated, soluble products of growth of the tubercle bacillus (Mycobacterium tuberculosis). This solution is adjusted to the standard potency by addition of glycerin and isotonic sodium chloride solution. Its final glycerin content is approximately 50%. Old tuberculin, in diluted form suitable for injection, is prepared in a buffered diluent.

In the preparation of this product, tubercle bacilli are grown in broth medium for 8 weeks. Afterward, the culture is boiled, the organisms are filtered and discarded, and the filtrate is evaporated to one-tenth its volume. The final product is a clear brownish liquid that is readily miscible with water and has a characteristic odor.

Old tuberculin should be stored at a temperature between 2 and 8° C. The expiration date of the undiluted old tuberculin is up to 5 years, but the expiration date of the diluted form is not more than 1 year after the date of manufacture or the date of issue.

USE AND DOSE. Old tuberculin is a diagnostic immunologic aid in testing patients suspected of having tuberculosis. Because of the glycerin, peptones, and mineral salts present in the final product, false-positive reactions may occur. The usual dose of old tuberculin is 0.1 ml containing 10 tuberculin units, intradermally. A positive test consists of an area of inflammation and definitely palpable induration or edema at least 5 mm in diameter. It appears in 6 to 8 hours, reaches its maximum in 24 to 48 hours, and usually disappears in 6 to 10 days.

PRESCRIPTION PRODUCTS. Tuberculin, Old, Human for Mantoux Test; Tuberculin Mono-Vacc Test®; Tuberculin Old, Tine Test®.

PURIFIED PROTEIN DERIVATIVE OF TUBERCULIN

Purified protein derivative of tuberculin or tuberculin P.P.D. is a sterile, soluble, partially purified product of growth of the tubercle bacillus *(Mycobacterium tuberculosis)* prepared in a special liquid medium that is free from protein.

The tubercle bacilli are cultured in a synthetic medium until the desired growth is obtained. The filtered active tuberculin material is purified by precipitating with trichloracetic acid. It is composed of tuberculo-protein and is usually supplied as tablets in which lactose may be present.

The expiration date is not later than 2 years after date of manufacture or date of issue.

USE AND DOSE. Purified protein derivative of tuberculin is an immunologic diagnostic aid. It is used to test patients suspected of having tuberculosis; it is not used to treat the disease. Usual dose is 5 tuberculin units intradermally. The test is read 48 to 72 hours after administration, and a palpable induration measuring 10 mm or more is considered positive.

PRESCRIPTION PRODUCTS. Aplisol®, Tubersol-Connaught®, Aplitest®, SclavoTest-PPD®, Sterneedle®.

HISTOPLASMIN

Histoplasmin is a sterile, standardized liquid concentrate of the soluble growth products developed by the fungus *Histoplasma capsulatum* when grown in the mycelial phase on a synthetic medium. It is employed in skin tests to determine the presence of histoplasmosis, a disease that affects the reticuloendothelial system and usually results in enlargement of the liver, spleen, and lymph nodes.

Histoplasmin is of no value in treating this disease; it is used only to aid the physician in determining whether the patient is harboring the fungal organisms.

This biologic should be preserved at a temperature between 2 and 8° C. The expiration date is not later than 2 years after date of manufacture or date of issue.

USE AND DOSE. Histoplasmin is a diagnostic aid (dermal). The usual dose is, intradermally, 0.1 ml of a 1:100 dilution.

Persons who suffer from histoplasmosis

always respond positively to the skin test; however, some individuals without any disease symptoms may also show a positive reaction, indicating a subclinical exposure or a cross-reaction of the fungal extract with other fungus organisms in the body. Histoplasmin skin test is seldom used because it may increase the complement fixation titer, which is the preferred method used to diagnose an active infection of histoplasmosis.

COCCIDIOIDIN

Coccidioidin is a sterile solution containing the antigens obtained from the by-products of mycelial growth or from the spherules of the fungus *Coccidioides immitis.* Coccidioidin should be stored at a temperature between 2 and 8° C. The expiration date is not later than 3 years after the date of issue.

Coccidioidomycosis is a dust-borne disease that is caused by *C. immitis* and is indigenous to the arid regions of the southwestern United States. This disease may infect any part of the body. Approximately 60% of the cases are asymptomatic and identifiable only by a positive skin test; most of the remaining cases evidence moderate to severe symptoms of respiratory infection.

USE AND DOSE. Coccidioidin is a diagnostic aid in detecting cases of coccidioidomycosis. The usual dose, intradermally, is 0.1 ml of a 1:100 dilution.

PRESCRIPTION PRODUCT. Spherulin®.

MUMPS SKIN TEST ANTIGEN

Mumps skin test antigen is a sterile suspension of formaldehyde-inactivated mumps virus prepared from the extra-embryonic fluids of the mumps virus-infected chicken embryo. It is concentrated and purified by differential centrifugation and diluted with isotonic sodium chloride solution so that each ml contains not less than 20 complement-fixing units. It should be stored between 2 and 8° C and has an expiration date of 18 months.

The mumps intradermal skin test is utilized to define an individual's previous experience with mumps virus. In about 75% of the cases, infection with the mumps virus is followed by skin sensitivity to the organism. The mumps skin test antigen is particularly helpful during and after adolescence as an aid in identifying those who should be protected against the disease.

A control test is not necessary, and an area of erythema at least 1.5 cm in diameter, with or without induration, that develops 24 to 36 hours after injecting the antigen is indicative of probable immunity.

USE AND DOSE. Mumps skin test antigen is a diagnostic aid, and the usual dose, intradermally, is 0.1 ml.

TOXINS AND TOXOIDS

Toxins are bacterial waste products that are considered poisonous to the animal body. Notwithstanding, they act as antigens owing to their power of stimulating certain cells of the body to produce antibodies called antitoxins. In practice, toxins are modified to inactivate the toxicophore group of the molecule, leaving the antigenic group unchanged.

When toxins are excreted from the bacterial cells producing them and are dissolved in the surrounding culture medium, they are referred to as **exotoxins.** In other cases, when they are retained within the bacterial body, they are called **endotoxins.**

To produce a solution of exotoxins commercially, the highly virulent organisms are cultured in beef broth medium and then killed by appropriate means. The organisms are removed by filtration through a bacterial filter, and the filtrate that contains the toxins and other products of growth is standardized on a suitable animal to determine the minimum lethal dose. This dose represents the smallest amount of the toxin that will kill a majority of a series of guinea pigs within 96 hours after subcutaneous administration. Commercial toxins serve as a starting point for the manufacture of antitoxins as described below.

The source of "the most poisonous poison" is *Clostridium botulinum*, a microorganism generally unable to grow in the body of a warm-blooded animal but capable of causing death if its exotoxins are ingested. Thus, botulism is a matter of food poisoning. When the toxins produced by this bacterium are compared with other types of protein poisons (diphtheria toxin and snake venom), their potencies range from 10 to 1000 times higher. Five kinds of neurotoxins have been determined; food poisoning in man commonly is produced by types A, B, and E.

Treating exotoxins with formaldehyde reduces or eliminates the toxic properties without affecting the antigenic properties. These products, detoxified in this manner, are called **fluid toxoids,** and they are used to induce artificial active immunity in susceptible individuals. By precipitating or adsorbing the fluid toxoid with alum, aluminum hydroxide, or aluminum phosphate, an **adsorbed toxoid** is produced which, when administered, results in a slower release of the antigen from the site of injection and a subsequent production of higher and more prolonged antibody titers. However, the adsorbed toxoids are more prone to produce local reactions at the site of injection than are fluid toxoids. To avoid this, adsorbed toxoids should be administered by deep intramuscular injection, whereas the fluid toxoid may be administered subcutaneously.

Both fluid and adsorbed toxoids are used to produce active immunity against diphtheria and tetanus. They are used alone and in combination. In young children, diphtheria and tetanus toxoid combined with pertussis vaccine is often used, and the combination is commonly known as triple antigen or DTP.

Repeated immunization with diphtheria and tetanus toxoids may result in increasingly severe local reactions. Diphtheria antigen in adsorbed diphtheria and tetanus toxoids for adult use (Td) is therefore 4- to 10-fold less than in adsorbed diphtheria and tetanus toxoids for pediatric use (DT) and in DTP. Also, a lower frequency of booster immunization for tetanus is now recommended (Table 13–2).

The toxoids alone and in combination with pertussis vaccine should be stored at a temperature between 2 and 8° C. The expiration date is not later than 2 years after the date of issue.

ANTITOXINS

Antitoxins are prepared from the blood of animals, usually horses, that have been immunized by repeated injections of specific bacterial exotoxins. The toxin, in constantly increasing doses, induces the formation of antitoxin in the blood of the injected animal. After tests have been conducted to determine the antitoxin titer of the serum, the animal is bled, the clot is permitted to form, and the clear supernatant serum is separated for processing.

In the past, diphtheria antitoxin consisted of unprocessed serum which, when injected, often caused numerous cases of sensitivity to horse serum proteins. Today, depending on the manufacturer, either of 2 methods of processing is employed. The first involves a series of precipitations using varying concentrations of ammonium sulfate. During this process, the euglobulin and fibrinogen fractions are initially "salted" out, followed by the

Table 13–2.   Therapeutically Important Toxoids

Agent	Indication for Use	Dosage Schedule	Products Available
Adsorbed Diphtheria Toxoid (Pediatric)	Active immunization against diphtheria in infants and children under 7 years of age.	For primary immunization, 2 injections of 0.5 ml given intramuscularly 6 to 8 weeks apart, and a third dose of 0.5 ml given 1 year later. Booster dose of 0.5 ml should be given at 5- to 10-year intervals.	generic
Tetanus Toxoid (Fluid)	Active immunization against tetanus.	For primary immunization, 3 injections of 0.5 ml given subcutaneously 3 to 4 weeks apart, and a fourth dose of 0.5 ml given 1 year after third injection. Booster dose of 0.5 ml should be given every 10 years.	generic
Adsorbed Tetanus Toxoid	Active immunization against tetanus and preferred agent over Tetanus Toxoid (Fluid) for primary immunization and booster doses.	For primary immunization, 2 injections of 0.5 ml given intramuscularly 4 to 6 weeks apart, and a third dose of 0.5 ml given 1 year later. Booster dose same as Tetanus Toxoid (Fluid).	generic
Diphtheria and Tetanus Toxoids (Fluid for Pediatric Use)	Indicated when it is inadvisable to give triple antigen containing pertussis vaccine to children less than 6 years of age.	For primary immunization, 3 injections of 0.5 ml given subcutaneously at intervals of 4 to 6 weeks, and a fourth dose 1 year after primary series. Booster dose of 0.5 ml at 5 years of age, then every 10 years thereafter.	generic

Table 13–2. Therapeutically Important Toxoids (continued)

Agent	Indication for Use	Dosage Schedule	Products Available
Adsorbed Diphtheria and Tetanus Toxoids for Pediatric Use (DT)	Same as for Diphtheria and Tetanus Toxoids (Fluids for Pediatric Use)	For primary immunization, 2 injections of 0.5 ml given intramuscularly at interval of 4 to 8 weeks. A reinforcing dose is given 6 to 12 months later. Booster dose of 0.5 ml at 5 years of age, then every 10 years thereafter.	generic
Adsorbed Diphtheria and Tetanus Toxoids for Adult Use (Td)	Primary active immunization in adults and for wound management. It contains the same amount of tetanus toxoid as in DT but only 10% to 25% of the diphtheria toxoid.	For primary immunization and booster dose, the same as for DT. For wound management of all wounds, whether tetanus-prone or not, and in cases where the immunization status of the patient is unimmunized, uncertain, incomplete, or last booster dose administered longer than 10 years ago, a single 0.5 ml dose of either DT or Td should be administered intramuscularly.	generic
Adsorbed Diphtheria and Tetanus Toxoids and Pertussis Vaccine (DPT)	Active immunization of infants and children under 7 years of age against diphtheria, tetanus, and whooping cough.	For primary immunization, administer at the age of 6 weeks to 3 months with 3 0.5-ml doses injected intramuscularly at 4- to 8-week intervals with a reinforcing dose given 1 year after the third injection. Booster dose of 0.5 ml administered when child is 3 to 6 years of age. For booster doses thereafter, Td should be used.	Tri-Immunol® Triogen® Triple Antigen®

pseudoglobulin fraction, which contains the antitoxin. The later fraction is redissolved, dialyzed, and filtered. The second method utilizes a pepsin solution to digest the plasma, thus removing up to 80% of the protein; however, a loss of about 20% in antitoxin content occurs also. The digested material is then treated with ammonium sulfate solution, redissolved, dialyzed, and filtered. Both of these methods aim to eliminate the proteins of horse serum and the resulting serum sickness.

Antitoxins are standardized in terms of "antitoxin units." The International unit of diphtheria antitoxin is the same as that of the American or National Institutes of Health unit: that amount of antitoxin that is contained in 1/6000 g of a certain dried, unconcentrated horse serum antitoxin which has been maintained since 1905 at the National Institutes of Health, Bethesda, Maryland. On the other hand, the International unit of tetanus antitoxin is equivalent to only one-half the potency of the American or National Institutes of Health unit: that amount of antitoxin that is contained in 0.00015 g of a dried, unconcentrated horse serum antitoxin maintained since 1907, 3000 International units being equivalent to 1500 American units.

No antitoxin, antivenin, or antiserum prepared from horse serum should be given without carefully inquiring about prior exposure to horse serum or about allergic response upon exposure to horses. Whenever these products are administered, a syringe containing epinephrine injection (1:1000) and a tourniquet should be available to counter an anaphylactic reaction. Also, sensitivity testing should be performed before administration either by injecting intracutaneously 0.02 ml of a 1:100 dilution of the product to be administered or by instilling a drop of 1:100 dilution of the product into the conjunctival sac. A drop of sodium chloride injec-

tion, USP, placed in the opposite eye, provides a control.

The hypersensitivity reactions that can arise from the injection of biologics prepared from horse serum can range in severity from acute anaphylaxis and death occurring almost immediately after injection to serum sickness, which may arise hours to weeks following treatment. Typical manifestations of serum sickness include fever, urticaria, adenopathy, and arthritis.

DIPHTHERIA ANTITOXIN

Diphtheria antitoxin is a sterile, nonpyrogenic solution of the refined and concentrated proteins, chiefly globulins, containing antitoxic antibodies obtained from the blood serum or plasma of healthy horses, that have been immunized against diphtheria toxin or toxoid. It has a potency of not less than 500 antitoxin units per ml.

The expiration date with a 20% excess of potency is not later than 5 years after the date of manufacture or of issue. Diphtheria antitoxin should be stored at a temperature between 2 and 8° C.

Uses and Dose. Diphtheria antitoxin is a passive immunizing agent capable of inducing passive immunity against diphtheria. It is a valuable curative agent when used in sufficient amount to neutralize the pathogenic effects of the toxin formed in the patient. This is especially true when the antitoxin is used early in the disease and before the detrimental effects are too far advanced. Any person with clinical symptoms of diphtheria should receive the antitoxin at once without waiting for bacteriologic confirmation. Usual dose, intramuscularly or intravenously, prophylactic, is 1000 to 10,000 units; therapeutic, 20,000 units to 80,000 units.

Although penicillin and other antibiotics kill the diphtheria organisms, they have no effect on the toxins.

TETANUS ANTITOXIN

Tetanus antitoxin is a sterile, non-pyrogenic solution of the refined and concentrated proteins, chiefly globulins, containing antitoxic antibodies obtained from the blood serum or plasma of healthy horses, that have been immunized against tetanus toxin or toxoid. It has a potency of not less than 400 antitoxin units per ml.

Tetanus antitoxin should be stored at a temperature between 2 and 8° C. The expiration date of the liquid antitoxin is not later than 5 years after the date of manufacture or issue with a 20% excess of potency.

Uses and Dose. Tetanus antitoxin is employed in the treatment and prophylaxis of tetanus if tetanus immune globulin is not available. It creates passive immunity to tetanus. Like diphtheria antitoxin, it is a valuable therapeutic agent when used early in the disease. Prophylactic doses should be given to individuals who have had 2 or less injections of tetanus toxoid and who have tetanus-prone injuries that are more than 24 hours old. Tetanus toxoid should also be administered at a different site on the patient. Usual dose, intramuscularly or subcutaneously, prophylactic, is 3000 to 10,000 units; therapeutic, 40,000 to 100,000 units or more.

BOTULISM ANTITOXIN

Botulism antitoxin is a sterile, non-pyrogenic solution of the refined and concentrated antitoxic antibodies, chiefly globulins, obtained from the blood serum or plasma of healthy horses that have been immunized against the toxins produced by both the type A and type B and/or type E strains of *Clostridium botulinum*. This antitoxin contains not more than 20% of solids and should be stored at a temperature between 2 and 8° C. The expiration date is not later than 5 years after the date of issue.

This multivalent antitoxin is used to treat all cases of toxemia caused by the types of botulinus bacteria used in its preparation. A multivalent antitoxin is advantageous because the prescribing physician is not required to wait for a determination of the type of the causative organism.

Use and Dose. Botulism antitoxin is classed as a passive immunizing agent to be used in the treatment of botulism. The usual dose is, intravenously, 20,000 units, repeated at 2- to 4-hour intervals, as necessary.

VENOMS AND ANTIVENINS

Venoms are poisonous excretions produced by animals; they can be compared with the toxic waste products (exotoxins) of bacteria. The detrimental effects developed in humans and animals following the bite of poisonous snakes (rattlesnake, copperhead, moccasin, cobra, others) have been known for many years. About 10,000 people are bitten by poisonous snakes every year in the United States. Poisonous snakebites often cause severe pain and can lead to tissue necrosis, amputation, and death. The venom of the rattlesnake is a complex mixture, chiefly proteins, many of which have enzymatic activity and a nonenzymatic neurotoxic fraction. Similarly, the venoms of the tarantula, scorpion, black widow spider, honeybee, wasp, and other arthropods produce various deleterious effects depending on the amount, time of year, and other conditions. Chemical examinations of the poisons of toads have revealed that both skin and glandular secretions possess toxic substances called bufotoxins. The chemical structures of the bufotoxins are somewhat similar to those of the aglycones of the cardiac glycosides;

in fact, the bufotoxins appear to have a similar pharmacologic effect.

Snake venins or venoms are obtained by holding a poisonous snake over a conical glass container covered with a sheet of thin rubber (Fig. 13–9). The snake strikes the rubber and penetrates it with its fangs, whereupon the semiliquid venom is ejected into the container.

Mixtures of venins from the poisonous snakes of a locality, country, or continent are prepared and used in the preparation of polyvalent antivenins (antisnakebite serums).

Treatment of snakebite is controversial, but most authorities believe that early ad-ministration of antivenin is the therapy of choice.

ANTIVENIN (CROTALIDAE) POLYVALENT

Antivenin (Crotalidae) polyvalent or North and South American antisnakebite serum is a sterile, nonpyrogenic preparation derived by drying a frozen solution of specific venom-neutralizing globulins obtained from the serum of healthy horses immunized against venoms of 4 species of pit vipers. These are *Crotalus atrox* (Western diamondback), *C. adamanteus* (Florida diamondback), *C. durissus terrificus* (South American rattlesnake) and

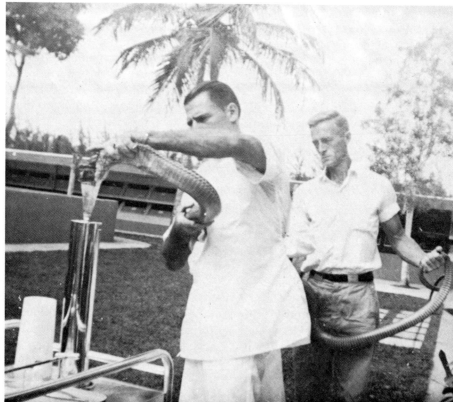

Fig. 13–9. Cobra being "milked" for its venom by Mr. Haast of the Miami Serpentarium. (Photo, courtesy of Hynson, Wescott and Dunning.)

Bothrops atrox (South American fer-de-lance) (Fam. Crotalidae).

This antivenin is standardized by biologic assay on mice in terms of venom neutralization. It should be protected against exposure to excessive heat. The expiration date for antivenin (Crotalidae) polyvalent with a 10% excess of potency is not more than 5 years after date of issue.

USE AND DOSE. Antivenin (Crotalidae) polyvalent is a passive immunizing agent in treating snakebite of the species indicated. Its usual dose, intramuscularly, is 10 ml of reconstituted antivenin; or intravenous infusion, as a 1:10 dilution of antivenin in sodium chloride injection or 5% dextrose injection, after testing for sensitivity to horse serum.

In general, antivenins are prepared in the same manner as antitoxins. The specific venin is injected into horses in gradually increasing doses until the blood titer reaches the desired strength. The animal is then bled, and the blood serum subjected to the required processing. Antivenins have been prepared for use in many parts of the world. In addition to antivenin (Crotalidae) polyvalent, univalent or bivalent antivenins are available to protect against the copperhead *(Agkistrodon)* alone, or combined with the rattlesnake *(Crotalus)* in the United States and with other snakes in other countries, such as the bushmaster and palm vipers of tropical America and the boomslang, cobra, puff adder, and gaboon viper of Africa.

Antivenin *(Micrurus fulvius)* or North American coral snake antivenin is the sterile, nonpyrogenic preparation derived by drying a frozen solution of specific venom-neutralizing globulins obtained from the serum of healthy horses that have been immunized with the venom of *Micrurus fulvius*, the eastern coral snake. This preparation also neutralizes the venom of *M. fulvius tenere* (Texas coral snake), but does not neutralize the venom of *Mic-*

ruroides euryxanthus (Arizona or Sonoran coral snake).

SPIDER-BITE ANTIVENIN

Antivenin *(Latrodectus mactans)* or black widow spider antivenin is prepared from the serum obtained from horses immunized against the venom of black widow spider *(Latrodectus mactans)*. It is available in a lyophilized form and is recommended as a specific treatment of the effects of venom from the bites of this spider. It may be given intramuscularly or intravenously over a 15-minute period when diluted in 10 to 50 ml of saline solution.

ANTISERUMS

Antiserums are biologics prepared in a manner similar to that for antitoxins and antivenins except that bacteria or viruses are used to stimulate the production of specific antibodies in a healthy animal such as the horse. Viral or bacterial cells, as found in vaccines, serve as the antigenic substances; these are introduced into the animal body in gradually increasing doses and are continued until the proper antibody titer of the blood serum is achieved. The destruction of the injected cells by phagocytes liberates antigenic materials with the subsequent development of corresponding antibodies. Antiserum against rabies is an example of this type of immunizing agent.

The therapeutic effectiveness of antiserums is based on their production of artificial passive immunity. Thus, each antiserum is a specific biologic employed to provide a supply of ready-made antibodies to combat the disease. Antiserum against rabies is useful in modern therapy, but many antiserums against bacteria that were formerly employed in therapy have been replaced by antibiotics.

ANTIRABIES SERUM

Antirabies serum is a sterile, non-pyrogenic solution containing antiviral substances obtained from the blood serum or plasma of a healthy horse that has been immunized against rabies by means of vaccine.

In 1953, a new concept in the immunization treatment of rabies was introduced consisting of the administration of antirabies serum in conjunction with rabies vaccine. Evidence that this method of treatment was superior to that of vaccine alone gradually was accumulated. At the present time, rabies immune globulin is preferred for this combined therapy; however, if it is not available, antirabies serum can be used after testing for sensitivity to horse serum.

Use and Dose. Injection of antirabies serum provides the patient with immediate protection against rabies. The biologic should bear an expiration date not later than 2 years after the date of manufacture. It is available in containers of 1000 units. The usual single dose is, intramuscularly, not less than 1000 units per 40 pounds of body weight. Part of the serum dose should be infiltrated into the tissue around the wound whenever feasible.

IMMUNE GLOBULINS

Immune globulins are immunizing biologics that contain specific antibodies derived from the blood of humans who have survived an attack of a specific disease or who have been immunized in some other manner. Chances of sensitization are less with human serum derivatives than with immune serums from animal sources.

Immune globulins may be obtained from the plasma or serum pool of a large number of random donors or from a limited number of individuals who have been hyperimmunized against a specific antigenic material. Preparations derived from a large, random source contain a general spectrum of antibodies and may be used for many diverse purposes. Standardization of the globulin fractions for specific antibodies provides specialty preparations of specific utility. Preparations such as mumps immune globulin, pertussis immune globulin, and tetanus immune globulin, which are obtained from hyperimmunized sources, contain high titers of specific antibodies and are intended for specific use.

This type of preparation should be stored at a temperature between 2 and 8°C. The expiration date is usually not more than 3 years after the date of issue. Serum globulins offer immediate protection (artificial passive immunity) and are administered intramuscularly.

IMMUNE GLOBULIN

Immune globulin, immune serum globulin (human), or gamma globulin is a sterile, nonpyrogenic solution of globulins and contains many antibodies normally present in adult human blood. Each lot of immune globulin is prepared by pooling approximately equal amounts of material (source blood, plasma, serum, or placentas) from at least 1000 individuals.

Immune globulin that has been standardized for measles (rubeola) antibody and/or poliomyelitis antibody is available. These specialty preparations can be used for prophylaxis of the corresponding infections. Immune globulin also has some prophylactic value in chicken pox, infectious hepatitis, rubella, and other diseases. In many instances, serum globulin offers no benefit after onset of disease symptoms. However, measles can be modified by using this preparation.

Use and Dose. Immune globulin is a passive immunizing agent. The dosage is based on body weight and varies with the intended use. The usual intramuscular dose is 0.25 ml per kg for measles prophylaxis, 0.05 ml per kg for measles modification, and 0.02 to 0.04 ml per kg for prophylaxis against infectious hepatitis. It is also given to treat gamma globulin deficiency for the prevention of recurrent infections. It is injected intramuscularly once a month in a dose of 20 to 40 ml for children and 30 to 50 ml for adults.

PRESCRIPTION PRODUCTS. Gamastan®, Gammagee®, Immu-G®, Immuglobin®, Gammar®.

MUMPS IMMUNE GLOBULIN

Mumps immune globulin is a sterile solution of the globulins derived from the blood of healthy adult human donors who have been previously hyperimmunized with mumps virus vaccine. This immune globulin is used for prevention and treatment of mumps in adults and children.

USE AND DOSE. Mumps immune globulin is a passive immunizing agent. The intramuscular prophylactic dose varies with body weight and is usually 1.5 ml for weights up to 40 kg, 3 ml between 40 and 64 kg, and 4.5 ml over 64 kg. Larger doses, which may be repeated at 24- to 48-hour intervals, are used in treatment of the disease.

PRESCRIPTION PRODUCT. Hyparotin®.

PERTUSSIS IMMUNE GLOBULIN

Pertussis immune globulin or pertussis immune globulin (human) is a sterile, nonpyrogenic solution of globulins derived from the blood plasma of adult human donors who have previously been immunized with pertussis vaccine.

USE AND DOSE. Pertussis immune globulin is used in the prophylaxis and treatment of pertussis. The usual intramuscular prophylactic dose is 1.25 to 2.5 ml, repeated in 1 or 2 weeks as necessary. The

therapeutic dose range is the same, but administration is repeated in 1 or 2 days as necessary.

PRESCRIPTION PRODUCT. Hypertussis®.

TETANUS IMMUNE GLOBULIN

Tetanus immune globulin or tetanus immune globulin (human) is a sterile, nonpyrogenic solution of globulins derived from the blood plasma of adult human donors who have been immunized with tetanus toxoid.

This immune globulin is especially useful for passive immunization against tetanus in individuals with wounds that may have been contaminated with tetanus microorganisms. It is intended particularly for persons who have not previously received tetanus toxoid for active immunization. Because it is derived from humans, tetanus immune globulin is much safer than tetanus antitoxin, which is also available (see page 417).

USE AND DOSE. Tetanus immune globulin is employed in the prophylaxis and treatment of tetanus. The usual intramuscular prophylactic dose is 250 units as a single injection. The therapeutic dose range is 3000 to 6000 units.

PRESCRIPTION PRODUCTS. Homo-Tet®, Hu-Tet®, Hyper-Tet®, Immu-Tetanus®, T-I-Gammagee®, Ar-Tet®.

RABIES IMMUNE GLOBULIN

Rabies immune globulin is a sterile, nonpyrogenic solution of antirabies gamma globulin concentrated by cold alcohol fractionation from plasma of donors hyperimmunized with rabies vaccine.

Rabies immune globulin is indicated for passive protection against rabies in persons suspected of exposure to rabies, particularly in cases of severe exposure. Its use is the same as antirabies serum (see page 420); however, because it is of human origin, it possesses the added advantage of removing the risk of serum sickness.

USE AND DOSE. It is recommended that rabies immune globulin be used in combination with rabies vaccine as the best postexposure prophylaxis. The usual dose is a single administration of 0.133 ml per kg of body weight at the time of the first vaccine dose. Up to half the dose should be used to infiltrate the wound and the rest administered intramuscularly.

PRESCRIPTION PRODUCT. Hyperab®.

HEPATITIS B IMMUNE GLOBULIN

Hepatitis B immune globulin is a sterile, nonpyrogenic solution of immunoglobulin prepared from pooled plasma obtained from donors with high titers of antibody to hepatitis B surface (HBs) antigen. Administration is indicated for postexposure prophylaxis following accidental exposure to hepatitis B surface antigen. The exposure can be either parenteral, through direct mucous membrane contact, or through oral ingestion. The materials most often involved are blood, plasma, or serum that is positive for HBs antigen.

Injections should be given intramuscularly not later than 7 days after exposure, and the recommended dose is 0.06 ml per kg of body weight, repeated 25 to 30 days after the first dose.

PRESCRIPTION PRODUCT. H-BIG®.

RH$_0$ (D) IMMUNE GLOBULIN

Rh$_0$ (D) immune globulin is a sterile, nonpyrogenic concentrated solution of globulins derived from human blood plasma containing antibody to the erythrocyte factor Rh$_0$ (D). This antibody neutralizes the antigen in Rh-positive blood, which sensitizes Rh-negative women and results in Rh hemolytic disease of the newborn in subsequent pregnancies.

This preparation is recommended for administration to unsensitized Rh-negative women who give birth to Rh$_0$ (D)- or D^u-positive infants. It should be administered within 72 hours of delivery, and the usual dose is the entire content of 1 vial (containing 300 μg of antibody), intramuscularly. The antibody neutralizes any antigen introduced into the mother as a result of mixing of fetal and maternal blood during childbirth and thus prevents sensitization.

PRESCRIPTION PRODUCTS. Gamulin Rh®, HypRho-D®, RhoGAM®, D-Imune®.

BIOLOGICS RELATED TO HUMAN BLOOD

A number of human blood products that have no immunizing property or function are considered as biologics. These products include whole blood, red blood cells, and various blood fractions. Such blood derivatives as various antihemophilic preparations have specialized application. Albumin human and plasma protein fraction serve as blood-volume supporters, and the radio-iodinated serum albumins are diagnostic aids. Fibrinolysin, which is obtained from human blood plasma, is used for its enzymatic action (see page 293). Recent years have been characterized by an increasing sophistication in the availability and use of blood products, and further developments, such as the common use of granulocyte and platelet fractions for granulocytopenia and thrombocytopenia, may be forthcoming.

A blood-related biologic from nonhuman sources is thrombin.

WHOLE BLOOD

Whole blood or whole blood (human) is blood that has been drawn from a selected donor under rigid aseptic conditions. It contains citrate ion or heparin as an anticoagulant. It should be stored at a constant temperature between 1 and 6° C. The expiration date is 21 days after the date of bleeding if the anticoagulant is citrate dextrose solution or citrate phosphate dextrose solution, 35 days if the anticoagulant is citrate phosphate dextrose adenine solution, and 48 hours if the anticoagulant is heparin. It is used as a blood replenisher. It is administered intravenously, usually in a volume of 1 unit or 500 ml, as necessary.

RED BLOOD CELLS

Red blood cells is whole blood from which plasma has been removed. Red blood cells may be prepared at any time during the dating period of the whole blood from which it is derived by centrifugation or undisturbed sedimentation. It contains a portion of the plasma sufficient to insure optimal cell preservation or contains a cryophylactic substance if it is used for extended manufacturers' storage at $-65°$ C or colder. The expiration date for unfrozen red blood cells is not later than that of the whole human blood from which it was derived. The expiration date for frozen red blood cells, stored at $-65°$ C or colder, is not later than 3 years after the date of collection of the source blood. This preparation is used as a blood replenisher. It is particularly useful in cases of anemia when the additional volume of plasma is undesirable. The usual dose is the equivalent of 1 unit of whole blood.

ANTIHEMOPHILIC DERIVATIVES

Concentrates of the antihemophilic factors in human plasma are available for control of 2 types of hemophilia. Details in the preparation of the various available products differ, but basically, human plasma is fractionated to eliminate many proteins that lack antihemophilic properties. The products are available in a lyophilized form and are standardized for antihemophilic activity. They are administered intravenously and offer the advantage of reducing the volume of fluid that must be injected.

Antihemophilic factor is a sterile, freeze-dried concentrate of human antihemophilic factor (prepared from the factor VIII-rich cryoprotein fraction of human venous plasma) for use in the therapy of hemophilia A (classic hemophilia) by accelerating the abnormally slow clotting time. Factor VIII is needed for the transformation of prothrombin to thrombin by the intrinsic pathway.

It should be stored at a temperature between 2 and 8° C, and the expiration date is not later than 1 or 2 years from the date of manufacture or date of issue.

Dose. Intravenous, 10 to 20 units per kg of body weight, 1 or 2 times a day, or as necessary to maintain a proper blood level of Factor VIII.

Prescription Products. Factorate®, Hemofil®, Humafac®, Koate®, Profilate®.

Antihemophilic factor IX complex is a dried plasma fraction comprising coagulation factors IX (plasma thromboplastin component), II (prothrombin), VII (proconvertin), and X (Stuart-Prower factor). This preparation is indicated to prevent a dangerous bleeding episode or to perform surgery whenever one or more of these specific coagulation factors is absent in the blood of a patient.

Dose. The dose depends on the patient and the circumstances.

Prescription Products. Konyne®, Proplex®.

ALBUMIN HUMAN

Albumin human or normal serum albumin (human) is a sterile, nonpyrogenic preparation of serum albumin obtained by fractionating material (source blood, plasma, serum, or placentas) from healthy, human donors. This material is then tested for the absence of hepatitis B surface antigen. Not less than 96% of its total protein is albumin. It is a solution containing in each 100 ml, 25 g of serum albumin osmotically equivalent to 500 ml, or 5 g equivalent to 100 ml, of normal human plasma.

Albumin human is a blood-volume supporter. The usual dose, intravenously, is a volume equivalent to 25 g of albumin.

PRESCRIPTION PRODUCTS. Albumisol®, Albuspan®, Pro-Bumin®, Albutein®, Buminate®, Albuminar®.

PLASMA PROTEIN FRACTION

Plasma protein fraction or plasma protein fraction (human) is a sterile solution of selected proteins derived by fractionating material (source blood, plasma, or serum) from healthy human donors and testing for the absence of hepatitis B surface antigen. It contains not less than 4.5 g and not more than 5.5 g of protein per 100 ml, of which not less than 83% is albumin, and not more than 17% is alpha and beta globulins. This substance is a human blood fraction that is indicated for restoration of blood volume when the patient is in a state of shock caused by burns, crushing injuries, and any other causes where loss of plasma fluids, not loss of red blood cells, is predominant.

USE AND DOSE. Plasma protein fraction is a blood-volume supporter. The usual dose is 250 to 500 ml by intravenous infusion at a rate not exceeding 10 ml per minute.

PRESCRIPTION PRODUCTS. Plasmanate®, Protenate®, Plasma-Plex®, Plasmatein®.

RADIO-IODINATED SERUM ALBUMINS

Preparations are available containing human serum albumin that has been iodinated using mild conditions with either ^{125}I or ^{131}I. The iodination is controlled to introduce not more than 1 gram-atom of iodine for each gram-molecule (60,000 g) of albumin.

Preparations of iodinated albumin are sterile, buffered, isotonic solutions prepared to contain not less than 10 mg of radio-iodinated normal human albumin per ml, and adjusted to provide not more than 1 millicurie of radioactivity per ml. These solutions must be labeled to indicate the radioactivity, expressed in microcuries or millicuries per ml, at a specified time.

Iodinated ^{125}I albumin injection and iodinated ^{131}I albumin injection are diagnostic aids for determining blood volume and cardiac output. The usual dose is 5 microcuries intravenously. Correction for radioactive decay must be made in dosage calculations. The radioactive half-life of ^{125}I is 60 days, and the half-life of ^{131}I is 8.08 days. The expiration date for preparations of radio-iodinated serum albumin is 120 days after completion of iodination if ^{125}I is used and 30 days if ^{131}I is used. A preparation of **iodinated ^{131}I aggregated injection** is also used as a diagnostic aid for determination of pulmonary clearance.

THROMBIN

Thrombin is a sterile protein substance prepared from prothrombin of bovine origin through interaction with added thromboplastin in the presence of calcium. It can, without the addition of other substances, cause the clotting of whole blood, plasma, or a solution of fibrinogen. Its activity is expressed in units on the basis of clotting a standard fibrinogen solution. Thrombin is available as a lyophilized solid and has an expiration date of not more than 3 years after the date of issue. Solutions should be used within a few hours after preparation.

Thrombin is a local hemostatic. It is used to control blood oozing from capillaries and small venules when the area is accessible. It is useful in dental surgery, laryngeal and nasal surgery, plastic surgery, and skin grafting procedures. It may be applied as a powder or as a solution containing 100 to 2000 NIH units per ml in sodium chloride irrigations or sterile water for injection.

READING REFERENCES

Arnold, R. E.: *What to Do About Bites and Stings of Venomous Animals*, New York, Macmillan Publishing Co., Inc., 1973.

Barrett, J. T.: *Textbook of Immunology*, 3rd ed., St. Louis, C. V. Mosby Co., 1978.

Bellanti, J. A.: *Immunology II*, Philadelphia, W. B. Saunders Co., 1978.

Benacerraf, B., and Unanue, E. R.: *Textbook of Immunology*, Baltimore, Williams & Wilkins Co., 1979.

Bücherl, W., Buckley, E. E., and Deulofeu, V., eds.: *Venomous Animals and Their Venoms*, Vol. I, New York, Academic Press Inc., 1968.

Bücherl, W., and Buckley, E. E., eds.: *Venomous Animals and Their Venoms*, Vols. II and III, New York, Academic Press, Inc., 1971.

Caras, R. A.: *Venomous Animals of the World*, Englewood Cliffs, New Jersey, Prentice-Hall, Inc., 1974.

Fenner, F. J., and White, D. O.: *Medical Virology*, 2nd ed., New York, Academic Press, Inc., 1976.

Fudenberg, H. H., Stites, D. P., Caldwell, J. L., and Wells, J. V., eds.: *Basic and Clinical Immunology*, 2nd ed., Los Altos, California, Lange Medical Publications, 1978.

Golub, E. S.: *The Cellular Basis of the Immune Response*, Sunderland, Massachusetts, Sinauer Associates, Inc., 1977.

Howard, B. D., and Gundersen, C. B., Jr.: Effects and Mechanisms of Polypeptide Neurotoxins that Act Presynaptically, Ann. Rev. Pharmacol., 20:307, 1980.

Joklik, W. K., and Willet, H. P., eds.: *Zinsser Microbiology*, 16th ed., New York, Appleton-Century-Crofts, 1976.

Litman, G. W., and Good, R. A., eds.: *Immunoglobulins*, New York, Plenum Publishing Corp., 1978.

McCollough, N. C., and Gennaro, J. F.: Treatment of Venomous Snakebite in the United States, Clin. Toxicol., 3 (3):483, 1970.

Minton, S. A., Jr.: *Venom Diseases*, Springfield, Illinois, Charles C Thomas, 1974.

Parrish, H. M., and Hayes, R. H.: Hospital Management of Pit Viper Venenations, Clin. Toxicol., 3 (3):501, 1970.

Rose, N. R., Milgrom, F., and Van Oss, C. J., eds.: *Principles of Immunology*, 2nd ed., New York, Macmillan Publishing Co., Inc., 1979.

Sela, M., ed.: *The Antigens*, Vols. I–V, New York, Academic Press, Inc., 1973–1979.

Tu, A. T.: *Venoms: Chemistry and Molecular Biology*, New York, John Wiley & Sons, Inc., 1977.

Turk, J. L.: *Immunology in Clinical Medicine*, 3rd ed., New York, Appleton-Century-Crofts, 1978.

Waldman, R. H., ed.: *Clinical Concepts of Immunology*, Baltimore, Williams & Wilkins Co., 1979.

Chapter 14

Allergens and Allergenic Preparations

Allergy has been a medical specialty for more than 50 years, although symptoms of allergic diseases have been recognized for centuries. Probably the first reference to allergic diseases was found in the Papyrus Ebers in which asthma and diseases owing to "autointoxication" were mentioned. The writings of Hippocrates record at least 12 instances of asthma; the first case of hayfever symptoms was recorded by Herodotus. The term **allergy** was first defined in 1906 by von Pirquet in describing a changed or altered reaction in the body. When an individual develops an unusual response to a substance or condition that is harmless to others, the individual is said to be **allergic.** According to published figures, approximately half the population of the United States suffers from some sort of allergic syndrome; however, it is estimated that only one person in 10 develops symptoms sufficiently severe to require the services of an allergist or a physician who specializes in allergic diseases (Fig. 14–1).

The exact cause of allergy is still undetermined, and much investigative research is devoted to this fascinating subject. The reasons why certain individuals exhibit an allergic response to ragweed pollen and others do not are not understood. Based on genetic studies, medical and immunologic investigators generally agree that the tendency to be allergic is hereditary (Fig. 14–2). However, at the present time, it is impossible to predict whether a newborn infant will be allergic or not. Perhaps future research into the pathophysiology of allergy will reveal the answers.

Allergens are antigenic substances capable of sensitizing the body in such a way that unusual responses occur in hypersensitive individuals. Almost any substance, whether of biologic, chemical, or synthetic origin, may prove to be **allergenic.** In addition, numerous other factors are allergy-producing, such as emotional factors, atmospheric factors, psychosomatic factors, and chronic types of infection. However, because most allergens are composed of

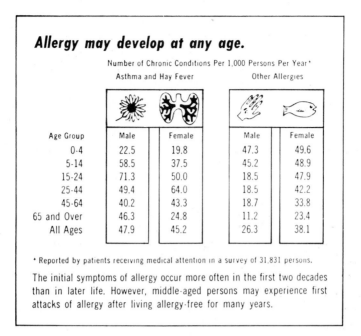

Fig. 14–1. Chart showing comparison of incidence of allergic response in males and females. (Courtesy of Burroughs Wellcome & Co., Inc.)

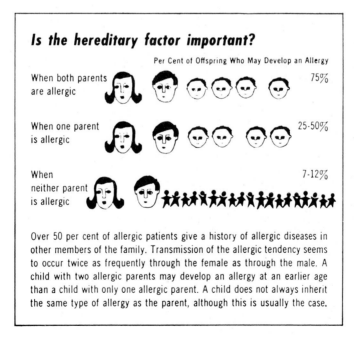

Fig. 14–2. Chart showing probability figures for inheriting a tendency toward allergy. (Courtesy of Burroughs Wellcome & Co., Inc.)

plant or animal matter, they merit consideration in a treatise on natural products.

The allergen concerned with the patient's symptoms must be **antigenic;** that is, it must be capable of eliciting an antibody response. The antigenic fraction of ragweed pollen, for example, causes a susceptible person's body to produce special protein molecules **(antibodies),** some of which circulate in the blood (**circulating** antibodies) and others which become attached to the cells of the nasal membranes (**fixed** antibodies). These particular antibodies have a special affinity for the chemical components of ragweed pollen and of related pollens in the ragweed family, but they cannot combine with the antigenic molecules in unrelated pollens, in foods, or in other allergenic substances. Thus, antibodies are considered **specific,** and, because allergenic substances do produce specific antibodies, each type of allergy is constitutionally different from other types.

When the body is first subjected to the allergen (antigen), the condition is referred to as the **primary exposure.** Because no antibodies have been formed previously, no symptoms of the allergy are produced during the primary exposure. However, during the subsequent exposures, the allergen contacts the fixed antibodies and an **antigen-antibody reaction** occurs.

Predisposing factors that may make some persons susceptible to allergy are: (1) hereditary tendency to allergic response, (2) dysfunction of the endocrine glands, (3) increased excitability of sympathetic and parasympathetic nervous systems, (4) absorption of toxic metabolic and catabolic substances, (5) hepatic dysfunction, and (6) psychic influences.

The antigen-antibody reaction causes a liberation of **histamine** and other mediators of allergic symptoms, including **leukotriene C** or **SRS** (slow-reacting substance) and **bradykinin** (from the cells of certain tissues and organs referred to as the

shock tissues or **shock organs**). If the state of shock is confined to the area of the introduction of the allergen, the condition is a localized reaction; if its effects extend beyond this area, it may be a generalized or constitutional reaction. The constitutional reactions produced in some patients by injections of penicillin preparations are extremely uncomfortable and sometimes dangerous—even fatal.

The types of symptoms depend on the shock organ affected by the particular allergen and its path of entry into the body. Substances that are distributed in the atmosphere and contact the nasal or buccal mucosa during respiration are **inhalant** allergens; those that occur in foodstuffs and are swallowed are **ingestants;** those that may be present in solutions intended for parenteral administration are **injectants;** and those that come into direct contact with the epithelium are **contactants.**

Still other types are represented by the metabolic wastes and growth products of pathogenic microorganisms **(infectants)** and of parasitic microorganisms in or on the body **(infestants).** In addition to these material allergens, allergies may be caused by heat or cold (physical allergy), changes in climate (environmental allergy), anger or frustration (psychosomatic allergy), and others.

In an attempt to discover the causative factors of a patient's symptoms, the allergist records a complete case history including a review of possible allergies shown by other members of the patient's family. The type of symptoms, whether gastrointestinal, bronchial, or epidermal, whether localized or general, whether seasonal or perennial, afford a starting point for the allergist's diagnosis.

INHALANT ALLERGENS

If the symptoms are restricted to the nasal mucosa and are manifested by sneezing, lacrimation, itching, and swelling of nose and eyes, an inhalant allergen is usually indicated. (However, certain food allergens also cause such symptoms.) The condition is known as **sinusitis** or **hayfever.** The term "hayfever" was originated by John Bostock in England over a century ago because he believed that the odor emanating from new-mown hay was responsible for the "fever" or stuffiness of the nasal passages. Occurrence of the symptoms during certain months of the year indicates **seasonal** hayfever. Because this condition is usually associated with the release of pollen grains from certain plants, the term **pollinosis** is often used. **Nonseasonal** hayfever, more commonly called **perennial rhinitis,** may be caused by inhalants other than pollens: mold spores, dust, animal epidermis or dander, feathers, cotton linters, volatile oils, and countless other factors.

In the case of seasonal hayfever, determination of the exact dates within which symptoms occur frequently gives a clue to the type of pollen grains responsible for the allergy. In all but the extreme southern and southwestern states, 3 well-defined pollen seasons exist: (1) the tree season in spring, extending from February until June; (2) the grass season in late spring and early summer, principally from April until August; and (3) the ragweed season in late summer and early fall, beginning the first week in August and continuing until mid-October. Variations in the pollinating periods of these plants are directly related to geographic locations, severity of winters, and similar factors. Published sources are available that divide the United States into different regions. Additional authentic information is distributed by the American College of Allergists, the American Academy of Allergy, and the Allergy Foundation of America.

Because of their heterogeneous nature, pollen grains can be distinguished and identified without difficulty. Pollen grains may be round, oval, angular, square, rectangular, or otherwise shaped, depending on whether the grains are contracted or fully expanded. Most pollen grains are single entities, but some may be 2-compound, 3-compound, tetrads, and so forth. They may either have no **germinal apertures** as such (acolpate), have many pores (multicolpate), or range between (dicolpate, tricolpate, tetracolpate). The outer wall is known as the **exine** and the inner wall as the **intine.** The surface appearance of the exine is characteristic and is a determining factor in identification; it may range from smooth (psilate) to spiny (echinate) with various intervening gradations (reticulate, granulate, lophate).

Atmospheric pollens are liberated chiefly by **anemophilous** (wind-pollinated) plants and are usually small (15 to 45 μ in diameter), light, nonadhesive, and relatively smooth (Fig. 14–3). Trees (oak, walnut), grasses (Bermuda grass and timothy), and weeds (ragweed, plantain) are examples of plants having anemophilous flowers. In contrast, pollens of **entomophilous** (insect-pollinated) plants are usually larger (up to 200 μ in diameter), heavier, adhesive, and may be somewhat spiny. Plants with scented, colored flowers (clover, hollyhock, honeysuckle, rose) are entomophilous. Wind-pollinated flowers are rarely colored and are generally not fragrant because they do not need to attract insects for the pollination process.

Nonseasonal hayfever, as the name indicates, cannot be related to a seasonal trend. The allergic symptoms may be manifested throughout the entire year or perhaps at several periods during the year but with no regularity. Often inhalant allergens may occur in the home, at the place of employment, or in some particular locale frequented by the patient. In the home, cotton pillowcases, sheets, and blankets usually shed "linters" or fragments of cotton

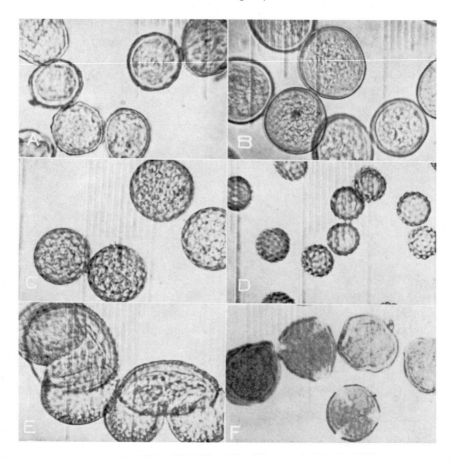

Fig. 14–3. Photomicrographs of pollen grains. *A*, American elm; *B*, orchard grass; *C*, lamb's quarters; *D*, giant ragweed; *E*, pine; *F*, white oak. All magnified to same scale: each space on micrometer scale equals 3.2 microns.

fibers that are light enough to float in the air. The pillows, if made of feathers, may be a source of the allergen, particularly if the pillows are old and the feathers are disintegrating. If a person has a sensitivity to feathers, he should use a foam rubber pillow or should cover the feather pillow with a plastic dust-free cover. Sometimes a pet canary or parakeet may cause a feather sensitivity.

Odors and perfumes are a major factor in nonseasonal allergy. The increased desire for unusual scents in toiletries and cosmetics has led manufacturers to use volatile oils from many new plant sources as ingredients in their formulations. For example, sandalwood oil is an ingredient in some men's toiletries; however, photoallergy to sandalwood oil has been reported in the medical literature. Many other volatile oils are allergenic. Removal of the allergens by substituting nonscented cosmetics brings relief (see page 433).

Animal epidermis or **animal dander** (epithelial scales) is a frequent source of allergenic matter. Cats, dogs, guinea pigs, and other pets are occasionally responsible for a patient's cough, wheeze, or asthmatic attack. Treatment with dander extracts does not always result in a significant number of improved cases, and the therapy of choice is avoidance of exposure. Sometimes patients are affected by the odors of the animals rather than by the dander. Any type of furniture stuffed with horsehair or other animal material should also be investigated as a cause of nonseasonal hayfever.

The allergen present in castor beans is often the cause of severe allergic reactions. The allergen is not removed with the oil when the seeds are expressed, but it does cause difficulty in the processing plant. Because this allergen is air-borne and wind-borne, persons living in the vicinity of industrial factories that make or use castor bean pomace may exhibit allergic reactions.

Much of the nonseasonal hayfever is thought to be caused by fungous spores, especially of such molds as *Alternaria* (Fig. 14–11). *Helminthosporium, Hormodendrum (Cladosporium)*, and *Aspergillus*. Mold spores are almost constantly present in the atmosphere, even during winter, and have been traced as the contributing factors to many cases of perennial rhinitis. *Aspergillus, Penicillium,* and other molds abound in moist places and occur in cellars and in damp cupboards.

Persons allergic to mold spores are usually allergic to dust as well. Dust is almost indefinable because it differs from one place to the next, but it probably is composed of mold spores, cotton linters, animal danders, sizing from rugs and carpets, and innumerable other allergenic particles. Various types of mites have also proved to be a major allergen in house dust, particularly the acarine mite, *Dermatophagoides*, and specifically its species, *D. pteronyssinus*.

Several years ago, the Allergy Research Laboratory of Northwestern University reported that nearly 30% of patients with symptoms of asthma or hayfever are sensitive to disintegrating bits of insect dust inhaled from air and soil; thus, a clinical diagnosis of "sensitivity to dust" is inadequate.

INGESTANT ALLERGENS

Food allergens ordinarily cause gastrointestinal symptoms, but they may also cause skin rash, puffed lips and tongue, migraine, rhinitis, or other more serious effects, such as bronchial asthma. Severe cases of eczema of the hands have been caused by allergenic foods. In food allergy, the activity of the allergen is not localized in one organ or area of the body, but is transferred to other organs by the blood. Thus, an **atopic dermatitis,** such as a tomato rash, strawberry rash, or that caused by eating oranges, chocolate, or shellfish, is developed by the patient. No doubt, many persons who exclaim, "Cucumbers don't agree with me!" have discovered the hard way (trial and error) that they have an allergy to certain foods. Such persons may not know that they have an allergy, but they do know that eating certain foods leads to dire consequences.

Some of the most common allergens ingested by children are foods considered essential to proper diet and growth, such as cow's milk, orange juice, cod liver oil, or other vitamin-containing fish liver oils. Colic may sometimes be an allergic manifestation to a food substance, just as dermatitis may indicate a hypersensitivity to other foods. Hundreds of extracts of foodstuffs are commercially available as single or multiple units for use by the allergist as diagnostic skin test materials; however, they have little or no value in therapy. The most satisfactory method of combating food allergies is elimination of the offending substance from the diet.

Milk allergy is a specific immunologic, antigen-antibody response owing partially to a lactalbumin. Because heating or boiling alters this protein, evaporated milk may be used as an effective substitute for cow's milk. Milk allergy may result in severe dermatitis, recurrent rhinorrhea, bronchitis, and asthma. Various commercial milk substitutes that are prepared from soybean isolates offer a milk-free formula claimed to be devoid of antigenicity. Two of these soybean products are Soyalac® and Prosobee®.

It has been definitely determined that coffee can produce allergic response. The principal water-extractable allergenic component of green coffee is chlorogenic acid (3-caffeoylquinic acid). Some authorities disagree about the allergenic properties of chlorogenic acid, claiming that the coffee-roasting process alters its structure. Various symptoms of coffee allergy have been reported: severe migraine, gastroenteritis, and widespread hives.

INJECTANT ALLERGENS

Allergic reactions to penicillin injections are well known to most of the lay public. More attention has been called to the allergies following penicillin injections than has been given to all other allergies produced by the injection method. It is estimated that anaphylactic reactions to penicillin occur with a frequency of 1 to 5 per 10,000 patient-courses of penicillin. Once a patient has suffered a penicillin reaction, he is keenly concerned about the next injection he may receive. Skin testing for penicillin allergy is of definite value, but tests must be conducted under controlled conditions.

6-Amino penicillanic acid (6-APA) and 7-aminocephalosporanic acid (7-ACA), as well as the semisynthetic penicillins and cephalosporins, cause positive intracutaneous reactions in most susceptible patients. For this reason, such antibiotics as the cephalosporins and semisynthetic penicillins should be used with caution by physicians treating patients that are sensitive to penicillin G.

In addition to penicillin products, other injectables may cause allergies—liver extract, antitoxins, and the glandular products. The symptoms in each case are similar to those of the antibiotic; itching of the palms of the hands and the soles of the feet, erythema, and peeling of the skin are characteristic.

Because bees, hornets, and wasps actually "sting" instead of "bite," such insects are considered as a source of injectant allergens. Stings of such insects can induce severe local and constitutional reactions, sometimes causing death. In fact, it has been estimated that more people die annually from bee stings and wasp stings than from snakebites. Such patients can be immunized by using injections of antigens because one antigen is common to all bees and wasps (see page 436); however, each species has its own additional distinct antigen(s).

Considerable research is being conducted on this subject at the present time. Immunologic comparisons of the effects of insect venoms, venom sac extracts, and whole insect extracts have been made to determine the optimal method of treatment. Not only are the hymenopterous insects being studied, but many of the "biting" arthropods are the subjects of clinical investigations. Among these forms are spiders, mites, lice, chiggers, ticks, sand flies, stable flies, horse flies, scorpions, centipedes, and numerous others indigenous to the geographic area of the investigators.

CONTACTANT ALLERGENS

Many substances and products have been recognized as the cause of contact allergies. One of the most important of these is the well-known poison ivy, *Toxicodendron radicans* (L.) Kuntze. Other allergenic species of the genus *Tox-icodendron* (formerly *Rhus*) include *T. diversilobum* (T. & G.) Greene (known as western poison oak), *T. quercifolium* (Michx.) Greene (known as eastern poison oak), and *T. vernix* (L.) Kuntze (known as poison sumac, poison elder, or poison dogwood). All of these contain the same nonvolatile, phenolic principle, **urushiol,** and all produce allergic symptoms in hypersensitive individuals. Watery blisters associated with pruritus are indicative of this affliction which can become quite distressing if not properly treated. The blisters break open, and the exuding fluid forms new blisters that spread quite rapidly.

Other plant excitants of contact dermatitis are: asparagus, buckwheat, buttercups, catalpa leaves, chrysanthemums, daffodils, English ivy, ginkgo leaves, lobelia, marigolds, mayapple, osage orange, flowering spurge, snow-on-the-mountain, smartweeds, and dozens of others. Occasional contact dermatitis has been caused by **aeroallergens,** such as the various pollen grains that contain oils, hairs from different kinds of leaves and flowers, and even small fragments of plant tissue carried by smoke emanating from brush fires, grass fires, and burning leaves. A number of cosmetic manufacturing companies have removed certain known irritants and allergens from their beauty products and consequently use the term **hypoallergenic cosmetics** to denote this fact. Products bearing the brand names of Ar-Ex, Allercreme, Almay, and Marcelle are examples of hypoallergenic cosmetics. Orris root, an ingredient in "violet" talcum powders, is a chief contact allergen. Dibromofluorescein, commonly used in indelible lipsticks, is another. Because perfumes can be allergenic, many hypoallergenic products are unscented; in others, the perfuming agents are carefully screened to eliminate possible allergens.

Frequently, individuals cannot tolerate wool in clothing, blanklets, or even in the form of wool fat (lanolin) in cosmetics. Soaps and soap powders, plain detergents and enzyme detergents, nail polishes and nail polish removers, and hair dyes and hair sprays are listed among the numerous major causes of contact dermatitis.

INFECTANT ALLERGENS

Numerous living organisms may cause allergy through the products they release during their metabolism in the human body. Some individuals harbor certain types of bacteria, protozoans, molds, helminths, and other parasitic forms which, by their continual presence in the body, are responsible for chronic illness. The patient may or may not be aware of this infection because it may or may not manifest recognizable symptoms. Metabolic products of growth of these organisms may be of such nature that the individual becomes sensitized.

The chronic bacterial infection of the bronchioles, known as bronchiectasis, wherein the constant presence of bacterial wastes may sensitize the allergic individual, is an example. Thus, the person may exhibit allergic symptoms but does not respond positively to skin tests for inhalant allergens. In this case, the bacterial metabolic wastes are considered as infectant allergens.

INFESTANT ALLERGENS

In a manner somewhat similar to the infectants, parasitic organisms may sensitize the human body. Invasions of hookworms, tapeworms, pinworms, threadworms, dermatophytes, and other forms have caused allergic response in susceptible individuals. Growth products and metabolic wastes of these parasites are constantly present in the body and are referred to as infestant allergens.

CASE HISTORY

To determine the circumstances surrounding the patient's allergy, the allergist must record all details regarding the allergic attacks, including data on the type of occupation and the familial background. Information concerning the place, time, and mode of onset of past symptoms, as well as those causing the most recent attack, is recorded in the case history or allergic history of the individual. As stated on a typical case history report, the entries include:

    name and sex
    marital status
    occupation
    chief complaint
    present illness
      age of onset
      date of first attack
      place, time, and mode of onset
      seasonal variation
      duration
      what relieves attacks
    present attack
      date of onset
      place of onset
      mode of onset
      sneezing
      nasal discharge
      wheeze
      cough
      headache
    symptoms affected by
      meals
      drugs
      exertion
      excitement
      weather changes
      wind
      smoke or fumes
      time of day

    mowing lawn
    rain
    working in garden
    automobile rides
    playing golf
    riding horse
    feeding stock
    cleaning house
    change of season
    change of environment
    change of occupation

Other points of information include the types of medication the patient may be taking and the conditions of the home environment (heating system, type of floor covering, presence of household pets, kinds of cosmetics used, nature of bed covers and pillows, and numerous other details). A past medical history may be requested. Allergic symptoms of the paternal and maternal relatives are frequently a clue.

A complete case history includes both a physical and a laboratory examination, the latter to include reports on urine, blood, sputum, and nasal smears. In addition, results of a radiograph and an electrocardiogram are customary. Following or concurrent with the laboratory examination, the allergist makes his diagnosis and attempts to confirm it by the use of skin tests.

SKIN TESTS

Skin tests are conducted in 2 principal ways: (1) by **scratch tests** administered similar to a smallpox vaccination, i.e., scratching the skin and introducing an extract of the allergenic substance (Fig. 14–4); or (2) by **intradermal (intracutaneous) tests** in which a small quantity of the extract is injected between the layers of the skin.

Allergenic extracts are stable preparations of various antigenic substances and are used for diagnosis, preseasonal

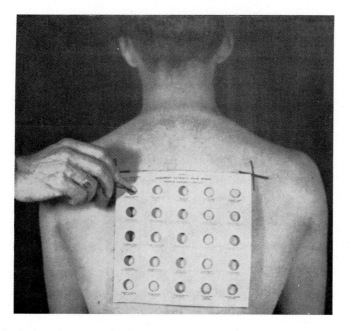

Fig. 14–4. Method of conducting multiple skin tests on patient. (Photo, courtesy of Hugh Graham, Inc., Dallas, Texas.)

prophylaxis, and treatment of allergies (except food allergies).

In each case, the allergenic extract represents a solution of the chief constituents of the tested material. (Preparation of extracts involves the use of one of several standard extracting fluids: Coca's fluid, normal saline solution, purified water, dilute glycero-dextrose solution, and others.) By injecting a small amount, usually 0.1 ml, into the arm of the patient, the allergist can observe the resulting reaction within 20 minutes and classify it using the scheme shown in Table 14–1.

A skin test, then, is actually a localized reaction that determines whether the patient responds to that particular allergen. Although not infallible, skin tests are quite useful in determining sensitivity to inhalants, injectants, contactants, and some ingestants, although the reactions with the ingestants are less reliable than with the other allergens.

Ordinarily, contactants are applied as a

Table 14–1. Clinical Designations of Skin Reactions

Designation	Symbol	Characteristics
Negative	−	No reaction or no different than control
Doubtful	±	No appreciable difference from control other than slight erythema
One-plus	+	Erythema smaller than 20 mm in diameter
Two-plus	+ +	Erythema larger than 20 mm but no wheal
Three-plus	+ + +	Definite wheal with surrounding erythema
Four-plus	+ + + +	Wheal with definite pseudopods and erythema

patch test, where the material is applied directly to the skin which is neither scratched nor penetrated with a needle. As a general rule, patch tests require a much longer time for the reaction to occur—at least 48 hours but sometimes 4 or 5 days. The offending allergen need not be extracted for applications to the skin in this type of test.

Other tests, such as the ophthalmic test, passive transfer (Prausnitz-Küstner) test, and microscopic examination of nasal secretions, may be employed by the physician as occasion demands.

TREATMENT

If the patient has a case history of allergy and exhibits a positive reaction to ragweed pollen extract, the allergist will probably resort to the **hyposensitization** method of treatment. At regular intervals, a measured amount of the greatly diluted extract is injected subcutaneously. The dose is gradually increased until the patient can withstand the inhalation of the normal seasonal atmospheric concentration of ragweed pollens with little ill effect. Complete freedom from symptoms is rarely accomplished because of the inadequacy of the extracting fluids; in addition, because the identity of the allergenic fraction has not been definitely established chemically, it cannot be assayed in the completed extract.

Pollen extracts are made on a weight-volume basis using defatted pollen and are standardized according to the number of pollen units, protein nitrogen units, or total nitrogen units, depending on the laboratory policy. One pollen unit (called a **Noon unit**) represents the activity in 0.001 mg of pollen. The strength of protein extracts is expressed in terms of mg of protein nitrogen per ml; however, some laboratory workers utilize the number of mg of total nitrogen per ml, and others refer to the weight-volume formula used in extracting the allergen. At the present time, no standard is generally recognized although measurement of protein nitrogen is perhaps the most accepted method.

Most of the research on pollens has been concentrated on those of ragweed. More is known about ragweed pollens than about any others, but a great deal must still be learned. Although highly active materials have been extracted from ragweed pollens, the identity and properties of these substances have not been positively determined. By using gel diffusion methods, 6 to 8 different antigens have been demonstrated in ragweed pollens, but it is not definitely known which of these are of greatest significance in human allergy.

Numerous investigators are studying the allergenic fractions of ragweed and other pollens. Much of this research involves the use of more selective extracting fluids, the preparation of alum-precipitated and ammonium sulfate-treated extracts, the application of chromatographic and electrophoretic means of analysis, and a comparison of the effectiveness of repository therapy with effectiveness of the usual hyposensitization method of treatment. Although these studies will undoubtedly result in a more efficient means of treating the individual, some researchers claim that all patients do not react in a similar manner to a specific allergenic extract because of the number of individual allergenic components in the extract.

If the treatment is conducted prior to the time of pollination of the plants, it is termed **preseasonal;** if it is maintained throughout the year for some allergies, it is called **perennial;** if the treatment is instituted during the symptomatic period, it is known as **coseasonal** (the least satisfactory method).

Rapid hyposensitization of certain allergic patients in a single day has proved feasible, safe, and highly effective. The method has proved particularly successful with bee and wasp venom allergies. The patient is given small injections every 20 or 30 minutes for at least several hours; immunity is developed in from 10 to 14 days.

The hyposensitization treatment is particularly useful for counteracting allergies caused by inhalants and some contactants. When food allergies are encountered, the patient is advised to avoid the offending food in his diet—"elimination diet." Similarly, a change in environment often provides relief from inhalant allergies. A substitution of foam rubber pillows for feather pillows frequently ends symptoms that occur on retiring. Because the allergic reaction depends on an antigen-antibody reaction, one can readily see that absence of allergen contact with the tissues of the patient provides satisfactory results.

As previously stated, studies on repository allergens are in progress. For such preparations to be free of ill effects, the antigen must be completely emulsified. A large dose of the antigen, when completely emulsified in an oil and buffered saline solution, is slowly absorbed into the system. One injection may be sufficient for an entire season.

The use of alum-precipitated extracts has also been suggested as a means of therapy. Nondefatted pollen is mixed with pyridine, resulting in extraction of lipid material as well as the water-soluble fraction. Alum is then added, thereby precipitating an antigenic complex. Pyridine and alum are removed by washing, and the precipitate is suspended in buffered saline solution. Alum-precipitated allergenic extracts are administered subcutaneously in the same manner as are aqueous extracts and emulsified extracts.

Several advantages are claimed for alum-precipitated extracts: delayed absorption of allergen permits the administration of fewer yearly injections, and

treatment permits the administration of larger amounts of the allergen per injection with less possibility of systemic allergic reaction; in addition, extracts are available commercially, suitably standardized, and relatively easy to administer. Allpyral® is an example of an alum-precipitated extract.

The allergist may elect to administer antihistaminic drugs orally in addition to using the allergenic extract. Although the antihistamines cannot prevent the antigen-antibody reactions, they do prevent the shock damage normally caused by the release of histamine. The pharmacist should be capable of advising the physicians about the many antihistaminic drugs and should know the chemical nature, the therapeutic advantages and disadvantages, and the generic and trade-marked names of each drug. The pharmacist, as a drug specialist, should be familiar with the products. Moreover, the pharmacist should warn customers about the potential dangers of continued promiscuous use of the antihistamines during self-medication.

PLANTS CAUSING HAYFEVER

To determine whether certain plants liberate air-borne pollens, one must sample the atmospheric content of the area. The gravity (Durham sampler) method of exposing slides, roto-rod, roto-bar sampler, fly-shield rotobar, flag sampler, volumetric impinger, Wells air centrifuge, Erdtman air filter, and many other methods have been devised by investigators in the field of aerobiology.

To ascertain whether certain plants are significant in seasonal pollinosis, a series of postulates was devised by authorities in the field of allergy to serve as definite criteria:

1. The pollen must contain an excitant of hayfever.

2. The pollen must be anemophilous, or wind-borne, as regards its mode of pollination.
3. The pollen must be produced in sufficiently large quantities.
4. The pollen must be sufficiently buoyant to be carried considerable distances.
5. The plant producing the pollen must be widely and abundantly distributed.

The Durham sampler method of determining the pollen count is the gravity method in which a microscope slide is rubbed with a petrolatum mixture (white petrolatum 75%, liquid petrolatum 25%) and is exposed in a standard exposure device (Figs. 14–5 and 14–6) for a 24-hour period. At the end of that time, the slide is examined microscopically by staining with Calberla's solution,* adding a 22-mm square cover glass, and counting the different kinds of pollen grains under the entire cover glass area. The pollen count represents the number of pollen grains per square centimeter of slide surface.

The chief advantages of the various aforementioned air-sampling devices are the ease of determining hour-by-hour pollen counts and the relationship of pollen occurrence to air volume.

Although such counts have little or no value insofar as individual hayfever sufferers are concerned, they are of great importance in national surveys. When a person wishes to change his place of employment, he can easily learn which parts of the country are relatively free from ragweed or other pollens. For instance, a ragweed hayfever victim should know that Portland, Oregon is preferable to St. Louis, Chicago, or Milwaukee because the pollen counts in the latter cities are exceedingly high. Again, a vacation at the eastern seashore or at the western national parks may provide a more comfortable time for a person suffering from ragweed allergy.

The American Academy of Allergy, through its Pollen and Mold Committee, has established a chart for the ragweed index of the principal cities.

In the New England, middle Atlantic, central, plains, and Pacific northwest states, the pollinating seasons of trees, grasses, and weeds are rather clearly defined. For example, in the middle Atlantic states, a seasonal hayfever occurring between February 9 and May 20 is undoubtedly caused by pollens from one or more trees, that between May 30 and July 4 is probably owing to grass pollens or to a few

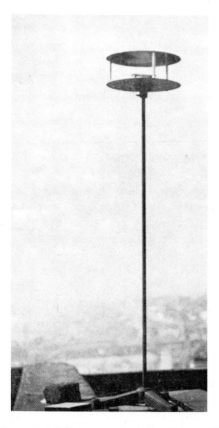

Fig. 14–5. Pollen exposure apparatus in position on roof.

*Calberla's solution: glycerin, 5 ml; alcohol (95%), 10 ml; distilled water, 15 ml; saturated aqueous solution of basic fuchsin, q.s. to a cherry red color.

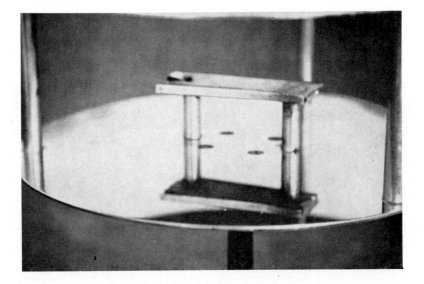

Fig. 14–6.   Enlargement of slide holder with slide in place.

early flowering weeds, and that between August 10 and October 1 is undoubtedly the result of ragweed pollens.

Thus, in most of the United States, 3 pollen seasons may be easily differentiated: (1) the spring, or tree season; (2) the early summer, or grass and early weed season; and (3) the later summer-early fall, or true weed season (often referred to as the ragweed season).

TREES

Although some species may overlap, the spring-flowering trees may be subdivided into those of early spring and those of late spring.

Early Spring Pollinating Trees:

Ulmus americana L.
   (American elm)
Ulmus rubra Muehlenb.
   (slippery elm)
Acer saccharinum L.
   (silver maple)
Acer rubrum L.
   (red maple)

Populus deltoides Marsh.
   (necklace poplar)
Populus tremuloides Michx.
   (quaking aspen)
Populus canadensis Moench.
   (Carolina poplar)
Alnus rugosa (Du Roi) Spreng.
   (speckled alder)
Alnus serrulata (Ait.) Willd.
   (common alder)

Later Spring Pollinating Trees:

Betula papyrifera Marsh.
   (paper birch)
Betula lenta L.
   (sweet birch)
Broussonetia papyrifera (L.) Vent.
   (paper mulberry)
Juglans cinerea L.
   (butternut)
Juglans nigra L.
   (black walnut)
Quercus alba L.
   (white oak)
Quercus rubra L.
   (red oak)

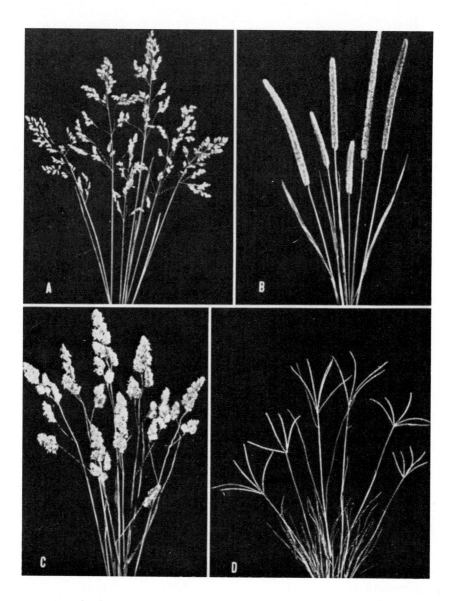

Fig. 14–7.   Common hayfever grasses. *A*, bluegrass or June grass; *B*, timothy; *C*, orchard grass; *D*, Bermuda grass. (Feinberg, *Allergy in Practice*, courtesy of Year Book Publishers, Inc. and O. C. Durham.)

Quercus velutina Lam.
  (black oak)
Platanus occidentalis L.
  (buttonwood)
Platanus acerifolia (Ait.) Willd.
  (London plane)

Significant allergenic pollens are liberated also from trees that may not adhere to these time schedules: the Australian pines, *Casuarina* species, common in Florida; the blue gum trees, *Eucalyptus* species, naturalized in California; the Rocky Mountain juniper, *Juniperus scopulorum* Sarg., occurring throughout the Rocky Mountain range; the mountain cedar, *Juniperus mexicana* Spreng., extending into Texas; the orange, lemon, and related species of citrus; and a number of others. It is interesting to note that although pine trees, *Pinus* species, produce considerable quantities of wind-borne pollen, they are not generally considered to be allergenic.

GRASSES

The most important grasses of the United States that shed allergenic pollens are:

  Cynodon dactylon (L.) Pers.
    (Bermuda grass) (Fig. 14–7)
  Sorghum halepense (L.) Pers.
    (Johnson grass)
  Dactylis glomerata L.
    (orchard grass) (Fig. 14–7)
  Phleum pratense L.
    (timothy) (Fig. 14–7)
  Poa pratensis L.
    (Kentucky bluegrass) (Fig. 14–7)
  Agrostis alba L.
    (redtop)
  Anthoxanthum odoratum L.
    (sweet vernal grass)

In the southern and southwestern states, grasses pollinate throughout the year and no particular season is apparent. It is prob-

able that many other grasses are factors in grass pollinosis.

WEEDS

Among the early flowing weeds, certain members of the Chenopodiaceae, Polygonaceae, Plantaginaceae, Amaranthaceae, and Compositae are responsible for a number of cases of allergy each year. Other members of these families pollinate later in the summer; in fact, depending on geographic location, they may extend into late fall. *Plantago major* L. (common plantain) and *Plantago lanceolata* L. (English plantain) (Fig. 14–8) are causes of widespread early summer weed pollinosis. Pollen grains of the plantains are rather small, averaging appoximately 24 μ, but they are

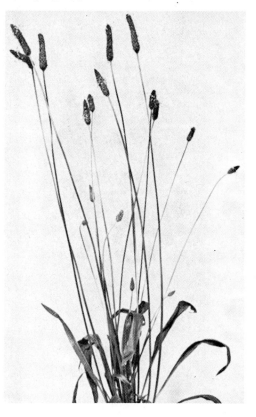

Fig. 14–8. English plantain. (Tuft, *Clinical Allergy*, Lea & Febiger.)

easily identifiable because of the protuber-
ances arising from the exine.

Other important hayfever weeds are:

Rumex crispus L.
  (yellow dock)
Rumex acetosella L.
  (sheep sorrel)
Chenopodium album L.
  (lamb's quarters)
Chenopodium ambrosioides L.
  (Mexican tea)

Amaranthus palmeri Wats.
  (Palmer's amaranth)
Amaranthus retroflexus L.
  (pigweed)
Acnida tamariscina (Nutt.) Wood.
  (western water hemp) (Fig. 14–9)
Salsola kali L. var. tenuifolia Mey.
  (Russian thistle) (Fig. 14–9)
Iva xanthifolia Nutt.
  (marsh elder)
Franseria tomentosa Gray
  (false ragweed)

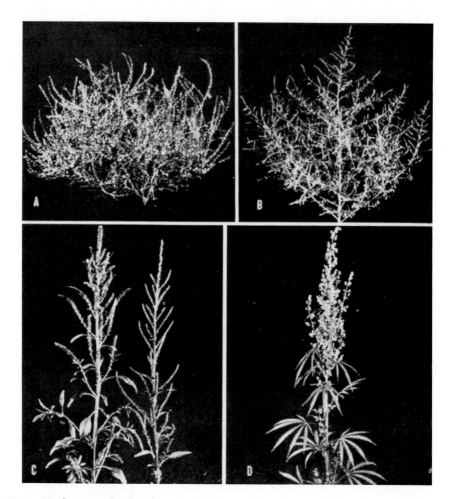

Fig. 14–9. Hayfever weeds of midwestern and western states. A, Russian thistle; B, burning bush or Mexican fireweed; C, western water hemp; D, hemp or marihuana, not related botanically to western water hemp. (Feinberg, *Allergy in Practice*, courtesy of Year Book Publishers, Inc.)

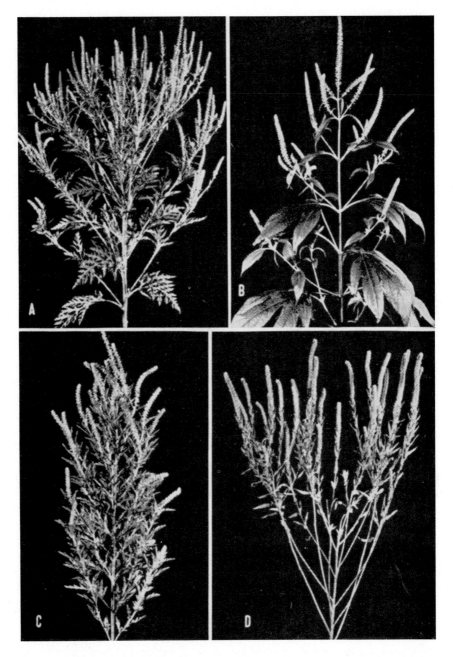

Fig. 14–10. Prominent members of the ragweed family. *A*, short or common; *B*, giant; *C*, western; *D*, southern or lanced-leaved. (Feinberg, *Allergy in Practice*, courtesy of Year Book Publishers, Inc.)

Artemisia ludoviciana Nutt.
(western mugwort)
Artemisia tridentata Nutt.
(sagebrush)
Ambrosia species
(ragweeds) (Fig. 14–10)
Kochia scoparia (L.) Schrad.
(burning bush) (Fig. 14–9)

The genus *Ambrosia* is responsible for about 90% of the pollinosis in the United States. Four species are widespread over the eastern, southern, central, and southwestern states. Only the west coast and the Pacific northwest states have ragweed pollen counts ranging from zero to only a few grains. The 2 species that may be found in greatest abundance are the **giant** or **great ragweed** and the **dwarf** or **common ragweed.** Although these vary considerably in height, leaf structure, and general habit, their pollens are practically indistinguishable. They range in size from 18 to 21 μ, are uniformly rounded, are tricolpate, and have a somewhat spiny exine.

Ambrosia trifida L., the giant ragweed, is a coarse annual that sometimes attains a height of 5 m. The staminate flowers are borne in terminal spikes or racemes at the base of which are the pistillate flowers. The leaves are oppositely arranged and long-petioled and are usually 3-lobed, although occasionally they are 5-lobed or entire-margined. The lower leaves are generally more uniform in appearance than those on the upper stems. Both stems and leaves are rough to the touch because of the stiff hairs.

Ambrosia artemisiifolia L. var. *elatior* (L.). Descourtils, the dwarf ragweed, is sometimes referred to merely as *Ambrosia elatior* L. It is a much-branched annual that occasionally grows 2 m high. It is characterized by its numerous staminate spikes or racemes and by its fernlike leaves which are bipinnatifid. The leaves are extremely variable and sometimes those of the flowering branches are undivided. As a rule, the leaves are alternate, and like the giant ragweed, the plant is hairy. Both of these ragweeds occur chiefly in the northeastern, middle Atlantic, and central states.

In the southern and western plains states, *Ambrosia bidentata* Michx., the southern ragweed, is an important species. It has alternate leaves that are lanceolate, partly clasping, and nearly entire except for a short lobe on each side near the base. In the western and southwestern states, *Ambrosia psilostachya* DC., the western ragweed, is the most abundant species. It is a branched perennial with thick 1-pinnatifid leaves; the plant is rough and hoary with short stiff hairs.

MOLDS CAUSING ALLERGY

Mold allergy is an exceedingly important cause of perennial rhinitis or non-seasonal hayfever. Atmospheric determinations conducted in much the same manner as pollen counts have revealed that the most common mold genera are: *Alternaria* (Fig. 14–11), *Macrosporium, Helminthosporium, Hormodendrum (Cladosporium), Aspergillus, Penicillium, Mucor, Rhizopus, Syncephalastrum, Curvularia, Brachysporium, Pullularia, Pleospora,* and others. Because of the difficulty in distinguishing between the spores, it is helpful to expose Petri dishes containing a mycologic medium specifically designed to encourage the growth of molds and yeasts but to inhibit bacterial colonies. Thus, each colony of the mold that develops is assumed to be the outgrowth of one spore; the vegetative characters of the mycelium and the methods of sporulation are employed to aid in identification of the mold. It is interesting to note that present investigators hold the

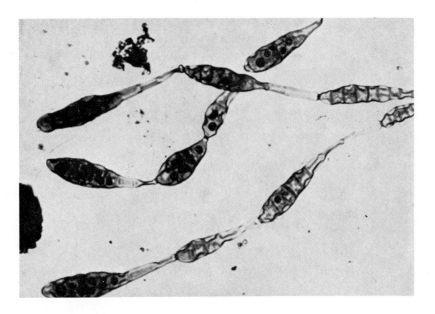

Fig. 14–11. Alternaria spores seen on exposed slide. (Tuft, *Clinical Allergy*, Lea & Febiger.)

imperfect fungi chiefly responsible for mold allergies.

PLANTS CAUSING DERMATITIS

Rhus toxicodendron or poison ivy is composed of the fresh leaflets of *Toxicodendron radicans* (L.) Kuntze, formerly known as *Rhus radicans* L. (Fam. Anacardiaceae), a woody vine common throughout the United States. The plant either trails over the ground, climbs by means of aerial roots, or remains shrublike. The common climbing type is shown in Figure 14–12. The leaves are 3-foliate, and the leaflets are ovate, acuminate, nearly entire, inequilateral, 3 to 20 cm long and have short stalks. They are inodorous and slightly astringent, saline, and acrid in taste. The flowers are green and occur as loose axillary panicles. The fruit is a globular, glabrous, grayish drupe.

A phenolic oily resin named **toxicodendrol** is present in all of the poisonous *Tox-icodendron* species and contains a complex active principle that is known as **urushiol.** One of the components of urushiol is **3-pentadecylcatechol.** Toxicodendrol is not volatile and is soluble in alcohol and in oils. It is nonnitrogenous, has phenolic groups, gives a blue-green reaction with iron, and absorbs bromine readily. It is precipitated by lead acetate solution and is gradually oxidized by exposure to air, losing its activity.

Toxicodendrol and urushiol occur in the sticky sap of the plant, which exudes when the plant is injured. It causes dermatitis on penetration of the epidermis of the skin. It may be conveyed by the hands or clothing from one person to another. Toxicodendrol can be transmitted readily from place to place by many different carriers, both animate and inanimate. Shoes, gloves, and clothing can retain the toxicity of urushiol for months. Dogs, cats, and farm animals frequently become contaminated, and their hairs may be the source of human

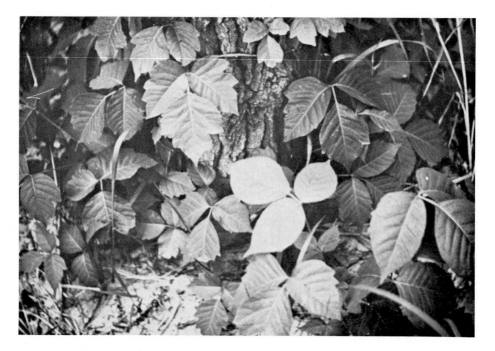

Fig. 14–12. Variation in the leaflets of poison ivy *(Toxicodendron radicans)*. The lobed leaflets are sometimes called poison oak.

contamination. Smoke from brush fires may carry leaf particles; such particles can produce cases of ivy poisoning when they contact the human skin.

Toxicodendrol is not infective and apparently does not enter the blood. Minute quantities (0.001 mg) on the epidermis can cause dermatitis.

***Toxicodendron vernix* (L.) Kuntze,** commonly known as **Poison Sumac, Poison Elder, or Poison Dogwood,** is allergenic, like *Toxicodendron radicans,* and contains the same principles. It is a shrub or small tree, found in swamps in the United States and Canada (Fig. 15–6). The leaves are 7- to 13-foliate, with obovate or oval, acuminate, entire leaflets; the flowers are small, green, and in axillary panicles; the fruit resembles that of poison ivy.

Other species of *Toxicodendron* are also poisonous, as the **western poison oak** *(T. diversilobum)* of the Pacific coast, and the **Japanese lacquer** or varnish tree *(T. verniciferum)*. The lacquer trees grow wild in both China and Japan, where they are also cultivated. The specific name *vernix* means "varnish." The lac is obtained by incising and removing the bark with a pointed spatula. The grayish white emulsion, which contains toxicodendrol, is strained and, when exposed to air, changes to brown and finally becomes black. This change is owing to the oxidizing enzyme, laccase.

In a series of tests on thousands of student volunteers, injections of 3-pentadecylcatechol (one of the constituents of urushiol) reduced sensitivity to poison ivy dermatitis and created immunity in some cases. The compound is a standard allergen used in patch tests to determine sensitivity to the poison ivy plant.

One of the products developed for the prevention and treatment of poison ivy dermatitis is an alum-precipitated, pyridine extract of *Toxicodendron radicans*. This product is, in reality, a purified extract of urushiol suspended in isotonic saline solution and is intended for subcutaneous administration. The antigen is slowly absorbed, thereby providing a continuous stimulation of antibodies for a long period of time. It should be stored at a temperature between 2 and 10° C. A commercial product that combines extracts of poison ivy and poison oak is Ivyol®. Two oral preparations, Poisonivi-oral® and Poisonok®, are apparently effective in building immunity against poison ivy.

OTHER CAUSES OF ALLERGY

No treatise on allergy would be complete without a consideration of other types of allergic conditions, such as **bacterial allergy, drug allergy, atmospheric allergy, occupational allergy, physical allergy,** and **psychosomatic allergy.** Because all of us are in daily contact with microorganisms, both externally and internally, it is not unthinkable that persons may become sensitized to bacteria. Indeed, it is difficult to distinguish between some forms of bacterial infections, particularly of the nasal and bronchial mucosa, and some forms of bacterial allergy.

Many drugs produce an allergic response in hypersensitive individuals. Penicillin allergy has already been discussed on page 432 and sensitivity to biologics prepared from horse serum has been mentioned on page 413. Numerous other drugs elicit symptoms characteristic of inhalant, ingestant, injectant, and contactant allergens.

Acetylsalicylic acid may cause allergic manifestations, not only in hypersensitive patients who ingest it, but also in susceptible community pharmacists who may use it in compounding. It may affect manufacturing pharmacists who work with it in quantity in formulating medicinal products. Frequently, the aspirin produces lacrimation and sneezing; occasionally, it causes dermatitis. Cases are recorded of allergic reactions to trypsin, insulin, sulfa drugs, antibiotics, and even to antihistamines and cortisone!

The primary cause of physical allergy is problematic although conceivably shock tissues are involved. Cold water, extreme pressure, or other conditions may produce erythema or configurations on the skin. Medical records indicate that emotional complexes of children and adults may produce certain types of allergies; often extreme anger, sorrow, or jealousy will be sufficient cause for asthma, dermatitis, or other allergies to become apparent. It is not definitely known if these allergies are the result of specific antigen-antibody reactions.

It is believed that one allergy may potentiate the action of another. A person who can tolerate ragweed pollen without sneezing may begin such a reaction only after eating allergenic foods such as shrimp or chocolate bars. Similarly, a person who normally suffers no gastrointestinal allergy after eating tomatoes may develop diarrhea, extreme abdominal pain, or exhibit a skin rash during a certain pollinating season.

The subject of allergy is exceedingly complex, but by the same token, it is usually interesting. The future holds the answer to the cause of allergenic reactions and their prevention and cure.

READING REFERENCES

Berrens, L.: *The Chemistry of Atopic Allergens*, Basel, S. Karger, 1971.

Brown, F. R., and Wolfe, H. I.: Observations of Animal Dander Hyposensitization, Ann. Allerg., 26(6):305, 1968.

Doskotch, R. W., and Hufford, C. D.: Damsin, the Cytotoxic Principle of *Ambrosia ambrosioides* (Cav.) Payne, J. Pharm. Sci., 58(2):186, 1969.

Frazier, C. A.: *Insect Allergy—Allergic and Toxic Reactions to Insects and Other Arthropods*, St. Louis, Warren H. Green, Inc., 1969.

Goodman, D. H., Harris, J., and Miller, S.: Extraction of Ragweed Pollen Antigens by Water Organic Soluble Solvents, Ann. Allerg., *26*(9):463, 1968.

Harris, M. C., and Shure, N.: *All About Allergy*, Englewood Cliffs, New Jersey, Prentice-Hall, Inc., 1969.

Kallos, P., and Waksman, B. H.: *Progress in Allergy*, White Plains, Albert J. Phiebig Books, 1968.

Lampe, K. F., and Fagerström, R.: *Plant Toxicity and Dermatitis*, Baltimore, The Williams & Wilkins Co., 1968.

Levine, B. B., and Zolov, D. M.: Prediction of Penicillin Allergy by Immunological Tests. J. Allergy, *43*(4):231, 1969.

Newmark, F. M.: Pollen Aerobiology—The Need for Research and Compilation, Ann. Allerg., *26*(7):358, 1968.

Patterson, R.: *Allergic Diseases*, Philadelphia, J. B. Lippincott Co., 1972.

Pepys, J., Chan, M., and Hargreave, F. E.: Mites and House Dust Allergy, Lancet (7555):1270, 1968.

Prince, H. E., and Morrow, M. B.: A Logical Approach to Mold Allergy, Ann. Allerg., *27*(2):79, 1969.

Rapaport, H. G., and Linde, S. M.: *The Complete Allergy Guide*, New York, Simon and Schuster, 1970.

Serafini, U., Frankland, A. W., Masala, C., and Jamar, J. M., eds.: *New Concepts in Allergy and Clinical Immunology*, Amsterdam, Excerpta Medica, 1971.

Sherman, W. B.: *Hypersensitivity Mechanisms and Management*, Philadelphia, W. B. Saunders Co., 1968.

Stanley, R. G., and Linskens, H. F.: *Pollen: Biology, Biochemistry, Management*, New York, Springer-Verlag, 1974.

Stanworth, D. R.: *Immediate Hypersensitivity*, Amsterdam, North-Holland Publishing Co., 1973.

Stewart, G. T., and McGovern, J. P., eds.: *Penicillin Allergy*, Springfield, Illinois, Charles C Thomas, 1970.

Swinney, B., Swinney, B., Jr., and Hicks, R.: A simple Improved Pollen Sampler, Ann. Allerg., *26*(11):605, 1968.

Wodehouse, R. P.: *Hayfever Plants*, 2nd ed., New York, Hafner Publishing Co., 1971.

Poisonous Plants

The separation of scientific fact from fiction is extremely difficult in the study of poisonous plants. Examination of the pertinent literature reveals considerable confusion that tends to mask an even greater amount of ignorance. Indeed, almost any plant may be judged as toxic, questionable, or edible, depending on the reference consulted. For example, perhaps the most famous cookbook in the world, *Larousse Gastronomique,* once declared that rhubarb leaves could be "eaten like spinach," but well-documented fatalities resulting from their ingestion, both by human beings and by animals, have long been known to the medical profession.

J. M. Kingsbury, who has written extensively on the subject, points out that compilers dealing with poisonous plants often felt obligated to carry a plant into newer literature even though uncertain of the original authority. He concludes that only about one half of the names in current American compilations are based on domestic experimental or case evidence. The remainder have been copied from European sources which, in some cases, date back to Dioscorides (first century A.D.).

S. B. O'Leary cites an incident in which "teenage soldiers in Hawaii" were fatally poisoned by oleander juice from sticks used as toasting forks. This passage may actually refer to the death of 8 French soldiers who cooked their meat ration on oleander sticks during the Napoleonic campaigns in Spain in 1808.

Unbelievable chaos reigns in the area of plant identification and nomenclature as applied by nonspecialists. In certain localities, poison dogwood refers not to a species of *Cornus,* but to poison sumac (*Toxicodendron vernix*). Deadly nightshade is a common pharmaceutic synonym for *Atropa belladonna,* but in the Pacific Northwest it is often applied to *Solanum dulcamara.* Deadly nightshade is also known as European bittersweet, not to be confused with *Celastrus scandens* or *Euonymus* species, which are also called bittersweet. On the other hand, belladonna may designate not only the *Atropa* species of that name, but also an *Amaryllis* species. One can only guess whether a reported case of poisoning by elephants-ears refers to a species of *Caladium, Colocasia, Dieffenbachia,* or to mandrake, a name

449

applied to some elephants-ears and to *Podophyllum peltatum* and *Mandragora officinarum* as well. When it comes to the application of common names to mushrooms, which were probably not identified correctly in the first place, the situation becomes almost hopeless.

This field is where the practicing pharmacist, in his ever-expanding clinical role of adviser to both the physician and the layman, can make an outstanding contribution to public health and community welfare. No other professional in the health field has so extensive a background in both the botany and chemistry of plants as does the pharmacist. By virtue of his scientific training in these areas, the pharmacist is the only readily available authority on matters of identification and nature of the principles responsible for the toxic effects of accidentally ingested vegetable materials.

In smaller communities, where poison control centers do not exist, the pharmacist may be the only knowledgeable person in this field. The opportunity to function as a professional adviser to a poison control center offers even greater opportunities for the utilization of professional knowledge. Many of the most dangerous higher plants are cultivated species that exist in numerous varieties. Those found in any given community will vary according to climate, geography, and proximity to certain seed houses or nurseries. To serve to best advantage, the pharmacist should endeavor to become thoroughly familiar with both the indigenous and the cultivated flora of his community.

Poison antidote kits contain ipecac syrup as well as activated charcoal to be used as directed by the physician to counteract the effects of poisonous substances. Each kit contains a one-half-ounce bottle of ipecac syrup and a 5-gram container of activated charcoal packaged in a plastic box.

The following outline of the most important toxic plants found in the United States can serve as an important basic reference to this field. Because of the space limitations inherent in any textbook that must cover a broad area, the listing is neither complete nor excessively detailed. Many poisonous plants that are of primary interest as forage crops for animals are not mentioned. Students desiring to develop additional competence are urged to consult the specialized books and monographs on poisonous plants in the selected reading list.

HIGHER PLANTS

Abrus precatorius Linné **(jequirity)** is a climbing shrub common to tropical and subtropical countries of both hemispheres. *Abrus* is Greek and means graceful, in allusion to the flowers; *precatorius* is from the Latin *precor*, meaning to pray, because the seeds are used as beads in rosaries. The seeds are ovoid, globular, from 5 to 9 mm in length, hard, smooth and shining. They are 2 distinct colors. The lower or hilum portion is purplish black and has a large lenticular scar: the upper portion is scarlet red; and the testa is shell-like and encloses a light yellowish brown embryo that has 2 large cotyledons and an incurved radicle (Fig. 15–1). The seed contains **abrin** (jequiritin), an agglutinating phytalbumin resembling ricin in its physiologic action. It is toxic, is soluble in a solution of sodium chloride, and has a melting point of 295°C.

Because jequirity seeds are colorful and attractive and because they are made into rosary beads, decorative table pads, necklaces, and other types of jewelry, they frequently are handled by small children. One must remember that these seeds contain the extremely toxic principle, abrin, which has caused death on numerous occasions.

Aconitum spp. **(aconite, monkshood)** are not commonly implicated in poisoning

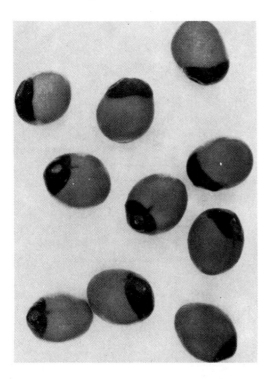

Fig. 15–1. Jequirity seed, magnified 3 times.

cases in the United States. They contain highly toxic diterpenoid alkaloids, including the well-known aconitine.

Aleurites fordii Hemsley **(tung-oil tree)** is a small tree cultivated along the Gulf Coast that produces brown, pendant, nearly spheric fruits. Commercial tung oil is obtained from the seeds which also contain uncharacterized toxic principles. Ingestion of a single seed can produce severe gastroenteritis in a human being.

Alocasia macrorhiza (Linné) Schott and other species of *Alocasia* are tropical herbs that generally have arrow-shaped leaves and are grown for their ornamental, often variegated foliage. The plant is an irritant poison owing to the raphides of calcium oxalate contained in the sap as well as to an additional unknown toxic ingredient.

Atropa belladonna Linné **(deadly nightshade)** contains tropine alkaloids, especially hyoscyamine (see page 201).

Blighia sapida Koenig **(akee)** is a small tropical tree, widely cultivated in Florida, that produces clusters of straw-colored to reddish fruit. The fleshy arils of ripe fruits are commonly eaten after parboiling and frying, but the fruit wall and seeds are toxic. Ingestion of the fruit, especially by children, produces a condition known as "vomiting sickness," which is characterized by marked hypoglycemia. The mortality rate is high, ranging from 40 to 80%.

Two toxic principles, hypoglycin A and B, have been isolated from the fruit. Hypoglycin A has been characterized as β-methylene-cyclopropyl-L-α-aminopropionic acid, and hypoglycin B is a dipeptide formed of hypoglycin A and glutamic acid. No specific antidotes for these toxins have been found; therefore, treatment of akee poisoning is primarily symptomatic.

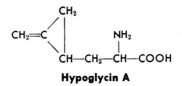

Hypoglycin A

Cicuta spp. **(water hemlock)** include a number of species of the genus *Cicuta*, especially *C. maculata* Linné. They constitute the most violently poisonous plants in the North Temperate Zone. The toxic principle, cicutoxin, an unsaturated higher alcohol (*trans*-heptadeca-8,10,12-triene-4,6-diyne-1,14-diol), has been isolated from *C. virosa* Linné. It is a violent convulsant that acts directly on the central nervous system.

Water hemlock has tuberous roots that are often mistaken for edible wild parsnips or wild artichokes. Such confusion may provoke disaster and emphasizes the folly of uninformed persons who attempt to collect wild plants for food.

$$HO-CH_2-(CH_2)_2-(C{\equiv}C)_2-(CH{=}CH)_3-\underset{\underset{OH}{|}}{CH}-(CH_2)_2-CH_3$$

Cicutoxin

Colchicum autumnale Linné **(autumn crocus)** contains colchicine (see page 254).

Colocasia antiquorum Schott and *C. esculenta* Schott **(elephants-ear)** are tropical plants widely cultivated for their large showy leaves. They contain large amounts of calcium oxalate.

Conium maculatum Linné **(poison hemlock)** is a large herb indigenous to Europe and naturalized in North and South America and in various parts of Asia. The plant resembles wild carrot (*Daucus carota* Linné), but does not possess its hairy stem and leaves. Poison hemlock also has a characteristic "mousey" odor. Its fruits were formerly used in medicine.

All parts of the plant are toxic because of the presence of several nicotinelike alkaloids, especially coniine, N-methylconiine, γ-coniceine, conhydrine, and pseudoconhydrine. The juice of poison hemlock constituted the famous hemlock potion of the ancient Greeks and was used to put their criminals to death. It is commonly believed that Socrates was executed by means of a decoction of this plant.

Because of its occurrence as a weed in many parts of the United States and the relative attractiveness, especially to children, of its leaves, fruits, and root, this toxic plant should be recognized by every pharmacist. It is particularly important to be able to differentiate poison hemlock from other members of the family Umbelliferae, both edible and toxic, that bear a close resemblance.

Convallaria majalis Linné **(lily-of-the-valley)** contains cardiac glycosides, especially convallatoxin (see page 180).

Daphne mezereum Linné **(mezereon)** is a small deciduous shrub with alternate leaves, purple flowers, and scarlet fruits. This plant and related species of *Daphne* are widely cultivated as ornamentals. Apparently, all parts of all species are toxic, but the drupes are particularly attractive to children. A few of these so-called "berries" can kill a child. Identity of the toxic principle was equivocal for many years, but recently daphnetoxin, a diterpene, was characterized.

Datura spp. **(stramonium, thornapple, Jamestown weed, jimson weed)** contain tropine alkaloids, especially hyoscyamine (see page 207 and Fig. 8–7).

Delphinium spp. **(larkspur)** include a large number of annual plants occurring as wild species throughout the United States, especially in the West but also widely cultivated in American gardens. They contain a number of toxic polycyclic diterpenoid alkaloids that account for their frequent involvement in the poisoning of livestock and human beings, especially children.

Dicentra cucullaria (Linné) Bernhardi **(Dutchman's breeches),** *D. canadensis* (Goldie) Walpers **(squirrel corn),** and other species of *Dicentra* commonly referred to as **bleeding heart** are herbaceous, spring-flowering plants with pendant, bilaterally symmetric flowers whose petals are prolonged into 2 spurs. About a dozen species are cultivated or occur naturally in North America. The plants contain a large number of isoquinoline alkaloids, and protopine has been found in all species examined. However, the degree of toxicity of the individual alkaloids requires clarification.

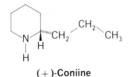

(+)-Coniine

Dieffenbachia seguine Schott and *D. picta* Schott **(dumbcane)** are common ornamental house plants that grow up to 2 meters in height and have large entire leaves that are either uniformly green or, more commonly, mottled with white, yellow, or other shades of green. Ingestion of the leaves results in severe corrosive burns of the oral cavity, esophagus, and stomach caused by calcium oxalate and by a proteolytic enzyme, dumbain.

Digitalis purpurea Linné **(foxglove)** contains cardioactive glycosides, digitoxin, gitoxin, and others (see page 172).

Eupatorium rugosum Houttuyn **(white snakeroot or richweed)** is a showy, herbaceous, erect perennial, attaining a height of more than 1 meter. It has opposite, ovate to cordate leaves borne on long petioles and white flowers, small in composite heads, and grouped in open terminal corymbs. Positive identification of this plant is difficult. The disease known as "milk sickness," common among the early settlers in the United States, has been traced to the ingestion of dairy products derived from animals poisoned by this plant. An incompletely characterized, unstable alcohol that is designated tremetol and occurs in combination with a resin acid is apparently the toxic principle (Fig. 15–2).

Euphorbia spp. **(spurge)** number more than 1000 and range from herbs or shrubs

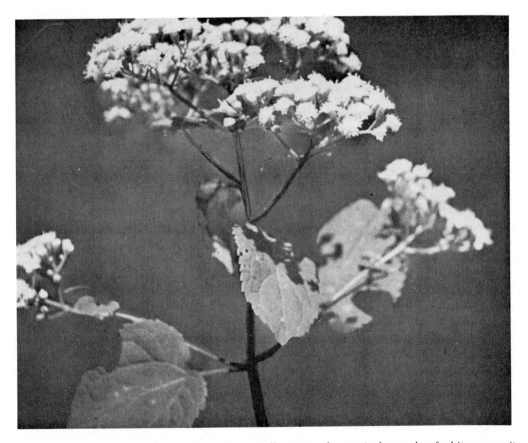

Fig. 15–2. *Eupatorim rugosum* (white snakeroot) illustrating the terminal corymbs of white composite flowers.

to more or less succulent trees. All contain a latex that exudes when the plant is damaged. The latex is highly irritating and often produces vesication from contact and emesis and purgation from ingestion. These effects are attributed to an acrid principle believed to be present in the latex resin. One of the best-known species is *Euphorbia pulcherrima* Willdenow, the common **poinsettia,** which is a favorite house plant during Christmas because of its bright red bracts.

Gelsemium sempervirens (Linné) Aiton **(yellow jasmine)** is a perennial woody evergreen climber growing in the moist woodlands of the southeastern United States. Its dried rhizome and roots constitute the crude drug gelsemium, formerly employed as a central nervous system depressant. Ingestion of sufficient quantities of the plant may lead to respiratory failure. Children have been poisoned by tasting the nectar of the flowers, and honey prepared by bees feeding on the nectar has caused fatalities. The active principles are indole alkaloids, especially gelsemine and sempervirine (Fig. 15–3).

Hedera helix Linné **(English ivy)** is the well-known cultivated vine commonly employed as an external decoration on buildings. Ingestion of the berries by children has resulted in fatalities. Their toxicity is attributed to hederin, a saponin glycoside.

Hippomane mancinella Linné **(manchineel tree)** is a small tropical tree occur-

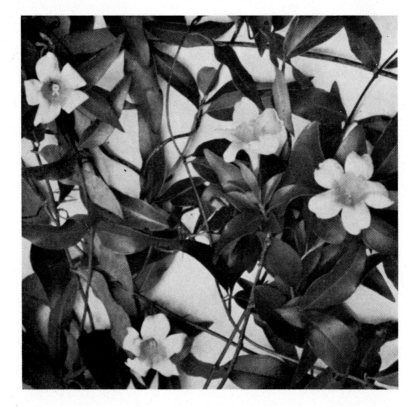

Fig. 15–3. Yellow jessamine or yellow jasmine *(Gelsemium sempervirens)* is a perennial woody climbing vine growing in the southeastern United States. (Photo, courtesy of Dr. Julia F. Morton, Director, Morton Collectanea, University of Miami.)

ring in the southern part of Florida. All parts of the plant contain an extremely caustic, milky sap whose active principles are designated hippomanin A and B. Hippomanin A, the main toxic constituent, is 2-galloyl-4,6-hexahydroxydiphenoyl-D-glucose.

Hyoscyamus niger Linné **(henbane)** contains hyoscyamine and scopolamine (see page 206).

Ilex aquifolium Linné **(English holly)** and several related species of *Ilex* are small trees or shrubs with shiny green leaves and bright red berries. They are often used as Christmas decorations. Ingestion of the berries produces vomiting, diarrhea, and "mild narcosis." The active principle, ilicin, remains uncharacterized.

Ipomoea spp. **(morning glory)** are common, cultivated ornamental vines. The seeds of some species and varieties contain ergot alkaloids, especially ergine (see page 248).

Jatropha curcas Linné and *J. multifida* Linné **(physic nut)** are tropical shrubs or small trees occurring with several closely related species in Florida, Texas, Puerto Rico, and Hawaii. Closely related botanically to the castor plant, these plants produce seeds containing a purgative oil and, apparently, a phytotoxin.

Kalmia angustifolia Linné **(dwarf laurel)**, *K. latifolia* Linné **(mountain laurel)**, and certain other members of the Ericaceae, such as species of *Ledum*, *Pieris*, and *Rhododendron (Azalea)*, are widely occurring shrubs or small trees. All contain the same poisonous principle, andromedotoxin, a diterpene derivative. Andromedotoxin has been identified as the toxic agent in honey produced by bees that feed on these plants.

Laburnum anagyroides Medicus **(laburnum, golden-chain)** is a large ornamental shrub or small tree that is widely cultivated as a spectacular ornamental owing to its long hanging racemes of golden yellow flowers. The fruit, a legume pod containing up to 8 seeds, is commonly ingested by children. Laburnum seeds contain cytisine, a quinolizidine alkaloid resembling nicotine in its physiologic effects.

Lantana camara Linné **(lantana)** is an ornamental shrub, up to 1.5 meters in height, with aromatic leaves, orange or bright red flowers, and dark blue or black fruits (drupes). The plant is widely cultivated in California and the southern United States where cases of poisoning have occurred through ingestion of the fruit. A triterpene derivative, lantadene A, is the toxic principle.

Lobelia inflata Linné **(Indian tobacco)** and several related species of *Lobelia* contain piperidine alkaloids, especially lobeline (see page 200).

Melia azedarach Linné **(chinaberry tree)** is a small, thickly branched tree with large compound leaves, purple flowers, and smooth ovoid fruits (drupes) that are yellow when mature. The plant is common in the southern United States, Puerto Rico, and Hawaii. Poisoning most often results from ingestion of the fruits whose toxicity is associated with an uncharacterized resinous fraction. Severe irritation, nervous symptoms, and fatty degeneration of the liver and kidneys characterize the toxic effects.

Menispermum canadense Linné **(Canada moonseed)** is a high-climbing vine, indigenous to the northern United States and Canada, that has broadly ovate, cordate, 3- to 10-lobed leaves. Its fruits resemble small purple grapes and have been the cause of poisoning in children. The toxic principles are isoquinoline alkaloids, including dauricine which has a curarelike action.

Metopium toxiferum Krug et Urban **(poisonwood tree)** is a large shrub or small tree with compound leaves and fleshy fruits. It is common in areas south of

Miami, Florida, and frequently causes severe contact dermatitis. Presumably, the active principle is identical or at least similar to urushiol, the causative agent of poison ivy dermatitis.

Narcissus spp. **(narcissus, daffodil, jonquil)** are well-known cultivated plants. Ingestion of narcissus bulbs produces severe gastroenteritis and nervous symptoms apparently owing to the phenanthridine alkaloids contained therein.

Nerium oleander Linné **(oleander)** is an ornamental bush or shrub with coriaceous, sharply pointed, oblong-lanceolate leaves and showy pink or white blossoms. It is widely cultivated in the southern United States and California and is grown elsewhere as an indoor pot plant. The plant contains a complex mixture of cardiac glycosides derived from 6 different genins that are closely related chemically and physiologically to the digitalis glycosides (see page 180).

Nicotiana spp. **(tobacco)** contain alkaloids, chiefly nicotine (see page 199).

Papaver spp. **(poppy)**, the related *Argemone mexicana* Linné **(prickly poppy)**, and *Chelidonium majus* Linné **(celandine poppy)** contain isoquinoline alkaloids (see page 219).

Philodendron spp. are perhaps the most common house plants in the United States. Like certain other members of the family Araceae, they may contain irritant principles (calcium oxalate and others). Numerous cases of poisoning in cats, 50% fatal, have been reported.

Phoradendron villosum Nuttall and *P. flavescens* (Pursh) Nuttall **(mistletoe)** are woody perennial plants growing as parasites on oaks and other deciduous trees. The latter species is widely employed as a Christmas decoration. Berries of these plants are reputedly toxic, possibly owing to their content of phoratoxin, a disulfide bond-containing protein found in the genus.

Phytolacca americana Linné **(pokeweed, pokeberry)** is a tall, branched perennial herb that reaches a height of 3 meters. It has white or greenish flowers in racemes, and 10-celled, juicy, purple berries. Ingestion of the berries produces severe gastrointestinal disturbances accompanied by weakened respiration and pulse. Apparently, the seeds and the root are especially toxic, but the identity of the active principles has not been established (see page 493).

Podophyllum peltatum Linné **(American mandrake, mayapple)** contains resinous principles that produce dermatitis on contact and catharsis on ingestion (see page 146).

Poinciana gilliesii Hooker **(poinciana, bird of paradise)** is a shrub or small tree with showy terminal racemes of yellow flowers with red stamens. In the southern United States, it is cultivated as an outdoor perennial; elsewhere it is grown as a large indoor plant. The green seed pods are extremely irritating to the digestive tract. This plant should not be confused with *Strelitzia*, the florist's bird of paradise flower.

Primula obconica Hance **(primrose)** is a popular house plant that produces a severe contact dermatitis in sensitive individuals.

Prunus serotina Ehrhart **(wild cherry)** and related species and varieties (*P. virginiana* Linné, *P. laurocerasus* Linné, etc.) contain cyanogenetic glycosides (see page 71).

Ranunculus spp. **(buttercup, crowfoot)** are perennial or annual herbs with yellow flowers. Some of these species are the most common weeds in fields and marshy areas in the United States. The juice of these plants has vesicant properties owing to the presence of a highly unstable γ-lactone, protoanemonin.

Rheum rhaponticum Linné **(rhapontic rhubarb, common rhubarb)** contains large quantities of oxalic acid and its salts in the lamina of the leaf (see page 63).

Rhododendron spp., see *Kalmia angustifolia*.

Rhus spp., see *Toxicodendron radicans*.

Ricinus communis Linné **(castor bean)** contains ricin, a phytotoxin, in the seeds (see page 88).

Robinia pseudoacacia Linné **(black locust)** contains a toxic principle in the seeds, leaves, and bark. The toxin, robin, is a protein, related to abrin in jequirity.

Sanguinaria canadensis Linné **(bloodroot)** contains isoquinoline alkaloids, especially sanguinarine (see page 223).

Skimmia japonica Thunberg **(skimmia)** is an ornamental evergreen shrub with alternate simple leaves, small white flowers in terminal panicles, and bright red berries. All parts of the plant are toxic, but the attractive berries are most commonly ingested. The active principle is skimmianine, a furoquinoline alkaloid that acts as a muscle poison and may cause cardiac or pulmonary arrest.

Solandra spp. **(chalice-vine)** are woody, erect or climbing, tropical plants with large white to yellow, showy flowers. Species encountered in Florida and California include *S. grandiflora* Swartz, *S. hartwegii* N. E. Brown, and *S. longiflora* Tussac. The plants contain tropane alkaloids; atropine, hyoscyamine, and norhyoscyamine have been isolated from various species.

Solanum spp. **(nightshade)** are annual or perennial herbs and shrubs with alternate, simple or compound leaves and wheel-shaped or shallowly bell-shaped flowers, often showy in white, yellow, blue, and purple. The fruit is a berry that is often quite attractive. *Solanum dulcamara* Linné **(European bittersweet)**, *S. nigrum* Linné **(black nightshade)**, and related species, including *S. tuberosum* Linné **(potato)**, contain toxic steroidal glycoalkaloids (solanine, demissine, others) in the green shoots, leaves, and fruits. The toxicity of a single species varies widely according to the part used, the stage of development, and possibly the genetic factors. Following ingestion, the glycoalkaloids are not readily absorbed, but first undergo hydrolysis to release the free alkamines.

These are then absorbed, producing nervous symptoms characterized by dulling of the senses and stupefaction.

Taxus spp. **(Yew)** are evergreen trees and shrubs with linear leaves that are dark green on the upper surface and yellow-green on the lower, inconspicuous flowers, and berrylike red fruits composed of a stony seed nearly surrounded by a thick fleshy cup. All species of *Taxus* that have been investigated contain a complex mixture of toxic alkaloids designated taxine in the leaves, bark, and seeds but apparently not in the pulp of the fruit. Ingestion of 50 to 100 needles can produce death in the human being through cardiac and respiratory depression (see Fig. 15–4).

Thevetia peruviana Schumacher **(yellow oleander)** is a large, cultivated evergreen shrub or small tree with linear, sharply pointed leaves, fragrant, showy yellow flowers, and fruits that are fleshy drupes, broadly triangular, and black when ripe. The plant is cultivated as an ornamental in southern Florida and Hawaii. On the island of Oahu it is said to be the most frequent cause of serious poisoning in human beings. Yellow Oleander contains cardiac glycosides (cerebrin, neriifolin, thevetin) that produce digitalislike effects.

Toxicodendron radicans (Linné) Kuntze **(poison ivy)** as well as other species of the

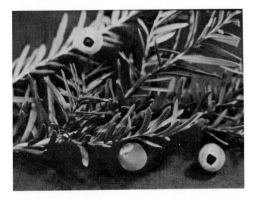

Fig. 15–4. *Taxus* sp. (yew) showing the leaves, berrylike fruit, and the dark stony seed surrounded by the fleshy cup-shaped aril of the fruit.

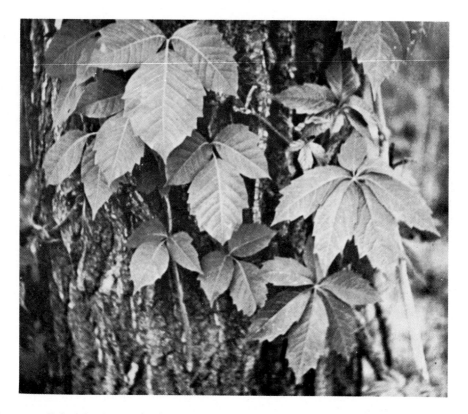

Fig. 15–5. Poison ivy *(Toxicodendron radicans)* is sometimes confused with Virginia creeper *(Psedera quinquefolia)*; the former *(left)* is 3-foliate and the latter *(right)* is usually 5- or more-foliate.

genus *Toxicodendron* (formerly *Rhus*), including *T. diversilobum* (Torrey et Gray) Greene **(western poison oak)**, *T. quercifolium* (Michaux) Greene **(eastern poison oak)**, and *T. vernix* (Linné) Kuntze **(poison sumac)**, all contain urushiol, a phenolic allergen that produces contact dermatitis (see page 445, also Figs. 15–5 and 15–6).

Veratrum viride Aiton **(green hellebore)** contains steroidal alkaloids (see page 250).

Wisteria spp. **(wisteria)** are ornamental woody vines with pinnate leaves and drooping terminal racemes of showy flowers, white, pink, blue, or purple in color, followed by fruit that are elongated pods, contracted at intervals. Ingestion of the seeds or pods produces mild to severe gastroenteritis, which has been attributed to the presence of sapotoxins.

Xanthosma sagittifolium (Linné) Schott **(malanga)** and related species of *Xanthosma* are large tropical aroids commonly grown as foliage plants. The leaves are extremely acrid owing to the presence of large amounts of calcium oxalate.

Zamia integrifolia Aiton **(Florida arrowroot)** and other members of the order Cycadales, including species of *Cycas* and *Macrozamia*, are primitive cone-bearing palmlike plants indigenous to the tropics but cultivated elsewhere as ornamentals. These cycads contain a carcinogenic and hepatotoxic glycoside, cycasin, which has been characterized as methylazoxymethanol-β-D-glucoside. In many tropical

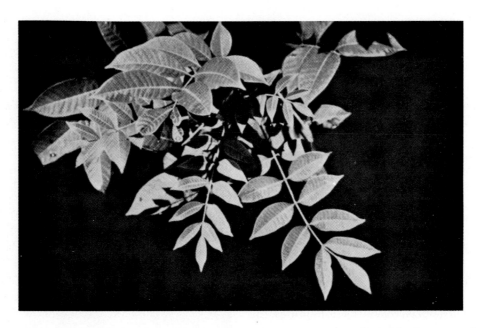

Fig. 15–6. *Toxicodendron vernix* (poison sumac) differs from the other toxic *Toxicodendron* species by its 7- to 13-compound leaves.

countries, the roots of cycads are employed for the preparation of edible flour, and most cases of poisoning result from the ingestion of an improperly prepared product. Acute intoxications resulting from a single ingestion of cycad roots or seeds are much less common.

$$CH_3-N=N-CH_2-O-C_6H_{11}O_5$$

Cycasin

Zigadenus spp. **(death camas)** are perennial herbs with grasslike leaves; underground bulbs or rhizomes; greenish white, yellow, or pink flowers; and capsular fruits. The plants contain steroidal glycoalkaloids, chemically and physiologically similar to those of *Veratrum viride*.

MUSHROOMS

Because the chemistry of the active principles in many poisonous mushrooms is still imperfectly known and positive botanic identification is often extremely difficult, these species must be classified on a physiologic basis, that is, according to the type of symptoms observed in human beings following ingestion. Four basic types of mushroom toxins, with several minor subdivisions, are generally recognized.

1. Protoplasmic poisons
   a. amanita toxins
   b. gyromitrin
   c. orellanine
2. Compounds exerting neurologic effects
   a. muscarine
   b. ibotenic acid-muscimol
   c. psilocybin and psilocin
3. Gastrointestinal irritants
4. Disulfiramlike constituents

All the known poisonous species contain one or more of these principles. The basic classification does not include poisonings from hypersensitivity to mushroom protein or from eating mushrooms partially decomposed by microbial action.

PROTOPLASMIC POISONS

Amanita Toxins. As the name implies, this mixture of peptide toxins was first detected in certain species of *Amanita*, a genus of mushrooms characterized by white spores, the presence of both an annulus and a volva, and typically free gills. More recently, certain of these toxins have been found in some species of *Galerina*, a genus typified by small nondescript carpophores with yellowish brown spores, whose species are distinguished principally on the basis of microscopic characteristics.

About a dozen related cyclopeptides, the most important of which are phalloidin, phalloin, and α-, β- and γ-amanitin, have been isolated from *Amanita phalloides* (Fries) Secretan **(deadly amanita)** of European origin. This particular mushroom is extremely rare in the United States, apparently existing only as an introduced species. Related species, including *Amanita bisporigera* Atkinson, *Amanita verna* (Fries) Vittadini, and *Amanita virosa* Secretan, are more common and also contain these toxins (Fig. 15–7). *Amanita brunnescens* Atkinson, long confused with *Amanita phalloides* in this country and still designated by some as a brown form of the latter, does not contain amanita toxins. Although its toxicity has not been scientifically verified, it does contain an unidentified alkaloid and is presumably poisonous.

Both α- and β-amanitin have been detected in *Galerina autumnalis* (Peck) Smith & Singer, *Galerina marginata* (Fries) Kühner, and *Galerina venenata* A. H. Smith. These species probably constitute a more serious health hazard than do the deadly amanitas because of the extreme difficulty in identifying them unequivo-

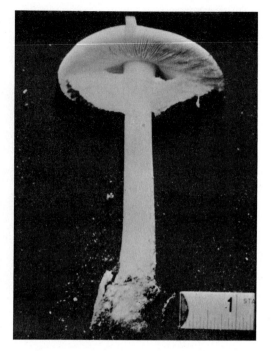

Fig. 15–7. *Amanita verna* (destroying angel) is one of the most deadly mushrooms known.

cally and because they often occur in lawns and other grassy areas.

Regardless of the species involved, poisoning by amanita toxins is characterized by a long latent period between ingestion of the mushrooms and onset of symptoms. An asymptomatic latent period lasting up to 24 hours precedes violent vomiting and diarrhea which may continue until death results. If the patient survives this initial phase through appropriate therapy, he may appear to recover for a short time but generally will relapse owing to progressive injury to the liver, kidneys, heart, and skeletal muscles. Death results in about 50% of the cases within 2 to 5 days.

Modern treatment of amanita toxin poisoning involves removal of the toxic material from the gastrointestinal tract, if necessary, followed by symptomatic and supportive therapy. Administration of corticosteroids, thioctic acid, cytochrome C, vitamins C, K, and B complex, and dextrose and sodium chloride injection have all been recommended. The compounds that have produced the greatest survival rate are penicillin G, chloramphenicol, phenylbutazone, and a combination of sulfamethoxazole and trimethoprim; however, at present, no antidote for amanitin intoxications is sufficiently established clinically for unequivocal recommendation.

Gyromitrin. A second type of protoplasmic poison, less dangerous than the amanita toxins but still capable of producing fatal results, occurs in certain **false morels,** especially *Helvella esculenta* Fries (*Gyromitra esculenta* Fries), *Helvella gigas* Krombholz (*Gyromitra gigas* Cooke), and *Helvella underwoodii* Seaver. These nongilled fungi are characterized by a pileus surface that varies from nearly smooth to strongly convoluted. However, it is never pitted (distinction from *Morchella* species—**morels**). Their pilei are nearly always lobed, usually more or less saddle-shaped.

The toxic principle of *Helvella* (*Gyromitra*) species was recently isolated, characterized as the N-methyl-N-formylhydrazone of acetaldehyde, and designated by the trivial name gyromitrin. It is essentially hepatotoxic but does exert additional effects on the hematopoietic system and the central nervous system. The compound is, therefore, classed as a protoplasmic poison, but differs markedly in its chemistry and toxicity from the amanita toxins.

Gyromitrin is volatile, which explains why species containing it may be rendered edible by extended drying or by parboiling. Whether the apparent irregular distribution of the compound in different collections of the same species is caused by the existence of different chemical races or may be attributed to other factors remains undetermined.

A minimum latent period of approximately 6 to 10 hours occurs between ingestion of the mushroom and the onset of symptoms that resemble those produced by amanita toxins but are generally less severe. Although cases of poisoning are common in Europe and often involve large numbers of people, fatal poisonings are rare in the United States. The mortality rate ranges between 2 and 4%. Treatment is similar to that recommended for amanita toxin poisoning.

Orellanine. Species of *Cortinarius*, a genus of agarics characterized by brownish to reddish brown spores and a cobweblike cortina, have long been considered as nonpoisonous, if not truly edible, mushrooms. It is now known that at least one species, *Cortinarius orellanus* Fries non Quélet, is definitely toxic and has been responsible for numerous poisoning cases in Poland during the past decades. The active constituent is a methanol-soluble, thermostable, crystalline compound that has been identified chemically as the bis-N-oxide of 3,3',4,4'-tetrahydroxy-2,2'-bipyridyl. It is commonly designated orellanine.

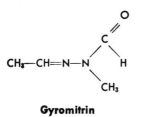

Gyromitrin

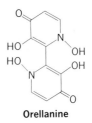

Orellanine

Orellanine poisoning is characterized by an extremely long latent period, varying from 3 to 14 days, between ingestion of the fungus and appearance of the symptoms. An intense burning thirst is first noted, followed by gastrointestinal disturbances, headache, pain in the limbs, spasms, and loss of consciousness. In severe cases, kidney damage occurs and may result in death after several weeks or longer. Recovery in less severe cases may be prolonged for months. About 15% of the recorded cases have proved fatal.

Because of the long latent period, treatment can only be symptomatic and supportive with particular attention to the maintenance of kidney function.

COMPOUNDS EXERTING NEUROLOGIC EFFECTS

Muscarine. Muscarine is a quaternary compound originally isolated from *Amanita muscaria* (Fries) Hooker, which occurs in that species and in the closely related *Amanita pantherina* (Fries) Secretan in small amounts. It is not, however, the principal toxic agent in either of these mushrooms. The compound has been re-

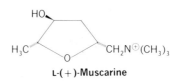

L-(+)-Muscarine

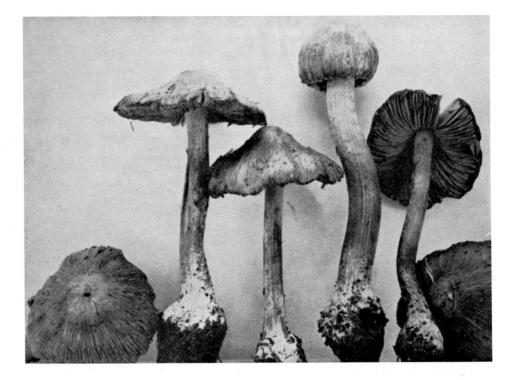

Fig. 15–8. *Inocybe napipes* J. Lange carpophores contain large quantities of muscarine. (Photo, courtesy of D. E. Stuntz.)

ported to occur in a number of species of *Boletus, Lepiota, Hebeloma, Russula,* but in many cases scientific verification is lacking. Certain species of *Clitocybe,* and especially *Inocybe,* contain muscarine in high concentrations, ranging in the latter species to more than 3% of dry weight when assayed physiologically. Both of these latter genera are readily recognized: *Clitocybe* by its typically white spores, fleshy central stipes, and broadly adnate to decurrent gills; *Inocybe* by its characteristic subconic to campanulate pileus, somewhat evanescent cortina, adnate or adnexed gills, and brownish spores (Fig. 15–8).

Symptoms of muscarine poisoning appear quite rapidly, usually 15 to 30 minutes after ingestion. Increased salivation, perspiration, and lacrimation, are fol-lowed by abdominal pain, severe nausea, and diarrhea. The pulse is slowed, the pupil is constricted, and breathing is asthmatic. The patient's mental processes remain clear. Death may result in severe cases from cardiac or respiratory failure, but it is infrequent. Treatment involves gastric lavage and administration of at-ropine, a specific antidote.

Ibotenic Acid-Muscimol. Ingestion of certain species of *Amanita (A. muscaria, A. pantherina)* produces symptoms that are not typical of muscarine, which is present in the species in small amounts, but resemble the central nervous system stimulation induced by atropine. Travelers in Siberia during the early part of the eighteenth century reported the use of the **fly agaric,** *Amanita muscaria,* as an intox-icant by tribes of the Kamchatkan Penin-

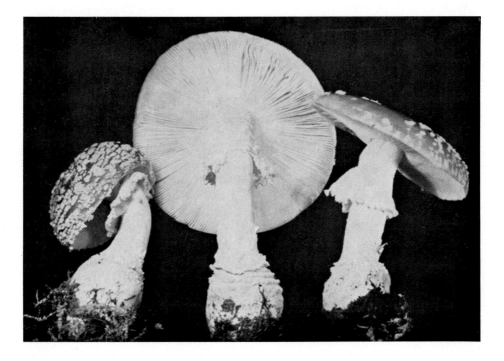

Fig. 15–9. Carpophores of *Amanita muscaria* (Fries) Hooker, commonly known as the fly agaric. This mushroom has been employed in Siberia as a hallucinogenic agent. (Photo, courtesy of D. E. Stuntz.)

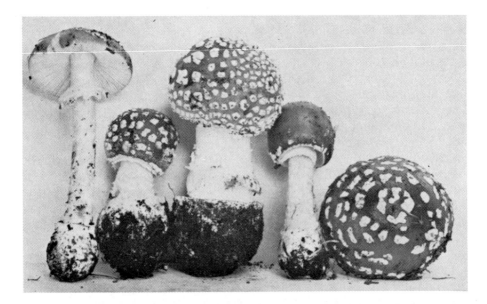

Fig. 15—10. Carpophores of *Amanita pantherina* (Fries) Secretan, the panther agaric. The brown pileus of this species readily distinguishes it from *Amanita muscaria* (red or orange pileus). (Photo, courtesy of D. E. Stuntz.)

sula. Vivid reports of orgies resulting from the use of this mushroom are found in the older literature (Figs. 15—9, 15—10).

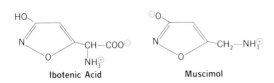

Ibotenic Acid   Muscimol

The active principle was ultimately identified as a mixture of 2 isoxazole derivatives, ibotenic acid and its decarboxylation product, muscimol. The compounds differ little in their qualitative effects, but quantitatively, muscimol is at least 5 times as active as ibotenic acid. These 2 psychotropic compounds are accompanied, at least in some specimens of *A. muscaria*, by a third active constituent, muscazone, which is an oxazole derivative.

Symptoms appear within 1 or 2 hours following ingestion. These are characterized by an initial state of excitement resembling alcoholic intoxication, followed by muscular twitching, depression, and, ultimately, loss of consciousness. Death is infrequent and recovery is ordinarily rapid. Treatment is largely symptomatic, employing mild depressants at first, followed by stimulants.

Psilocybin. Ingestion of certain small mushrooms not commonly employed as food can result in psychotropic manifestations in the human being. Most of them are species of *Psilocybe* and *Conocybe* [*P. cubensis* (Earle) Singer, *P. mexicana* Heim, *C. cyanopus* (Atkinson) Kühner] that have been used for many years by Indians in southern Mexico in magicoreligious ceremonies. Active members of both genera are brownish and somewhat nondescript in appearance (Fig. 15—11) but are readily characterized by the bluish stains that form, especially near the base of

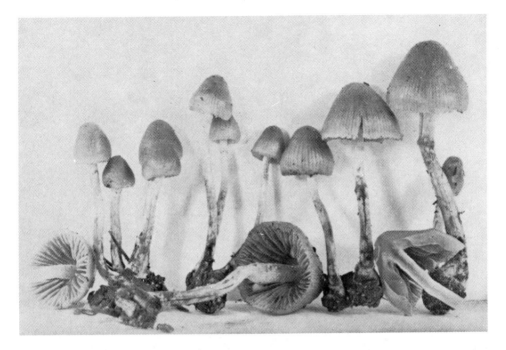

Fig. 15–11. Carpophores of *Psilocybe pelliculosa* A. H. Smith. This North American hallucinogenic mushroom contains psilocybin. (Photo, courtesy of D. E. Stuntz.)

the stipe, when the tissue is damaged or becomes aged. Chemical studies have revealed that 2 tryptamine derivatives, psilocybin and psilocin, are the active principles in these mushrooms. Psilocybin has been investigated clinically to determine its value in the treatment of psychiatric disorders.

Symptoms of psilocybin poisoning develop rapidly and continue for several hours. Anxiety and difficulty in concentration and in comprehension are common. Both elementary and true hallucinations may be experienced. Recovery is ordinarily spontaneous and complete after 5 to 10 hours.

GASTROINTESTINAL IRRITANTS

Mushrooms containing compounds that have an irritating effect on the gastrointestinal tract include such species as *Boletus satanas* Lenz, *Lactarius torminosus* (Fries)

Gray, *Paxillus involutus* (Fries) Fries, *Rhodophyllus lividus* (Mérat) Quélet (Fig. 15–12), *Russula emetica* (Fries) S. F. Gray, and *Tricholoma pardinum* Quélet. The chemical nature of the active principles of these species is not known, but they are generally presumed to be resinlike substances.

Symptoms are prompt in onset and include nausea, vomiting, and diarrhea, ranging from mild to extremely severe. Fatalities have resulted, especially among children. *Rhodophyllus lividus* also displays some hepatotoxic activity. In most cases, recovery is spontaneous and complete, but symptomatic care, bed rest, and light diet are indicated.

DISULFIRAMLIKE CONSTITUENTS

Ingestion of *Coprinus atramentarius* (Fries) Fries and the subsequent ingestion of alcohol give rise to symptoms resem-

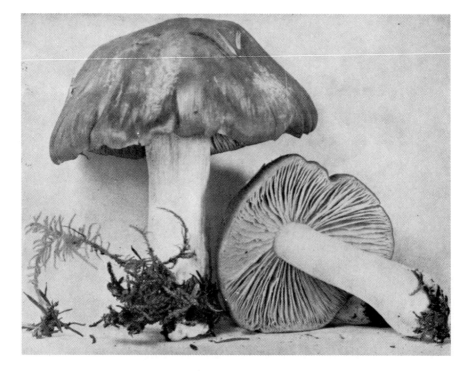

Fig. 15–12. *Rhodophyllus lividus* (Mérat) Quélet carpophores produce gastrointestinal upsets with associated hepatoxicity. (Photo, courtesy of D. E. Stuntz.)

bling those of the alcohol-disulfiram syndrome. This species is recognized by its black spores, smooth or minutely scaly grayish pileus, and free gills that deliquesce into a dark-colored fluid as the spores are discharged.

Because of the similarity in its physiologic action to disulfiram or cyanamide, the activity of the mushroom has been attributed to one or the other of these compounds. In 1975, two groups of scientists, one in the United States and the other in Sweden, independently isolated

Coprine

the toxic constituent, N-(1-hydroxy-cyclopropyl)-L-glutamine. This compound has been named coprine.

The compound is itself inactive, but breaks down partially in the body to form cyclopropanone hydrate. This interferes with the function of acetaldehyde dehydrogenase in the liver. Normal alcohol metabolism is thereby retarded and acetaldehyde concentrations in the blood remain abnormally high.

Symptoms, which occur within one-half to 2 hours following consumption of the mushroom and alcohol, include flushing, palpitations, dyspnea, hyperventilation, and tachycardia. Vomiting and diarrhea are usually absent. Recovery is ordinarily spontaneous and complete, but severe cases may require gastric lavage and symptomatic care.

READING REFERENCES

Baskin, E.: *The Poppy and Other Deadly Plants*, New York, Delacorte Press, 1967.

Benedict, R. G.: Mushroom Toxins Other Than *Amanita*. In *Microbial Toxins, Vol. VIII*, Kadis, S. A., Ceigler, A., and Ajl, S. J., eds., New York, Academic Press, Inc., 1972.

Blohm, H.: *Poisonous Plants of Venezuela*, Cambridge, Harvard University Press, 1962.

Brady, L., and Catalfomo, P.: Mushroom Toxicity and Medical Treatment. In *Mushrooms and Man*. Walters, T., Ed. Albany, Oregon, Linn-Benton Community College, 1977.

Christensen, W. I.: Milk Sickness: A Review of the Literature, Econ. Botany, 19(3):293, 1965.

Der Marderosian, A.: Poisonous Plants In and Around the Home, Am. J. Pharm. Ed., 30(1):115, 1966.

Dreisbach, R. H.: *Handbook of Poisoning*, 9th ed., Los Altos, Lange Medical Publications, 1977.

Everist, S. L.: *Poisonous Plants of Australia*, Sydney, Australia, Angus and Robertson (Publishers) Pty Ltd., 1974.

Evers, R. A., and Link, R. P.: *Poisonous Plants of the Midwest and Their Effects on Livestock*, Special Publ. 24, Urbana-Champaign, University of Illinois, 1972.

Fochtman, F. W., Manno, J. E., Winek, C. L., and Cooper, J. A.: Toxicity of the Genus *Dieffenbachia*, Toxicol. Appl. Pharmacol., 15(1):38, 1969.

Francis, D. F., and Southcott, R. V.: *Plants Harmful to Man in Australia*, Adelaide, Botanic Garden, 1967.

Hardin, J. W., and Arena, J. M.: *Human Poisoning from Native and Cultivated Plants*, 2nd ed., Durham, North Carolina, Duke University Press, 1974.

Hatfield, G. M., and Brady, L. R.: Toxins of Higher Fungi, Lloydia, 38(1):36, 1975.

Howard, R. A., DeWolf, G. P., Jr., and Pride, G. H.: Poisonous Plants, Arnoldia, 34(2):41, 1974.

Keeler, R. F.: Toxins and Teratogens of Higher Plants, Lloydia, 38(1):56, 1975.

Kingsbury, J. M.: *Poisonous Plants of the United States and Canada*, Englewood Cliffs, New Jersey, Prentice-Hall, Inc., 1964.

Kingsbury, J. M.: *Deadly Harvest*, New York, Holt, Rinehart & Winston, 1965.

Lampe, K. F., and Fagerström, R.: *Plant Toxicity and Dermatitis*, Baltimore, The Williams & Wilkins Co., 1968.

Lincoff, G., and Mitchel, D. H.: *Toxic and Hallucinogenic Mushroom Poisoning*. New York, Van Nostrand Reinhold Co., 1977.

McKenny, M., and Stuntz, D. E.: *The Savory Wild Mushroom*, rev. ed., Seattle, University of Washington Press, 1971.

Morton, J. F.: *Plants Poisonous to People*, Miami, Hurricaine House, Publishers, Inc., 1971.

Muenscher, W. C.: *Poisonous Plants of the United States*, New York, The Macmillan Co., 1951.

North, P. M.: *Poisonous Plants and Fungi*, London, Blandford Press, 1967.

O'Leary, S. B.: Poisoning in Man from Eating Poisonous Plants, Arch. Environ. Health, 9(8):216, 1964.

Rumack, B. H., and Salzman, E., eds.: *Mushroom Poisoning: Diagnosis and Treatment*. West Palm Beach, Florida, CRC Press, Inc., 1978.

Schwarting, A. E.: Poisonous Plants. In *Toxicology, Mechanisms and Methods*, Vol. II, Stewart, C. P., and Stolman, A., eds., New York, Academic Press Inc., 1961.

Schwarting, A. E.: Poisonous Seeds and Fruits, Prog. Chem. Toxicol., 1:385, 1963.

Smith, A. H.: *Mushrooms in Their Natural Habitats*, Portland, Oregon, Sawyer's Inc., 1949.

Smith, A. H.: *The Mushroom Hunter's Field Guide*, rev. ed., Ann Arbor, University of Michigan Press, 1971.

Tyler, V. E., Jr.: Poisonous Mushrooms, Prog. Chem. Toxicol., 1:339, 1963.

Walter, W. G.: *Dieffenbachia Toxicity*, JAMA, 201(2):154, 1967.

Watt, J. M., and Breyer-Brandwijk, M. G.: *The Medicinal and Poisonous Plants of Southern and Eastern Africa*, Edinburgh, E. & S. Livingstone, Ltd., 1962.

Wieland, T., and Wieland, O.: The Toxic Peptides of *Amanita* Species. In *Microbial Toxins*, Vol. VIII, Kadis, S. A., Ciegler, A., and Ajl, S. J., eds., New York, Academic Press, Inc., 1972.

Youngken, H. W., Jr., and Karas, J. S.: *Common Poisonous Plants of New England*, Washington, D.C., U.S. Department of Health, Education and Welfare, Public Health Service Publication No. 1220, 1964.

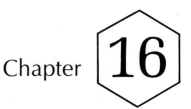

Chapter 16

Herbs and "Health Foods"

LEGALITY OF SALE

Recently, the American public has renewed its interest in the self-treatment of disease states or less-than-optimal health conditions with various products of natural origin which, for reasons to be explained later, are referred to as herbs or "health foods" but not as drugs or medicinal agents. This interest has resulted in the development of a large number of retail outlets and mail-order houses specializing in the distribution of these and related commodities. Their sales amounted to $1.1 billion in 1978. This enormous development took place while most crude vegetable drugs were disappearing from the stocks of pharmacies and from the purview of pharmacists. The causes of this seemingly anomalous situation are found in the laws and regulations that apply to the marketing of drugs in the United States today.

The 1938 Federal Food, Drug, and Cosmetic Act, which had initially required all drugs sold in this country to be proved

safe, was amended in 1962 following an extensive Congressional investigation of the drug industry led by the late Senator Estes Kefauver. The 1962 Drug Amendments (commonly referred to as the Kefauver-Harris Amendments) required that drugs marketed after 1938 be proved both *safe* and *effective*. This requirement led to a new era of drug regulation.

Drugs introduced after 1938 had been proved safe by a procedure known as a New Drug Application (NDA). To determine the effectiveness of such drugs, the Food and Drug Administration (FDA) turned for help in 1962 to the National Academy of Sciences—National Research Council. That group, in turn, organized a "Drug Efficacy Study," which was completed and submitted to the FDA in 1969. Then, in 1972, the FDA proposed an additional review of all drugs available for self-selection by the patient. Only a small number of these over-the-counter (OTC) drugs had been included in the original NAS-NRC study. But the problem, from the regulatory viewpoint, was how to make this review apply to some of the older products that had been "grandfathered" under the 1962 and the 1938 laws because they came under the jurisdiction of the original 1906 Food and Drugs Act. All such drugs were seemingly immune from the "effective" requirement.

The FDA reached these "grandfathered" drugs by what can only be characterized as an extremely innovative application of administrative law. The agency declared that a drug would be considered misbranded if the manufacturer made any claims for it that were not in accord with the findings of 1 of 17 panels set up to review the efficacy of the active ingredients of all OTC drugs. In other words, the drug, even though exempt from proofs of safety and efficacy under existing laws, was barred from commerce if any part of the labeling claimed that the drug was "good" for anything, that is, "effective" for the treatment of a disease state. Substantive evidence of efficacy must be available to permit a labeling claim of therapeutic utility. Statistically designed, clinical, double-blind crossover studies are rarely available to support claims for crude plant materials. The pharmaceutic industry has shown little interest in sponsoring such studies and has not submitted alternate types of supporting data in most cases.

This has led to the curious situation in which essentially all of the old-time plant drugs have been removed from the shelves of pharmacies and from the supervision of knowledgeable pharmacists. Selling drugs that ostensibly have no use violates the ethical code of pharmacists. But such plant drugs have not ceased to be sold or used. Instead they have found their way into the stocks of the retail or mail-order health-food stores where, under the guise of herbs, teas, health foods, food supplements, nutritional products, or the like, they are labeled only with the name of the product. No claim of effectiveness for any condition appears on the label of such containers nor does it appear in any leaflet or advertisement that directly accompanies the drug because that would technically qualify as part of the labeling (Fig. 16–1). Sales staff generally avoid specific recommendations on use of a product to preclude potential charges of unlicensed

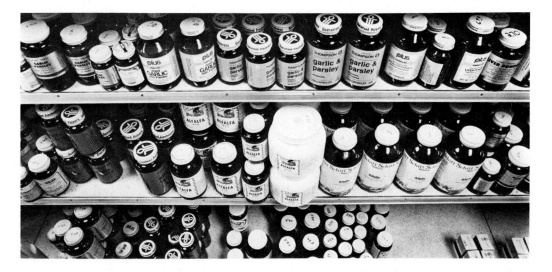

Fig. 16–1. A variety of herbal products in a "health-food" store. (Photo, courtesy of David Umberger.)

practice of medicine. However, if a customer wishes to know the use of a particular drug, the health-food store clerk or mail-order catalog will refer him to a large selection of books, pamphlets, and charts that list the drugs and provide the sought-for information. Some of these information sources are referred to as herbals, or as natural medicine or health-food books; others are devoted to a single drug; and still others employ a therapeutic classification, listing the disease state and describing the products recommended for treatment. In this way, the present laws and regulations requiring that drugs be proved safe and effective are circumvented. The situation encourages the consuming public to become its own medical counsel, a practice of questionable wisdom and acknowledged risk.

At least some of the drugs of natural origin that must, of legal necessity, be sold in this manner are safe and possess useful therapeutic properties. If this is true, why isn't an effort made to satisfy the appropriate federal requirements and to market these products in the normal manner? The answer lies in the economics of such efforts. A prospective pharmaceutic manufacturer or marketer must invest vast sums of money to conduct the tests needed to meet all of the requirements of a New Drug Application. Estimated costs of such exhaustive studies vary, but figures as high as $50 million have been advanced for an individual drug. Because patent protection for the natural drugs is difficult, if not impossible, to obtain, organizations are not willing to make such an investment. This situation is also disappointing because many of the older plant drugs, if investigated by modern methodologies, might yield novel therapeutic agents of considerable utility.

But even more disappointing from the scientific, professional, and economic viewpoints is the quackery that has been fostered by permitting useless and sometimes even dangerous drugs to be sold by nonprofessionals to individuals who hope that their conditions, not alleviated by recognized drugs, will yield to folkloric treatments of unproven value. For this reason alone, although there are many others, the knowledgeable pharmacist of today must have a working knowledge of these questionable herbal and nutritional remedies. The pharmacist must be able to provide as accurate information as possible to patients who, through ignorance or desperation, may be tempted to utilize such products. One must be alert to the need and opportunity to refer a patient for more traditional contemporary health care when indicated, but it is equally important to maintain credibility and lines of communication by avoiding demeaning or categoric "turn off" comments such as "that is old fashioned," "it is worthless," etc.

"NATURAL" AND "ORGANIC"

Before considering these so-called remedies on an individual basis, brief mention must be made of the misuse of the terms "natural" and "organic" when applied especially to certain foods and vitamins touted by their purveyors as superior to those not so categorized. The pharmacy student, because of his understanding of biology and biochemistry, immediately recognizes that there is no difference between, for example, vitamin C obtained from natural biosynthetic processes in rose hips and vitamin C obtained by synthetic processes in the laboratory. Thus, the word "natural," when applied to such materials, identifies only a source and not necessarily a degree of superiority or inferiority. In addition, it usually indicates that the purchaser may expect to pay 2 to 3 times the regular price for items so labeled.

The term, "organic," as commonly

applied to "health foods," implies that the produce was grown under conditions utilizing only natural fertilizers, such as manure, and that no pesticides of any type were applied. Plants cannot differentiate whether nutrients, such as nitrogen or potassium, are derived from organic or inorganic sources, providing they are in a form the plant can assimilate. They respond in the same way to equivalent quantities of each. Certain pesticide residues may pose health hazards if present in sufficient concentrations, but most are removed by proper cleansing, and appropriate limits of safety have been established for the others, e.g., environmental contaminants. Besides, the typical purchaser has absolutely no way of knowing whether the health-food item purchased is "organic" and "natural" as labeled except for the recognition that the seller has probably charged a substantial premium for items so designated. Thus, when used in the ways just defined, such terms are meaningless.

SAFETY AND EFFICACY CONSIDERATIONS

One final topic remains to be considered regarding the kinds of plants and products discussed in this chapter. If many of these products have little or no therapeutic value, and if others are actually harmful if used excessively, why do people insist on using them and why are they willing to pay high prices for such commodities? It is apparent that, in many such instances, certain beneficial effects may actually result owing to the so-called placebo effect, a medication action that is independent of, or minimally related to, the specific effects of the procedure or drug employed. The placebo effect operates through a psychologic mechanism.

Studies have demonstrated that, depending on the condition treated, placebos are effective in about 35% of the patients to whom they are administered. The benefi-

cial effects are most likely to be manifested when the desired end point of therapy is a change in behavior, a subjective sensation, or a response under endocrine or autonomic control. Because the majority of herbs and "health foods" are utilized with the hope of inducing such changes, e.g., to make one "feel better," it is obvious that the desired result will be attained with some frequency. Confidence is also a factor in achieving good response to therapy or medical manipulation, and the selection of plant materials is often based on a long family or ethnic tradition or on the recommendation of a respected friend or relative.

Use of the products does, however, present a number of hazards that must be made clear to any potential purchaser. Some of the products are definitely not safe for human use because they contain carcinogens or other toxic principles. Use of such self-selected nontherapeutic agents may prevent, or at least delay, the patient from seeking and obtaining needed medical treatment for a serious ailment. Because there are no applicable standards of quality, such products often do not consist, either partially or entirely, of the material specified on the label; they are, therefore, frequently misbranded. Even if properly identified from a qualitative viewpoint, they are usually not standardized with respect to the contained concentrations of active constituents. That is, the analytic data that are critical and necessary for informed dosage determination are lacking for plant materials marketed through herb stores. Finally, most of these products are relatively expensive, and their routine use may prove quite costly without resulting in any appreciable benefit to the user. For all of these reasons, prudent persons generally wish to avoid the indiscriminate use of herbs and "health foods."

In the following list, a number of so-called herbs, teas, health foods, food supplements, nutritional products, and the like, are treated monographically. Each will be discussed, in the light of the most recent objective scientific evidence, from the standpoint of its known safety and efficacy as well as from its probable potential therapeutic utility. Many of the value judgments rendered on this basis will vary appreciably from those presented in literature devoted to the promotion of the use of such drugs and related products. One must recognize that there is some degree of rationale for historic or folkloric uses of many plant materials, but their use may have been superseded in medical practice by more potent or effective therapeutic agents.

HERBS AND "HEALTH FOODS"

ALFALFA

The dried leaves, flowering tops, and seeds of *Medicago sativa* Linné (Fam. Leguminosae), commonly known as **alfalfa** or **lucerne,** are said to have stimulating properties when employed in the form of a tea. Alfalfa has been reputed to relieve arthritic conditions and to stimulate the appetite, thereby inducing an increase in weight. There is no reliable scientific evidence that alfalfa has any of these effects in human beings.

ANGELICA

Both the dried fruit and the dried root of *Angelica archangelica* Linné (Fam. Umbelliferae) contain approximately 0.5% of a volatile oil, which accounts for their use as flavoring agents. **Angelica** also has a history of use for a wide variety of medical purposes, including employment as an aromatic stimulant, a bronchial tonic, a carminative, a diaphoretic, a diuretic, an emmenagogue, and a treatment for rheumatism. Any efficacy associated with such

applications would be related presumably to the volatile oil fraction. No active constituent nor any specific pharmacologic response has been documented for angelica, and the plant is believed to lack major therapeutic utility.

APRICOT PITS

Kernels of varieties of *Prunus armeniaca* Linné (Fam. Rosaceae), commonly referred to as **apricot pits,** are sold in "health-food" stores throughout the United States as a source of laetrile or amygdalin, which exists to the extent of about 3%. Technically, laetrile and amygdalin are not synonymous; the former is supposedly (−)-mandelonitrile-β-glucuronoside. However, because the product now offered as an anticancer agent is primarily amygdalin, the 2 names can be used interchangeably.

Controversy of an emotional and political nature has raged in recent years regarding the effectiveness of laetrile in treating cancer patients, particularly those who are terminally ill. Its purported mechanism of action, a selective release of cyanide or a toxic cyanide-containing compound in the cancer cells without injury to other normal cells or tissues, has never been proved. The FDA banned laetrile from interstate commerce in 1971; however, a number of states have since declared that intrastate production and sale are legal. The American Cancer Society takes the position that it "does not have evidence that treatment with Laetrile results in objective benefit in the treatment of cancer in human beings."

Still the controversy continues, largely owing to the innate human desire to cure something that, at present, is incurable. Because of the federal ban, pure amygdalin for drug purposes is not readily available in the United States. As a consequence, patients have turned to the acquisition and use of apricot kernels as a source of a drug. This is a dangerous practice for, in addition to the amygdalin, the pits contain emulsin, an enzyme that hydrolyzes the glycoside, releasing toxic cyanide as detailed on page 70. Deaths have been reported from the ingestion of apricot pits. Although the emulsin may be inactivated by heating, complete inactivation is always uncertain. Even if inactivation is accomplished, the user may not realize that other sources of emulsin, e.g., almonds, must be avoided. Further, evidence now obtained from small-animal experimentation indicates that amygdalin alone, without the action of exogenous β-glycosidases, causes cyanide toxicity.

Because the treatment is doubtful and carries considerable potential danger, the use of apricot pits as an anticancer drug must be considered irrational. Failing proof of laetrile's efficacy and safety, its use should be avoided.

ARNICA

An alcoholic extract or tincture of **arnica,** the dried flowering heads of *Arnica montana* Linné and related *Arnica* species (Fam. Compositae), has been used widely as a counterirritant in the treatment of abrasions, bruises, and sprains. Small amounts of the extract have also been used to treat inflammation of the gums and as a gargle/mouthwash for sore throats. The plant material contains constituents with antibacterial properties, but its topical utility is attributed to 2 isomeric dihydric alcohols, arnidiol and faradiol, which act as irritants. Arnica extract can be toxic if ingested; unnecessary risks are associated with a continuation of the old European folkloric practice of using such a preparation internally for cardiac and circulatory purposes.

BLACK COHOSH

Black cohosh is the dried rhizome and roots of *Cimicifuga racemosa* (Linné) Nuttall (Fam. Ranunculaceae). The plant material has been used as an ingredient in bitter tonics to treat indigestion and loss of appetite, but its most common use has been related to its folkloric reputation for curing dysmenorrhea. It is also claimed to have value in treating bronchitis, coughs, and chronic rheumatism.

The drug contains 15 to 20% of resin, a bitter principle, saponins, and other glycosidic constituents, but knowledge of the chemical composition of black cohosh is incomplete. No pharmacologic evidence supports any therapeutic use of the plant material. Toxic reactions, including bradycardia, tremors, and vertigo, have followed ingestion of preparations that contain black cohosh. Prudence dictates that neither the drug nor preparations containing it should be consumed.

BLESSED THISTLE

Blessed thistle, the dried overground portion of *Cnicus benedictus*Linné (Fam. Compositae), contains cnicin, a bitter diterpenoid lactone. The plant material still finds limited use as a bitter tonic for appetite stimulation and for relief of flatulence and indigestion. It also has an old reputation of use in diseases of the liver and gallbladder, but no acceptable scientific evidence supports any therapeutic value for this plant.

BLUE VERVAIN

Blue vervain or wild hyssop is the dried tops of *Verbena hastata* Linné (Fam. Verbenaceae). The bitter-tasting material has been used as a diaphoretic, emmenagogue, expectorant, tonic, and tranquilizer. It contains verbenalin, a glucoside with weak parasympathomimetic activity. The plant material is nauseating when ingested in quantity and lacks practical therapeutic utility.

BONESET

Use of the bitter-tasting dried leaves and flowering tops of *Eupatorium perfoliatum* Linné (Fam. Compositae) or **boneset** was introduced to settlers by the American Indians. The plant material was once considered a panacea. Most uses were related to the diaphoretic response obtained on ingestion of a cupful of an infusion or tea prepared from a small amount of the material (2 to 4 g). The plant also has a laxative action and is an emetic in large doses.

Boneset is currently considered to lack therapeutic merit, and the discomfort associated with its ingestion obviates any use for nutritional purposes. The plant, although incompletely characterized chemically, is reported to contain eupatorin, a triterpenic saponin.

BORAGE

Borage, the dried leaves of *Borago officinalis* Linné (Fam. Boraginaceae), has an extensive folkloric reputation as a source of emotional courage and as a cure for melancholy. An infusion of the plant material (4 g) has been recommended for internal use as a demulcent, a diaphoretic, a diuretic, and an emollient; a poultice of fresh leaves is allegedly useful in treating inflammations. However, borage has no recognized therapeutic utility in modern medicine.

BRAN

Bran consists of the coarse outer coat or hull of the grain of wheat, *Triticum aestivum* Linné (Fam. Gramineae). Techni-cally, it comprises the pericarp, the integuments, and the nucellus of the seed. The product is valued in human nutrition for its high content of dietary fiber, that is, the food ingested by a monogastric animal that reaches the large intestine virtually unchanged. One series of analyses revealed 26.7% of dietary fiber in bran; in comparison, canned baked beans had 7.27%, boiled carrots 3.70%, and whole peaches 2.28%. The average American's diet provides a total of 2 to 5 g of fiber per day.

There is considerable evidence of an epidemiologic, clinical, and experimental nature that suggests that various disorders of the gastrointestinal tract are linked to inadequate dietary fiber intake. These conditions range from constipation and diverticulitis to tumors of the colon and rectum, and they include such seemingly unrelated problems as cardiovascular and gallbladder disease. The salubrious effects of sufficient amounts of bran or other sources of crude fiber in the diet are apparently due not only to its water-holding capacity, but also to its ability to adsorb such compounds as bile acids. This ability, in turn, modifies cholesterol metabolism.

The therapeutic value of bran (crude fiber) seems obvious, at least in the treatment of certain gastrointestinal disorders, such as constipation, appendicitis, and hemorrhoids. It has also brought about recent modifications in the recommended treatment of such conditions as ulcerative colitis and colonic diverticulosis. Preventive aspects of high-fiber diets for gastrointestinal and cardiovascular disorders are more speculative.

Some authorities now recommend that bran or other appropriate foods be included in the diet in sufficient amounts to provide 10 g of dietary fiber daily. This would be supplied by 2 to 4 tablespoons of natural unprocessed bran or one-half cup of All-Bran® cereal.

BROOM

The dried tops of *Cytisus scoparius* (Linné) Link (Fam. Leguminosae) are known as **broom or Scotch broom.** The plant contains up to 1.5% of sparteine as well as lesser quantities of cytisine and other alkaloids. Broom has a long history of use as a cardiac remedy, a cathartic, and a diuretic. The moldy, dried blossoms have recently gained a reputation as a hallucinogen when smoked.

Sparteine has been used therapeutically for its depressant action in cardiac arrhythmias and for its oxytocic effect. The therapeutic use of sparteine for cardiac irregularities ceased a number of years ago owing to the availability of better drugs. FDA approval for use of this alkaloid as an oxytocic was withdrawn in late 1978 because of an unfavorable benefit-to-risk ratio. Broom is not safe for self-medication.

BUCHU

Buchu is the dried leaves of *Barosma betulina* (Thunberg) Bartling et Wendland, *B. crenulata* (Linné) Hooker, or *B. serratifolia* (Curtis) Willdenow (Fam. Rutaceae). The plant material contains diosmin, a flavonoid glycoside, and a volatile oil. Diosphenol, a phenolic ketone, is the principal constituent of the volatile oil (see page 127).

The plants are indigenous to South Africa, and their medicinal use was introduced into Europe early in the nineteenth century. Although buchu functions as a diuretic and as a weak urinary antiseptic, more effective drugs are indicated for most conditions requiring these properties.

BURDOCK

Burdock or lappa, the dried first-year root of *Arctium lappa* Linné (Fam. Compositae), lacks known physiologically ac-

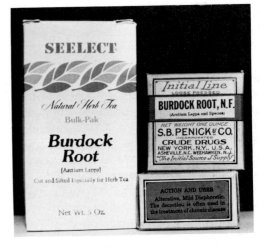

Fig. 16–2. Typical new (left) and old (right) packages of burdock root. (Photo, courtesy of Kathy Delvecchio.)

tive constituents, but it has had many uses in folk medicine. It has been used as a diuretic, diaphoretic, childbirth aid, and alterative for treatment of gout, rheumatism, and syphilitic disorders. Preparations of the root have also been used to stimulate hair growth and to treat chronic skin conditions, such as dandruff and psoriasis. No substantive evidence supports any of these historic uses. Burdock root currently enjoys some popularity as an herbal tea (Fig. 16–2).

CANAIGRE

In recent years, certain herb marketers have attempted to promote the sale of **canaigre,** the root of *Rumex hymenosepalus* Torrey, by labeling it as "wild red American ginseng" or "wild red desert ginseng." This plant, a member of the family Polygonaceae and native to the arid regions of Texas and Mexico, bears no botanic relationship to ginseng, which is classified in the family Araliaceae. No evidence for the presence in canaigre of active panaxosidelike saponin glycosides, such as occur in ginseng, has ever been obtained. Instead, the root contains 30 to 45% of tannins in addition to anthraquinones.

The medicinal uses of canaigre by Indians in the southwestern states and in Mexico relate to the root's astringent properties. They include topical use for skin irritations, treatment of sore throat, and prevention of diarrhea. No tonic, stress-relieving, or other adaptogenic properties of canaigre have been reported. Application of the name "ginseng" to canaigre is of recent origin.

As a result of an investigation conducted in 1978, the Herb Trade Association adopted a policy stating that any herb products consisting in whole or in part of *Rumex hymenosepalus* should not be labeled as containing ginseng. Although this action was directed toward solving a nomenclatural problem and did not deal with the relative benefits or risks of using canaigre, it is important to note the carcinogenic potential of the plant owing to its high tannin content. Canaigre may be a useful material for tanning leather and dying wool, but at present, it has no established place in therapeutics.

CATNIP

Catnip consists of the dried leaves and flowering tops of *Nepeta cataria* Linné (Fam. Labiatae), a perennial herb common in the United States. It was formerly an official drug in the *National Formulary* but was found lacking in therapeutic activity, excepting that of a mild aromatic, and was therefore deleted from that compendium. Many persons continued to employ catnip as a pleasant-tasting tea.

A resurgence of interest in the herb occurred recently when it was reported that smoking catnip, either by itself or in combination with tobacco, induced a mild euphoria. Apparently, the psychedelic effects are so mild that users question whether they occur at all. One recent volume on drugs of abuse starts its discussion of catnip with the words, "Does it or doesn't it?" The book indicates that a debate has continued for many years as to whether one can actually get "high" by using the herb. Any drug whose physiologic effects in human beings are as questionable as those of catnip is scarcely worth considering for any purpose.

CHAMOMILE

The dried flower heads of *Matricaria chamomilla* Linné (Fam. Compositae) constitute the drug known as **German chamomile** or **matricaria** (Fig. 16–3). A related plant, *Anthemis nobilis* Linné, known as **Roman chamomile,** contains

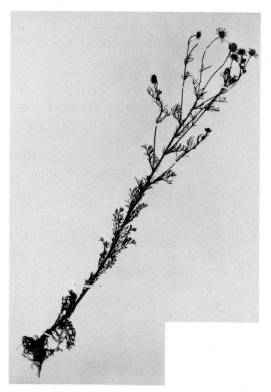

Fig. 16–3. Herbarium specimen of German chamomile *(Matricaria chamomilla).*

similar constituents and is similarly employed. Chamomile is extensively cultivated in Europe where it is widely utilized in folk medicine for its carminative, spasmolytic, and anti-inflammatory effects. The most common form of the drug is a tea, but various extracts and volatile-oil-containing preparations are also available. In fact, chamomile is so highly regarded and so extensively used that it might be labeled the "ginseng" of Europe. Recently, chamomile has become one of the most popular herbal teas in the United States.

One group of persons should be especially cautious in utilizing chamomile. The tea, prepared from pollen-rich flower heads, has caused contact dermatitis, anaphylaxis, and other severe hypersensitivity reactions in individuals allergic to ragweeds, asters, chrysanthemums, and similar plants. In fact, persons allergic to any member of the family Compositae should avoid this as well as other teas prepared from composite flower heads.

As might be expected, such a renowned plant has been the subject of a large number of botanic, agronomic, chemical, and pharmacologic studies. In essence, the latter have revealed definite anti-inflammatory properties in chamomile, owing primarily to constituents of (or formed in) the volatile oil, especially chamazulene and $(-)$-α-bisabolol. Flavonoids and coumarin derivatives are, without doubt, responsible for most of the spasmolytic effects. Various other effects of the drug are probably caused by these and other undetermined constituents.

Unfortunately, an infusion (tea) contains only about 10 to 15% of the volatile oil present in the plant material, and the ingredients in the volatile oil provide most of the anti-inflammatory activity. Whole plant extracts or preparations containing quantities of the volatile oil are certainly much more effective. In spite of the relatively low concentrations of lipid-soluble active ingredients in the tea, one authority believes that, when the tea is used over a long period of time, a cumulative beneficial effect may result. This belief is attested to by the centuries-old use of chamomile as a home remedy and healthful beverage in Europe and by its increasing popularity for these purposes among the laity in the United States.

CHAPARRAL

Chaparral is a relatively ambiguous term that refers to a number of low shrubby plants growing wild in the arid regions of the southwestern United States and Mexico. As currently employed in "health-food" circles, the name designates the leaflets of Larrea tridentata (De Candolle) Coville (Fam. Zygophyllaceae), a plant more properly referred to by the common name, creosote bush. It is a strongly scented, olive-green bush that may attain a height of more than 3 meters. It grows from California to Texas and in Mexico.

The drug has been employed in the treatment of bronchitis and similar conditions related to the common cold. It is also said to be useful in the alleviation of rheumatic pain. Chaparral does not contain active principles known to be safe and effective in the treatment of either of these ailments. The leaflets do yield up to 20% of a resin that is an effective antioxidant because of the presence of an appreciable quantity of nordihydroguaiaretic acid.

CHICORY

Chicory, the dried rhizome and roots of Cichorium intybus Linné (Fam. Compositae), is probably best known as an additive that enhances the bitterness, color, and body of coffee. It also has a history of use as a diuretic, laxative, and tonic and as a treatment for gallstones, hepatic disorders, and indigestion. Chicory contains the bitter sesquiterpenoid lactones, lactucin and lactucopikrin, as well as cichoriin (a coumarin glucoside), maltol (a simple pyrone), and taraxasterin (a triterpene).

The crude drug has no recognized therapeutic utility, but maltol, a constituent that also occurs in roasted malt and several other plant materials, has the potentially useful property of intensifying the sweetness of sugar.

COCILLANA

Cocillana is the dried bark of *Guarea rusbyi* (Britton) Rusby (Fam. Meliaceae). It is obtained from a tree indigenous to the Bolivian Andes where the bark is employed by natives for its cathartic and emetic properties. The plant material was used medicinally as a nauseating expectorant in some cough syrups, but the use of this ingredient has been discontinued.

COLLINSONIA

Collinsonia or stoneroot is the dried rhizome and roots of *Collinsonia canadensis* Linné (Fam. Labiatae). The plant material, which contains mucilage, resin, and tannin, has been used as an astringent, a diuretic, a diaphoretic, and a tonic. It is still used as an ingredient in a hemorrhoidal product, but therapeutic merit of the plant material is questionable.

COLTSFOOT

Farfara or coltsfoot may consist either of the dried flower heads or of the leaves of the plant *Tussilago farfara* Linné (Fam. Compositae). Curiously, the flowers develop first, and the broad leaves begin to appear only after the flowers have withered. Both parts of the plant contain large quantities of mucilage, which accounts for their popular use as demulcents and expectorants, particularly in the treatment of coughs.

Recent studies have shown that the young flowers of the plant are carcinogenic, producing a high incidence of hemangioendothelial sarcoma of the liver when fed to rats. The probable causative agent is senkirkine, a hepatotoxic pyrrolizidine alkaloid. Although the alkaloid was identified only in coltsfoot flowers, the only part studied for carcinogenicity, it probably occurs in leaves as well (such is the case in a closely related plant, *Senecio kirkii* Hooker filius). The ingestion of any portion of the coltsfoot plant as an herbal remedy is highly inadvisable.

COMFREY

Symphytum officinale Linné (Fam. Boraginaceae) or **comfrey** is an ancient herbal remedy with a reputation as a cure for ulcerations of the external and internal organs following topical or systemic administration. The healing action of the rhizome, roots, and leaves has been attributed to their allantoin content, which ranges from 0.6 to 1% in the underground parts but exists only in traces in the leaves. At the present time, comfrey is one of the most common herbal teas sold to the American public (Fig. 16–4).

Unfortunately, at least some specimens of the plant also contain a number of pyrrolizidine alkaloids that are highly hepatotoxic. One of these alkaloids, lasiocarpine, has produced liver cancer in rodents fed diets containing only 50 ppm of the alkaloid. Additional studies incorporating 0.5% comfrey leaves in the feed of rodents produced malignant tumors of the liver and bladder. Based on these findings, the herb definitely cannot be recommended as a medicinal agent and, indeed, possesses considerable likelihood of causing harmful effects in those utilizing it in-

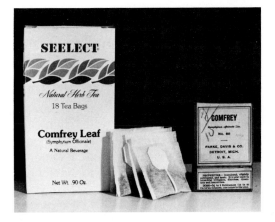

Fig. 16–4. New (left) and old (right) packages of comfrey. (Photo, courtesy of Kathy Delvecchio.)

ternally. In addition, deaths have been reported among amateur herb collectors who confused comfrey with digitalis (*Digitalis purpurea*) and mistakenly drank teas brewed from leaves of the latter species.

CUCURBITA SEED

The seed of various *Cucurbita* species (Fam. Cucurbitaceae), especially that of *C. pepo* Linné (pumpkin and summer squash), *C. maxima* Duchesne (Hubbard, Turban, Marblehead, and Sibley squashes), and *C. moschata* Duchesne (crookneck and China squashes), has been widely employed as a relatively effective teniafuge. Ordinarily, a beverage prepared from at least 60 g of **cucurbita seed** is administered in divided doses; however, some authorities recommend a total dose of as much as 500 g.

An unusual amino acid, 3-amino-3-carboxypyrrolidine (cucurbitin), found only in the seeds of certain *Cucurbita* species, is the active principle. The fact that a relatively large dose is required and the finding that the cucurbitin content is quite variable even within seeds of the

same species probably explain certain literature reports of the lack of effectiveness of cucurbita seed as a teniafuge. Toxicity or other adverse side effects from this drug have apparently not been reported.

DAMIANA

Damiana consists of the leaves of the subtropical shrub *Turnera diffusa* Willdenow var. *aphrodisiaca* Urban (Fam. Turneraceae) native to the southern United States and Mexico. The drug is said to have been highly regarded as an aphrodisiac by the ancient Aztecs. At the turn of the century, various proprietary damiana preparations were marketed in the United States, but their physiologic activity was probably caused by their high ethanol content (usually 50%) or by the addition of other drugs, such as coca. One such preparation, Nyal's Compound Extract of Damiana, contained all of these ingredients plus nux vomica and phosphorus. Damiana was listed in the *National Formulary* until 1946.

Modern popular writers on drugs indicate that ingesting an infusion of damiana or alternatively smoking the leaves produces in the user a feeling of euphoria, characterized by relaxation and increased imagination. These reactions are said to be especially pronounced in women. It is stated that excessive use of the drug is deleterious to the liver. A damiana-containing cordial is produced in Mexico, but it is believed to contain too little of the drug to produce any physiologic effects.

Chemical studies of damiana have resulted in the isolation of 0.2 to 0.9% of a volatile oil, some of the constituents of which have been characterized, in addition to resin, tannins, gum, etc. The report of the presence of caffeine in the drug requires verification. No principle responsible for the purported activity of damiana as an aphrodisiac has been identified nor have any scientific studies of the drug's physiologic effects been reported. Until this information is obtained, there is no proper basis for its use by human beings.

DEVIL'S CLAW

The secondary storage roots of *Harpagophytum procumbens* DeCandolle, a South African plant belonging to the family Pedaliaceae, are now widely sold in both Europe and the United States under the name **Devil's Claw** (Fig. 16–5). An aqueous extract (infusion or decoction) is recommended in the treatment of a large number of conditions, particularly rheumatism. The anti-inflammatory effects of the drug have been attributed to 3 iridiod glycosides—harpagoside, harpagide, and procumbide.

Pharmacologic tests in small animals

and clinical studies in human beings conducted in Europe have reported that devil's claw possesses an anti-inflammatory and analgesic activity comparable to that of phenylbutazone. The clinical trials also revealed that the plant reduced elevated cholesterol and uric acid levels in the subjects. These promising findings have not been verified in this country, and devil's claw has not been approved (that is, proved safe and effective) for medicinal use in the United States.

The allegation that devil's claw possesses oxytocic properties requires verification. It apparently is based on a misinterpretation of statements by Watt and Breyer-Brandwijk that indicate that the drug is used by African natives to alleviate pain in pregnant women and especially in those anticipating a difficult delivery.

ECHINACEA

As used in the United States, the terms **echinacea, cone flower, and purple cone flower** refer to the dried rhizome and roots of *Echinacea angustifolia* De Candolle (*E. pallida* Nuttall). This plant is a perennial herb of the family Compositae and is native to the midwestern states. In Europe, the entire fresh, flowering plant is employed medicinally as is another species, *E. purpurea* (Linné) Moench. Both species are said to have the same properties.

Echinacea was introduced into American medicine in 1885 by Dr. H. C. F. Meyer, who recommended it as a "blood purifier." He probably gained his knowledge of the plant from the early settlers and the Indians. Both groups valued it highly as a remedy against various types of infections, in treating bites of poisonous reptiles and insects, as a palliative agent in malignant conditions, and for its wound-healing properties. The drug continues to be used in this country as a folk medicine in the treatment of these same conditions, but

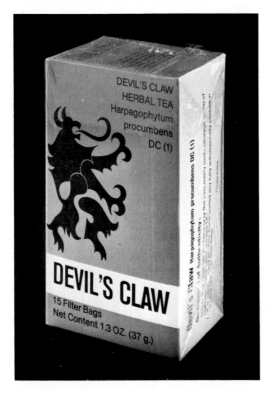

Fig. 16–5. A package of devil's claw tea bags.

particularly to increase resistance to infections. Echinacea is taken either in powdered form, as an infusion or decoction, or as an alcoholic tincture or extract. In Europe, it is used primarily in lotions and cosmetics for its wound-healing action.

The bacteriostatic principle, echinacoside, a caffeic acid glycoside, has been isolated from the drug. Echinacea's wound-healing effects are attributed to a polysaccharide, echinacin B, which apparently forms a complex with hyaluronic acid that is resistant to attack by hyaluronidase. A hydrocarbon obtained from the root oil, (Z)-1,8-pentadecadiene, possesses in vivo antitumor activity. However, neither these nor any of the other numerous constituents that have been identified in echinacea may be said to account for its folkloric reputation as a truly outstanding medicinal agent. Further research is required to determine the therapeutic value of this drug and the chemical identity of its active constituents.

ELEUTHERO

Acanthopanax senticosus (Ruprecht et Maximowicz) Harms, also known as *Eleutherococcus senticosus* Maximowicz (Fam. Araliaceae), is a tall shrub native to eastern Siberia, Korea, and the Shansi and Hopei Provinces of China. It yields the drug known as **eleuthero** or **Siberian ginseng.** Apparently, eleuthero consists of the root of the plant, and most of the chemical studies have been devoted to that morphologic part, although the leaves, indeed the entire plant, may be employed. It is not always possible to determine which parts are actually used because the whole drug is not ordinarily an article of commerce; an extract is usually exported from the Soviet Union or from China.

Eleuthero, like ginseng, is a member of the family Araliaceae. It also contains a series of saponin glycosides, known in this case as eleutherosides, which accounts for its reputation as an adaptogen or antistress agent. The stimulant and tonic effects of eleuthero are said to be greater and longer acting than those of ginseng. This may, however, be related to the lesser variation in its concentration of active principles, at least in comparison to the extremely variable ginseng. One author believes that the enthusiasm shown for the drug in the Soviet Union is owing to its great abundance and ready availability there.

Because the commercial form of eleuthero is a powder (variously described as root or bark) that is either sold as such or as capsules, the extract is apparently mixed with a suitable diluent prior to marketing in the United States. The caveats expressed in the subsequent discussion of ginseng also apply to this drug. Lack of standardization, relatively high cost, the potential of an abuse syndrome with such saponin-containing natural products, and unproven clinical effects in human beings all militate against the indiscriminate medicinal use of eleuthero.

EYEBRIGHT

Eyebright or the dried flowering tops of *Euphasia officinalis* Linné (Fam. Scrophulariaceae) has a popular reputation for use in various eye conditions, including black eyes, blepharitis, conjunctivitis, eye strain, and styes. It has also been used in the treatment of hay fever. The plant contains a tannin that could conceivably be beneficial, but the material is generally acknowledged as lacking therapeutic merit.

FENUGREEK

Fenugreek consists of the dried ripe seeds of *Trigonella foenumgraecum* Linné (Fam. Leguminosae). The plant has hypoglycemic properties and, in addition, has been used as a demulcent, an emollient, and a treatment for indigestion. Originally, fenugreek was the principal ingredient, other than alcohol, in the well-known proprietary remedy, Lydia Pinkham's Vegetable Compound. Fenugreek contains trigonelline and a mucilagenous hydrocolloid. Although the seeds are not recognized as useful in the therapeutic control of hypoglycemia, they are employed as a flavoring agent in imitation maple syrup and as a poultice and an emollient in veterinary practice.

FO-TI-TIENG®

Fo-ti-tieng® is said to consist of a mixture of the leaves and stems of *Centella asiatica* (Linné) Urban var. *minor* (Fam. Umbelliferae), meadowsweet, and cola nut. Meadowsweet, in this instance, refers to the plant *Gillenia trifoliata* (Linné) Moench (Fam. Rosaceae) and cola (kola) is the dried cotyledon of *Cola nitida* (Ventenot) Schott et Endlicher (Fam. Sterculiaceae) or related species. Apparently, little kola is contained in the mixture, which consists mainly of a diminutive variety of the tropical plant that yields gotu kola (q.v.). The name Fo-ti-tieng® is a registered trademark. It should not be confused with fo-ti, an entirely different drug derived from *Polygonum multiflorum* Thunberg (Fam. Polygonaceae).

Advocates maintain that the drug contains vitamin X, a principle alleged to exert a marvelous rejuvenating effect on the brain cells and endocrine glands. Supposedly, the regular use of Fo-ti-tieng® permitted a Chinese herbalist to live 256 years, surviving 23 wives in the process.

The active constituents of Fo-ti-tieng® are probably identical to those of gotu kola. They confer some sedative, anti-inflammatory, and wound-healing activities on the drug. No scientific evidence supports the allegations that Fo-ti-tieng® promotes

longevity nor has its safety or efficacy been documented.

GARLIC AND ONION

An appreciable body of folklore and a much smaller amount of scientific evidence indicate that the ingestion of relatively large quantities of the bulbs of **garlic** (*Allium sativum* Linné) or of **onion** (*Allium cepa* Linné), both members of the family Liliaceae, results in a variety of physiologic effects, including stimulation of bile production, lowering of blood sugar and blood lipids, reduction of hypertension, acceleration of wound healing, and curing of the common cold. Recent controlled studies in human beings showed that those persons on a garlic- and onion-free vegetarian diet or on a diet involving the consumption of only small amounts of those foods (less than 10 g of garlic and 200 g of onion per week) had significantly higher serum triglycerides and *beta* lipoproteins than those eating more than 600 g of onion and 50 g of garlic per week.

Chemical studies long ago revealed the presence of a potent antibacterial principle in garlic. This principle, designated allicin, was diallyldisulfide-S-oxide. Unfortunately, it is also the compound responsible for the characteristic odor of garlic, decomposing readily in the presence of air and water to yield diallyldisulfide and other similar odorous sulfides. Recently, prostaglandin A_1, which has a hypotensive action on injection, was isolated from onions. This was the first reported occurrence of prostaglandins in higher plants and may facilitate our eventual understanding of the physiologic activity long attributed to this species.

Further chemical and pharmacologic research is needed to determine the real value of garlic and onion for the many conditions in which they are reputed to be effective. The isolation of a potent prostaglandin from onion further supports the speculation that both of these closely related species possess considerable potential value as therapeutic agents.

GENTIAN

Gentian or gentian root is the dried rhizome and roots of *Gentiana lutea* Linné (Fam. Gentianaceae), a plant indigenous to central and southern Europe and to Asia Minor. Commonly used as a medicine in the Middle Ages, gentian has been employed in modern times as a bitter tonic in anorexia and dyspepsia. Its current popularity in the United States is limited, but it is still widely used in Europe as an ingredient in alcoholic beverages valued for their stomachic properties.

High-quality gentian (yellowish brown to yellowish orange internal color) contains about 2% of gentiopicrin, a bitter glucoside. Slow drying of the root permits enzymatic hydrolysis of gentiopicrin and yields a darker reddish brown product that is inferior for use as a medicinal bitter.

GINSENG

Ginseng is the root of the perennial herbs *Panax quinquefolius* Linné and *Panax pseudoginseng* Wallich (*P. ginseng* C. A. Mey, *P. shinseng* Nees) (Fam. Araliaceae). The former grows in rich woods in the eastern United States and Canada, and the latter is indigenous to the mountainous forests of eastern Asia. The roots are gathered from 3- to 6-year-old plants and carefully cleaned and dried (Fig. 16–6).

Over 350,000 pounds of ginseng, valued at more than $25 million, were exported from the United States in 1978. Most of the drug was shipped to Hong Kong.

American ginseng has been collected from wild plants and from cultivated stands and has been exported to China

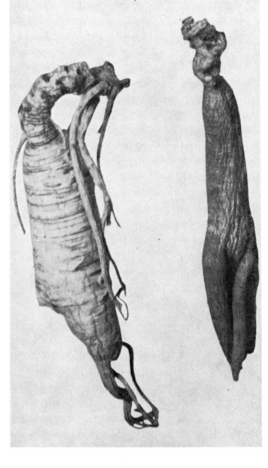

Fig. 16–6. Tuberous root of ginseng. The root on the left is a fresh specimen and was grown in the United States. The root on the right was purchased at a Chinese bazaar. It is translucent, yellowish brown, and has the characteristic shape and markings considered desirable by the Chinese. The markings on the upper segment of the specimen are stem-scars and are usually found on old roots. The translucent appearance is caused by the manner of treatment.

since the early 1700s. A ship sailed from Boston for China in 1773 with 55 tons of ginseng. The plant is now an endangered species in the United States. Its collection and sale are subject to registration, permits, reports, and an official ginseng season. Collector education is also mandatory. Cultivated ginseng is produced in

Korea, Japan, the Soviet Union, and the United States, primarily in Wisconsin.

Ginseng contains a complex mixture of triterpenoid saponins. These glycosides have been categorized into 3 series, the panaxosides, the ginsenosides, and the chikusetsusaponins. One or more of these groups of glycosides appear to account for the biologic properties of ginseng.

Ginseng is a favorite remedy in Chinese medicine and is considered to have tonic, stimulant, diuretic, and carminative properties. It reportedly reduces the blood sugar concentration and acts favorably on metabolism, the central nervous system, and the endocrine secretion. It is employed in the Orient in the treatment of anemia, diabetes, insomnia, neurasthenia, gastritis, and, especially, sexual impotence.

Recently, Western interest in the drug has vastly increased, and ginseng has become widely available in "health-food" outlets. Indeed, it is estimated that, at present, 5 to 6 million people use the herb in the United States alone. Such widespread use has been accompanied by a veritable deluge of literature pertaining to the product and its purported activity.

Pharmacologically speaking, ginseng is classified as an adaptogen because some studies in animals suggest that it may help the body to adapt to stress and to correct adrenal and thyroid dysfunctions. Such effects, if real, are quite subtle, but are apparently a function of the panaxoside saponin glycosides contained in the root. Ginseng is also heavily promoted as an aphrodisiac. The drug is administered in such forms as powders, extracts, and teas, usually in quantities ranging up to 15 g of root per day but averaging about 3 g.

Because of the relatively high cost of ginseng products and almost total lack of quality control in the "health-food" industry, studies recently performed have shown great variations in the panaxoside glycoside content of various preparations. Indeed, 60% of the products in one sampling were judged "worthless," and 25% of those sampled contained no ginseng whatsoever.

Perhaps even more disturbing, however, have been the results of some preliminary studies that seem to point to a definite ginseng-abuse syndrome in human beings utilizing the drug. Long-term use was associated with hypertension, nervousness, and sleeplessness in some subjects, but had the opposite effects, hypotension and a tranquilizing effect, in others. These apparently contradictory findings may result from products containing different quantities of the various active glycosides.

Taken as a whole, the symptoms observed in ginseng abuse mimic those of corticosteroid poisoning, suggesting a steroid mechanism of action operating through the adrenal cortex or the pituitary gland. Although the effects are neither uniformly negative nor uniformly predictable, long-term ingestion of large amounts of ginseng should be avoided. In addition, the FDA found no evidence of enhanced sexual experience or potency resulting from its use.

GLYCYRRHIZA

Glycyrrhiza or licorice (see page 68) has a long history of folkloric use for a wide variety of purposes. Some of these applications evolved into the medicinal use of licorice extracts in products for treating coughs and colds. Other uses are consistent with scientific evidence that suggests therapeutic potential in treating some inflammatory conditions and peptic ulcers, but many of the alleged benefits of this plant material as a cure-all have no basis in fact. Glycyrrhiza is distinct from anise and other anethole-containing plant materials that have a licoricelike flavor.

GOLDENSEAL

Goldenseal is the dried rhizome and roots of *Hydrastis canadensis* Linné (Fam. Ranunculaceae). It has been used to soothe inflamed eyes and mucous membranes and as a hemostatic in intestinal and uterine bleeding, a uterine stimulant, and a vasoconstrictor. The plant contains berberine and hydrastine; these alkaloids are astringents and have weak antibiotic properties (see page 223).

Medicinal uses of goldenseal have been discontinued except for the use of berberine in eye washes. Some heroin addicts undergoing treatment in methadone programs have claimed that goldenseal, used as an herbal tea, impairs the detection of morphine in the urine. Scientific studies have shown that this allegation is totally false. The plant material neither obscures the analysis of morphine nor does it facilitate urinary excretion of that alkaloid.

GOTU KOLA

The leaves and stems of *Centella asiatica* (Linné) Urban (Fam. Umbelliferae) constitute the drug known as **gotu kola.** It is also referred to in the literature as **hydrocotyle** and **indian pennywort.** Native to the warmer regions of both hemispheres, this slender, creeping plant is especially abundant in the swampy areas of India and Sri Lanka, in South Africa, and in the tropical regions of the New World. In addition to its use as a diuretic, as a "blood purifier," in promoting the healing of skin conditions, and in treating leprosy, gotu kola has been promoted as a body strengthener and revitalizer that can promote longevity. It is widely sold for this latter purpose.

Studies have shown that in large doses the drug has a definite sedative effect that resides in 2 saponin glycosides, brahmoside and brahminoside. Another glycoside, madecassoside, exhibits anti-inflammatory activity, and still another, asiaticoside, exerts a wound-healing action by stimulating mitosis. As yet, no evidence supports the use of gotu kola as a longevity promoter, nor does any substantive data exist on its safety or efficacy.

Common names often cause nomenclatural difficulties; the kola portion of the appellation gotu kola has caused some writers to confuse this drug with kolanuts, the dried cotyledon of *Cola nitida* (see page 257). The 2 drugs are not related. Caffeine, the active constituent of kolanuts, has not been identified in gotu kola.

HAWTHORN

Dried flowers, fruits, leaves, and twigs of *Crataegus monogyna* Jacquin and related *Crataegus* species (Fam. Rosaceae) have been used in folk medicine since the Middle Ages. **Hawthorn** currently has no recognized medicinal application in the United States, but therapeutic use of an extract of the flowers or of powdered fruits has increased in Europe during the last 25 years. The plant product has a slow onset of action. It acts on cardiac or circulatory problems by causing dilation of blood vessels, especially the coronary arteries, and by causing some reduction in blood pressure; it is used prophylactically in angina pectoris. Claims of digitalislike or cardiotonic activity are apparently false. Toxicity from ingestion of hawthorn preparations is uncommon and is associated only with high doses.

Hawthorn contains neither cardiotonic glycosides nor alkaloids. It does contain a number of saponins, the aglycones of which are triterpenic acids, and it is rich in flavonoid glycosides. The flavonoid glycosides are thought to be the active constituents.

Angina pectoris and hypertension are serious conditions not readily amenable to self-treatment. The use of hawthorn or any other drug for therapeutic treatment of such serious ailments should be undertaken only on the advice of a physician.

HEDGE HYSSOP

Hedge hyssop, the dried tops of *Gratiola officinalis* Linné (Fam. Scrophulariaceae), has a long history of use as a cathartic, diuretic, and emetic. Although it is still employed in folk medicine for treatment of chronic ailments of the liver and spleen, no scientific evidence supports its effectiveness. The known constituents of the plant include betulinic acid, a triterpenic acid, and gratiolin, a triterpenic saponin.

HIBISCUS

The dried, dark-red flowers of *Hibiscus sabdariffa* Linné (Fam. Malvaceae) are infused to prepare **hibiscus** or **Sudanese tea.** Relatively large concentrations of oxalic, malic, citric, tartaric, and hibiscic acid (the lactone of hydroxycitric acid) are present in the flowers. They impart to the beverage a refreshing aromatic taste and a mild laxative action.

HONEY

Honey or mel is a saccharine secretion deposited in the honeycomb by the bee, *Apis mellifera* Linné (Fam. Apidae). Dextrose and fructose, in equimolar quantities, are the major constituents of honey. Some sucrose, small quantities of other carbohydrates, volatile oils, pigments, and pollen grains are also present.

Honey is a useful nutrient and sweetener. Therapeutically, it has a long tradition of use as a demulcent in cough preparations, and many special claims for the virtues of honey are found in the records of folkloric remedies. No scientific evidence supports any of the special medical claims that are sometimes advanced for honey, including specific wildflower honeys. The demulcent and nutrient properties of honey are not significantly superior to those of less expensive carbohydrate products, such as liquid glucose (see page 28).

HOPS

Hops or humulus consists of the dried strobile of *Humulus lupulus* Linné (Fam. Moraceae), which bear glandular hairs. These hairs, known as **lupulin,** contain most of the bitter principles that account for the use of the product in brewing and in medicine. The plant is a perennial herbaceous climber, extensively cultivated in England, Germany, various parts of the United States, South America, and Australia. Hops are collected in September when they are ripe, are carefully dried by means of artificial heat, and are packed into bales or bags.

The principal constituents of hops are contained in a volatile oil fraction (0.3 to 1%) and a resinous fraction (30%) which combine to produce the drug's characteristic taste and aroma. β-Myrcene (30 to 50%), humulene (15 to 25%), esters of myrcenol, linalool, and numerous other minor constituents comprise the volatile oil. Chemically unstable phloroglucinol derivatives, such as humulone and lupulone, are found in the resinous fraction. These latter components isomerize to produce principles whose bitter taste and bacteriostatic properties account for the use of hops in the brewing process.

Since the Middle Ages, when it was observed that hop pickers tired easily, the drug has been reputed to have a sedative effect. The active principles responsible for this activity are, in all probability, the bitter acidic compounds, such as humulone and lupulone, or closely related conversion compounds, but their action is erratic owing to instability toward air and light. Further, different varieties of hops seem to vary considerably in their sedative effects.

In spite of the fact that scientific proof is lacking for central-nervous-system depressant effects of hops in human beings, extracts of the drug are widely employed in OTC sedative preparations marketed in Europe. Hops are also marketed in "health-food" stores in the United States, not only for the preparation of a sedative tea but also as a legal intoxicant. Because the plant is rather closely related to marihuana, hops is said to produce a mild sensation of euphoria when smoked. This practice is definitely not recommended because prolonged use produces side effects, including dizziness, intoxication, and jaundice.

HOREHOUND

Horehound is the dried leaves and flowering tops of *Marrubium vulgare* Linné (Fam. Labiatae). The material has been widely used as an expectorant and flavoring agent in cough preparations. It is said to be the most popular of the herbal cough remedies. A volatile oil fraction and marrubiin, a hydroxyditerpenoid lactone bitter principle, contribute the distinctive taste to horehound preparations (Fig. 16–7).

HYDRANGEA

The dried rhizome and roots of *Hydrangea arborescens* Linné (Fam. Saxifragaceae), an old Cherokee Indian remedy, has an extensive folkloric reputation as a diuretic and a treatment for kidney stones. **Hydrangea** is also said to have cathartic properties. Leaves of *H. paniculata* Siebold var. *grandiflora*, the

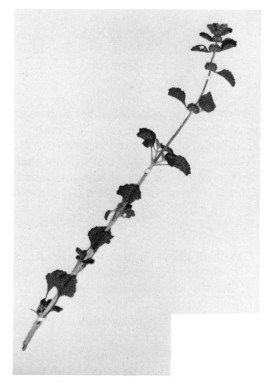

Fig. 16–7. Dried leaves and flowering top of horehound (*Marrubium vulgare*).

hydrangea commonly cultivated in gardens, have been smoked to induce a kind of intoxication. They have also been recommended as a non-nutritive sweetener in hot beverages.

The plant contains, among other constituents, a cyanogenic glycoside that renders its consumption in any form unsafe and unwise. Vertigo and other toxic effects have been recorded following the use of hydrangea. There is no valid justification for its consumption.

HYSSOP

Hyssop, the dried leaves and young tops of *Hyssopus officinale* Linné (Fam. Labiatae), is a volatile-oil-containing plant with a biblical record. The plant is used occasionally as a flavoring agent, and a decoction has been employed in folkloric medicine for a variety of purposes, such as catharsis, chronic catarrh, diseases of the chest, fevers, and rheumatism. A poultice of the decoction reputedly removes discoloration from black eyes. The volatile oil fraction of hyssop contains such constituents as cadinene, α-pinene, $(-)$-pinocampheol, and pinocamphone. No pharmacologically active constituent that might account for the plant's medicinal reputation has been identified.

KELP

The term **kelp** is applied to a group of brown algae with large, flat, leaflike fronds that usually grow attached to rocks by means of a holdfast. They belong to the order Laminariales and include species of *Macrocystis* and *Nereocystis*, which are native to the Pacific coast, and *Laminaria*, which grows on the Atlantic coast of North America. The plants serve as a source of sodium alginate (see page 47).

Powdered kelp is employed in folk medicine primarily for its content of minerals, especially iodine. The concentration of iodine in kelp is extremely variable, depending on the species used, the age of the plants, and the time of harvest. It may range from less than 0.1% to more than 0.5% on a dry-weight basis. If a kelp preparation is to be useful, its iodine content should be standardized or at least determined and expressed on the label. Potassium is also present in kelp in relatively large amounts, but unfortunately, the sodium concentration is also high. Ingestion of kelp should consequently be avoided by those who must restrict their salt intake.

For many years, kelp has enjoyed a reputation as a useful agent in the control of obesity. Once again, this role is attributed to its iodine content, which, it is postulated, stimulates the production of the iodine-containing thyroid hormones (see page 268). This applies only when the person suffers from a deficiency of iodine, an unlikely event in this age of iodized salt. The RDA of iodine in adults does not exceed 150 μg. Because the ability of the thyroid gland to utilize iodine is limited, administration of moderate quantities beyond the saturation point has essentially no effect. Even if it were effective, the use of increased quantities of endogenous or exogenous thyroid hormones for weight reduction is not recommended.

Some persons claim that atherosclerosis is also amenable to treatment with the iodine-containing kelp. Those who recommend such treatment claim that kelp "cleanses" and "gives tone" to the walls of the blood vessels. Treatment of atherosclerosis with iodine is controversial and is not recommended. When iodine is used, precise doses, not available in the unstandardized kelp, are employed.

The use of kelp for any condition presents no advantages over conventional therapy. In addition to all other problems associated with the product, kelp tastes bad.

LECITHIN

Lecithin is a mixture of phosphatides that yield, on hydrolysis, α- or β-glycerophosphoric acid, fatty acids, and choline. The role of lecithin in choline biosynthesis is illustrated on page 315. Although lecithin occurs in a variety of natural sources, including eggs, brain tissue, and many vegetable oils, the principal commercial source today is soybeans.

The daily ingestion of relatively large amounts of lecithin (10 g) is recommended by some "health-food" enthusiasts in the treatment of such conditions as gallstones, atherosclerosis, and various skin and nerve disorders. Such treatments are apparently based on the lipotropic properties of lecithin and on its utility, in vitro, as an emulsifying agent. Proof of its effectiveness, in vivo, for any of these conditions is either insubstantial or completely lacking.

LIFE ROOT

The dried plant of *Senecio aureus* Linné (Fam. Compositae) is known as **life root or golden ragwort.** This plant has been used medicinally, primarily as an emmenagogue, but is considered without value in conventional medicine. The chemistry of the plant has not been studied thoroughly. It reportedly lacks the toxicity of most *Senecio* species, but its use presents an unnecessary risk.

LINDEN FLOWERS

The flowers and leaves of several *Tilia* species (Fam. Tiliaceae) have been employed as a folkloric remedy for colds, headache, indigestion, and nervousness. **Linden flowers** contain flavonoid glycosides but are reportedly free of xanthine bases. Although the plant material has no substantiated medical utility, it is useful as a caffeine-free tea.

LOVAGE

Lovage, the dried rhizome and roots of *Levisticum officinale* Koch (Fam. Umbelliferae), contains several coumarins and up to 1% of a volatile oil. The plant material has been used as a mild stomachic, but its most common application is as a diuretic. Lovage is an example of the large number of volatile-oil-containing plants that are weak diuretics; the diuresis is caused by mild irritation of the renal tubules which retards slightly the normally efficient resorption processes. Such herbs are not a replacement for more potent diuretics that are prescribed for cases of congestive heart failure and hypertension.

MARIGOLD

Marigold is the dried ligulate florets of *Calendula officinalis* Linné (Fam. Compositae). It contains bitter principles, carotenoids, flavonoids, and a saponin. An infusion of the plant material has been applied locally as a vulnerary in chronic skin ulcers, contusions, cuts, hemorrhoids, sprains, and warts; it has also achieved some popularity as an aromatic bitter, a hair rinse, and a diaphoretic bath. The plant material has no current, recognized utility beyond its use as a weak aromatic tonic. Because pollen grains are present, the allergenic potential of marigold cannot be overlooked.

MISTLETOE

The mistletoes are generally classified into 2 types, American and European, but, because of the similarity of their active constituents, they may be discussed together. Botanically, the common **American mistletoe** is *Phoradendron tomentosum* (De Candolle) Engelmann subspecies *macrophyllum* (Cockerell) Wiens. It is synonymous with *P. serotinum* (Rafinesque-Schmaltz) M. C. Johnston and *P. flavescens* (Pursh) Nuttall. **European mistletoe** is *Viscum album* Linné, also a member of the family Loranthaceae. Three subspecies are commonly recognized: *album*, growing on broad-leaf trees; *abietis* (Wiesbaur) Abromeit, growing on *Abies alba*; and *austriacum* (Wiesbaur) Vollmann, growing on various *Pinus* and *Picea* species.

Although the berries of both types of these parasitic shrubs have long been considered poisonous, the leaves, used in the form of a tea, have a considerable reputation as home remedies. Oddly enough, the 2 plants reputedly have somewhat opposite effects. American mistletoe is said to simulate smooth muscles, causing a rise in blood pressure and an increase in uterine and intestinal contractions. European mistletoe has the reputation of reducing blood pressure and acting as an antispasmodic and calmative agent.

Scientific studies have now shown that the stems and leaves of both plants contain similar toxic proteins, designated phoratoxin, when isolated from *Phoradendron* species, and viscotoxins, when obtained from various subspecies of *Viscum album*. Both types are small basic proteins having the same molecular size (molecular weight approximately 5000) and the same number of amino acid residues (46). Six cystine residues occupy the same position in the chains. The biggest difference between phoratoxin and the viscotoxins is in the C-terminal part of the chain where tryptophan and histidine appear in phoratoxin but not in the viscotoxins.

Contrary to the folkloric reputations of the respective plants containing them, phoratoxin and the viscotoxins produce similar physiologic effects when intravenously injected in mammals. These include hypotension, bradycardia, negative inotropic effect on the heart muscle, and vasoconstriction of vessels in skin and skeletal muscle. The LD_{50} of phoratoxin administered intraperitoneally to mice was 0.57 ± 0.05 mg per kg of body weight. It exhibited no antibiotic effect against bacteria or fungi. The effects of these toxins following oral administration in human beings remain uninvestigated.

Another hazard observed with certain Australian mistletoes (species of *Phrygilanthus*, *Dendrophthoe*, and *Amyema*) growing on oleander plants is the uptake by the parasite and the storage in its leaves of certain, potentially toxic, cardiac glycosides from the host. This activity also extends to mistletoes parasitizing other host plants containing extractable toxic constituents, such as certain solanaceous alkaloids in *Duboisia myoporoides* R.

Brown. Thus, the identity of the host is of considerable significance in the case of mistletoes intended for medicinal use.

Mistletoe tea is widely recommended by many of the popular writers on herbs and "health foods" as a treatment for a variety of conditions ranging from anxiety to cancer. In fact, during the period of high coffee prices, some people promoted mistletoe as a pleasant common beverage. Results of the scientific investigations previously summarized emphasize the toxic nature of plant material derived from various types of mistletoe. The indiscriminate use of these products as home remedies should definitely be avoided.

MORMON TEA

Mormon tea consists of the stems and branches of *Ephedra nevadensis* Watson, (Fam. Gnetaceae), a small, erect shrub with divergent branches. This shrub occurs widely in the arid regions of the western and southwestern United States and in adjacent regions of Mexico. It is variously known as **Mexican tea, teamster's tea, squaw tea,** and, in Mexico, as **popotillo.**

Frontiersmen and Mexicans of the old West prepared a strong infusion (tea) from the plant, which was highly regarded in the treatment of syphilis and gonorrhea. The drink is quite astringent because of its high tannin content and has been regarded as a pleasant substitute for caffeine-containing ordinary tea and coffee. This latter usage probably accounts for the name Mormon tea.

Unlike certain other medicinally used species of *Ephedra*, Mormon tea does not contain ephedrine. It does have a mild diuretic effect and is also slightly constipating, probably owing to the contained tannins. No therapeutic utility for Mormon tea has been established. Terry's statement concerning the drug is still as applicable today as when it was made more than 50 years ago, "Outside of its domestic use [as a pleasant beverage], very little may be said in its favor."

MUIRA PUAMA

Considerable confusion exists in the literature as to the botanic origin of **muira puama** or **potency wood.** It has been said to derive from *Liriosma ovata* Miers or *Acanthea virilis* (nom. nudum), but it is now believed to consist of the wood, stem bark, and root of 2 Brazilian shrubs of the family Oleacaceae, *Ptychopetalum olacoides* Bentham and *Ptychopetalum uncinatum* Anselmino. The drug has a long history of use in Brazilian folk medicine as a remedy for impotence.

Various "authorities" on herbs in this country recommend muira puama as an aprodisiac and nerve tonic, indicating that the contained resin has a strong stimulating effect on the central nervous system. An aqueous decoction or alcoholic extract is administered internally, but the effect is also said to be obtained by bathing the genitals with a concentrated extract of the drug. The root bark is considered especially active.

Chemical studies have identified lupeol in the bark, but not in the wood, of *P. olacoides*. Lesser amounts appear in *P. uncinatum*. Campestrol and β-sitosterol have also been identified. None of these constituents accounts for the purported action of muira puama nor have any controlled clinical studies been conducted to determine its efficacy. Until an active principle can be identified chemically or physiologically, the reputation of this drug must be viewed with considerable skepticism.

OREGANO

Oregano or wild marjoram is the dried leaves and flowering tops of *Origanum vulgare* Linné (Fam. Labiatae). It is widely used as a culinary flavoring agent. The herbal literature lists many reputed uses of this plant material; the most common use involves the treatment of toothaches and oral inflammations. It is also recommended as a carminative, a diaphoretic, an emmenagogue, and a tonic, as well as for the relief of arthritic joints and nervous headaches.

The plant material contains a volatile oil whose most distinctive ingredient is carvacrol. This phenolic terpene may induce minor beneficial effects in some of the alleged health-related uses of the plant, but oregano has no significant therapeutic merit.

PANGAMIC ACID (CALCIUM PANGAMATE)

The exact composition of **pangamic acid** or **vitamin B$_{15}$** varies with the brand. One such product was found to be a mechanical mixture of 61.5% of calcium gluconate and 38.5% of dimethylglycine and was misrepresented as a single compound, the calcium salt of pangamic acid. It has been claimed to increase tissue respiration by the stimulation of glucose oxidation, particularly in the cardiac muscle, where it also is alleged to restore impaired metabolism in the myocardium, to dilate the venous blood vessels, and to exhibit a lipotropic function. Promoters therefore recommend it as a remedy for heart disease, but also think it may be useful in treating blood abnormalities, asthma, emphysema, alcoholism, diabetes, and fatigue.

None of these activities has been scientifically proved. Pangamic acid is not recognized as essential in human nutrition and is, therefore, not a vitamin. Further, there is no evidence that pangamic acid is either safe or effective as a drug. In fact, dichloracetate, found as a component of some pangamic products, has caused adverse reactions in diabetic patients, including mild sedation and increased serum uric acid levels. Based on present knowledge, pangamic acid must be considered as totally without merit.

PARSLEY

The leaf, root, and fruit of **parsley,** *Petroselinum crispum* (Miller) Nyman (Fam. Umbelliferae), have been used for centuries in folk medicine, primarily as diuretics and stomachics. The leaf of this common garden herb, cultivated throughout the world, is also widely employed as a culinary garnish. Although eaten infrequently, parsley is a rich, natural source of carotene, ascorbic acid, iron, and other minerals.

Medicinal use of the plant as a diuretic is based primarily on its volatile oil content, which varies from less than 0.1% in the root, to about 0.3% in the leaf, and to 2 to 7% in the fruit. Several chemical races of parsley are known; some yield oils rich (60 to 80%) in apiol. In other races, apiol is largely replaced by myristicin. Both apiol and myristicin are uterine stimulants, accounting for the use of parsley oil as an emmenagogue and its misuse as an abortifacient. There is no satisfactory evidence that it possesses any significant therapeutic value.

PASSIFLORA

Use of the dried flowering and fruiting tops of *Passiflora incarnata* Linné (Fam. Passifloraceae), known as **passiflora** or **passion flower,** has a long history in folk medicine as a calmative agent for nervous unrest and as a sedative. The herb is usually administered in the form of a tea; an extract is also employed in a number of pharmaceutic specialty products marketed in Europe. The constituents responsible for its depressant effect remain unidentified, although harman has been isolated from the plant.

As of 1978, the FDA stated that it had not received valid scientific evidence to support the use of passion flower extract as a sedative or nighttime sleep-aid. Therefore, the FDA classified passiflora as a product that could not be generally recognized as safe or effective.

PENNYROYAL

The dried leaves and tops of *Hedeoma pulegioides* (Linné) Persoon (Fam. Labiatae) are known as **pennyroyal** or **American pennyroyal** (Fig. 16–8). The plant material was employed in a number of ways by the American Indians, including the treatment of headaches. It has a

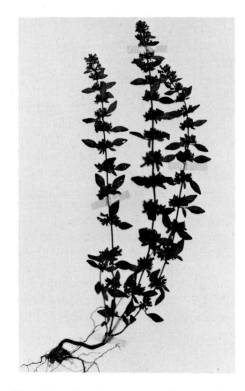

Fig. 16–8. American pennyroyal plant *(Hedeoma pulegioides).*

long history of medical use as an aromatic stimulant, a carminative, a diaphoretic, and an emmenagogue. The medical uses of the plant were presumably related to the contained volatile oil whose principal constituents include (−)-menthone, (+)-isomenthone, and pulegone.

Formal therapeutic use of the plant material and its volatile oil has been abandoned. No substantive evidence supports any claims for the use of pennyroyal as an emmenagogue or as a headache remedy.

POKE ROOT

Poke root is the dried root of *Phytolacca americana* Linné (Fam. Phytolaccaceae). It is a large, much-branched perennial herb that occurs abundantly in all parts of the United States and also grows spontaneously in southern Europe and northern Africa. The plant bears racemes of flowers that develop into clusters of dark purple,

almost black, shining, compound berries (Fig. 16–9).

Various herbals promote the use of poke root for its emetic and cathartic properties, for the treatment of dyspepsia, and especially for chronic rheumatism. It is also claimed to be effective in a variety of conditions, ranging from dysmenorrhea to ringworm.

Actually, poke root is quite toxic; children have died and adults have been hospitalized from the gastroenteritis and diminished respiration induced by ingesting it or other parts of the plant. Extracts of poke are also mitogenic; therefore, the use of gloves is recommended when handling the plant. Employment of the young shoots as pot herbs, a widespread practice in some areas, is also not recommended.

The Herb Trade Association issued a policy statement in May, 1979 declaring that poke root should not be sold as an herbal beverage or food. It further recom-

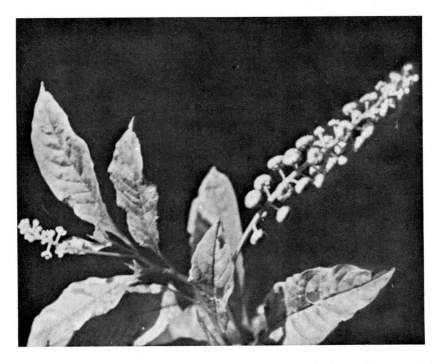

Fig. 16–9. *Phytolacca americana* (pokeweed, pokeberry) showing the leaves, flowers, and fruits.

mended that all packages containing poke root carry an appropriate warning statement regarding the product's toxicity and its potential danger when taken internally.

POLLEN

Pollen consists of the microspores of seed-bearing plants. The pollen available in "health-food" outlets in the form of tablets, capsules, extracts, and the like, consists of mixtures of the pollens of various entomophilous species. However, because collection techniques do not necessarily utilize the bee, this may not always be the case.

Promoted as a health food and general tonic, pollen contains small amounts of vitamins and minerals, as well as protein, carbohydrates, lipids, enzymes, and other constituents. Unfortunately, many pollens are highly allergenic when inhaled, and even entomophilous pollens may induce allergic responses when ingested. Because the product is potentially harmful and because its useful nutrients can be obtained more easily and more cheaply from other sources, its employment as a food supplement or a medicine cannot be recommended.

PROPOLIS

Propolis or bee glue is a brownish resinous material collected by bees from the buds of various poplar and conifer trees and used by the insects to fill cracks or gaps in the hive. It is commercially available in the form of capsules, either as such or mixed half and half with bee pollen. The product is advertised as a natural antibiotic that can build body health and protect against harmful bacteria. No scientific evidence supports such claims, and propolis has no recognized therapeutic value. It is of some utility in sealing openings in bee hives.

RED BUSH TEA

Red bush or rooibos tea consists of the dried flowering twigs of *Aspalathus linearis* (Burman filius) R. Dahlgren (Syn.: *Borbonia pinifolia* Marloth) (Fam. Leguminosae). The plant is native to the mountainous regions of South Africa. It contains no xanthine bases and little tannin; therefore, the tea is claimed to be useful as a stomachic without adverse cardiac or gastrointestinal effects. One such product is marketed under the name Kaffree® Tea.

ROSE HIPS

Although fresh **rose hips,** the fruit of *Rosa canina* Linné (Fam. Rosaceae), contain concentrations of ascorbic acid ranging from 0.5 to 1.7%, the actual vitamin content of the commercially available, dried fruit is highly dependent on the exact botanic variety employed, its habitat, the climate where grown, time of collection, and method of drying. As a matter of fact, many of the marketed samples no longer contain detectable quantities of vitamin C.

Even if one assumes that commercial rose hips contain the relatively high ascorbic acid concentration of 1% and further assumes that all of the vitamin is extracted in preparing the tea, jam, soup, or other preparation that is to be ingested, the cost of vitamin C from this source would be about 25 times that of the synthetic product. Because neither of the mentioned assumptions is necessarily valid and because the natural vitamin is not intrinsically superior to the synthetic, rose hips are not an economical source of vitamin C. Commercial preparations, such as vitamin tablets that contain rose hips in combination with synthetic ascorbic acid, rarely state the proportion of vitamin derived from the natural source. In most cases, the proportion is probably insignificant.

ROYAL JELLY

The milky white, highly viscous secretion from the paired salivary glands of the worker honey bee, *Apis mellifera* Linné (Fam. Apidae), is known as **royal jelly.** It constitutes the sole food of all bee larvae for the first 3 days of life, and future queens continue to be nurtured with the product which is, in some way, responsible for their development into mature female insects.

Royal jelly contains proteins, lipids, fatty acids (including 10-hydroxy-Δ^2-decenoic acid and 9-oxo-Δ^2-decenoic acid), and vitamins of the B complex, especially pantothenic acid (100 μg per g of fresh material). Although various claims have been made for it, almost the only undisputed biologic action of royal jelly is in the differentiation of queen bees from workers. It is available commercially in almost all forms, including lotions, creams, soaps, capsules, and injections. A "hair restorer" containing royal jelly proved so popular in Hungary that fights broke out among the men waiting in line to purchase a bottle.

There is no scientific evidence that royal jelly affects the growth, longevity, or fertility of experimental animals. Likewise it does not exhibit estrogenic activity. Its use as a general tonic, to ward off the effects of old age and to ease suffering from degenerative diseases, is without foundation.

SARSAPARILLA

Sarsaparilla is the dried root of various *Smilax* species (Fam. Liliaceae). *S. aristolochiaefolia* Miller, *S. regelii* Killip et Morton, and *S. febrifuga* Kunth are known in commerce as Mexican, Honduran, and Ecuadorian sarsaparilla, respectively (Fig. 16–10). Sarsaparilla has been used as an alterative, an antirheumatic, a pectoral, and a tonic. It also has had a reputation as a "blood purifier" and as a specific for syphilis. Sarsaparilla is currently recognized as having potential value only as a flavoring agent and as a source of sarsasapogenin and smilagenin, steroidal aglycones used as precursors for the semisynthetic production of cortisone and other steroidal drugs (see page 183).

SASSAFRAS

Sassafras albidum (Nuttall) Nees (Fam. Lauraceae), a small tree indigenous to eastern North America, yields a root bark known as **sassafras** or **sassafras bark** which is widely used in the preparation of a tea employed as a spring tonic and "blood thinner." This is owing primarily to the 5 to 9% of highly aromatic oil contained in it, of which about 80% is safrole, a phenolic ether. Safrole has been recognized since the early 1960s as a carcinogenic agent in rats and mice. Both sassafras oil and safrole are presently prohibited by the FDA from use as flavors or food additives (Fig. 16–11).

Nevertheless, sassafras is still sold by "health-food" outlets, and writers of popular accounts of herbs continue to praise its virtues as an unexcelled home remedy. The town of Vernon in Jennings County, Indiana, even hosts an annual sassafras festival in the spring to publicize the aromatic root.

At present, it is estimated that a safrole dose of 0.66 mg per kg may prove hazardous to human beings. One cup of tea prepared from 2.5 g of sassafras could yield as much as 200 mg of safrole (equivalent to 3 mg per kg), depending on the exact method of preparation and the amount consumed. In spite of the drug's pleasant flavor and its folkloric reputation as a useful tonic, prudent people will avoid using sassafras because of its potentially harmful properties.

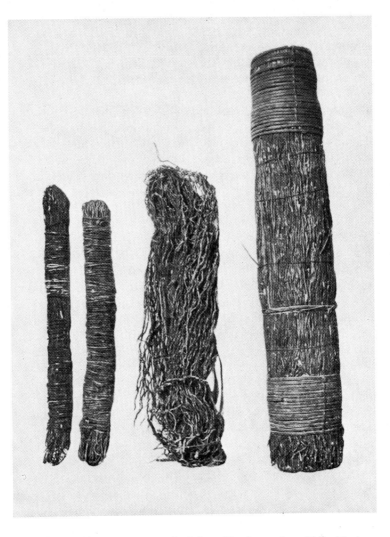

Fig. 16—10. Bundles of sarsaparilla, the 2 on the left are Honduran, the middle, Mexican, and the right, Paran, from a state in northern Brazil. (About ⅛ natural size.)

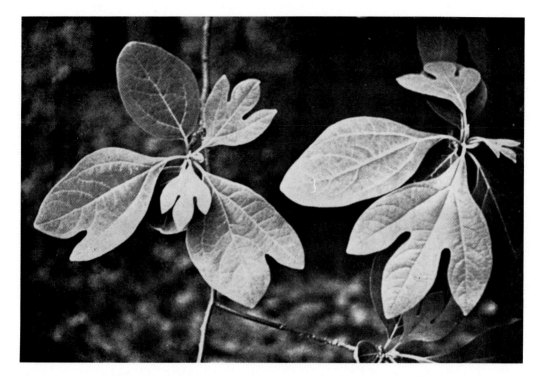

Fig. 16–11.   Sassafras leaves showing considerable variation in shape.

For those who wish to enjoy a somewhat modified flavor of sassafras without the health hazard, an extract from which the safrole has been removed is available on the market. Unfortunately, however, recent studies have shown two thirds of the rats treated with a safrole-free ethanolic extract of sassafras produced tumors. Ingestion of sassafras in any form cannot be recommended.

selenium are essential to animal health, no direct evidence supports any prophylactic benefit (reduction in cancer risk) from supplemental ingestion of the drug.

Selenium is toxic; the daily intake, including dietary sources, should not exceed 200 μg for the average adult. Use of selenium supplementation at this time is best left to controlled investigational situations.

SELENIUM

Trace quantities of **selenium** reputedly possess anticancer properties. An inverse correlation has been claimed between dietary intake of selenium and age-corrected mortalities from leukemia and from cancer of the breast, large intestine, lung, ovary, prostate, and rectum. Although traces of

SENEGA SNAKEROOT

Senega snakeroot is the dried root of *Polygala senega* Linné (Fam. Polygalaceae). The plant material containing triterpenic saponins has been used as an expectorant (approximately 1-g dose). Larger doses may cause vomiting and purging.

SENNA

Senna or senna leaves, the leaflets of one or more *Cassia* species (see page 64), are readily available for use as an herbal tea. These leaflets contain dimeric anthrone glycosides, which are a potent laxative. Ingestion of senna tea can result in diarrhea, dehydration, and related complications. Use of the tea presents unnecessary risks, and it should be avoided. If the laxative properties of senna are desired, an appropriately standardized OTC product with adequate dosing and precautionary labeling should be selected.

TAMARIND

Tamarind is the partially dried ripe fruit of *Tamarindus indica* Linné (Fam. Leguminosae) that has been deprived of the outer layer of pericarp and preserved with sugar. The plant material is rich in citric and tartaric acids. It has a reputation of usefulness in dysentery and fevers. Tamarind (15 g) has been used medicinally as a laxative, but it has been replaced for this purpose by other drugs.

TARRAGON

Tarragon, the dried leaves and flowering tops of *Artemisia dracunculus* Linné (Fam. Compositae), is usually employed as a flavoring agent, especially in vinegar. It has been described as an aromatic bitter, a diaphoretic, an emmenagogue, and a mild sedative. The plant material contains a volatile oil and the coumarin derivatives, aesculetin dimethyl ether and herniarin. The therapeutic need for an aromatic bitter is questionable, and no scientific evidence supports the other medicinal uses of tarragon.

TIENCHI

Tienchi, also known as **tienchi-ginseng and sanchi,** is the root of *Panax notoginseng* (Burkholder) F. H. Chen (Fam. Araliaceae), a perennial shrub cultivated in the Yunnan and Kwangsi regions of China. It contains the same type of saponin glycosides found in ginseng, and its physiologic activity and use are comparable to that drug. A number of tienchi products, including whole and powdered root, are currently marketed.

L-TRYPTOPHAN

The time-honored method of inducing sleep by drinking a glass of warm milk at bedtime has gained some credence in recent years as a result of clinical studies indicating that administration of **L-tryptophan** in a dose of 1 g reduced sleep latency (time taken to fall asleep) in both normal human beings and in mild insomniacs. Doses larger than 1 g did not produce any increased effects. "Health-food" outlets, quick to recognize a potential article of commerce, promptly marketed 500-mg tablets of the amino acid at relatively high prices.

Advocates of the treatment have pointed out that most persons ingest from 0.5 to 2 g of L-tryptophan in their normal daily diet so it can be thought of as a food substance rather than as a drug. This position is somewhat questionable because the probable mechanism of action of the relatively large single dose of the pure amino acid is an increase of serotonin in the serotoninergic neurons of the brain. No safety studies have been conducted. In view of the lack of such information, L-tryptophan may be regarded as a potentially useful drug in sleep-onset insomnia, but its use certainly cannot be recommended.

TURMERIC

Turmeric or curcuma is the prepared rhizome of *Curcuma longa* Linné (Fam. Zingiberaceae). The fresh plant material is treated by scalding or boiling prior to drying. Used primarily as a coloring agent and condiment in curry powders, prepared mustards, and pickles, turmeric has also been employed to stimulate biliary secretions and to treat gallstones. The plant material contains bitter principles, curcumin (a yellow pigment), and a volatile oil. Curcumin has some broad-spectrum antimicrobial activity, but turmeric lacks recognized therapeutic utility.

UVA URSI

Leaves of **uva ursi** (see page 77) are readily available in the form of herbal teas. The plant material is a diuretic and a weak urinary antiseptic, but more effective drugs than uva ursi are known for most conditions requiring these properties.

VALERIAN

Valerian consists of the dried rhizome and roots of *Valeriana officinalis* Linné (Fam. Valerianaceae), although other species of the genus, such as *V. mexicana* De Candolle, also contain active constituents (Fig. 16–12). The drug has been employed as a calmative in nervousness and hysteria for at least 1000 years.

Recent chemical studies of valerian resulted in the isolation of a series of water-insoluble, acid- and alkali-labile active constituents, collectively designated as valepotriates. These principles possess mild but definite tranquilizing activity in mice, cats, and human beings. Such effects are not synergistic with those of alcohol

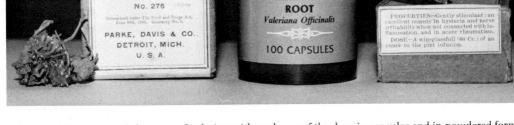

Fig. 16–12.   Roots and rhizomes of valerian with packages of the drug in capsules and in powdered form. (Photo, courtesy of Kathy Delvecchio.)

and barbiturates. This fact is particularly significant in view of the problems often encountered with these agents and the synthetic tranquilizers.

A large number of valerian products, often in combination with other sedatives of plant origin, is produced, marketed, and widely utilized in Europe. Valerian tincture is available in the United States, as is the powdered crude drug that is often administered in sweetened water. No official evaluation of the safety and efficacy of valerian has been made in this country, but its long and continued widespread use abroad seems to proclaim its utility.

WILD LETTUCE

The dried milky juice of **wild lettuce,** *Lactuca virosa* Linné (Fam. Compositae), and of several other species of *Lactuca*, has been thought to possess soporific properties since remote antiquity. This belief was probably based on the similarity between the white milky juice exuded when the plant is incised and that yielded by the opium poppy. Claims for the presence of active principles, such as morphine or hyoscyamine, were made during the last century but were never verified. Wild lettuce ceased to be employed in conventional medicine in the 1920s.

Interest in the product was revived during the past decade when experimenters, searching the literature for legal intoxicants, encountered some uncritical statements concerning its purported physiologic activity. The placebo effect and a considerable amount of wishful thinking prompted various authors of drug-abuse books to advocate the smoking of wild lettuce. Fulton has provided a more accurate estimate of the lack of virtues of the drug, "Modern medicine considers its sleep-producing qualities a superstition, its therapeutic action doubtful or nil."

WORMWOOD

Wormwood, the dried leaves and flowering tops of *Artemisia absinthium* Linné (Fam. Compositae), has a history of use as an aromatic bitter for flatulence and indigestion, as a diaphoretic, and as a flavoring agent in alcoholic beverages where it allegedly had a "narcotic" action for relief of general weakness. The plant material is not a narcotic pharmacologically, and its volatile oil is no longer a flavoring component in absinthe liqueur.

The plant material contains approximately 0.5% of a volatile oil with bitter substances such as absinthin, a diterpenic lactone that is an azulene derivative. The volatile oil is composed of (+)-thujone, thujyl alcohol, esters of thujyl alcohol, and other terpenoid compounds (see page 127).

The volatile oil has been associated with both acute and chronic toxicity, presumably owing in significant part to its thujone content. The toxic response may be characterized by trembling, stupor, and convulsions; dementia or even death may occur. Legal restrictions in most countries now prohibit the use of wormwood or wormwood oil in preparations intended for human consumption. The plant material must be considered hazardous and should not be consumed.

YARROW

The flowering tops of *Achillea millefolium* Linné (Fam. Compositae), a perennial herb common in both the United States and Europe, comprise the drug **yarrow** or **milfoil.** Both flowers and leaves contain an aromatic volatile oil which, like that of chamomile, is blue in color owing to the presence of chamazulene. This also accounts for the use of yarrow, usually in the form of a tea, for the same purposes as chamomile. Other bitter and astringent principles are also present in the plant.

Most of the statements made about the properties and application of chamomile also apply to yarrow. Persons who are allergic to any member of the family Compositae should be cautioned about its use.

YOHIMBE

Yohimbe is the dried bark of *Pausinystalia yohimbe* (K. Schumann) Pierre (Fam. Rubiaceae) a tree native to some of the tropical areas of west Africa. The bark contains up to 6.1% of a mixture of alkaloids, principally yohimbine.

Both yohimbe and yohimbine have been employed in folk medicine as aphrodisiacs. Shavings of the inner bark are boiled in water for one-half hour to yield a decoction that is drunk. Yohimbine hydrochloride is available as a prescription drug in a variety of solid dosage forms, often in admixture with such drugs as strychnine, thyroid, and/or methyltestosterone. Some authors recommend sniffing the drug to achieve both stimulant and mild hallucinogenic effects.

The drug dilates the peripheral blood vessels and lowers blood pressure. Alleged aphrodisiacal effects are attributed to the enlargement of blood vessels in the sexual organs and increased reflex excitability in the sacral region of the spinal cord. Yohimbe is a monoamine oxidase inhibitor, and appropriate dietary and drug restrictions should be observed when it is administered. Its use is contraindicated for persons suffering from hypotension, from diabetes, or from heart, liver, or kidney disease.

READING REFERENCES

To avoid confusion, reading references are divided into 2 groups:

1. Authoritative literature, which presents information on these products generally deemed factual by the scientific community.

2. Advocacy literature, which consists of modern herbal writings listing these materials and describing their uses in a largely uncritical fashion. These works are so numerous that only a limited sampling can be included here.

AUTHORITATIVE LITERATURE

Abramowicz, M., ed.: Toxic Reactions to Plant Products Sold in Health Food Stores, Med. Lett. Drugs Ther., 21(7):29, 1979.

Harlow, D. R.: The FDA's OTC Drug Review: The Development and an Analysis of Some Aspects of the Procedure. Food, Drug, Cosmetic Law J., 32(6):248, 1977.

Hoppe, H.: *Drogenkunde*, 8th ed., Vol. I, Berlin, Walter de Gruyter, 1975.

Lewis, W. H., and Elvin-Lewis, M. P. F.: *Medical Botany*, New York, John Wiley & Sons, 1977.

List, P. H., and Hörhammer, L., eds.: *Hagers Handbuch der Pharmazeutischen Praxis*, 4th ed., Vols. II–VI, Berlin, Springer-Verlag, 1969–1979.

Morton, J. F.: *Major Medicinal Plants*, Springfield, Illinois, Charles C Thomas, 1977.

Osol, A., and Farrar, G. E., Jr., eds.: *The Dispensatory of the United States of America*, 25th ed., Philadelphia, J. B. Lippincott Co., 1955.

Penna, R. P., Corrigan, L. L., Welsh, J., and Rasmussen, M. T., eds.: *Handbook of Nonprescription Drugs*, 6th ed., Washington, D. C., American Pharmaceutical Association, 1979.

Rosengarten, F., Jr.: *The Book of Spices*, rev. ed., New York, Pyramid Books, 1973.

Schrauzer, G. N., White, D. A., and Schneider, C. J.: Cancer Mortality Correlation Studies. III. Statistical Associations with Dietary Selenium Intakes, Bioinorg. Chem., 7(1):23, 1977.

Steinegger, E., and Hänsel, R.: *Lehrbuch der Pharmakognosie*, Berlin, Springer-Verlag, 1972.

Youngken, H. W.: *Textbook of Pharmacognosy*, 6th ed., Philadelphia, The Blakiston Co., 1948.

ADVOCACY LITERATURE

Adams, R., and Murray, F.: *Health Foods*, New York, Larchmont Books, 1975.

Coon, N.: *Using Plants for Healing*, Emmaus, Pennsylvania, Rodale Press, 1979.

Fielder, M.: *Plant Medicine and Folklore*, New York, Winchester Press, 1975.

Gibbons, E.: *Stalking the Healthful Herbs*, field guide ed., New York, David McKay Co., Inc., 1970.

Hall, D.: *The Book of Herbs*, New York, Charles Scribner's Sons, 1972.

Hylton, W. H., ed.: *The Rodale Herb Book*, Emmaus, Pennsylvania, Rodale Press, Inc., 1974.

Law, D.: *The Concise Herbal Encyclopedia*, New York, Saint Martin's Press, 1973.

Lucas, R.: *Nature's Medicines*, No. Hollywood, California, Wilshire Book Co., 1966.

Lucas, R.: *Common & Uncommon Uses of Herbs for Healthful Living*, New York, Arco, 1978.

Mitton, F., and Mitton, V.: *Mitton's Practical Modern Herbal*, London, W. Foulsham & Co. Ltd., 1976.

Pond, B.: *A Sampler of Wayside Herbs*, Riverside, Connecticut, The Chatham Press, Inc., 1974.

Rose, J.: *Herbs & Things*, New York, Grosset & Dunlap Workman Publishing Co., 1972.

Simmonite, W. J., and Culpeper, N.: *The Simmonite-Culpeper Herbal Remedies*, New York, Universal-Award House, Inc., 1957.

Thomson, W. A. R., ed.: *Medicines from the Earth*, New York, McGraw-Hill Book Co., 1978.

Veninga, L., and Zaricor, B. R.: *Goldenseal/Etc.*, Santa Cruz, California, Ruka Publications, 1976.

Wren, R. C., and Wren, R. W.: *Potter's New Cyclopaedia of Botanical Drugs and Preparations*, new ed., Hengiscote, England, Health Science Press, 1975.

Index

Page numbers in *italics* refer to illustrations; page numbers followed by t refer to tables.